Adaptation to environment:

essays on the physiology of marine animals

Adaptation to environment:

essays on the physiology of marine animals

Edited by R. C. Newell, D.Sc.
Institute of Biology, University of Odense, Denmark

BUTTERWORTHS
London – Boston
Sydney–Wellington–Durban–Toronto

THE BUTTERWORTH GROUP

UNITED KINGDOM

Butterworth & Co (Publishers) Ltd
London: 88 Kingsway, WC2B 6AB

AUSTRALIA

Butterworths Pty Ltd
Sydney: 586 Pacific Highway,
Chatswood, NSW 2067
Also at Melbourne, Brisbane, Adelaide and Perth

SOUTH AFRICA

Butterworth & Co (South Africa) (Pty) Ltd
Durban: 152–154 Gale Street

NEW ZEALAND

Butterworths of New Zealand Ltd
Wellington: 26–28 Waring Taylor Street, 1

CANADA

Butterworth & Co (Canada) Ltd
Toronto: 2265 Midland Avenue,
Scarborough, Ontario, M1P 4S1

USA

Butterworths (Publishers) Inc
Boston: 19 Cummings Park
Woburn, Mass. 01801

First published 1976

ISBN 0 408 70778 X

Library of Congress Cataloging in Publication Data
Main entry under title:

Adaptation to environment.

Includes bibliographies and indexes.
1. Marine fauna—Physiology. 2. Adaptation (Physiology) I. Newell, Richard Charles.
QL121.A24 591.5′2636 75-33894
ISBN 0-408-70778-X

Photoset by Amos Typesetters, Hockley, Essex
Printed in Great Britain by
Cox & Wyman Ltd, London
Fakenham and Reading

Preface

This book contains a series of essays each of which is intended as a review of the special adaptations of marine organisms to the particular environmental conditions which they are likely to encounter in the natural habitat. Emphasis is placed throughout the text on recent developments in the subject and on new approaches to the study of the adaptations of marine organisms. With this in mind, the term 'Physiology' has been interpreted in its widest sense to include all aspects of the functioning of the organism from the behaviour of animals to the mode of function of enzymes. For this reason structural adaptations have been reviewed in detail only where their functional role is understood and where they constitute a specific adaptation to defined environmental conditions.

As might be expected in a multi-author work of this kind, the approaches to the subject and styles of presentation are rather different from one another and in some cases similar data have been referred to independently in more than one of the chapters. Rather than interrupt the continuity of each review, I have preferred to regard each chapter as complete in itself, and to provide cross-references to other chapters where this was necessary. I have also found it refreshing to foster the differences in style of presentation for they reflect the individuality which each scientist brings to research problems, and perhaps give the reader some insight into the conceptual framework behind some of the experimental work which is reviewed here.

All of the figures have been drawn specially for this book, and the sources from which they are taken are acknowledged in the legend. There is a comprehensive bibliography at the end of each chapter, and cross-referencing is aided by author and subject indexes at the end of the book.

We hope that this series of reviews will place recent developments in some aspects of the physiology of marine animals into perspective, and in particular stimulate further work in this rapidly developing subject.

R.C.N.

Contents

One

Adaptations to intertidal life

R. C. NEWELL
Institute of Biology, University of Odense, 5000-Odense, Denmark

1.1 THE NATURE OF THE INTERTIDAL ENVIRONMENT

Before we consider the physical and chemical conditions which characterise the intertidal environment, it is worth reminding ourselves that the sea-shore represents a rather special type of environment which contrasts sharply with conditions that prevail elsewhere in the sea. The total area represented by the intertidal zone is also minute compared with that occupied by the oceans as a whole. The oceans, for example, cover some 361 million square kilometres (139 × 10^6 square miles) which corresponds with approximately 71% of the entire surface of the globe. By comparison, the area occupied by the sea-shore is insignificant. Nevertheless its interest to the biologist lies in the special adaptations which are required by organisms which live in an environment which is alternately marine and terrestrial. This unusual habitat, and its accessibility for study, undoubtedly accounts for what is perhaps a disproportionate amount of work which has been carried out on intertidal animals compared with those of deeper waters.

Broadly speaking, the oceanic environment is characterised by a great stability of physical and chemical conditions. The surface temperature of the sea, for example, rarely shows a diurnal fluctuation of as much as 1°C and below 10 metres in depth even this small variation is eliminated. Again, seasonal changes which may amount to as much as 15°C between summer and winter values at the surface of the ocean, are reduced to less than 1°C at 100 metres depth (Sverdrup, Johnson, and Fleming, 1946). In much the same way, the uniform chemical composition of oceanic water results in a medium whose osmotic pressure and pH have great stability. In contrast, the organisms of the sea-shore experience wide and largely unpredictable variations in temperature, salinity and water loss (for review, *see* Newell 1969; 1970) which call for a broad spectrum of structural, physiological and behavioural adaptations.

Even those factors which show a spatial variation in the ocean, do so in a predictable fashion. The most important of these, as is discussed in Chapters 8 and 9, are associated with the fact that the pressure increases by one

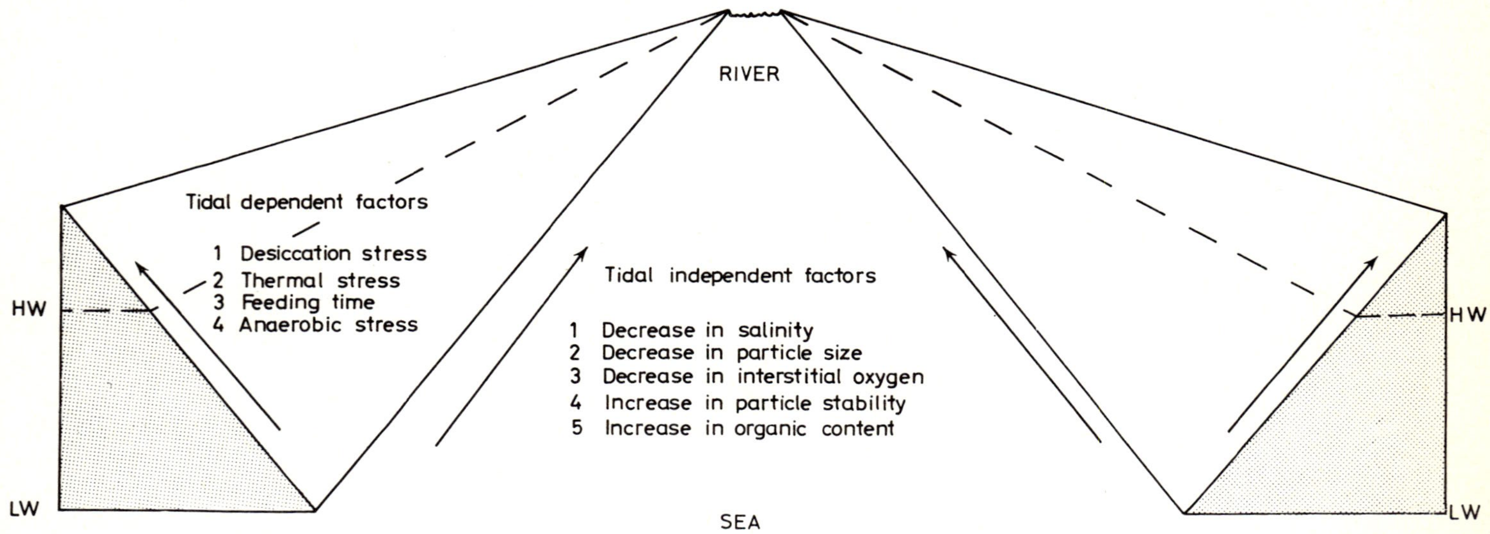

Figure 1.1 *Diagram illustrating the main groups of environmental factors likely to influence the distribution of organisms on the sea-shore*

atmosphere for each 10 metres in depth and that light, especially at the red end of the spectrum, is rapidly absorbed in the surface layers of the sea. Pelagic organisms of the deep sea are thus structurally and functionally adapted to life in darkness and at great pressure. Again, because primary production is confined to the surface layers, deep sea animals are adapted to exploit limited food supplies with minimal energy expenditure (Denton and Marshall, 1958; Denton, 1961; Marshall, 1965). On the sea-shore, however, there is little evidence of a regular change in the environment. Instead conditions in the algae, rockpools, crevices, sands and rock surfaces which characterise the habitat give rise to a discontinuous pattern of adaptations which make broad generalisations from isolated experimental data difficult. Despite these problems, it is possible to define what part of the environment we mean by the 'intertidal zone' and then to recognise common physico-chemical features to which the organisms must be adapted. Some of these are illustrated in *Figure 1.1*.

1.1.1 Simple models of a generalised sea-shore

At first sight it may seem a simple enough task to predict the type of conditions which organisms living on the sea-shore are likely to experience. In the first instance we know that there are generally two tides per 24 h so that a typical organism living on the sea-shore would be expected to experience a twice-daily cycle of exposure to air and immersion in seawater. Clearly, organisms living at the extreme high water mark would be exposed to air for much of the time whilst those at the lower part of the shore would experience primarily aquatic conditions. Organisms living at mid-tide level would be expected to experience about 50% of aquatic and aerial conditions. The important prediction from any such model is that all intertidal animals 'by definition' would be wetted twice per 24 h even if this is for short periods only.

The type of environmental situation which would be predicted by a model of this kind is illustrated in *Figure 1.2(a)*, and the regular gradation of aquatic through to aerial conditions forms a conceptual background to many of the studies on the graded tolerances of intertidal animals which have been carried out in the past (for review, *see* Newell, 1970). Indeed, it remains true that whether the shore is complex or not, both the magnitude and the duration of the physical stresses are greater on the open rock surfaces at high tidal levels than lower ones. Davies (1970), for example, has recorded the body temperatures of high and low level *Patella vulgata* during the summer. The data are illustrated in *Figure 1.3* from which it will be noticed that the tissue temperature of the upper shore limpets reached approximately 32°C for as much as six hours whereas a maximum tissue temperature of 26°C was recorded for only one hour in the lower shore limpets. These data illustrate well the kind of differences which must exist on a wide variety of shores regarding both temperature and desiccation stresses.

Unfortunately as far as such predictions are concerned, there is also a cycle of tides of maximum amplitude (Spring Tides) occurring at new and full moon alternating with tides of minimum amplitude (Neap Tides). This

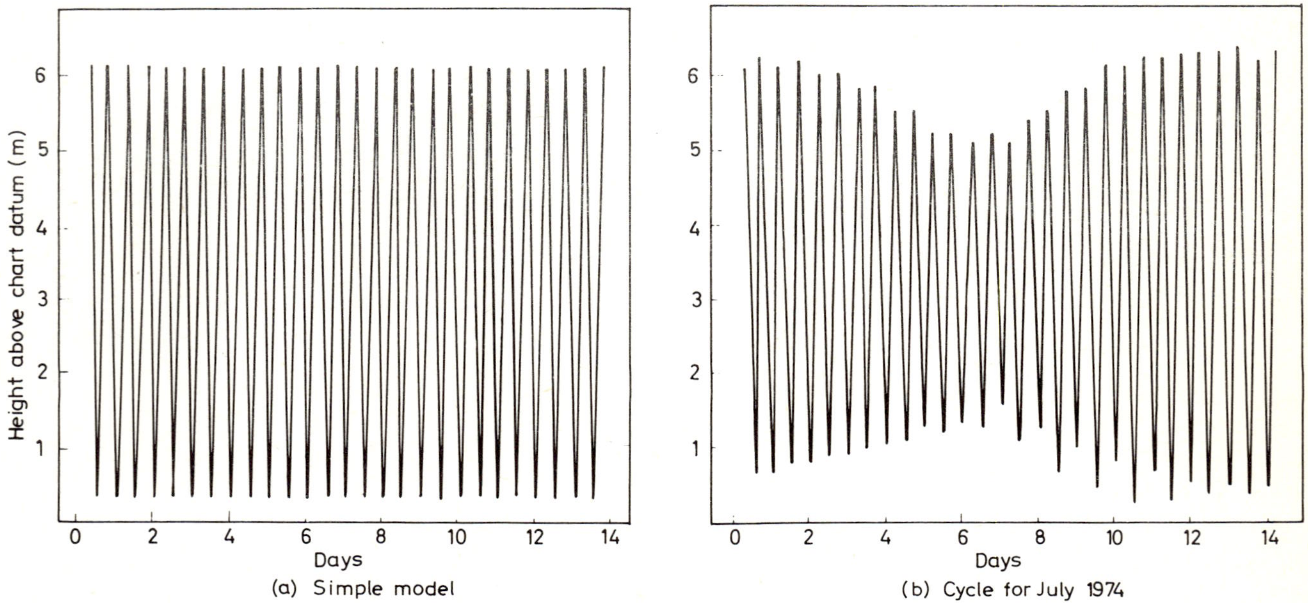

Figure 1.2 *Graphs showing the tidal oscillation in (a) a simple semi-diurnal system and (b) an actual semi-diurnal tidal cycle showing Spring and Neap Tides in July 1974 on the North Kent Coast.*

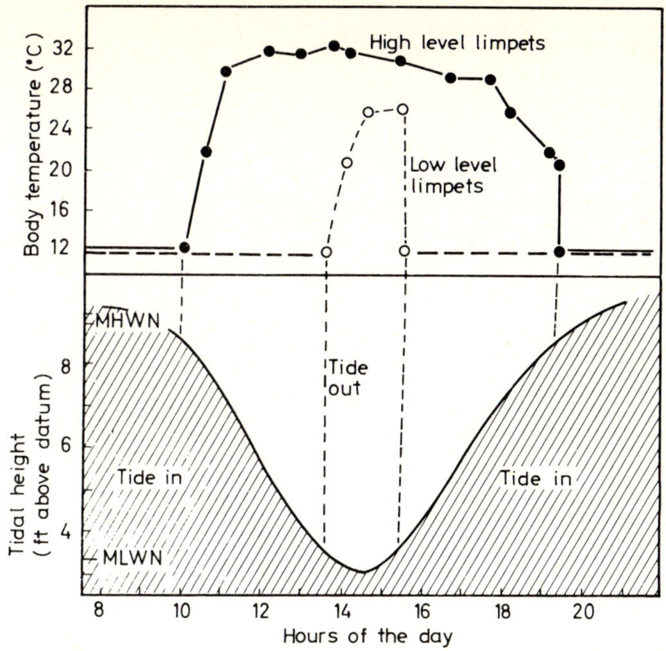

Figure 1.3 Graphs showing the body temperature of the upper shore limpets (Patella) *(closed circles) and lower shore limpets (open circles), during one tidal cycle on a hot day in the summer. (After Davies, 1970; courtesy Cambridge University Press)*

fortnightly cycle is illustrated in *Figure 1.2(b)* and imposes a major constraint on the model outlined above for, as emphasised by Lewis (1964), organisms living at the top of the shore may not be reached by the tide except during the Spring Tide period. This has profound implications for our definition of environmental conditions in the intertidal zone. It means that organisms of the upper shore may require terrestrial adaptations which last them for several days, or even for two weeks. Conversely, animals living on the lower shore may not be uncovered during the period of Neap Tides and may thus experience permanently aquatic conditions for all but a few hours each fortnight. A comparison between the physical conditions which would be expected from the two models is shown in *Figure 1.4(a and b)*.

We may therefore redefine the sea-shore, or intertidal zone, not in terms of an area which is covered or uncovered twice each 24 h, but as the zone between the extreme high water and extreme low water of Spring Tides. These features of the intertidal zone are illustrated in *Figure 1.5*, which shows that the only group of organisms to experience a twice daily exposure/immersion cycle would be those living near the mid-tidal level. From these considerations it would also be predicted that organisms below mid-tide level would be marine organisms adapted primarily to resist short periods of exposure to unfavourable environmental conditions in air. In contrast, organisms above the mid-tide level would be highly specialised to survive, feed and reproduce under aerial conditions. In practice it is at this

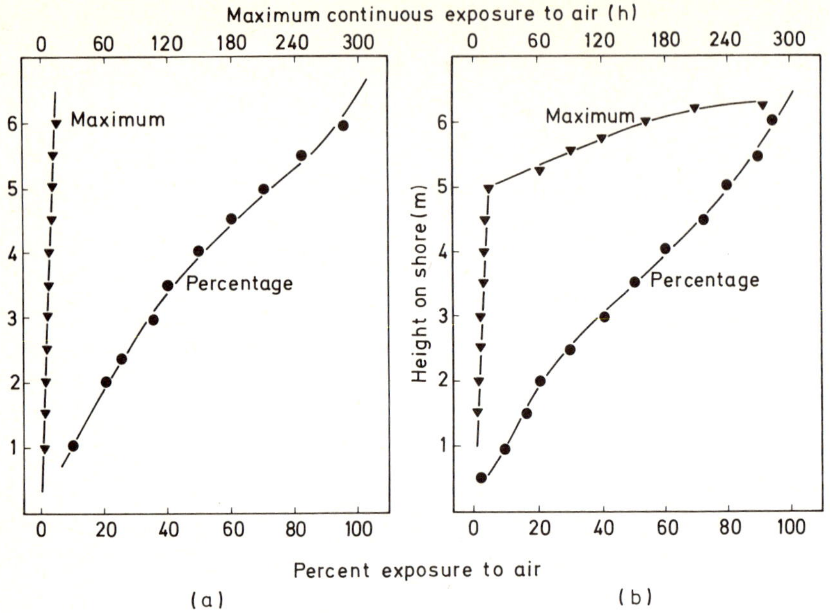

Figure 1.4 *Graphs showing the percentage exposure to air (•–•) and maximum duration of aerial exposure (▾–▾) in (a) a simple semi-diurnal oscillating tidal situation and (b) in a tidal situation where Spring and Neap Tides are superimposed on the semi-diurnal rhythm*

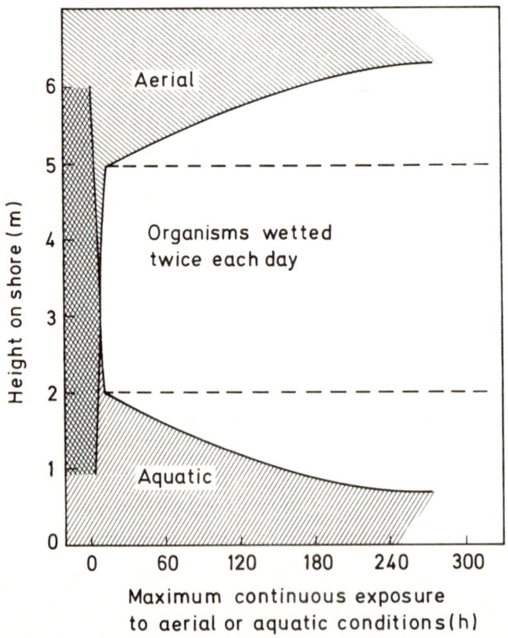

Figure 1.5 *Graphs showing the duration of aerial and aquatic conditions in relation to height on the shore*

point that a major break in the nature and abundance of the organisms occurs and this reflects the rigorous environmental conditions to be faced on the upper shore. It is part of the interest of comparative studies on intertidal organisms to show (a) how marine organisms of the lower shore manage to escape the competition of the subtidal zone and yet evade the severe physico-chemical conditions of the upper shore, and (b) what special features are required by organisms confined to the upper part of the intertidal zone.

1.1.2 Towards a more complex model

Both of these simplistic models have assumed that the sea-shore may be represented by a uniform gradient of constant composition. Whilst under idealised conditions we can find sloping rock surfaces or man-made sea walls which approach this situation, it is obviously much more commonplace to find that the sea-shore consists of varying slopes, boulders and rockpools. It is also often covered with algae and barnacles all of which may profoundly modify the local physico-chemical environment and allow survival of organisms which would not normally be capable of life under those conditions.

A good example of the way in which the physical environment may vary according to local conditions is shown in *Figure 1.6.* This illustrates the temperature profiles in the vicinity of a saline pool on an intertidal saltmarsh in Kent during July 1973 and is based on data from Marsden (1975). The temperature on the surface of the marsh varied from an afternoon maximum of 30°C to a minimum of approximately 15°C. The seawater temperature was approximately 15°C but was warmed to approximately 17-18°C during its passage over the marsh, so that during immersion by the tide in the morning, the temperature of much of the surface of the marsh was approximately 17°C. When the tide had ebbed the temperature rapidly rose to 30°C and then decreased as the heat of the sun declined during the afternoon and evening. By the time the tide flowed over the marsh again, its effect was to raise slightly the temperature of the substratum compared with the night temperature and the cycle was repeated on the following morning. The water in the pools showed a less violent diurnal cycle and the temperature amongst the vegetation also shows that a good deal of protection is afforded by the plants. The maximum temperature amongst the latter, for example, was 23°C and the minimum was 15°C which gives a temperature flux of only 8°C compared with 15°C on the bare surface. In much the same way the temperature 1 cm below the surface on the mud in the pools showed a diurnal variation of only 14-21°C whilst amongst the roots of the vegetation the diurnal change was only 2°C from 15.5 to 17.5°C. It is thus clear that not only could the stresses associated with desiccation be evaded by an organism taking shelter from aerial conditions in pools or amongst moist vegetation, but that temperature extremes could be largely minimised in organisms capable of burrowing into the substratum.

Burrowing into the substratum also forms a principal mechanism by which

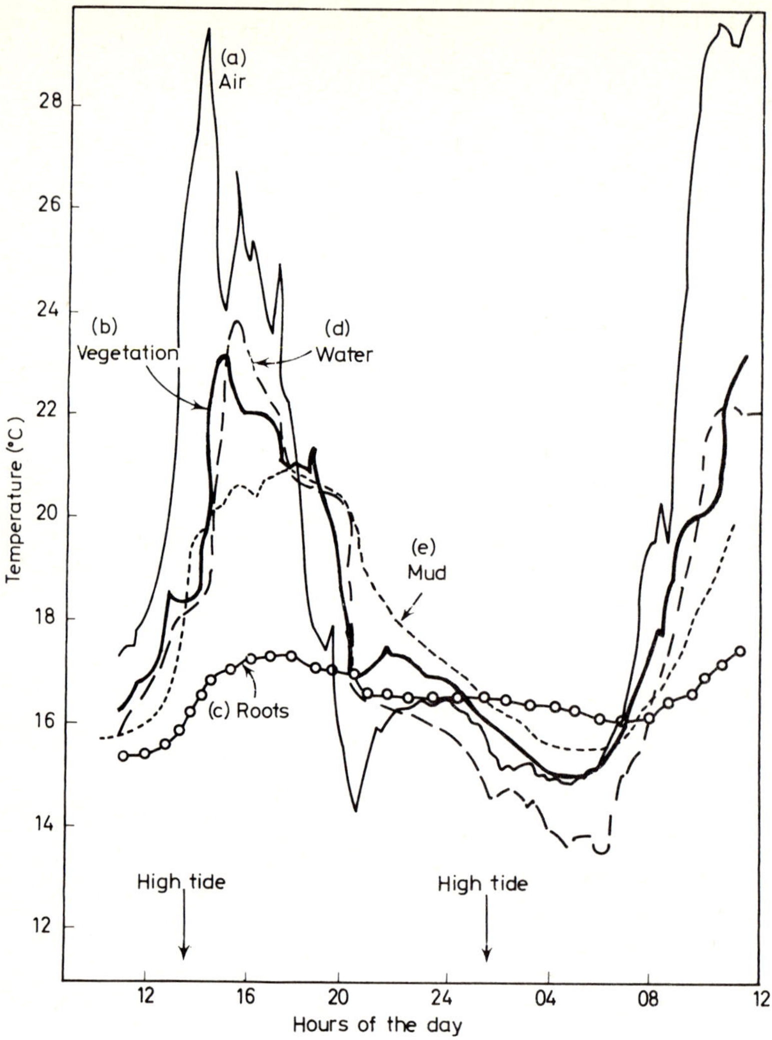

Figure 1.6 Graphs showing the temperature profiles in the vicinity of a saline pool on a salt marsh in North Kent during July 1973. (a) Air temperature (b) vegetation temperature (c) root temperature (d) water temperature in pools (e) mud temperature at the bottom of pools. (After Marsden, 1975)

many organisms living in other parts of the intertidal zone could evade the stresses associated with life on the sea-shore. Jansson (1967) has shown that the effects of even quite marked diurnal temperature fluctuation are small at a depth of 25 cm below the surface of sediments. During May 1964, for example, the maximum surface temperature recorded on a dry sandy beach at Askö was 43°C and fell to a minimum of approximately 6°C during the night. This gives a diurnal variation of as much as 37°C. This very severe thermal stress, however, was rapidly reduced to a diurnal variation of only

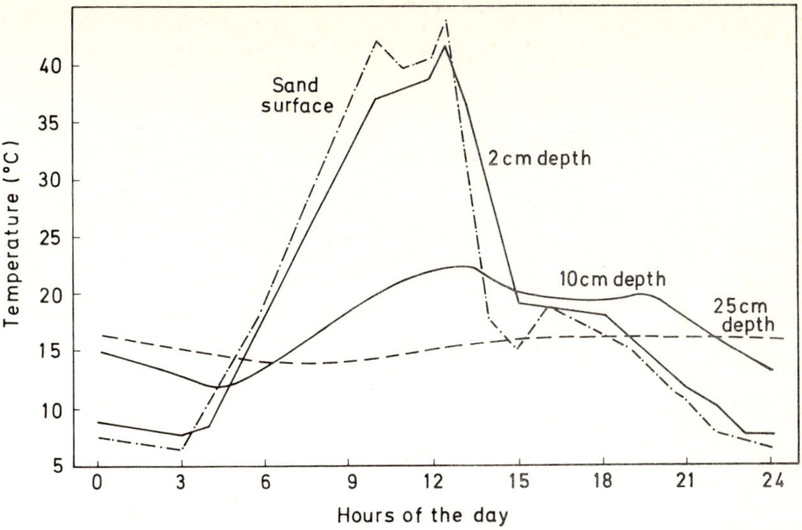

Figure 1.7 Graphs showing the diurnal variations of temperature on a beach as Askö, Sweden in May 1964. (After Jansson, 1967; courtesy Ophelia, Marine Biological Laboratory)

10°C at 10 cm depth as is shown in *Figure 1.7*. Again, the possibilities for evasion of environmental stress are obvious for organisms capable of burrowing. The mechanisms by which this can be accomplished in a variety of marine invertebrates is reviewed by Trueman and Ansell (1969).

The work of Glynne-Williams and Hobart (1952), Morton (1954), Kensler and Crisp (1965) and Kensler (1967) on factors controlling the distribution of crevice dwelling species has also shown that to a large extent crevices protect the organisms from the extremes of temperature and desiccation which occur on the exposed rock surfaces. Species capable of survival on open rock surfaces as well as in crevices are thus able to colonise higher shore levels in the protected environment of crevices than outside (Glynne-Williams and Hobart, 1952). There is also a distinct zonation in the desiccation resistance of organisms inhabiting intertidal crevices, those of the outer regions being more resistant than those occupying the moist inner region of the crevices.

Important studies have also been made on the physical and chemical features of the rockpool environment but in this case the situation is considerably more complex than merely protecting organisms from the extremes of the environment encountered on the open shore. Apart from the early work of Stephenson, Zoond and Eyre (1934), Järnefelt (1940), Lindberg (1944), Pyefinch (1943) and Naylor and Slinn (1958), much of which is summarised in Newell (1970), the most detailed work has been carried out in a series of studies by Ganning (for review, *see* 1971). In general it is true that organisms living in such pools are able to evade some of the physical stresses associated with life on the sea-shore such as desiccation, but in so doing also encounter additional variables such as pH fluctuation and oxygen depletion which are set up by the relative abundance of animals and plants in the pools. They also still experience much of the diurnal fluctuation of temperature to which their counterparts on the open rock surfaces must be adapted.

As has been shown by Clark (1968), the level of the pool on the shore and the regularity of its inundation by the sea largely determines the magnitude of the differences in the environment from that of seawater itself. The salinity and temperature are also affected by evaporation and precipitation as well as by ice formation which may result in a pronounced stratification in the pools (Ganning, 1971a). There are also several factors which show a marked diurnal fluctuation. As in the salt marsh pools described above, there tends to be a diurnal temperature cycle whose magnitude is dependent upon the tidal level of the pool and the season of the year. But in addition, the relative abundance of algae, especially *Enteromorpha,* imparts a cycle of

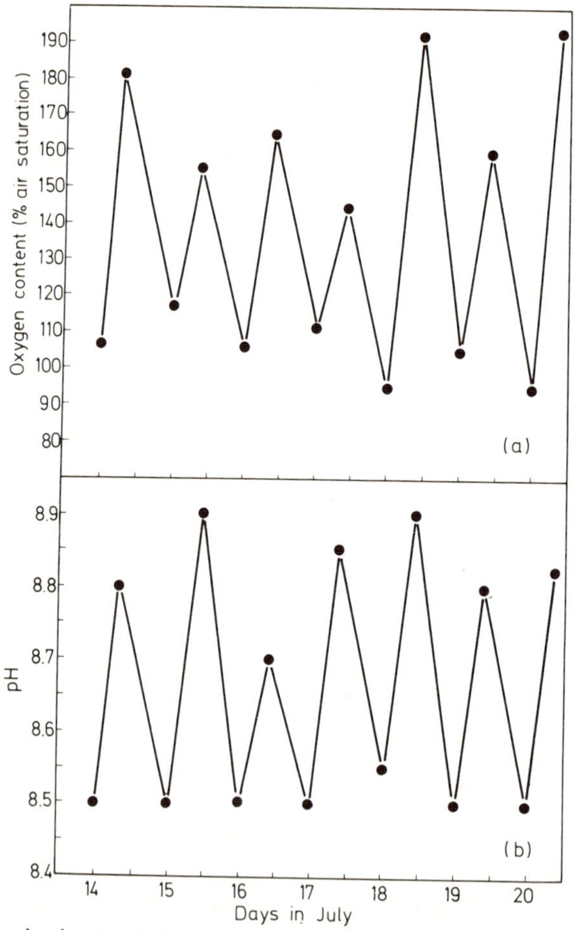

Figure 1.8 Graphs showing daily variations in (a) the oxygen content and (b) the pH of a rockpool during July. (From Newell, 1970; after Pyefinch, 1943; courtesy Paul Elek (Scientific Books) Ltd

oxygen content which reaches a maximum in the day (Pyefinch, 1943; Stephenson, Zoond and Eyre, 1934; Utinomi, Yamizi and Ikeri, 1950; Ganning, 1971a, b). The midday maximum may exceed 100% of oxygen saturation due to algal photosynthesis but at night, when algal respiration is added to that of the animals, the oxygen content falls to low values, especially near the sediments at the bottom of the pool. At the same time the pH may vary from high values at midday to much lower values at night or where biodegradation of organic deposits is taking place (*Figure 1.8*).

On the lower shore, therefore, where frequent tidal inundation results in less prolonged variations in the physico-chemical environment from the mean values, the rockpool environment is one which allows typical marine organisms to extend their range upwards into the intertidal zone. But the rather severe abiotic conditions which occur in upper shore rockpools result in the occurrence of an increasingly specialised assemblage of organisms. Such species, not surprisingly, are rather few in variety and like their counterparts in other parts of the intertidal zone, show adaptations which are of particular interest to the ecophysiologist.

1.2 STRATEGIES OF ADAPTATION FOR SURVIVAL IN THE INTERTIDAL ZONE

From this brief account of the nature of the sea-shore environment it is clear that a variety of strategies of adaptation are available to enable survival in the intertidal zone. We may regard these as falling into three main categories:

1. Evasion of adverse environmental conditions by selection of a suitable microhabitat within the intertidal zone.
2. Structural adaptations to allow colonisation even under the severe conditions which occur on the surface of the sea-shore.
3. Physiological adaptations to allow survival under the conditions likely to prevail at any particular time on the sea-shore.

1.2.1 The evasion of environmental stress

The ability to select suitable microhabitats within the intertidal zone plays a dominant part in controlling the distribution of organisms on the shore. In the case of sessile organisms such as serpulid polychaetes, barnacles and organisms with limited powers of locomotion, an irreversible choice is made at the time the larvae settle from the plankton. The mechanisms by which this is accomplished are diverse, and largely outside the scope of this review. Nevertheless they commonly include a hierarchy of generalised responses to light and gravity which bring the larvae into the vicinity of a suitable substratum. Then this initial exploratory behaviour is replaced by a site-selection response involving a chemoreception of a suitable substratum such as algae, or more commonly of substances characteristic of adults of the same species. This chemical tactile sense allows a final assessment to be made of the suitability of the environment and is followed by a complex spacing behaviour and finally settlement (for review, *see* Chapter 2 and Crisp, 1969; Newell, 1970; Grant and Mackie, 1974).

In organisms which are capable of movement, it becomes possible for them to actively evade potentially damaging environmental situations. The sand shrimp *Crangon septemspinosa*, for example, is able to detect and avoid the anoxic conditions which may occur in estuaries (Haefner, 1969; 1970; 1971). Again, the isopod *Sphaeroma rugicauda* can avoid potentially lethal temperatures when placed in a temperature gradient (Marsden, 1973a). Other small crustaceans are also capable of showing a preference for particular environmental conditions when offered a choice (Ganning and Wulff, 1966), although in rockpools where salinity and temperature changes affect the whole environment it seems likely that the limits of physiological tolerances may have more ecological significance than escape responses (Wulff, 1972). An avoidance response to salinity discontinuities is also well documented on zoae larvae of *Pisidia longicornis* (Lance, 1962), *Homarus americanus* (Scarratt and Raine, 1967) and *Pagurus longicarpus* (Roberts, 1971) as well as in trochophore larvae of *Mercenaria* (Turner and George, 1955; *see also* Chapter 6). The ability of hermit crabs to survive in the intertidal zone is also determined to a major extent by evasion of environmental stresses within the microhabitat of gastropod shells (Reese, 1969).

Amongst the intertidal trochid gastropods there is a good deal of evidence that the overall pattern of intertidal zonation itself is partly controlled by seasonal migration in response to temperature (Micallef, 1966; 1968; 1969). Lewis (1954) noted a similar downward movement of limpets on the shore in spring and summer with an upward movement in winter. Temperature stresses of less than the lethal values may also play a part in controlling the distribution of littorinids on the shore (Sandison, 1966, 1967; for review, *see* Newell, 1970). This conclusion is supported by the work of Bock and Johnson (1967) who have shown that the vertical distribution of littorinids including *Littorina planaxis* and *L. scutulata* are controlled by responses to gravity which are induced by immersion and inhibited by desiccation, thermal stress and the presence of suitable algae.

Many intertidal animals not only maintain themselves in one particular zonational position but also undertake moderately extensive migrations in search of food when suitable conditions prevail and retreat to protected situations at other stages of the tidal cycle. In the case of many terrestrial organisms extending their range down the shore, feeding occurs principally when the tide has ebbed and the animals retreat into the air pockets trapped in crevices when the sea covers the intertidal zone. Conversely, the aquatic component of the fauna feeds mainly from the plankton when the tide is in and shelters in the moist conditions of the crevice when the tide has ebbed (Glynne-Williams and Hobart, 1952). This avoidance of adverse environmental conditions during certain phases of the tidal cycle is especially noticeable in some gastropods such as *Cerithium* which aggregates during the intertidal period (Moulton, 1962). A similar gregarious behaviour is often also seen in *Littorina littorea* and results in a reduction in the temperature and desiccation stresses to which the group is subjected. In some animals the feeding excursions made during the optimal phase of the tidal cycle may be extensive and a good deal of work has been carried out on the mechanisms by which intertidal animals are able to find their way back to a suitable environmental situation to allow survival during the unfavourable part of the tidal cycle.

The behaviour of the snail *Olivella biplicata* is a good example of a relatively simple mechanism which restricts the intertidal distribution of the animal to a zone where the environmental stresses are within the limits of physiological tolerance of the animal. Edwards (1969) showed that the upper shore was colonised by large specimens of *Olivella* whilst the low shore supported a dense population of small animals (*Figure 1.9*).

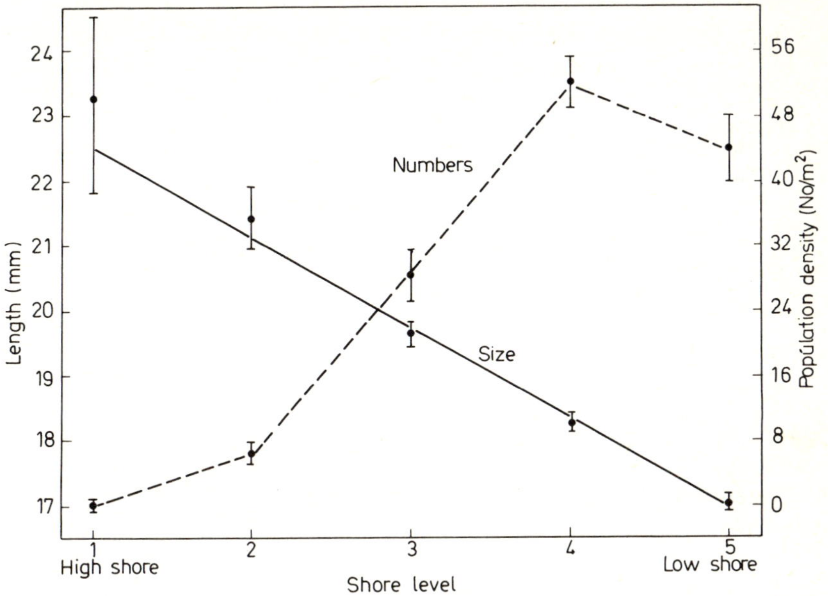

Figure 1.9 Graphs showing the relationship between the size of the gastropod Olivella *(continuous line) and density (broken line) to level on a sandy beach. (After Edwards, 1969; courtesy Editor, American Zoologist)*

Experimental studies suggested that this was brought about by differences in the response of large and small individuals to light. Large animals tend to crawl more actively than small ones especially in the dark, and bury themselves in the sand under the illuminated conditions of the upper shore. This behaviour results in an accumulation of large animals on the upper shore where they are least active. It seems likely that this response carries the larger individuals away from the intense intra-specific competition on the lower shore and allows new food supplies to be exploited. Interestingly, Edwards (1969) also showed that the physiological tolerances of large individuals, especially to desiccation stress, was greater than the small snails so that the behaviour restricts the small individuals to a level on the shore where the physiological stresses are minimised.

This example shows how a non-directional response to light can restrict distribution to certain zones on the shore; but many molluscs orientate in a directional fashion to the sun, or to gravity. The sign of the response is then reversed after a time so that the animals return to approximately the position from which they started. This behaviour allows feeding under moist conditions on the shore and yet prevents the gradual dispersal from the zonational position which would occur if feeding movements were at random. Directional orientation to light has been reported in the stenoglossan *Urosalpinx* (Carriker, 1955), in the winkle *Littorina littorea* (Newell, 1958a, b; Burdon-Jones and Charles, 1958; Charles, 1961), in *Littorina punctata* (Evans, 1961) and more recently in *Nerita plicata* (Warburton, 1973). Warburton (1973) showed that on a beach in Kenya specimens of *Nerita* on the lower shore were photonegative in the morning and photopositive in the afternoon so that the animals tended to migrate away from the sea. It seems likely that in this case the behaviour minimises dislodgement by wave action. The possibility of desiccation at high shore levels is reduced by the retention of a large volume of seawater under the shell when the animal attaches itself to the substratum. During the night, when desiccation stress is minimal, the snails make random browsing movements whilst the tide is out and return to higher shore levels by orientation to the sun during the day.

The ecological implications of such responses are, however, not always as clear as they are in *Olivella* and *Nerita*. Some bivalves, including *Macoma balthica, Cardium edule* and *Venus striatula* have also been observed to make looped tracks in the sand (Brafield and Newell, 1961; Swennen, 1969; Hulscher, 1973). It is difficult in these instances to ascribe a functional basis for the behaviour since at all times the animals in the deposits are protected from desiccation and thermal stress. Brafield and Newell (1961) suggested that in *Macoma* the response was a mechanism for utilising new feeding areas. But food is rarely limiting in the muds in which the bivalve lives*, and in any event a similar crawling also occurs in the suspension-feeding cockle *Cardium edule.* Swennen (1969) and Hulscher (1973) have both noted that in *Macoma* a high proportion of individuals which crawl are also infected by trematode parasites. Swennen (1969) suggests that the parasite might induce crawling behaviour in *Macoma* and thus increase the chance of detection and predation by birds so that the parasite can complete its life cycle.

Other molluscs have combined responses to light and gravity which enable the animal to return to a microhabitat which is sheltered from the rigours of intertidal life. The chiton *Lepidochitona cinereus*, for example, is very susceptible to desiccation and makes random browsing excursions over the surface of stones only when covered by the tide. But when the tide ebbs and the light intensity increases, the chitons become positively geotactic and crawl rapidly in bright light down to the humid conditions under stones (Evans, 1951). The bivalve *Lasaea rubra* also uses a combination of

*Recent evidence suggests however that in the case of *Hydrobia* grazing may significantly reduce the population of larger diatoms and that competition for food may then occur (Fenchel and Kofoed, 1976).

responses to light and gravity to secure a position which is protected from thermal stress and desiccation. Morton (1960) showed that if displaced from its normal zonational position high on the shore, *Lasaea rubra* is negatively geotactic. This provides a coarse adjustment which brings the animal into the vicinity of the high shore crevices in which it usually lives. This response is overridden by a negative phototaxis so when a crevice is encountered the bivalve tends to crawl away from light into the crevice. Finally, this latter response is in turn overridden by a response to contact (thigmotaxis) which causes the animals to aggregate in narrow regions where displacement by wave action is less likely.

In other cases responses to light and gravity have been combined in tidal areas to produce a complex behaviour pattern which results in both an evasion of physical stress as well as utilisation of feeding areas outside the normal habitat which the animals occupy. The small gastropod *Hydrobia ulvae*, for example, normally lives in muddy estuarine situations and when the tide has ebbed feeds on the deposits making looped tracks much as occur in the molluscs referred to above. After a time, however, by a combination of responses to light and gravity, the animals float themselves by means of a mucous raft from the surface of the water between the ripple marks. The raft is continuously secreted and at the same time the snail eats the particles trapped in the mucus which thus acts as a food net and enables the animal to extend its feeding over the whole tidal cycle. Later, when the tide ebbs, the snails re-attach themselves to the substratum and the cycle is completed (Newell, 1962; 1965). This sequence is illustrated in *Figure 1.10*.

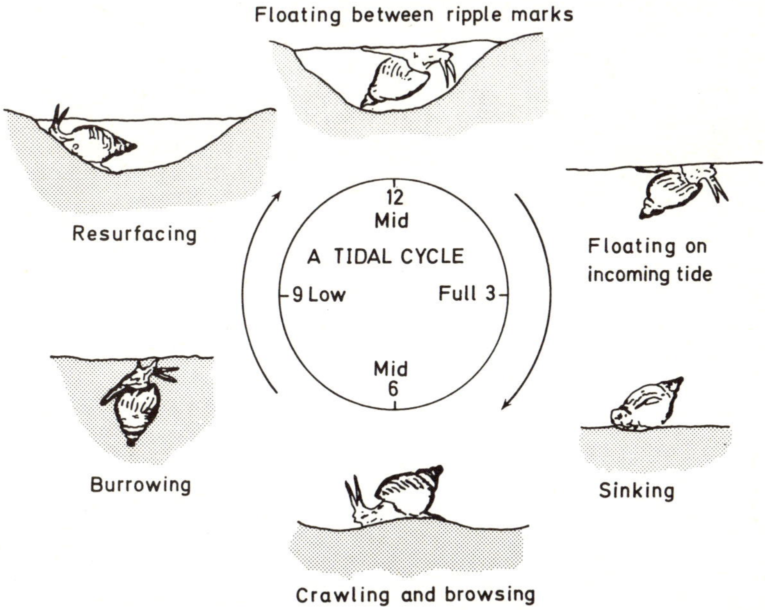

Figure 1.10. Diagram summarising the behaviour of Hydrobia ulvae *during one tidal cycle on the shore on the North Kent Coast. (After Newell, 1970; from Newell, 1962; courtesy Paul Elek (Scientific Books) Ltd)*

The responses of intertidal crustaceans such as fiddler crabs of the genus *Uca* and the sand hopper *Talitrus saltator* are perhaps the best documented examples of organisms whose complex behaviour ensures survival in the intertidal zone. The sand hopper *Talitrus saltator* lives in burrows in sand above the high water mark where it is protected from both temperature and humidity stresses. Under humid conditions when the tide has ebbed or at night time the sand hoppers migrate seaward to scavenge amongst the moist algae of the strandline and later return to the safety of the sand above the high water mark. Pardi and Papi (1952; 1953; 1961), Papi and Pardi (1953; 1959) and Pardi (1960) have shown that seaward and landward migration is made possible by the use of solar navigation and that in the absence of direct sunlight, the hoppers are able to respond to the plane of polarisation of the light as in many other crustaceans (for review, *see* Waterman, 1961). It also seems likely that such orientation is aided by a response to the slope of the shore (Ercolini and Scapini, 1974) and that landward migration might also occur in response to the silhouette of the shoreline (Williamson, 1953). The animals also have an internal time mechanism which allows compensation for the movement of the sun in navigation (for review, *see* Pardi and Papi, 1961) and this may also be of importance in allowing the buried hoppers to predict the environmental conditions without constant reference to them (Bregazzi and Naylor, 1972; *see also* Chapter 7); emergence can then be made at night when optimal humidities prevail.

Aerial exposure on the beach can modify the behaviour of sand hoppers and drying the animals causes a complete reversal of the landward migration of *Talitrus* (Pardi and Papi, 1961). It also influences the sign of phototaxis in other arthropods (Pertunen, 1963). Fiddler crabs belonging to the genus *Uca* live in burrows in the sand where they are protected from desiccation and during the low tide period the animals emerge from the sand and migrate down into the intertidal zone. As in *Talitrus,* navigation is principally by celestial orientation but other factors including responses to the configuration of the shoreline play a part in guiding the animals back up the shore to the safety of the burrow. As mentioned above, the response of a particular individual is modified by other factors such as the degree of desiccation. Edney (1961; 1962) for example, showed that on some occasions the surface temperature of the sand reached 44.5–46°C near a colony of *Uca annulipes.* This is well above the heat lethal temperature of 42°C for the crab. Under these conditions, brief feeding excursions were made from the burrow and evaporative water loss reduced the body temperature to 34–38.7°C. The crabs then returned to their humid burrows at frequent intervals to restore evaporative water losses before another feeding excursion was made. More recently Smith and Miller (1973) have shown that lethal body temperatures may be approached in both *Uca rapax* and *U. pugilator* during the year. Under these conditions, retreat into the burrow or moving into the shade were shown to be the most effective strategies for reduction of the body temperature, although other responses including changing colour, wetting the body and orientation to the sun or wind are each implicated in the maintenance of heat balance. In much the same way, the isopod *Ligia oceanica* seeks the protection of the humid conditions amongst stones and under vegetation but is able to lose heat by evaporative water loss when the temperature rises (Edney, 1953; *see also* p.26). A review of these and other adaptations to life on land shown by crustaceans is given by Bliss and Mantel (1968).

A much more precise orientation mechanism is required in those animals which undertake feeding excursions from a very restricted microhabitat. Many limpets, for example, live on irregular rock surfaces which the shell fits accurately. Water loss is greatly reduced if the limpets return to the same 'limpet scar' from which they started (Davies, 1969). Homing behaviour of this kind had been reported for *Acmaea scabra* (Hewatt, 1940; Jessee, 1968), in *Acmaea digitalis* and *Lottia gigantea* (Galbraith, 1965) and in *Patella* (Orton, 1929; Cook *et al.,* 1969). The pulmonate limpet, *Siphonaria,* also undertakes feeding excursions when first exposed by the ebbing tide and also when first covered by the flowing tide, retiring each time to a fixed limpet scar (Ohgushi, 1954; Cook, 1969, 1971). Rather little is known of the precise way in which such limpets return to their scar but at least in the case of *Siphonaria normalis,* the limpets appear to use chemoreception to detect the mucous trail left on the outward excursion. Cook (1969) showed that solar navigation and silhouette responses such as have been described above for many intertidal invertebrates, could not apply in the case of *Siphonaria.* Experimental animals were able to return home even when the rocks were rotated 90° in the horizontal plane or 180° in the vertical plane while the limpets were away from the home rock.

Figure 1.11(a) shows the result of an experiment in which each of 46 limpets was allowed to lay a mucous trail on a slide and was then removed. Each animal was then replaced on the slide with its head next to the trail and the long axis perpendicular to the trail. The subsequent movements of the limpet were then recorded and the percentage of the original trail that was retraced was calculated. Of the 46 limpets used, 40 retraced 90-100% of their original tracks. In a control series of experiments, the limpets were placed on the reverse side of the slide from the original mucous trail and as can be seen from *Figure 1.11(b),* there is no evidence that the animals were responding to other features of the environmental situation. Several species of *Patella* may also use a similar series of chemical clues for homing (Funke, 1968) and other gastropods may also be able to respond to mucous trails (Crisp, 1969; Wells and Buckley, 1972). The ability to respond to the chemical nature of the substratum and especially to mucopolysaccharides, is well known in studies of the settlement responses of marine invertebrates (Williams, 1964; for review, *see* Newell, 1970) and may therefore be of general occurrence where precise orientation is required.

These examples show that many intertidal organisms which are apparently ill-equipped to survive the rigours of the intertidal environment have managed to do so by synchronisation of their behaviour with optimal phases of the tidal cycle. In some cases terrestrial organisms which have invaded the upper part of the intertidal zone retreat to the air spaces within crevices when the tide has covered the shore. Alternatively many marine organisms, including fishes (*see* Gibson, 1969), which are susceptible to water loss, have evolved complex behavioural mechanisms to allow both survival in suitable

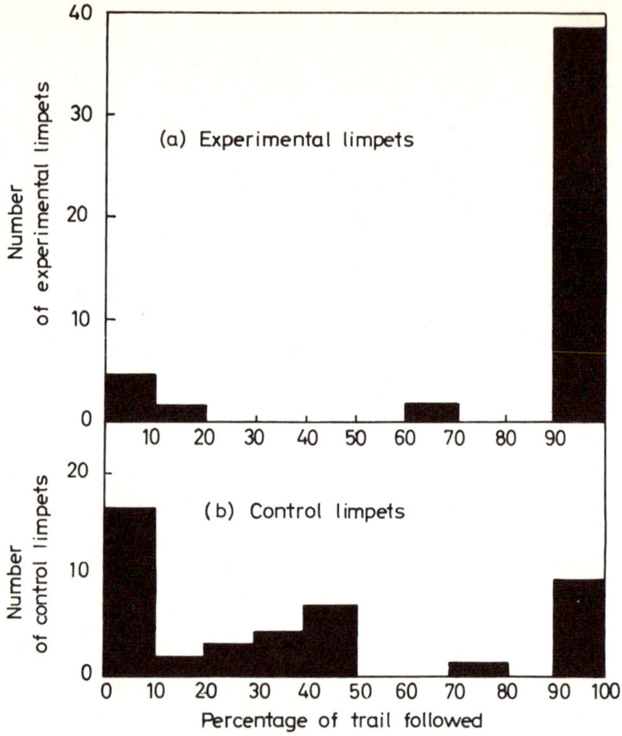

Figure 1.11 Histograms showing the ability of the limpet Siphonaria alternata *to follow a mucous trail. (a) The percentage of trail followed by 47 limpets placed with their long axis at right angles to the trail. (b) The percentage trail followed when the limpets were placed on an inverted slide in the same position as in (a) but the mucous trails were absent. (After Cook, 1971; courtesy Editor, Biological Bulletin)*

microhabitats and the utilisation of the rich food resources of the intertidal zone. Several different mechanisms of site-selection exist. These range from generalised responses to light and gravity which are sufficient to define a broad zone in which the organism is likely to be able to survive. More specific site-selection involves a hierarchy of responses in which increasingly precise environmental stimuli are used to initiate settlement. Responses to humidity, particle size and contact with the walls of crevices are all used in the detailed choice of microhabitat. But chemotactile responses as are shown by the larvae of many marine invertebrates, as well as in a variety of limpets, represent the most precise definition of conditions which are likely to be suitable for life in the intertidal zone.

1.2.2 Structural and behavioural maintenance of heat balance

We have seen that the ability of intertidal organisms to evade stresses associated with life on the sea-shore is one of the principal mechanisms which allows colonisation of the intertidal environment by aquatic organisms. Equally, a second component of organisms, which characteristically have colonised the upper shore, display a variety of structural and behavioural mechanisms to withstand the stresses associated with temperature and water loss. It is axiomatic that most intertidal organisms which are capable of colonising open rock surfaces of the sea-shore possess some means of excluding the environment during unfavourable phases of the tidal cycle. In some prosobranch gastropods, such as the limpets, there is a thick impermeable shell which can be clamped tightly against the substratum and so prevent water loss. Many other gastropods have an operculum which is often of a quinone-tanned protein associated with micropolysaccharides and is in some cases calcified (*see* Vovelle, 1969a, b; 1970; 1973). This structure is used to close the aperture of the shell and in high level species tends to be more impermeable and tight-fitting than in low-level gastropods (Micallef, 1966). Resistance to desiccation in barnacles also appears to be related at least partly to structural features. Newman (1967) showed that the relative rates of desiccation of barnacles could be correlated with the permeability of the integument, more thick shelled barnacles such as *Balanus balanoides, Chthamalus stellatus* and *Elminius modestus* being able to survive higher on the shore than *Balanus improvisus* which has a thin more permeable shell. Again, although most intertidal bivalves seek the protection of crevices and deposits, those such as the mussels *Mytilus edulis* and *Modiolus demissus* are able to live in the intertidal zone at least partly because they can close the shell valves and exclude desiccation stress.

It is only relatively recently, however, that a systematic survey has been carried out of the implications of shell shape on the survival of intertidal gastropods. Vermeij (1971a, b; 1973) has made a detailed study of the distribution, shape and temperature relationships of a variety of tropical intertidal molluscs. His important work suggests that within the relatively simple body plan of shelled gastropods, many of the structural features are related to strategies for the maintenance of heat balance. Vermeij (1973) also showed that shell shape in tropical gastropods is partly a reflection of adaptation to temperature and desiccation stress in an upshore direction, and partly to increased mechanical stress by wave action in a downshore direction. Some species which have a narrow vertical range of distribution can be adapted to either one or other of these groups of stresses. In those with a wide vertical range on the shore, however, intraspecific gradients in shell size and shape reflecting adaptations to both groups of stresses with shore level may occur.

The energy exchange between such animals and their external environment depends on a balance between two main components. First, there is heat gained from the environment by radiation absorbed by the animal's surface, by conduction from the substratum plus endogenous heat from metabolic processes. Secondly, there is heat loss by evaporation and convection which in turn are influenced greatly by humidity, wind speed and the difference between the body temperature of the organism and that of the environment. In a steady-state situation (which is rarely reached under natural conditions) the general equation for heat balance would be of the form:

$$\text{Radiation} + \text{Conduction} + \text{Metabolic Heat} = \text{Convection} + \text{Evaporation} + \text{Emission}$$
$$(\text{HEAT GAIN}) = (\text{HEAT LOSS})$$

For a perfect radiator (a black body) of unit area in a uniform environment the energy exchange is a constant, but very few materials even approach being a black body. They are poor radiators but better reflectors and shell colour will greatly influence the energy loss side of the equation. The importance of these factors in the heat balance of a variety of animals is discussed by Parry (1951), Edney (1953), Porter and Gates (1969), Newell (1970), Smith and Miller (1973) and Vermeij (1973). Clearly, from the general equation for heat balance outlined above, the heat of upper shore animals can be minimised by (1) a reduction in heat gain from the environment or (2) an increase in heat loss from the animal.

1. Heat gain can be minimised by one or more of the following strategies:
   (a) A reduction in the total surface area relative to volume of the organism since this will reduce heat gain by radiation.
   (b) A reduction in the surface area in contact with the substratum since this will reduce conduction.
   (c) A reduction in the metabolic rate.
2. Equally, organisms can increase heat loss from the tissues by:
   (a) The possession of strong shell sculpturing in upper shore species which increases heat loss by convection.
   (b) The ability to lose water by evaporation over the period of intertidal exposure, which thus increases evaporative heat loss.
   (c) The possession of a light coloured shell which increases the emission relative to absorption.

Each of these terms is an independent variable, and in cases such as evaporative water loss, can be varied in one individual over a short period of time. It is thus clear that a great variety of strategies can be adopted by intertidal animals to maintain their heat balance and these dominate the structural adaptations which such organisms show to life on the sea-shore.

1.2.2.1 REDUCTION OF HEAT GAIN FROM THE ENVIRONMENT

One of the implications of the heat balance equation is that in tropical environments where organisms of the upper shore are subjected to intense heat stress, certain convergent patterns would be anticipated. Amongst the gastropods, for example, we might expect to find one or more of the following features: (a) An increase in relative size of upper shore individuals and genera compared with those on the lower shore where heat stress is less. This would reduce the relative surface area through which heat gain by radiation occurs. An increase in size from low to high shore levels would also minimise the rate of change of body temperature, since it takes longer for the tissues of a large animal to equilibrate with the environmental temperature during the low tide period. (b) A smaller area of foot through which heat gain by conduction can occur. (c) A reduced metabolic rate compared with lower shore animals.

Both inter- and intraspecific differences in the body size of gastropods with shore level is widespread and not confined to tropical environments. Smith and Newell (1955) showed that in *Littorina littorea* the initial settlement of juveniles is on the lower shore, upper shore levels being colonised later by the larger individuals. Equally, the occurrence of mainly large specimens of *Olivella* in the upper intertidal zone has already been noted (*See Figure 1.9* and Edwards, 1969). More recently, Davies (1969) showed that intra- and interspecific differences occur in the shell shape of limpets at different tidal levels. Large specimens with a steep shell occur on open rock surfaces at high tidal levels whereas small individuals, or those with a flattened cone, occur in damp situations and on the lower shore. Amongst the intertidal trochids, too, large genera such as *Monodonta lineata* occur at high shore levels and on open rock surfaces whereas their smaller relatives such as *Gibbula cineraria* and *G. umbilicalis* are confined to damper situations on the lower shore.

Vermeij (1973) has collected data for a wide variety of intertidal gastropods from tropical habitats. His principal data relate to widespread members of the families Littorinidae, the limpets and to the Neritidae. He showed that amongst the littorinids there was an increase in relative spire height and the degree of sculpturing both interspecifically and often intraspecifically from low to high levels on tropical shores. Similar trends were also apparent from high to low latitudes but the physical gradients on the shores in temperate regions were less distinct and this tended to obscure some of the more obvious trends seen on tropical shores. Similarly, the limpets show, as a general rule, an interspecific increase in shell height with shore level, but latitudinal trends are less clear than in littorinids. Finally, in neritids there is an interspecific increase in relative shell globosity from low to high shore levels. Upper shore species living in tropical environments have a globose shell which is strongly sculptured and these specialised species tend to disappear as one moves away from the tropics towards higher latitudes. As has been pointed out on p.20, an increase in size and in shell sculpturing would provide an effective means both of reduction of heat gain by radiation and increase of heat loss by convection. The correlation between these shell characteristics and both tidal-dependent and latitudinal gradients in environmental conditions is, as demonstrated by Vermeij (1972; 1973), a strong argument for the importance of structural features in the heat balance of intertidal gastropods.

The second general feature which might be anticipated from the general heat balance equation is that a reduction in heat gain by conduction from the environment could be achieved by a reduction of the area in contact with the substratum. A relative decrease in surface area by increase in size, as pointed out above, reduces both heat gain by radiation and the rate of equilibration of the tissues with environmental conditions when the tide ebbs. But an increase in body size without a change in other morphological characters would lead to an increase in the importance of conduction through the foot. It is interesting to note, therefore, that Vermeij (1971a; 1972; 1973; *see also*

Davies, 1969) has shown that there is a relative reduction in basal area amongst the neritids and limpets with increase in size. The area of contact between the tissues and the substratum is, however, large in spite of this, perhaps allowing the animals to survive in zones where the physical force of wave action would dislodge other organisms. Because of the large area of the foot in these species, it is not surprising to find that the tissue temperatures of limpets vary according to the absorptive and conductive properties of the substratum. Segal and Dehnel (1962) and Davies (1970), for example, have shown that at high shore levels the tissue temperatures of limpets on igneous rocks was higher than those on sandstone. Clearly, the thermal properties of the substratum become important in controlling the distribution of such animals on the upper shore and at these levels only the cooler types of substratum may be suitable for organisms with a large surface area in contact with the rock. But heat gain by conduction is less important on the lower shore and in these situations neritids and limpets appear to occupy a wider range of substratum types (Vermeij, 1971a).

An alternative strategy, and one which allows a greater independence from the substratum even at high shore levels, is adopted by organisms which remain attached to the substratum by a small foot, as in planaxids and some trochids such as *Monodonta labio.* In other organisms, such as some species of *Nerita* and in many littorinids (Vermeij, 1971a, b) as well as in the limpets *Acmaea digitalis* and *A. persona* (Wolcott, 1973), a further degree of independence from the substratum is gained by attachment to the substratum by means of a mucous film. Even on temperate shores during the summer, specimens of *Littorina littorea* living at high shore levels in full sunlight are to be seen hanging from vertical surfaces by means of a dried mucous sheet which attaches the front lip of the shell to the substratum. This occurs also in the gastropod *Hydrobia ulvae* when its floating movements carry it into an unfavourable part of the intertidal zone. The only point of contact with the substratum is the anterior shell lip so that heat gain by conduction from the substratum is virtually eliminated by this method. This strategy is clearly suitable only in organisms left high on the shore by the retreating tide, and capable of rapid reattachment when the incoming tide reaches them. Any individuals dislodged by the incoming tide must also be capable of regaining their zonational position by the appropriate responses to light and gravity (Newell, 1958a, b; 1962; for review, *see* 1970).

Finally, heat gain could be minimised by a reduction in metabolism of high level species compared with lower shore individuals. There is some evidence that this does occur, although whether the amounts of heat are significant compared with the heat gain from other sources is highly questionable. Parry (1951) showed that in the case of insects resting in direct sunlight, metabolic heat gain does not contribute significantly to the total heat balance. The heat gained by metabolism was also considered to be insignificant in the isopod *Ligia oceanica* by Edney (1951; 1953). In this case the oxygen consumption of an average individual in air at 25°C was 0.02 ml/cm^2/h. Since 1ml oxygen is equivalent to 4.775 calories, the energy gain contributed by metabolism in a typical *Ligia* was calculated to amount to only 0.11 milliwatts/cm^2. The small contribution made by metabolic heat to the overall heat balance of

Ligia is supported by the fact that prevention of evaporative heat loss in saturated air did not result in a marked gain of metabolic heat at high environmental temperatures. It therefore seems likely that under these conditions the contribution made by metabolic heat is insignificant, although at low environmental temperatures it may make a more important impact on the overall heat balance. The ability of upper shore organisms to suppress their level of activity during the intertidal period, and hence to reduce their metabolic rate is well known (for review, *see* Newell, 1970; Vermeij, 1973). It has also been shown that the metabolism of high level individuals of *Patella vulgata* may be depressed compared with lower shore individuals during the summer (Davies, 1966; 1967). Similar differences exist between upper shore and lower shore species of *Acmaea* (Baldwin, 1968). Nevertheless, for the reasons mentioned above, such inter- and intraspecific differences in metabolism in relation to tidal gradients are unlikely to be related to heat balance and are discussed in relation to problems of metabolic energy balance on p.55.

1.2.2.2 INCREASE OF HEAT LOSS FROM THE TISSUES

As pointed out on p.20, heat loss from the tissues is increased by features which facilitate convection, evaporation and heat emission from the organism. Heat loss by convection could be enhanced by greater shell sculpturing and this indeed appears to be the case in high level tropical gastropods (Vermeij, 1971a). In littorinids such ridges and grooves represent a considerable increase in surface area through which heat can be transferred to the environment, relative to the silhouette area which represents that through which heat gain occurs. Vermeij (1971a; 1973) has shown, for example, that in *Tectarius muricatus* and *Nodilittorina tuberculata,* both of which have strongly sculptured shells, the shell temperature is approximately 0.5°C lower than that of the substratum when the animals are exposed to direct sunlight. The shell surface temperature is the same as that of the substratum when the animals are in the shade. In contrast, the difference between the shell surface temperature and that of the substratum in weakly ribbed forms such as *Littorina lineata* is significantly less.

Again, the emissivity of an organism will be greatly increased if the shell and tissues are light in colour. Vermeij (1971a) has pointed out that many tropical gastropods living on the upper shore including *Littorina coccinea,* the New Zealand *L. unifasciata,* the Pacific *Nodilittorina plicata,* the Caribbean *N. peloronta* and the West Indian *Tectarius muricatus,* are all light in colour. This contrasts with the dark colour of many species characteristic of the lower shore in tropical environments. Smith and Miller (1973) have made a detailed study of the components of the heat balance equation in *Uca rapax* and *U. pugilator.* They were able to incorporate environmental and endogenous factors into a mathematical model which could then be used to predict the effects of a variety of strategies of heat loss in these animals. This approach is very similar to that adopted for predicting the effects of temperature, salinity and other factors on a survival, growth and metabolism in intertidal animals (*see* pp. 43 and 63). Both species of fiddler crab blanch the carapace during the middle of the day, *U. pugilator* undergoing the greatest change, and this results in an increase of the reflectance of solar radiation of about 50% between unblanched and blanched crabs.

Of all the potential methods of heat loss, that represented by evaporation is the most important in intertidal organisms. Each gram of water evaporated from the tissues at 33°C removes 544 calories of heat and although this value increases with temperature, a figure of 540–580 calories/gram would cover the normal tissue temperatures experienced by most intertidal animals. It is not surprising to find, therefore, that intertidal animals in general show several adaptations to capitalise on heat loss by evaporation, and can also control the excessive water loss which might occur under severe environmental conditions. (a) Many animals hold an extra-corporeal water reserve which increases the total volume from which evaporative cooling can take place and minimises changes in the ionic concentration of the body fluids. (b) Many upper shore animals, especially those living in tropical environments, have structural and behavioural adaptations to reduce the rate of water loss when this becomes necessary. (c) Nearly all intertidal animals are able to withstand desiccation to a remarkable extent despite the extensive changes in ionic concentration which might be anticipated from such strategy. This latter adaptation falls into the category of physiological tolerances which are discussed in more detail on p.30.

Amongst the molluscs the retention of water in the mantle cavity from which evaporative heat loss can occur is widespread amongst both tropical and temperate gastropods. In *Littorina littorea* and intertidal trochids such as *Monodonta lineata,* for example, water is retained for much of the intertidal period unless excessive water loss induces complete closure of the operculum. Similarly in *Nerita* (Vermeij, 1971a; Warburton, 1973) and in many limpets (Abe, 1931; Shotwell, 1950; Segal, 1956; Segal and Dehnel, 1962; Vermeij, 1971a) extra-corporeal water may play an important part in extending the period over which evaporation can take place. As pointed out by Wolcott (1973), since there is no osmotic barrier between the tissues and the extra-corporeal water, the total amount of water stored under the shell, including tissue water, is the significant measure of osmotic buffering ability. He concluded that differences in the ability of *Acmaea* species from different zones on the shore to withstand desiccation were not only correlated with the retention of relatively larger volumes of extra-corporeal water in the upper shore animals but also with the larger tissue volumes as well. As pointed out by Vermeij (1973), the larger globose form of neritids of the upper shore would, together with extra-corporeal water, confer a larger total reservoir of water since a sphere maximises the internal volume for any given surface area. In the case of limpets an increase in tissue volume, compared with the basal perimeter through which evaporation occurs, would require an increase in the relative shell height of upper shore limpets. Both intra- and interspecific differences in shell form have been reported in limpets (Davies, 1969). Again, in the high shore trochid genus *Monodonta,* there is a relatively high shell spire and small aperture, a shell morphology which might account for the high tolerance of desiccation shown by this animal (Sourie, 1954; Regis, 1969; Vermeij, 1971a).

In short, it is apparent that many of the structural features of intertidal animals, and gastropods in particular, are related to strategies for the maintenance of heat balance. Of these, adaptations to minimise heat gain by radiation and conduction interact with those which enhance heat loss by convection, emission and evaporation. Superimposed on this pattern of adaptation to life in the intertidal environment are structural requirements to resist the prolonged mechanical wave action of the lower shore as well as physiological differences both of which are largely independent of the problems of heat balance.

1.2.2.3 BEHAVIOURAL THERMOREGULATION

Although the adaptations reviewed above are of fundamental significance in permitting intertidal animals to survive on the upper part of the sea-shore, it is also true that one of the characteristics of the intertidal environment is that physical and chemical conditions are subject to great variation (*see* p. 3). Because the physical environment is not a steady state system, a prime requirement is for the organism to be able to manipulate the components of the heat balance equation to suit local environmental conditions.

In its simplest form, we can include the site selection and evasion behaviour outlined in Section 1.2.1, but many organisms, including sessile ones, adopt a more complex response to one or a combination of several different environmental factors. The sea-shore bristle-tail *Petrobius maritimus,* for example, can increase its heat gain from the environment during the night by utilising the heat accumulated during the daytime by insolation. Since the body temperature of *Petrobius* is close to that of the rock surface, the animal can maintain its activity level even in air temperatures which would normally inhibit activity (Makings, 1973). Again, the ribbed mussel, *Modiolus demissus,* is well adapted for intermittent air-gaping which allows both aerial oxygen consumption as well as suppression of the tissue temperature by evaporative heat loss (Lent, 1968; 1969). *Figure 1.12* shows the suppression of the body temperature which results from air-gaping by *Modiolus demissus* under experimental conditions at an environmental temperature of 22°C and a relative humidity of 60%. There is evidently a rapid initial decline in tissue temperature associated with water loss and the temperature then gradually approaches that of the environment during prolonged exposure. Presumably this latter effect occurs when desiccation has reduced the amount of water available for evaporative heat loss. The adaptive significance of such heat loss must be established by the use of two other criteria because even an inert body will lose heat by evaporation. First, it must be established that the organism actually facilitates such water loss under environmental conditions. Secondly, it must be demonstrated that the reduction in body temperature enhances survival under conditions which occur in the natural environment.

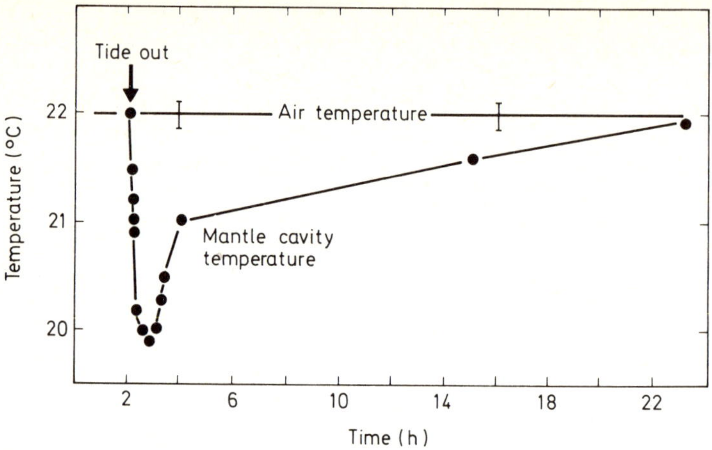

Figure 1.12 Graph showing the temperature of the mantle cavity of an individual Modiolus demissus *during a simulated tide. Air temperature 22°C (±2°C), relative humidity 60%. (After Lent, 1968; courtesy Editor, Biological Bulletin)*

In the case of *Modiolus,* this last criterion has not been clearly established and it remains open whether heat loss in this animal is merely an incidental corollary to air-breathing (*see* Lent, 1968). In *Ligia,* however, evaporation plays an important part in the heat balance of the animal. Edney (1951; 1953; 1954; 1960) has shown that the isopods adopt particular behaviour patterns in response to thermal stress and that the body temperature of *Ligia*

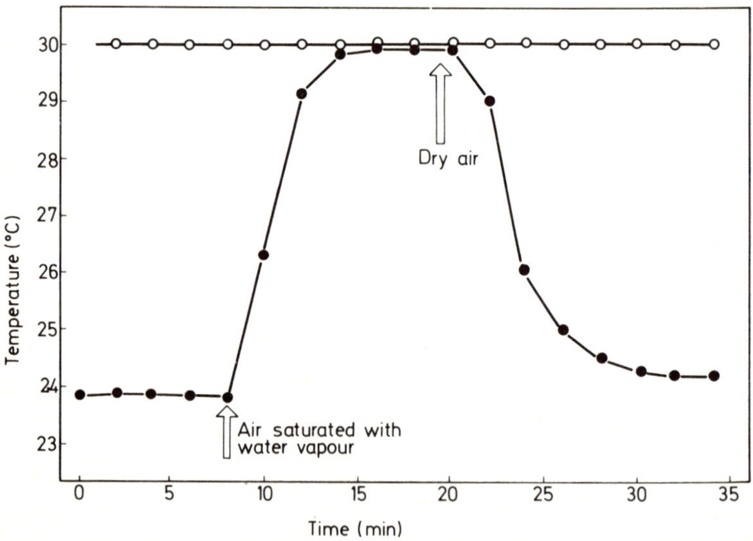

Figure 1.13 Graph showing the effect of evaporative water loss on the body temperature of Ligia. *The animal was first exposed to a slowly moving stream of dry air at 30°C (open circles) alternating with a stream of air saturated with water vapour at 30°C. (After Newell, 1970; from Edney, 1951; courtesy Paul Elek (Scientific Books) Ltd)*

in dry air may be several degrees lower than that of the environment. *Figure 1.13* shows the result of an experiment in which a specimen of *Ligia* was exposed to a slowly-moving stream of dry air at 30°C alternating with a stream of air saturated with water vapour at 30°C. A suppression of the body temperature by as much as six degrees occurred. This compares well with measured values under natural conditions of 8°C between the temperature of rock surfaces and that of the tissues.

The body temperature of fiddler crabs (Edney, 1961, 1962; Wilkens and Fingerman, 1965; Smith and Miller, 1973) and the shore crab *Carcinus* (Ahsanullah, 1969) is also related to their ability to migrate from water saturated microhabitats to those where evaporative cooling can occur. In both of these instances, as well as in *Ligia* (Edney, 1953) and possibly in *Modiolus demissus* (Lent, 1968), behavioural thermoregulation may result in a significant increase in survival at high temperatures. *Figure 1.14* shows

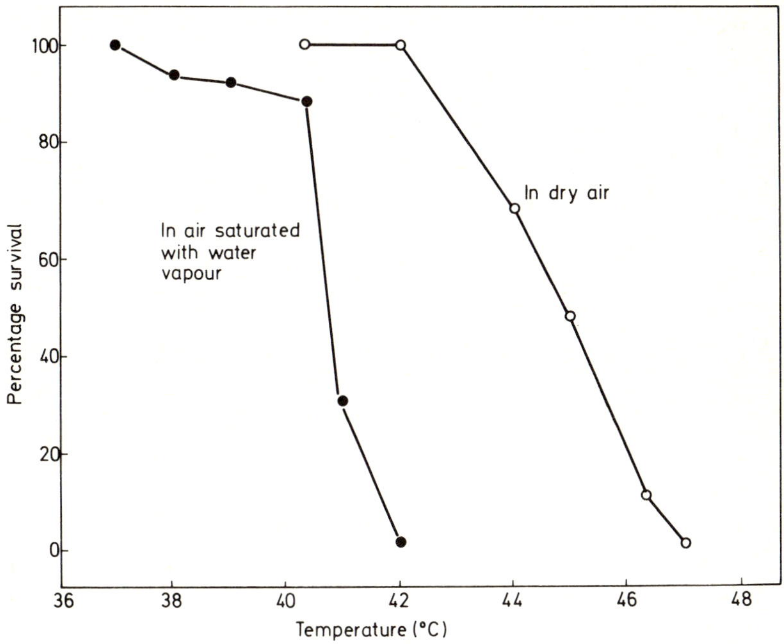

Figure 1.14 Graphs showing the percentage survival of the fiddler crab Uca pugilator *after one hour in dry air (open circles) and in air saturated with water vapour (solid circles). (After Newell, 1970; from Wilkens and Fingerman, 1965; courtesy Paul Elek (Scientific Books) Ltd)*

the percentage survival of *Uca pugilator* after one hour in dry air and in air saturated with water vapour. The temperature for 50% survival was only 41°C in water saturated air but as much as 45°C in dry air. The difference in these values is accounted for by the suppression of the body temperature made possible by evaporative heat loss in dry air. The shore crab *Carcinus maenas* also shows a greater tolerance of high temperatures in dry air than in

Table 1.1 THE DIFFERENT STRATEGIES OF ADAPTATION INVOLVED IN THE MAINTENANCE OF HEAT BALANCE IN INTERTIDAL ANIMALS LIVING IN REGIONS OF TEMPERATURE STRESS (FOR EXPLANATION, *SEE* TEXT)

Heat gain				*Heat loss*			
Energy source	*Adaptation*	*Example*	*Reference*	*Energy source*	*Adaptation*	*Example*	*Reference*
A. RADIATION	Increase in relative size with shore level	*Olivella*	Edwards, 1968	A. CONVECTION	Increased shell sculpturing at high shore levels	*Tectarius muricatus*	Vermeij, 1971a; 1973
		Littorina littorea	Smith and Newell, 1955			*Nodilittorina tubercutata*	
		Littorinids Limpets Neritids	Vermeij, 1971a: 1973	B. EMISSIVITY	Light colour in upper shore forms	*Littorina coccinea* *L.unifasciata* *Nodilittorina plicata* *N.pelorata*	Vermeij, 1971a
B. CONDUCTION	1. Reduce relative area of foot at high shore levels	*Patella*	Davies, 1969				
		Neritids Limpets	Vermeij, 1971a; 1972; 1973			*Uca rapax* *U.pugilator*	Smith and Miller, 1973
	2. Reduce contact with substratum by mucus	Littorinids *Acmaea*	Vermeij, 1971a, b; Wolcott, 1973				
	3. Behavioural thermo-regulation (at low temperatures)	*Petrobius*	Makings, 1973				
		Uca	Smith and Miller, 1973				

C. METABOLISM	Reduce metabolic rate on upper shore in warm environments. (Probably insignificant in heat balance compared with A and B).	*Patella*	Davies, 1966; 1967
		Acmaea	Baldwin, 1968

C. EVAPORATION	1. Increase water store	*Nerita*	Vermeij, 1971a; 1973
			Warburton, 1973
		Limpets	Segal, 1956; Segal and Dehnel, 1962; Vermeij, 1971a
	2. Reduced perimeter	*Monodonta*	Vermeij, 1971a; Sourie, 1954; Regis, 1969
		Patella	Davies, 1969
	3. Intermittent air gaping	*Modiolus demissus*	Lent, 1968; 1969
	4. Behavioural thermo-regulation	*Ligia*	Edney, 1951; 1953
		Uca	Edney, 1961; 1962
			Wilkens and Fingerman, 1965; Smith and Miller, 1973
		Carcinus	Ahsanullah, 1969

water and, like *Ligia,* exposes itself to dry conditions when environmental temperatures rise towards lethal levels.

The different strategies of adaptation involved in the maintenance of heat balance in intertidal organisms are summarised in *Table 1.1.* It is clear that the ability to regulate evaporative water loss, and above all, to tolerate dehydration of the tissues, represents a major factor controlling colonisation of the sea-shore. The relevance of gradations in the physiological tolerances of intertidal organisms to their distribution on the shore is discussed in more detail in Section 1.2.3.

1.2.3 Physiological limits of survival

We have seen that to a large extent structural and behavioural mechanisms may minimise the stresses to which the tissues of intertidal organisms are subjected. Nevertheless, it remains true that despite these adaptations, animals living on the upper shore will experience greater stresses, and for a longer period of time, than their counterparts on the lower shore. A good deal of the earlier literature has been concerned with determining to what extent the tolerances of animals to environmental stresses are related to gradients of physical conditions on the shore. There has also been the problem of whether the differences in the tolerances of intertidal animals to environmental stress are sufficient to account for the zonation which occurs on most shores throughout the world. Tidal-dependent factors which might be expected to limit the distribution of intertidal animals include temperature, desiccation and a combination of these two variables. In some habitats such as high-level rockpools, salinity stress may acquire an ecological significance (Hagerman, 1969; Ganning, 1971) and this may be associated with marked fluctuations in environmental temperature. Interactions of this kind between the effects of temperature and salinity on invertebrates are now well documented and have been reviewed by Kinne (1963; 1964).

1.2.3.1 TOLERANCE OF TEMPERATURE STRESS

Early work of Huntsman and Sparks (1924) and Henderson (1929) showed that the upper limit of thermal tolerance of a variety of marine invertebrates was correlated with the temperature range experienced under natural conditions. Both latitudinal and vertical differences are apparent and even within one species, individuals from upper shore levels have a higher limit of thermal tolerance than lower shore individuals (Gowanloch and Hayes, 1926). The most detailed of these early studies relating the physical tolerances of intertidal organisms to zonational position on the shore was undoubtedly that of Broekhuysen (1940). He showed that the sequence of thermal death points in a series of six South African gastropods shows a general correspondence with their zonational position on the shore. *Littorina knysnaënsis,* whose upper limit extends to approximately 12.5 ft above datum, had an upper lethal temperature of 48.6°C whilst *Oxystele variegata,* which extends up to 9.75 ft above datum, had an upper lethal temperature of only 42.1°C. Again, *Thais dubia* extends up to 9.25 ft above datum and had an upper lethal temperature of 41.7°C whilst that of *Oxystele tigrina* which lives up to 8 ft above datum, was 39.5°C. Finally, the lower shore *Oxystele sinensis,* which lives up to 5.25 ft above datum, had an upper lethal temperature of 39.6°C which is similar to its neighbour *O. tigrina.*

Since that time there have been many studies which confirm and amplify these ecological sequences in thermal tolerance. Evans (1948) found a correlation between the upper limit of thermal tolerance and the normal temperature range occurring at particular sites from which the animals were collected. He concluded, however, that the topography of the shore was too complicated to allow a simple relationship between tidal level and thermal tolerance as demonstrated by Broekhuysen (1940). Much of this earlier work has been reviewed elsewhere (Gunter, 1957; Southward, 1958; Newell, 1970). More recently, Hardin (1968) and Wolcott (1973) have shown that in *Acmaea* both inter- and intraspecific differences exist with high shore individuals having a higher lethal temperature than lower shore specimens. Again, Vernberg and Vernberg (1970) have reviewed the zoogeographical significance of temperature and have shown that in general southern affinity species survived higher temperatures than northerly displaced species. Equally in species with overlapping distribution on the shore, differences in thermal tolerance were related to conditions in the microhabitats which they select. Sassaman and Mangum (1970) have also demonstrated that the southern distribution of three different species of North Atlantic sea anemones is correlated with their lethal temperature. The main problem in any interpretation of the ecological relevance of such studies is that:

1. The heat-lethal temperatures obtained experimentally appear to be much higher than the actual environmental temperatures recorded, which suggests that these tolerances may not limit distribution on the shore.
2. The environmental temperatures, or more strictly the tissue temperatures of the animals, are commonly not known in detail under natural conditions.
3. The upper lethal temperature of the animals may be different in air and in water as, for example, in chitons (Kenny, 1958), *Uca* (Wilkens and Fingermann, 1965) and in trochid gastropods (Micallef, 1966).
4. Large scale mortality of intertidal animals has only rarely been related causally to environmental and tissue temperatures of animals whose thermal tolerances are known (Orton, 1933; Hodgkin, 1959; Frank, 1965; Sutherland, 1970; Wolcott, 1973).

All the recent studies have been concerned with the establishment of what might be regarded as an 'ecologically relevant' measure of the heat-lethal temperature of the organism. This is affected by (a) the criterion of heat death. In some cases the temperature at which the animal is unable to resume normal activity when returned to low temperatures may be considerably less than the lethal temperature. Heat damage may thus operate in the environment at lower temperatures than those required to kill the animal outright. (b) The time of exposure to potentially lethal conditions. A long period of exposure to near lethal conditions may have a similar effect on an upper shore animal as a short exposure to a much higher temperature (*see also* Chapter 3). (c) the previous thermal history of the organism. Latitudinal and seasonal differences in thermal tolerances may be brought about by the ability of intertidal animals to adjust their limits of temperature tolerance to meet local environmental conditions. It is only when these additional factors are taken into account, and in particular when we have detailed data on environmental temperature and its effects on natural populations, that we can assess the ecological significance of temperature tolerance.

Orr (1955), Micallef (1966), Crisp and Ritz (1967a), Ritz (1968) and Foster (1969) have each taken the effect of exposure time into account in an assessment of the temperature tolerance of marine invertebrates. Fraenkel (1960) has also emphasised the importance of using proper criteria for the judgment of survival. He suggested that the resumption of normal behaviour when returned to controlled conditions, was the best criterion for the absence of thermal damage. This approach was also adopted by Sassaman and Mangum (1970). Typical time-temperature curves are obtained by plotting the time taken to 50% mortality (LT50) against exposure temperature (*Figure 1.15*). The curves obtained by Foster (1969) for a series of barnacles show that there is an exponential decline in survival time as

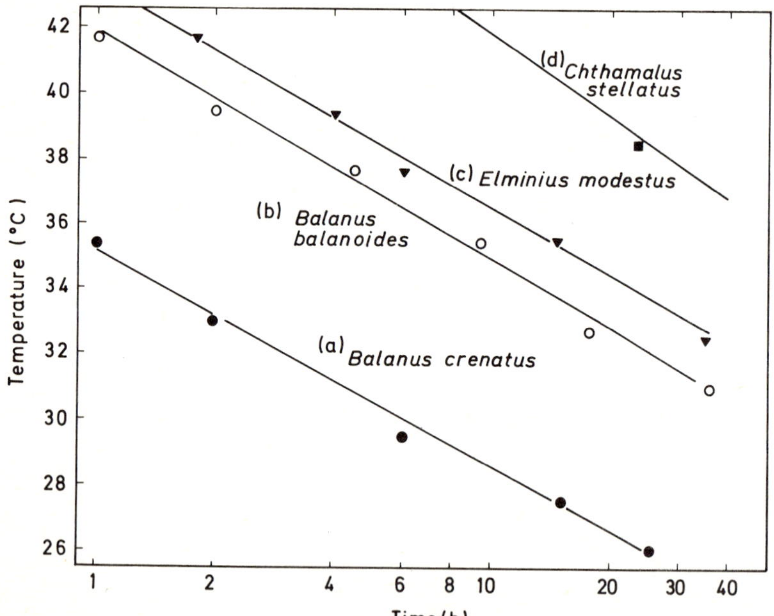

Figure 1.15 Graphs showing the effect of time on the median lethal temperature for (a) Balanus crenatus *(b)* B. balanoides *(c)* Elminius modestus *(d)* Chthamalus stellatus. *(After Foster, 1969; courtesy Editor, Marine Biology)*

exposure temperature increases. Clearly, the thermal tolerance of different organisms can be compared by means of the temperature required to cause 50% mortality in a given time period. Crisp and Ritz (1967a) and Ritz

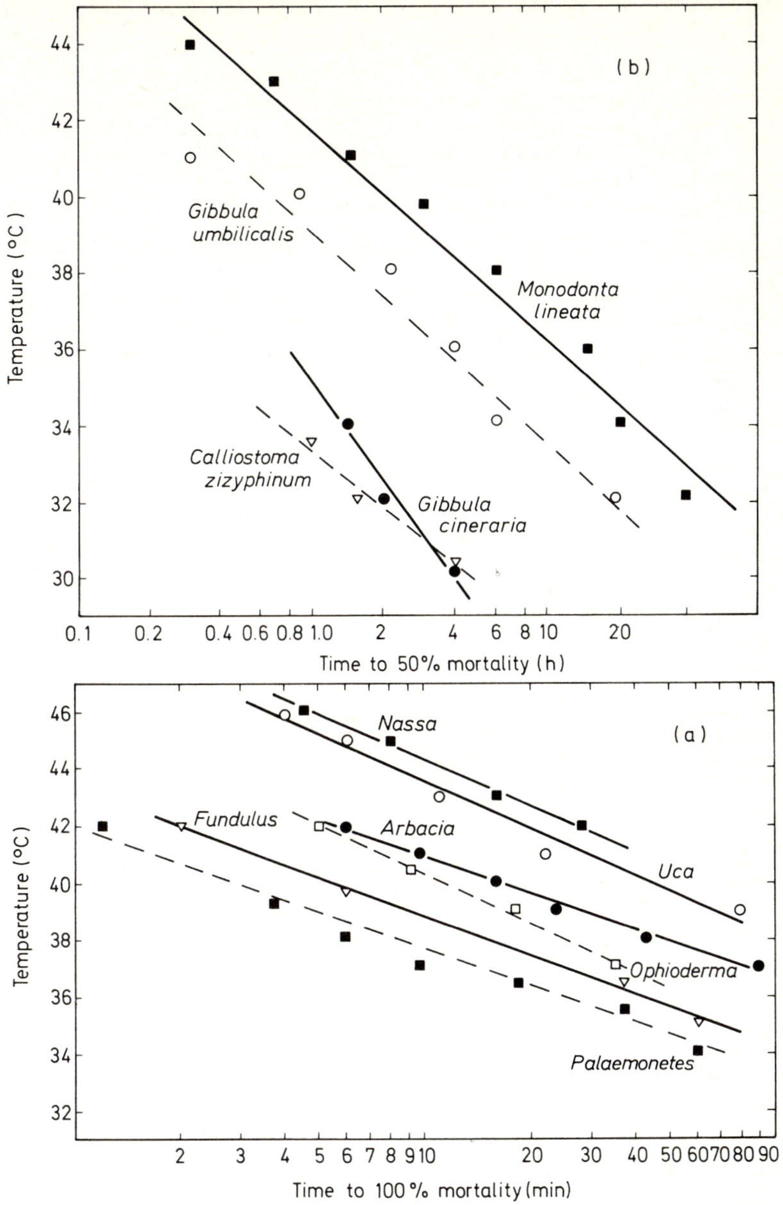

Figure 1.16 Graphs showing the thermal resistance of lines of various marine invertebrates in water. (a) The time taken for 100% mortality (data from Orr, 1955). (b) The time taken for 50% mortality in a series of trochid gastropods (data from Micallef, 1966). (After Newell, 1970; courtesy Paul Elek (Scientific Books) Ltd)

(1968) in a study of the cold tolerance of barnacles, used an 18 h period for comparison of the species. Orr (1955) has produced similar data for the survival of a variety of marine organisms as a function of time. His data are expressed in terms of the temperature for 100% mortality and are replotted on a semi-logarithmic scale in *Figure 1.16*.

Both Broekhuysen (1940) and Micallef (1966) gave details of the distribution of the animals they studied so that in this case the lethal temperature can be plotted against an index of zonational level (*Figure 1.17*). Although the absolute levels cannot be validly compared because of

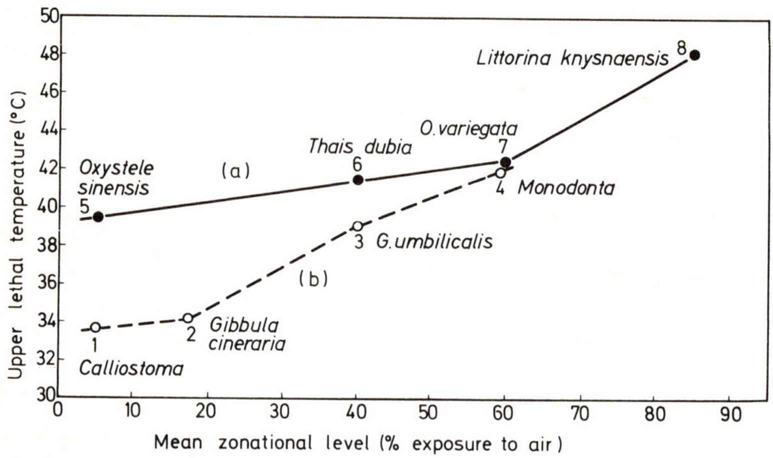

Figure 1.17 Graphs showing the relationship between zonational distribution and upper limit of thermal tolerance in (a) a series of gastropods from False Bay, South Africa (data from Brockhuysen, 1940) and (b) a series of trochid gastropods from Wembury, Devon (data from Micallef, 1966). (After Newell, 1970; courtesy Paul Elek (Scientific Books) Ltd)

the different experimental methods used, nevertheless the correspondence between the lethal limits and zonational position are striking. Clearly, one strategy might be for an organism to retain a fixed and species-specific temperature tolerance. There is a good deal of evidence, principally from the work of Ushakov and his co-workers (for review, *see* Troshin, 1967) that the protein thermostability of marine invertebrates is a relatively fixed feature. In organisms which are subject to a regular and predictable change in environmental conditions, however, the possibility of seasonal adjustment of the limits of thermal tolerance emerges. Such a response would be especially relevant to intertidal organisms where the increase of sea temperatures which occurs during the early summer could serve as an environmental stimulus to initiate changes in the upper lethal temperature and so allow survival when exposed to air. Conversely, where upper shore organisms such as barnacles and limpets are denied a predictable change in environmental conditions, the retention of fixed and relatively broad limits of thermal tolerance may be the rule.

Latitudinal and tidal-dependent differences in the thermal tolerance of intertidal organisms are commonly induced intraspecifically by thermal acclimation. Vernberg, Schlieper and Schneider (1963) showed that the thermal resistance lines for isolated gill pieces from the intertidal bivalves *Crassostrea* and *Modiolus* were raised in response to storage at 22–25°C compared with tissue from animals held at 10°C. Tissue from the subtidal bivalve *Aequipecten* showed no such increase of the thermal tolerance in response to thermal acclimation. Since that time there have been many studies carried out on the heat-lethal temperatures of intact intertidal organisms which show that intraspecific differences in relation to latitudinal and tidal-dependent gradients of environmental temperature can be induced by thermal acclimation. Kenny (1969a, b), for example, showed that the heat-lethal temperature obtained by gradually heating *Clymenella torquata* at a rate of 1°C per 5 min, was raised by storage for two weeks at temperatures from 5 to 15°C (*Figure 1.18*). These differences were similar

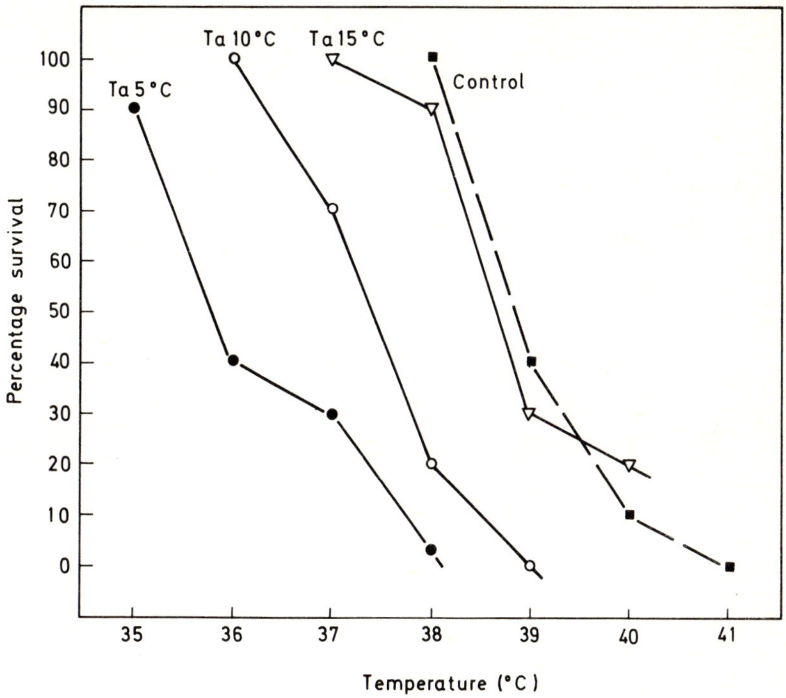

Figure 1.18 Graphs showing the influence of thermal acclimation (Ta) to 5, 10 and 15°C on the percentage survival of the polychaete Clymenella torquata *at various experimental temperatures. (After Kenny, 1969a; courtesy Editor, Marine Biology)*

to differences in the heat-lethal temperatures of animals collected in the winter and in the summer. It seems then, that this polychaete is able to increase its upper limit of thermal tolerance to meet the raised environmental temperatures which are likely to occur in the summer.

It is interesting to note that a relatively modest increase in acclimation temperature from 5 to 15°C was evidently sufficient to alter the survival of

Clymenella at high temperatures. Some animals, such as the rockpool copepod *Tigriopus californicus,* gain heat tolerance only after acclimation to temperatures above 20°C and lose it below that temperature (Kontogiannis, 1973). This animal may not experience the regular increase in sea temperature which could serve as an environmental cue to increase the thermal tolerance in preparation for summer conditions. In the winkle *Littorina littorea,* the situation is similar to that in *Clymenella,* an increase in acclimation temperature between 5 and 16°C having a major effect on the heat tolerance of the organism (Newell, Pye and Ahsanullah, 1971b). The data are summarised in *Figure 1.19* which shows that further acclimation to temperatures between 16 and 25°C resulted in little further enhancement of the heat tolerance.

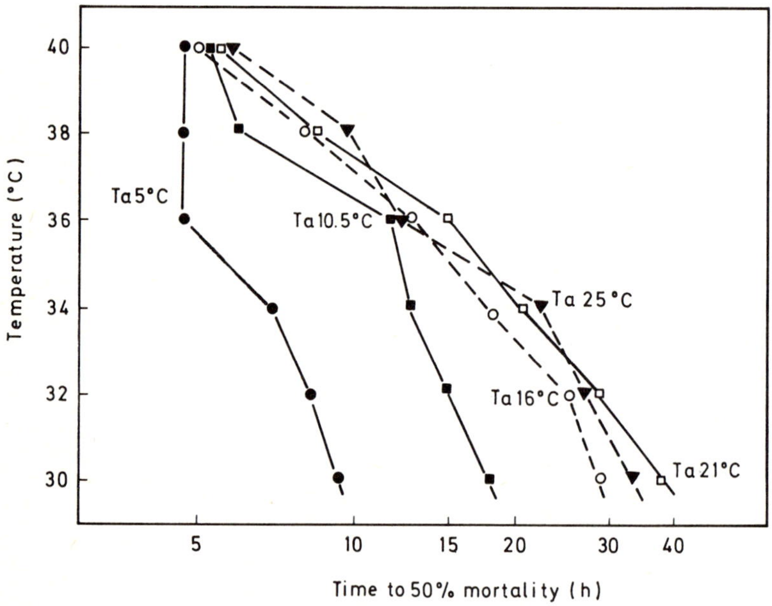

Figure 1.19 Graphs showing the influence of thermal acclimation (Ta) to 5, 10.5, 16, 21 and 25°C on the heat tolerance of the winkle Littorina littorea. *Note that thermal acclimation between 5 and 16°C was most effective in increasing the upper lethal temperature. (After Newell, Pye and Ahsanullah, 1971b; courtesy Dr. R. J. Skaer)*

Finally, there are those intertidal animals, such as *Acmaea,* which show little or no seasonal acclimation of the upper limit of thermal tolerance (Wolcott, 1973). Many barnacles seem to show little change in their upper limits of thermal tolerance in response to seasonal changes in temperature (Foster, 1969), although major changes in the rate of cirral beating occur in response to geographical or experimental changes in temperature (Crisp and Ritz, 1967b; Ritz and Foster, 1968). But there is some evidence of a loss of resistance to long periods of exposure to high temperatures in *Balanus balanoides* collected during the winter. This reduced tolerance in *B.*

balanoides coincides with an increase in its cold tolerance (Crisp and Ritz, 1967a; Ritz, 1968; Cook and Gabbott, 1970; Cook and Lewis, 1971). Animals which do not adjust their upper limits of thermal tolerance may thus be those which are denied a regular change in environmental temperature such as occur on the lower shore. In this case an alternative strategy might involve the maintenance of a fixed upper limit of thermal tolerance which is only marginally affected by seasonal adjustment to low temperatures. Clearly, a good deal more information is required before we are in a position to more than outline the basic strategies which might be involved in meeting the seasonal changes in environmental conditions which occur in the intertidal zone.

1.2.3.2 TOLERANCE OF DESICCATION STRESS

As pointed out in Section 1.2.2, the principal factor which controls the distribution of intertidal animals is their different abilities to withstand desiccation, for evaporative cooling is involved in the heat balance of nearly all the fauna. Apart from some isolated studies on the ability of the winkles *Littorina saxatilis* and *L. neritoides* (Colgan, 1910; Patané, 1933) and of the barnacle *Chthamalus stellatus* (Monterosso, 1930) to survive for long periods in a desiccator, the first systematic survey of intertidal organisms was made by Broekhuysen (1940). He established the correlation between zonational distribution and resistance to desiccation, and since then many studies have confirmed his conclusions. *Table 1.2* shows the general

Table 1.2 THE PERCENTAGE WEIGHT LOSS REQUIRED PER 50% MORTALITY IN A SERIES OF GASTROPODS FROM FALSE BAY, SOUTH AFRICA (DATA FROM BROEKHUYSEN, 1940)

Species	*Percentage exposure to air*	*% weight loss for 50% mortality at 14–17°C*	*% weight loss for 50% mortality at 39–40°C*
Littorina knysnaënsis	85	22.0	19.0
Oxystele variegata	58	17.5	13.0
Thais dubia	40	19.0	14.5
Oxystele tigrina	30	9.0	6.0
Cominella cincta	19	11.0	9.5
Oxystele sinensis	5	6.5	4.0

relationship between zonational level and weight loss in South African gastropods. The only exception to the rule appears to be *Oxystele tigrina* which, as pointed out by Broekhuysen (1940), normally lives in pools so that its high zonational position is little indication of the desiccation which it normally experiences. It was also shown that the relative humidity was remarkably similar over much of the intertidal zone, varying from 74 to 83%. It thus appears that it is the duration rather than the magnitude of desiccation which is the important tidal-dependent variable.

Micallef (1966) has also shown that amongst intertidal trochids there is a graded resistance to desiccation. The upper shore *Monodonta lineata* can survive for much longer in dry air than the lower shore species. *Gibbula umbilicalis* overlaps *Monodonta lineata* in distribution on the shore so the differences between the tolerances of the two genera are greater than one would expect on a basis of their respective zonational positions. In fact *Monodonta* lives on open rock surfaces whereas *Gibbula umbilicalis* is confined to damper situations so, as in the case of *Oxystele tigrina* referred to above, differences in local conditions are also of importance in an interpretation of the graded tolerances of intertidal animals. Kensler (1967) has studied the desiccation resistance of a variety of organisms which inhabit intertidal crevices. His data show that there is an interaction between temperature and desiccation in controlling the local distribution of the organisms. In general, however, there is a correlation between resistance to desiccation and the position the animal occupies in the crevice. Animals which occupy the inner parts of the crevice such as *Ovatella myosotis, Anurida maritima, Dynameme bidentata* and *Porcellana platycheles* are less resistant to desiccation than species living in the outer regions such as *Campecopea hirsuta, Lasaea rubra, Littorina saxtilis* and *Eulalia viridis*. Upper shore specimens of the bivalve *Lasaea rubra* were also more resistant to desiccation than those from lower shore levels. Some of these data are compared in *Figure 1.20*.

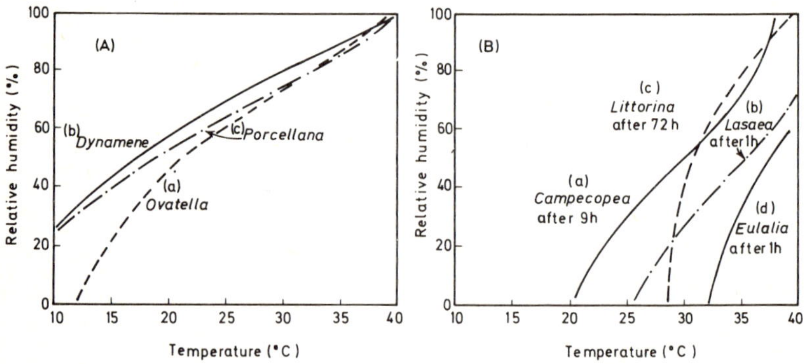

Figure 1.20 Graphs showing the contours of median lethal conditions for a series of crevice-dwelling animals. (A) Data for animals occupying the inner parts of the crevice after 1 h exposure to different combinations of temperature and humidity. (a) Ovatella *(b)* Dynamene *(c)* Porcellana. *(B) Data for species occupying the outer region of the crevice after various times of exposure to different combinations of temperature and humidity (a)* Campecopea *(b)* Lasaea rubra *(from Mid-tide level) (c)* Littorina *(d)* Eulalia. *(Data from Kensler, 1967; courtesy Blackwell Scientific Publications Ltd)*

In fact the ability of intertidal animals from high shore levels to survive water loss is very great indeed — far in excess of the losses which might be anticipated during one tidal cycle. *Patella,* for example, can withstand water losses of 30–65% (Davies, 1969), *Acmaea* can survive water loss of 70–80% (Wolcott, 1973) whilst chitons can tolerate 75% water loss (Boyle, 1969). These values compare well with those from the most extreme environments including deserts. The tsetse fly can lose up to 55% of its water (Bursell, 1959) whilst the desert amphibian *Scaphiopus* can tolerate a loss of 60% of its water (Thorson and Svihla, 1943). The explanation of this great tolerance of water loss shown by intertidal invertebrates is clear when we remember (a) that water loss is a fundamental strategy for heat loss in upper shore animals and (b) that the form of the fortnightly tidal cycle dictates a maximum exposure to air of as much as 13–14 days (*Figure 1.4* p. 6). The importance of this last factor has been demonstrated by Davies (1969). He showed that intraspecific differences exist both in the rate of water loss and in the amount of water loss which can be tolerated in upper and lower shore individuals of the limpet *Patella vulgata.* The large steep sided individuals of the upper shore had a relatively reduced perimeter through which water loss occurred. The flatter *Patella aspera* and small *P. vulgata* of the lower shore thus lost water at a faster rate than high level *P. vulgata* (*see also* p. 24).

The tolerance of water loss by high and low level *Patella vulgata* and by the lower shore *P. aspera* is shown in *Table 1.3*. Davies (1969) found that

Table 1.3 THE TOLERANCE OF WATER LOSS IN TWO POPULATIONS OF THE LIMPET *PATELLA VULGATA* AND IN THE LOWER SHORE *P. ASPERA*. NOTE THAT BOTH INTRA- AS WELL AS INTERSPECIFIC DIFFERENCES OCCUR IN THE TOLERANCE OF WATER LOSS (AFTER DAVIES, 1969)

	High level P. vulgata	*Low level* P. vulgata	P. aspera *(low level)*
% weight loss which all survive	60	44	24
% weight loss for 50% mortality	60–65	50–55	30–35
% weight loss for 100% mortality	65	55–60	40

specimens of *P. vulgata* on the sea-shore rarely showed evidence of experiencing dehydration amounting to 60% weight loss. In fact a value of 3-5% was common but the effect of size was shown to markedly affect this value. Thus under conditions where a 21 mm long high level *Patella vulgata* (5 g wet tissue weight) would lose 15% of its body weight, a small limpet of 15 mm shell length (0.15 g wet tissue weight) would lose as much as 65% of its body weight. Recovery of water following weight loss by desiccation was slow and it took as much as 4–5 h for recovery when more than 28% weight loss had occurred. The importance of this recovery time can be demonstrated if we imagine the situation at a high shore level which, let us assume, is covered for only 4 days per 14 day cycle. Let us further assume that a 3% weight loss per day occurs, then in 10 days there would be a total weight loss of 30%. During the next four days the limpet would be covered, say for 3 h per tidal cycle and this would be scarcely sufficient to restore the water levels in the tissues before the onset of the next period of continuous aerial exposure. This example assumes a low rate of water loss per day. Clearly, severe environmental conditions, especially if coupled with high temperatures, might result in water losses which approach the lethal values for the species.

Wolcott (1973) has recently pointed out that differences in the ability of graded series of intertidal limpets to survive water loss may not seem at first sight sufficient to account for their zonational distribution on the shore. But he showed that apparently minor differences in the desiccation tolerance of 80% water loss in upper shore specimens of *Acmaea* to 70% total water lost in lower shore *Acmaea* are not minor when the equivalent osmotic pressure of the body fluids is calculated. The value is not proportional to the percentage water lost but to the inverse of the percentage water remaining. In the case of *Acmaea* species, a 70% water loss is equivalent to an increase of tissue concentration to 333% seawater whereas the ability to survive an 80% water loss is equivalent to a tolerance of tissue osmotic pressures equal to that of 500% seawater. The ability of intertidal animals to survive water loss thus appears to be related to a truly remarkable ability to tolerate hyperosmotic body fluids which in many other animals would lead to an excretion of inorganic ions.

In much the same way as the magnitude of desiccation may be related to the duration of intertidal exposure and body size of the organism, the problem of whether environmental temperatures ever reach potentially lethal values probably hinges on complex interactions between exposure time and the lethal temperature of the organism. Comparatively minor differences in the heat-lethal temperature of organisms may acquire an ecological significance following prolonged periods of exposure to near lethal temperatures. Equally, the effects of concentration of the body fluids by water loss may interact with the effects of temperature to produce a lethal situation within the zone of tolerance for each factor independently. Some of the possible interactions between the effects of temperature and salinity are discussed below.

1.2.3.3 TOLERANCE OF SALINITY STRESS

The effects of external salinity change make themselves felt on both the survival and growth rates of many marine organisms. We have seen above that the ability to withstand temperature stress in animals exposed to direct insolation is partly dependent upon mechanisms for facilitating evaporative heat loss. Equally, this strategy for evasion of thermal stress requires a tolerance of hyperosmotic conditions which is truly remarkable compared even with organisms from the most extreme environments. The ability of intertidal animals such as *Acmaea* (Wolcott, 1973) to survive in hyperosmotic solutions is therefore largely a reflection of their desiccation resistance rather than some specific adaptation to high external salt concentrations. In general, external osmotic stress is not a physical gradient which varies regularly with shore level and does not appear to be a significant factor in controlling the distribution of organisms which live on open rock surfaces. Some studies such as that of Seelemann (1968) have, however, shown that salinity tolerance appears to increase with shore level amongst some intertidal gastropods. Most intertidal animals are osmotic conformers (*see* Chapter 6), but they evade contact with the medium by burrowing (Kinne, 1964) or can close shell valves as in barnacles and bivalves (Krogh, 1939; Freeman and Rigler, 1957). Some exclude the medium by closure of the operculum as in littorinids (Mayes, 1962; Avens and Sleigh, 1965) or by clamping down against the substratum as in *Patella* (Milne, 1940; Arnold, 1957, 1959), *Acmaea* (Segal, 1956; Segal and Dehnel, 1962; Wolcott, 1973) and *Siphonaria* (McAlister and Fisher, 1968), a response which tends to exclude short term changes in salinity. Such differences as do exist in the abilities of intertidal organisms to tolerate hypo- and hyperosmotic conditions occur in the aquatic component which inhabits upper shore rockpools compared with those of the lower shore. Gradients in osmotic conditions also occur independently of tidal level in estuaries and it is in these two aquatic habitats that the most detailed comparative studies have been made (*see* Chapter 6).

The physical environment of rockpools is largely determined by the number of times they are inundated by the tide. Clearly, those of the upper shore experience wider and more prolonged fluctuations in salinity, temperature, pH and oxygen content than those of the lower shore. Salinity variations in rockpools have been recorded by Klugh (1924), Pyefinch (1943), Naylor and Slinn (1958) and Ganning (1967) and more recently by Clark (1968). Much of this work is summarised in Newell (1970) and Ganning (1971a). Hagerman (1969) has shown that in small isolated rockpools the salinity may vary from 0.5 to 40% and that specialised organisms such as the ostracod *Hirschmannia* are well adapted to survive and reproduce under such conditions. Ganning (1966; 1970; 1971a) and Clark (1968) have also shown that other characteristic components of the rockpool ecosystem, including ostracods such as *Heterocypris, Cypridiopsis* and *Loxoconcha,* harpactidoids such as *Tigriopus, Mesochra* and *Nitocra,* as well as the mite *Hyadesia fusca,* are each well adapted to survive the marked changes in salinity which occur in high level rockpools.

Such adaptations are not, however, confined to mere tolerance of extreme variations in temperature and salinity. Ganning (1971b) has shown that the fauna must also be able to capitalise on suitable conditions for the short time they prevail. Thus short life cycles and rapid development to sexual maturity, as well as the ability to reproduce asexually, all play a part in enabling the animals to colonise rapidly a temporary pool found at high shore levels. The production of eggs which are resistant to desiccation also aids in the survival of the species when the pool dries (Ganning, 1970; 1971a, b). Some of the inhabitants such as insects and gammarids may leave the rockpool ecosystem when conditions become too severe and seek protection in other microhabitats within the intertidal zone (Forsman, 1951; Pajunen and Jansson, 1969; Ganning, 1971b). All of these features, and the limited trophic levels in rockpool food webs (Clark, 1968; Ganning, 1971b), are highly specialised features which are not relevant to environmental conditions which prevail over the intertidal zone as a whole.

The importance of salinity in limiting the occurrence of the aquatic component of the fauna has been reviewed by Kinne (1963; 1964; 1966; 1967). He has shown that interactions between the effects of temperature and salinity frequently occur and that an organism may reduce the detrimental effects of salinity by seeking conditions of lower temperature stress. Both temperature and salinity have been implicated as factors controlling the distribution of estuarine isopods. Harvey, Jones and Naylor (1973) determined the lethal temperatures at various salinities for an overlapping series of isopods including the marine species *Campecopea hirsuta, Sphaeroma serratum, Dynamene bidentata* and the brackish water

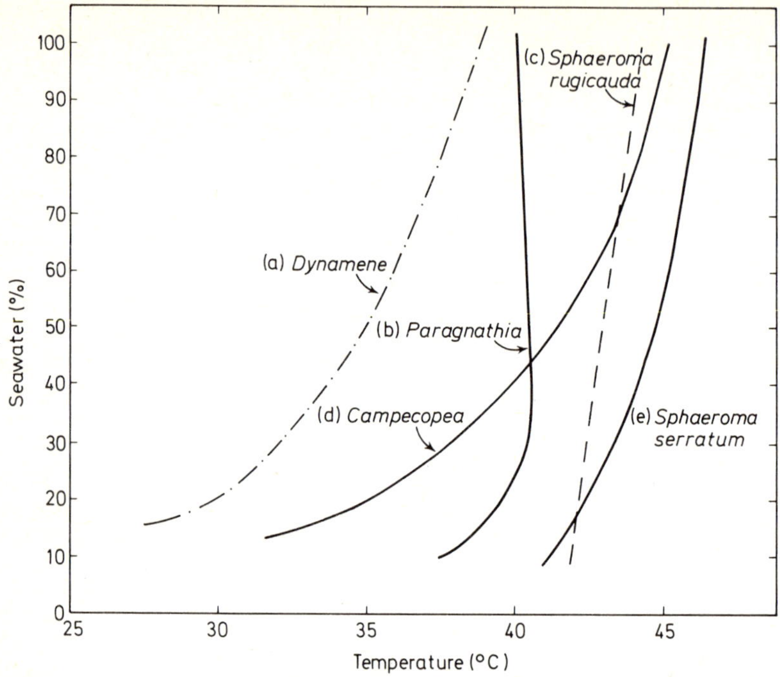

Figure 1.21 Graphs showing the lethal temperature of a series of isopods in relation to salinity. Lethal temperatures assessed in terms of the temperature required to produce 100% mortality following a temperature rise of 1 deg C for each 15 min. (a) Dynamene bidentata *(b)* Paragnathia formica *(c)* Sphaeroma rugicauda *(d)* Campecopea hirsuta *(e)* Sphaeroma serratum. *(After Harvey, Jones and Naylor, 1973; courtesy Academic Press)*

species *Sphaeroma rugicauda* and *Paragnathia formica*. The results are shown in *Figure 1.21* from which it is evident that the species surviving to the highest temperature was *Sphaeroma serratum*. This animal could tolerate 46.5°C in 100% seawater. In *Paragnathia, S. rugicauda,* and *S. serratum* salinity obviously had little effect on the temperature tolerance, whereas in *Dynamene* and *Campecopea* there was a more pronounced interaction between salinity and temperature. The different ability of overlapping species to survive salinity stress is also important in isopods belonging to the genus *Jaera* (Jones, 1972; *see also* Sjoberg, 1967).

Wiesepape, Adrich and Strawn (1972) have studied the combined effects of temperature and salinity on the survival of *Penaeus aztecus*. They showed that survival time was directly related not only to acclimation temperature, but that the thermal resistance of *Penaeus* varied also with salinity. A higher thermal resistance was shown in high test salinities of 25‰ than at lower ones of 5‰ or 15‰, perhaps indicating a reduction in the amount of osmotic work necessary at high salinities. Acclimation to low salinities also affected the relationship between survival and experimental conditions. Thus in this animal it is evident that a complex interaction between at least four environmental factors is of importance; these include acclimation salinity, experimental salinity, acclimation temperature and experimental temperature. The survival of *Sphaeroma rugicauda* and *S. hookeri* is also controlled by both temperature and salinity (Jansen, 1970, 1971; Marsden, 1973a). As in *Penaeus*, both acclimation salinity and acclimation temperature have been implicated in survival and in addition it has been shown that large and small individuals have a different range of tolerance. Interactions including body size thus need to be incorporated into an experimental analysis. The situation is further complicated by the fact that in many organisms, salinity and temperature affect not only the survival but may influence other indicator processes such as reproduction (Jansen, 1970) and activity (Marsden, 1973a; Rosenberg and Rosenberg, 1973). Complex effects of temperature and salinity on development have also been described in the land crab *Cardisoma guanhumi* (Costlow and Bookhout, 1968) and in the hermit crab *Pagurus bernhardus* (Roberts, 1971a).

An alternative approach to the analysis of the effects of environmental and endogenous factors on survival is to calculate a multiple regression equation which relates each experimental parameter such as body size, experimental salinity, acclimation salinity, experimental temperature, acclimation temperature and exposure time as well as combinations of these factors to an indicator process such as survival or growth (Ralston and Wilf, 1960). The multiple regression equation so obtained can then be used to calculate survival or growth curves for the organism under different experimental conditions. This kind of approach has been used by Lough and Gonor (1973a, b) in a study of the effects of temperature and salinity on larval development in the mussel *Adula californiensis*. A rather similar treatment of the data has been used by Haefner (1969; 1970) on the shrimp *Crangon septemspinosa*, as well as by Cain (1973) on the embryo and larvae of the clam *Rangia cuneata* and by Kennedy *et al.* (1974) on embryos and larvae of the bivalve *Mulinia*.

Haefner (1969; 1970) studied the combined effects of temperature and salinity on the survival of *Crangon septemspinosa*. He analysed the

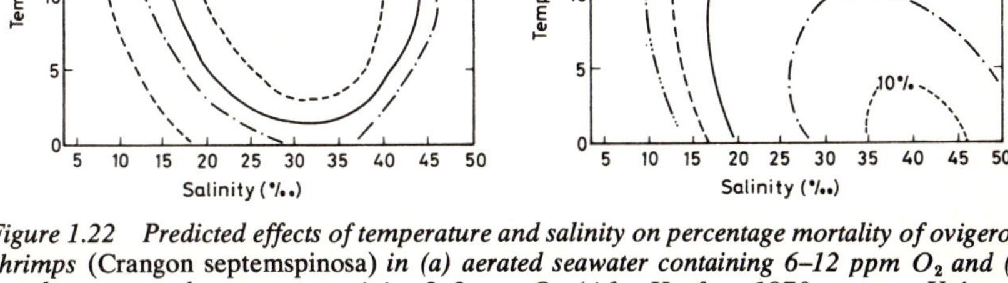

Figure 1.22 Predicted effects of temperature and salinity on percentage mortality of ovigerous shrimps (Crangon septemspinosa) *in (a) aerated seawater containing 6–12 ppm O_2 and (b) poorly oxygenated seawater containing 2–3 ppm O_2. (After Haefner, 1970; courtesy University of Chicago Press)*

percentage mortality data by the method of Box and Youle (1955) and Box (1956) and showed that the contours obtained could be shifted according to whether the females were ovigerous or not and also according to oxygen availability. *Figure 1.22* shows the response surfaces calculated under different combinations of salinity and temperature in (a) aerated seawater containing 6–12 ppm O_2 and (b) in poorly aerated water containing 2–3 ppm O_2. It is evident that a wider variety of temperatures and salinities could be tolerated in aerated water and that the additional stress of low oxygen availability affected the response to the other two variables. Equally, Lough and Gonor (1973a, b) have shown that the survival of larvae of *Adula* is affected not only by temperature and salinity but also by the age of the test organism. *Figure 1.23* shows the curves generated from computer analyses of their data. An increase in age results in an increase of salinity tolerance but a decrease in temperature tolerance of the larvae.

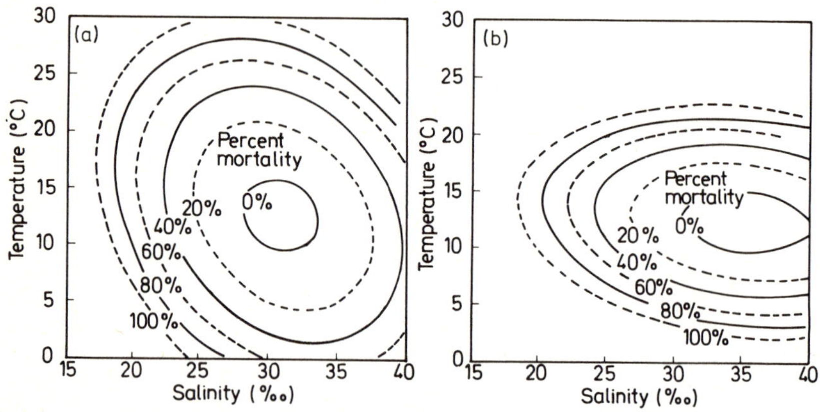

Figure 1.23 Graphs showing the predicted effects of temperature and salinity on mortality of larvae of the bivalve Adula californiensis *(a) after 3 days (b) after 15 days development at different combinations of temperature and salinity. (After Lough and Gonor, 1973a; courtesy, Editor, Marine Biology)*

An identical analytical technique was also used by Cain (1973) who studied the effects of temperature and salinity not only on survival but also on growth of larvae of the clam *Rangia cuneata.* Interactions of this kind between environmental and endogenous factors in controlling survival have also been analysed by stepwise multiple regression programs. Kennedy *et al.* (1974), for example, have studied the influence of time and temperature on survival of larvae of the bivalve *Mulinia lateralis.* This allowed the calculation of response surfaces which showed that both temperature and period of exposure controlled survival and that temperature tolerance increased with age.

This analytical approach has largely replaced the simple ecological sequences in which the effects of one factor are studied independently of others. In general, the shore environment is a complex one in which temperature and desiccation interact to produce stresses which are characteristic of the upper shore whilst temperature and salinity may be the predominant factors affecting survival in estuarine situations. The effects of these factors on survival are, however, also controlled by age and sex of the organism whilst other indicator processes such as growth may also be implicated in the effects of environmental factors on survival. It is only when experimental studies reflect such complex interactions between the organism and its physico-chemical environment that we can meaningfully extrapolate the results of comparative studies into the environmental situation. From past studies, however, it seems likely that the distribution of organisms on the upper shore is controlled at least partly by combinations of physical factors which may become lethal when time of intertidal exposure is taken into account. Most of the activities of the organism must be designed to function within the limits imposed by its tolerance of the physical and chemical environment and responses which promote successful competition with neighbouring species then determine the abundance of the organism. Some of these factors are considered in Section 1.3.

1.3 STRATEGIES IN THE COMPETITION FOR ENERGY IN THE INTERTIDAL ZONE

One way of assessing whether an organism is likely to be able to compete successfully with its neighbours within the limits of its physiological tolerances is to study the partitioning of energy which occurs in the population. Clearly, a net energy gain will result in enhanced growth and reproduction and this provides a useful index to compare with other species occupying a similar habitat. The well-known balanced energy equation of Winberg (1956) has been extensively applied to studies on the production of whole populations and all the components are expressed as kcal/m^2/year. Briefly, the energy consumed by a population is equal to the production plus losses due to metabolism, faeces and dissolved organic matter (Odum and Smalley, 1959; Petrusewicz and Macfadyen, 1970). The equation may be written:

$$C = (Pg + Pr) + R + F + U$$

Where C = the total amount of energy consumed by a population.
Pg = the energy addition by growth and recruitment.
Pr = the energy released as gametes.
R = the energy equivalent of metabolism.
F = the energy equivalent of faeces.
U = the energy equivalent of dissolved organic matter including nitrogenous compounds.

Kay and Brafield (1973) have studied the annual calorie flow through a population of the polychaete *Neanthes virens* and have quantified each of the major components of the energy balance equation outlined above. In this animal the major energy loss to the population was the mortality due to spawning, and that lost through metabolism. The contribution made by each component appears, however, to vary a good deal in different kinds of organisms. Miller and Mann (1973) have shown, for example, that there are large amounts of energy unaccounted for in the energy budgets of many marine benthic grazing animals. These losses may account for as much as 80% of the absorption in sea-urchins and appear to be due to the loss of dissolved organic matter by the animals.

One of the problems with the use of equations based on this concept of partitioning of energy is that they assume steady-state conditions. Where environmental conditions are uniform, and in particular, where food supplies are constant, this assumption is probably valid. But one of the characteristics of the sea-shore is that conditions are by no means constant. As emphasised on p. 6, both available food and physico-chemical characteristics are subject to extreme fluctuations. It thus becomes interesting to see how the organisms can adapt the major components of the equation to maintain a positive index of energy balance. The important point is that each component is an independent variable and hence many strategies are available. The equation for individual organisms may be written in the form:

$$A - (R + U) = P + G$$

Where A = the nett energy assimilated from the food ration (i.e. input, C, minus faeces production, F).
R = the energy equivalent of oxygen consumption.
U = the energy equivalent of excretory and other dissolved organic matter losses.
P = the energy equivalent of growth.
G = the energy equivalent of gametes (Crisp, 1971).

As pointed out by Bayne, Thompson and Widdows (1973), the index of energy balance may be positive, in which case there is 'scope for growth and reproduction' (*see also* Warren and Davis, 1967). Alternatively when utilisation of energy exceeds the energy input, the index becomes negative and under these conditions body reserves must be utilised (Gabbott and Bayne, 1973; Thompson, Ratcliffe and Bayne, 1974). The maintenance of a positive index of energy balance is, of course, in the long term essential to the survival of the individual and the species as a whole. Large size achieved by a positive index of energy balance is, as we have seen on p. 20, one important strategy for the maintenance of heat balance in upper shore animals. Energy available for production of gametes is also essential for the survival of the species and for its effective competition with neighbouring organisms.

When the tide ebbs there is a loss of food availability to both suspension feeders and many browsing organisms, for browsing cannot take place under conditions of desiccation. There is also an increase of environmental temperature in many intertidal habitats and this would be expected to increase the metabolic energy losses just at the time when energy input is minimal. Under these circumstances we can envisage at least three strategies for the maintenance of energy balance. There may be: (a) An increase of energy input during favourable parts of the tidal cycle to compensate for reduced food availability at other times. (b) The use of aerobic pathways for converting assimilated food into energy rich phosphates. This is an important way of reducing the amount of food reserves which are expended on metabolism. (c) A reduction in the amount of metabolic work which is performed by the organism. This may be brought about by a reduction in activity, and by a suppression of the effects of temperature increase during the intertidal period. When we remember that metabolism may account for as much as 88% of the energy loss by populations of *Nerita* (Hughes, 1971), it is clear that this third strategy may represent the most important means of maintaining a positive index of energy balance in intertidal organisms.

1.3.1 Compensation in the rate of energy input

The availability of food may vary seasonally in suspension feeding animals which are permanently covered by the sea, and semi-diurnally with the ebb and flow of the tide in intertidal animals. Much of the earlier literature on factors affecting the rate of suspension feeding in bivalves has been summarised by Jørgensen (1966). More recently Vahl (1972a, b; 1973a, b, c) has studied the relationship between water transport and particle retention in a series of bivalves including the mussel *Mytilus edulis,* the queen scallop *Chlamys opercularis* and the cockle *Cardium edule.* He showed that marked differences exist in the retention efficiency of *Chlamys* and *Mytilus.* The latter is able to retain fine particles more efficiently and the queen scallop compensates for the loss of these fine particles by a high pumping rate. It was also shown that in both *Cardium* and *Mytilus* the metabolism increases faster with body size than does pumping rate (Vahl, 1973a, b; Winter, 1969). Thus the energy available for growth and reproduction decreases with body size and it is not surprising to find that the growth rate therefore decreases with size in these animals.

As well as interspecific differences in the particle retention by different bivalves, feeding is also influenced by temperature and food availability. Winter (1969) and Ali (1970) have reviewed the effect of food concentration and temperature on filtration in bivalves. Their results have been confirmed and amplified by Walne (1972), McLusky (1973) and Tenore and Dunstan (1973). In general it has been found that the amount of food removed from suspension by bivalves may vary both with temperature and food availability and that marked differences may exist in the effects of these two factors. Thompson and Bayne (1972) and Bayne, Thompson and Widdows (1973) have made a detailed study of the components of an energy budget in *Mytilus* held at different temperatures and levels of food ration. They showed that at high food ration levels the index of energy balance was relatively independent of temperature over the range 10–20°C. Above 20°C, however, there was a marked decline in the scope for growth and reproduction. This was due to an increase in the rate of oxygen consumption at 25°C coupled with a reduction in filtration rate.

The availability of food also greatly affects the index of energy balance in *Mytilus.* The assimilated ration (A) minus the energy loss (R) gave negative values at low ration levels of 0.91% of the body weight/day at all temperatures between 10 and 25°C. Mussels held at a higher ration of 1.52% of the body weight/day gave a negative balance only at 20 and 25°C. Finally, in mussels given a ration of 3.04% of the body weight/day were able to maintain a positive index of energy balance at all temperatures except 25°C. These results thus suggest that the feeding rate of *Mytilus* cannot be compensated for major variations in food concentration. A decline in available food or an increase in environmental temperature must then lead to a negative index of energy balance and a utilisation of metabolic reserves.

The situation is a good deal more complicated in those animals which experience long periods of exposure to air. Once again there is some evidence that in *Mytilus* there is a simple 'on/off' system with the bivalve pumping at a fixed rate irrespective of the duration of available feeding time. Segal, Rao and James (1953) have shown that the rate of water propulsion of *Mytilus californianus* collected from the mid-intertidal zone was rather slower than that of specimens from the lower shore. This is the reverse of that necessary to offset the reduced feeding time on the upper shore. Similarly Southward (1964) has shown a suppression of the cirral activity of high level populations of the barnacle *Chthamalus stellatus* compared with low level populations. Both of these responses may be the result of acclimation to the higher temperatures which occur on the upper shore. On the other hand, Jørgensen (1960) has not demonstrated any differences in the filtration rate of *Mytilus edulis* collected from different tidal levels. This lack of compensatory change in the feeding rate of *Mytilus edulis* suggests that the species may be limited on the upper shore by a predominantly negative index of energy balance, which yields little scope for growth or reproduction.

In contrast to this apparently simple 'on/off' feeding response when *Mytilus* is covered by the tide, some other bivalves are apparently able to compensate for the reduced feeding period on the upper shore by increasing their rate of food assimilation. Morton, Boney and Corner (1957) studied the filtration rate of the small crevice-dwelling bivalve *Lasaea rubra*. This animal may live in situations where it is covered for an average of only 1 h in 12 h, and may not be covered at all for 12 consecutive days during neap tides. On the other hand, lower shore individuals are covered for an average of 8 h per 12 h tidal cycle and are not exposed continuously for more than 12 h. Ballantine and Morton (1956) and Morton, Boney and Corner (1957) have shown that *Lasaea* is a suspension feeder and that upper shore animals differ from their lower shore counterparts in two important respects. First, they respond more rapidly to wetting and thus start to filter with minimal delay even when wetted by wave splash. Second, the rate of feeding during the first two hours of submersion is approximately double that of animals from the lower shore.

The time available for feeding may also be limited in browsing animals which require moist conditions for their activity. The winkle *Littorina littorea*, for example, can feed under moist conditions when the tide is out and orientates to light and gravity at this stage of the tidal cycle (Newell, 1958a, b; *see* p. 14). But during the summer the surfaces of boulders rapidly dry and then it is common for the winkles to close the operculum until moistened by the tide when they are able to emerge and feed. Animals on the upper shore then experience a reduced feeding period compared with lower shore individuals just as described above for *Lasaea rubra*. We were concerned that many of the studies of the responses of such organisms had been carried out following transport to the laboratory and often did not accurately simulate the sequences of events which might control feeding activity on the shore (Newell, Pye and Ahsanullah, 1971a). We placed a series of glass plates in flowing seawater for several days to allow a film of algae to develop on the surface of the glass. Then animals were taken from the lower shore where they were uncovered for only 2 h per tidal cycle, and were placed under water in an aquarium on the glass plate just as the incoming tide reached the natural population on the shore. The water was aerated and stirred and soon the animals started to rasp the algae from the glass plate by means of the radula. These radular movements could be counted after observation with a hand lens (*see also* Cornelius, 1972). Meanwhile the incoming tide reached another part of the shore where the natural population was uncovered for 5½ h per tidal cycle. Additional animals were collected from this position and again immersed in another aquarium of seawater in the laboratory. The feeding rate was recorded as before. Similar measurements were made as the incoming tide covered populations at approximately mid-tide level and as it finally reached an upper shore population uncovered for as much as 8 h per 12 h tidal cycle.

During this time recordings were made on all four sets of aquaria and the tide started to ebb. When the ebbing tide uncovered the highest population from which specimens were taken, the aquarium containing those animals

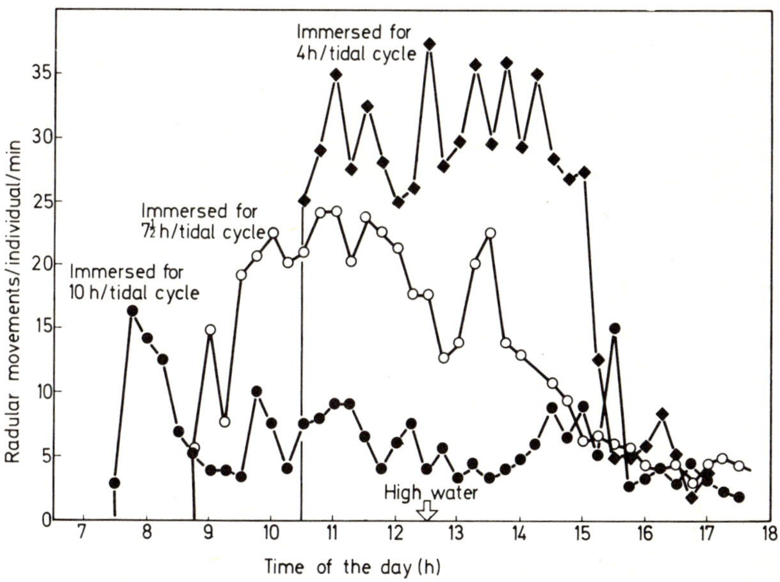

Figure 1.24 Graphs showing the mean activity of three groups of 50 winkles (Littorina littorea) *collected from different shore levels and measured in seawater at 18°C during the immersion time naturally experienced on the shore. Solid circles: animals normally covered for 10 h per 12 h tidal cycle. Open circles: animals normally covered for 7½ h per 12 h tidal cycle. Squares: animals normally covered for 4 h per 12 h tidal cycle. (After Newell, Pye and Ahsanullah, 1971a; courtesy Editor, Marine Biology)*

was drained and browsing soon ceased. Then as the tide ebbed further the aquaria were drained in turn and in each case the winkles became quiescent. The upper shore animals were thus covered for the shortest time and the experimental conditions were very similar to those actually occurring on the shore. The results are shown in *Figure 1.24* and it is clear that the upper shore winkles fed at a high rate for a short length of time compared with those from lower tidal levels.

Obviously, the immersion time multiplied by the mean rate of feeding gives the total potential energy input assuming that the amount of food is equal at all tidal levels. These data are summarised in *Table 1.4*. There is a

Table 1.4 THE FEEDING ACTIVITY OF *LITTORINA LITTOREA* COLLECTED FROM THE DIFFERENT SHORE LEVELS AND IMMERSED IN SEAWATER AT 18°C. THE MEAN WET TISSUE WEIGHT OF THE 50 INDIVIDUALS USED IN EACH EXPERIMENT ARE ALSO SHOWN (DATA FROM NEWELL *ET AL.*, (1971A)). FOR EXPLANATION, *SEE* TEXT

Tidal level from which the winkles were collected (Hour from low water of spring tides)	*Corresponding immersion time* (h)	*Mean wet tissue weight* (mg)	*Radular movements per animal per tidal cycle at 18°C*
1 h	10	486.3	3677
2¼ h	7½	391.2	6371
3¼ h	5½	409.5	6494
4 h	4	398.9	6811

remarkable correspondence between the total feeding activity carried out despite the shorter feeding time available to the upper shore animals. The only major discrepancy is in the extreme lower shore individuals and it is these which have been observed to make looped feeding excursions even during the low tide period under the moist conditions of the lower shore (Newell, 1958a, b). Perhaps this group has a longer potential feeding time than was calculated on a basis of the immersion period. More recently, Grahame (1973a, b) has shown that the reproductive cost of breeding in this species is offset by the longevity of the adults which ingest about 1.27% of their dry body weight daily. The gravimetric assimilation efficiency amounted to 57% which was equal to an 87% calorific efficiency of 45.6 cal/g dry body weight per day. This value is similar to that in *Ligia* which has an assimilation efficiency of 55–78% depending on the type of diet (Carefoot, 1973). It seems likely then that the compensatory changes in the rate of feeding of *Littorina littorea* from different tidal levels are sufficient to maintain an ingestion rate of about 0.63% of the dry body weight of the animal per tidal cycle, since there are two tides per day.

One obvious question is whether these responses reflect some genotypic variability in populations from the upper and lower shore. The larvae, however, are freely mixed in the plankton and settlement appears to be at random over the lower shore (Smith and Newell, 1955). It is therefore likely that the different rates of feeding are induced after site selection by the winkles and this can be shown to be true by a relatively simple experiment. Winkles were taken from the lower shore just before the incoming tide immersed them and some of the group were placed in an aquarium of

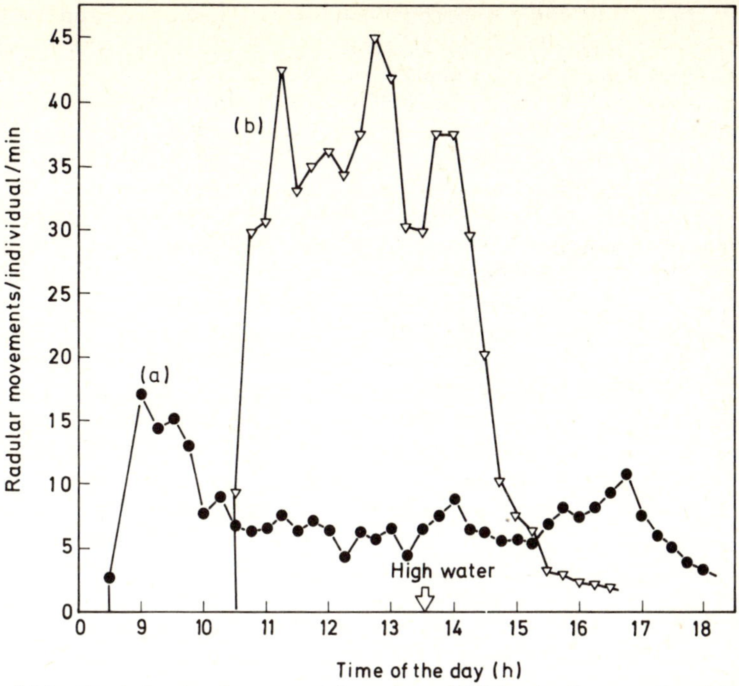

Figure 1.25 Graph showing the mean radular activity of 50 Littorina littorea *collected from the lower shore in July 1970 and immersed in seawater at 18°C (a) at the time the incoming tide covered the natural lower shore population (solid circles); (b) at the time the tide covered the upper shore population (open triangles). (After Newell, Pye and Ahsanullah, 1971a; courtesy Editor, Marine Biology)*

seawater in the laboratory and the feeding rate recorded as before. The other group of lower shore animals, however, were retained dry until the incoming tide reached the upper shore population. Then they were immersed in seawater and the feeding rate recorded. The results are shown in *Figure 1.25* from which it can be seen that their rate on immersion was similar to that of upper shore winkles. Upper shore animals can also take up the slower rate of lower shore animals by submersion for a long period in seawater. The tidal rhythm is thus controlled by the immersion sequence and its amplitude is governed by the period of exposure to air. Whether a lowering of metabolic reserves by starvation during the intertidal period induces the higher rate of feeding is not known. These experiments do show, however, that prolonged immersion of experimental animals in the laboratory prior to experimental studies on feeding rates would effectively mask any tidal-dependent compensation in the feeding rates which occur under natural conditions.

1.3.2 Maintenance of aerobic respiration

Despite the presence of alternative metabolic pathways which may enhance energy conversion under anaerobic conditions (Hochachka and Mustafa, 1972; *see also* Chapter 5), it remains true that the efficiency of conversion of energy from sugar into high energy phosphates is much lower than under aerobic conditions. Approximately 273 kcal of energy is captured out of the 686 kcal contained per mole of hexose sugar under aerobic conditions, which gives an efficiency of conversion of about 40%. Of this, only some 3–7% could be obtained under anaerobic conditions. Thus even a generous estimate of the efficiency of anaerobic pathways shows that about six times the metabolic reserves are burnt to yield the same amount of energy as could be obtained under aerobic conditions. It is thus obvious that a major contribution can be made to the maintenance of a positive index of energy balance by the retention of aerobic pathways even when the tide has ebbed.

Faced with a lack of aerated seawater, intertidal animals which live in deposits are often able to facilitate oxygen transfer and thus maintain aerobic metabolism even when the oxygen content of the interstitial water is low, by means of respiratory pigments (Mangum and Winkle, 1973; *see* Chapter 4). Alternatively, in those organisms which are not subject to intense desiccation stress the metabolic energy requirements may be met by aerial gas exchange through relatively unmodified gill structures. Many intertidal animals including polychaetes such as *Arenicola marina, Nereis diversicolor* and *Thoracophelia mucronata* (Wells, 1949; Dales, 1963), some bivalves such as the cockle *Cardium edule* (Boyden, 1972), the gastropod *Nassarius* (Kushins and Mangum, 1971) and intertidal fishes such as *Blennius pholis* (Daniel, 1971; Wallace, 1973a) are able to utilise atmospheric air at some stages of the tidal cycle as long as they are able to do so without incurring water loss. Finally, there is a series of animals which are able to maintain aerial gas exchange even under conditions of desiccation stress. These include terrestrial and semi-terrestrial crabs (for review, *see* Edney, 1960), many gastropods (Sandison, 1966; Micallef, 1966; Micallef and Bannister, 1967; Baldwin, 1968), bivalves (Kuenzler, 1961; Lent, 1968, 1969) and barnacles (Barnes, Finlayson and Piatigorsky, 1963; Grainger and Newell, 1965).

In an early study, Wells (1949) showed that the lugworm *Arenicola marina* may draw an air bubble in through the exit of the tail shaft and force it over the gills by a modification of the normal headward irrigation movements. *Nereis diversicolor* also draws bubbles over the body at low tide by means of normal undulatory irrigation movements. Another polychaete *Thoracophelia mucronata,* exposes the hind-end of the body through a funnel like depression in the sand and in this way is able to meet its metabolic energy requirements without recourse to anaerobiosis (for review, *see* Dales, 1963). More recently, Kushins and Mangum (1971) have shown that in *Nassarius obsoletus* gas bubbles are held in the mantle cavity and that the oxygen content is significantly different from that of the external environment. *Nassarius obsoletus* burrows in mud flats and hence it is protected from desiccation stress but the oxygen in the interstitial water is at a low level during the intertidal period. They concluded that a single average sized bubble held in the mantle cavity could supply the animal with oxygen for about 15 min. Since the snails may have as many as a dozen bubbles held in the mantle cavity, aerobic metabolism could be sustained for several hours even without renewal from the air.

A very similar response has been described in the cockle *Cardium* (=*Cerastoderma*) *edule* by Boyden (1972). This bivalve also lives in intertidal deposits so that aerial oxygen consumption need not involve an ability to survive extensive water loss. When the tide ebbs the bivalve becomes inactive and the heart rate is reduced (bradycardia) so that under these conditions the metabolic demand is minimal. Air is then taken into the mantle cavity and is intermittently replaced. When the tide covers the animals again, the gas bubble is released and normal aquatic oxygen consumption resumed. *Cardium edule* is thus able to maintain aerobic metabolism by a combination of reduced metabolic demand and aerial gas exchange. The rate of oxygen consumption in air is similar to the minimal rates recorded in water so it seems likely that aerial gas exchange is sufficient to meet the total metabolic demands of the inactive animal. In contrast, *Cardium glaucum* does not air breathe and is confined to lower shore levels where the period of exposure to air is small.

The situation is rather different in intertidal animals which are uncovered by the tide and hence experience varying amounts of desiccation stress. In some, aerial gas exchange can be maintained through relatively unmodified gill structures provided that conditions are moist, but in others both structural and behavioural adaptations are required to allow air-breathing at high tidal levels. Petersen and Johansen (1973) have shown that the giant chiton *Cryptochiton stelleri* is able to meet its metabolic energy requirements by aerial gas exchange. When uncovered by the tide the chitons choose shaded crevices and expose the gills to air. Under these conditions the aerial gas exchange is 4–5 times lower than in water which largely reflects the greater activity in water. There is no evidence of an oxygen debt being incurred. It seems probable that the ability of this animal to satisfy completely its metabolic oxygen requirements by aerial gas exchange is aided by the large surface area of the gills whose filaments are supported by connective tissue strands which prevent collapse of the filaments in air. In other molluscs the necessity for an increased area through which gas exchange can occur in air is met by vascularisation of the mantle edge. Deshpande (1957; for review, *see* Fretter and Graham, 1962) has shown that in a series of trochid gastropods ranging from the lower shore *Calliostoma zizyphinum* through *Gibbula cineraria* and *G. umbilicalis* to the high level *Monodonta lineata* this vascularisation is related to the tidal level at which the animals occur. It is also correlated with the ability of these animals to maintain high levels of activity during the period of exposure to air (Micallef, 1966; Micallef and Bannister, 1967). Air-breathing also occurs at a rate which is comparable to that in water in many littorinids (Sandison, 1966; Newell and Pye, 1971c) and limpets such as *Patella* (Davies, 1966, 1967). In both *Acmaea scabra* and *A. digitalis* the oxygen consumption in air is a good deal less than that in water or under moist conditions although these differences are again probably associated with the increased activity which occurs in water, rather than to a partial anaerobiosis which occurs under aerial conditions.

As has been pointed out on p.37, many of these gastropods have a high tolerance of water loss and only when survival is threatened by desiccation stress is anaerobiosis likely to occur. In most organisms, however, it is necessary for both water conservation and aerial gas exchange to be integrated into a common behaviour pattern. In many bivalves which live at high tidal levels this is accomplished by intermittent air-gaping which serves to replace the air in the mantle cavity and prevent excessive water loss. Air gaping has been reported in the mussels *Modiolus demissus* (Kuenzler, 1961; Lent, 1968, 1969), *Mytilus edulis* (Helm and Trueman, 1967; Colman and Trueman, 1971) and *Mytilus californianus* (Moon and Pritchard, 1970) and in *Isognomon alatus* (Trueman and Lowe, 1971). This behaviour is associated in most cases with quiescence and often with bradycardia much as occurs in some subtidal bivalves exposed to respiratory stress (Brand and Roberts, 1973). A reduction in activity associated with bradycardia and intermittent air gaping thus appear to be common features which allow intertidal molluscs to maintain aerobic metabolism even under conditions of increasing desiccation stress.

Amongst the crustaceans the adaptations which allow the maintenance of aerobic respiration are generally similar to those cited above for molluscs. One strategy, as in *Cryptochiton,* is for the animal to seek moist conditions and remain quiescent. Many intertidal crustaceans such as the isopod *Ligia oceanica* and the sand hopper *Talitrus* and *Orchestia,* for example, air-breathe in the moist conditions which occur amongst the deposits of the upper shore (Edney and Spencer, 1955; Bliss and Mantel, 1968; Hurley, 1968; Warburg, 1968). Again, the common shore crab *Carcinus maenas,* is able to maintain its oxygen consumption in air at a level which is approximately 75% of that in water (Wallace, 1972; Newell, Ahsanullah and Pye, 1972). Such differences as do exist between the aerial and aquatic oxygen consumption are probably related to differences in activity level in air and in water. The heart rate also shows little evidence of suppression when crabs are exposed to moist air even for periods as long as 6–7 h which suggests that this animal is well adapted to maintain aerobic metabolism during the intertidal period (Ahsanullah and Newell, 1971). In other crabs there is progressive reduction in the importance of gills as sites of gas exchange from those characteristic of aquatic through to terrestrial habitats which is rather similar to the sequence noted above in intertidal gastropods (Pearse, 1929; Ayres, 1938; Gray, 1953). In *Uca, Ocypode* and *Grapsus,* however, air is circulated through water which is retained in the branchial cavity so that an essentially aquatic method of gas exchange is used even under aerial conditions (for review, *see* Edney, 1960).

Intertidal barnacles show interesting patterns of adaptation to the maintenance of aerobic metabolism even though they are unable to evade the rigours of the intertidal environment. It has been known for a long time that the intertidal barnacles *Balanus balanoides* and *Chthamalus stellatus* are able to air-breathe. They do so through a small micropylar opening or pneumostome between the opercular valves and gas exchange may be facilitated by ventilation movements of the cirri (Darwin, 1854; Monterosso, 1930; Barnes and Barnes, 1957, 1958; Barnes, Finlayson and

Piatigorsky, 1963; Grainger and Newell, 1965). Barnes, Finlayson and Piatigorsky (1963) showed that the micropyle was of sufficient diameter to allow a diffusion of 350 μl of gas per hour. Since the oxygen requirement of a barnacle was found to be only 2.7 μl/h, it is obvious that diffusion through the micropyle is more than adequate to meet the metabolic requirements of the barnacle. When conditions are moist, a high proportion of barnacles on the shore have a micropylar opening, but with increasing water loss the upper shore animals reduce the size of the micropyle and eventually it is closed altogether (Barnes, Finlayson and Piatigorsky, 1963; Grainger and Newell, 1965). After this, anaerobiosis occurs but metabolism through aerobic pathways is probably predominant for much of the period of exposure to air.

The principal characteristic of upper shore animals is thus their ability to maintain aerial oxygen consumption under conditions which would involve excessive water loss in organisms with unspecialised organs of gas exchange. Control of water loss by intermittent air gaping in bivalves and barnacles coupled with an enhanced ability to withstand dehydration (*see* p. 37) then allows the food captured during limited phases of the tidal cycle to be converted through aerobic pathways into metabolic fuel with an efficiency far in excess of that available from anaerobiosis.

1.3.3 Reduction in the metabolic expenditure of energy

We have seen that of the principal components of the energy budget, both energy input and the efficiency of conversion of assimilated food into metabolic fuel is subject to feedback or control. This is important where both food availability and oxygen are not in a steady state. A further factor which can be used to adjust the balance of the energy equation outlined on p. 46 to yield a positive index of energy balance, is the level of energy expenditure. This can be measured in terms of the oxygen consumption of the organism and is affected by a variety of endogenous and environmental factors. The principal endogenous component affecting energy expenditure is activity level but other factors such as high environmental temperatures during the intertidal period may lead to a major utilisation of metabolic reserves in the absence of an increase in energy input. Principal strategies for reduction of energy expenditure thus involve (a) a reduction of activity level during periods of reduced food availability and (b) a suppression in the effects of temperature increase on metabolic processes, especially on the quiescent organisms during the low tide period, since it is at this time that food availability will be low and environmental temperatures at their maximum.

1.3.3.1 THE INFLUENCE OF ACTIVITY LEVEL

The amount of metabolic activity is, as one would expect, related to the work performed by the organism. In fishes, for example, it has been common practice to measure the rate of oxygen consumption as a function of swimming speed. This then allows an important distinction to be made between the 'active rate' at maximal swimming speeds and the 'standard rate' of oxygen consumption of the quiescent organism. There is also a variety of 'routine rates' which reflect the different activity levels between maximal and minimal rates of oxygen consumption (Spoor, 1946; Fry, 1947; Fry and Hart, 1948; Beamish and Mookherjii, 1964; Muir, Nelson and Bridges, 1965; Brett, 1971; Muir and Niimi, 1972). Rather surprisingly, a similar approach to the study of the metabolism of intertidal invertebrates has been adopted only comparatively recently. This is partly because the activity level of many invertebrates is difficult to quantify, but in some cases data which are directly comparable to that of fishes have been obtained. This allows a calculation of the saving of metabolic reserves which could be achieved by a reduction in activity during the intertidal period or at other times when food reserves are scarce.

McFarland and Pickens (1965) measured the oxygen consumption of the grass shrimp *Palaemonetes vulgaris* swimming at various speeds against a current of water. In this way they were able to obtain data for the active rate and they measured the minimal rate of undisturbed specimens to obtain a value which approached the standard rate. The difference between the active rate and the standard rate is defined in the 'scope for activity'. The values for shrimps acclimated to 20°C are shown in *Table 1.5.*

Although these values are extracted from graphs, and therefore can only be regarded as approximate, it is evident that an approximately three-fold reduction in metabolic cost could be achieved in this animal with the onset of quiescence. This is equivalent to a saving of between 1.4 and 3.57×10^{-3} cal/g/h. Further, the energy conservation is progressively greater at high temperatures which is likely to be a useful asset in organisms subjected to increased environmental temperature at times when food supplies are reduced.

Halcrow and Boyd (1967) have measured the swimming activity and oxygen consumption of the amphipod *Gammarus oceanicus*. Unfortunately, the maximum activity they were able to record corresponds with the routine level of activity in this animal. Nevertheless it is instructive to calculate the scale of energy conservation which might be involved with cessation of activity in this animal. The data from Halcrow and Boyd (1967) are summarised in *Table 1.6.*

Here the difference between the routine and standard rates in *Gammarus* is obviously less than the differences between the active and standard rates in *Palaemonetes vulgaris.* But even so, there is up to a 2.5-fold reduction in energy expenditure with the onset of quiescence. This leads to a saving of up to 0.5×10^{-3} cal/g wet weight/h in *Gammarus oceanicus* and clearly greater economies are achieved if the energy expenditure of maximum sustained performance were calculated.

Detailed studies have also been made of the relationship between ventilation rate and oxygen consumption in the mussel *Mytilus edulis* (Thompson and Bayne, 1970; Bayne, Thompson and Widdows, 1973; Widdows, 1973). In *Gammarus oceanicus* there is a linear relationship

Table 1.5 THE METABOLIC COST OF ACTIVITY IN THE GRASS SHRIMP *PALAEMONETES VULGARIS*. VALUES EXTRACTED FROM DATA OF McFARLAND AND PICKENS (1965) FOR ANIMALS ACCLIMATED AT 20°C. THE ENERGY EQUIVALENT OF OXYGEN CONSUMPTION IS CALCULATED ON THE ASSUMPTION THAT 1 ML O_2 IS EQUIVALENT TO 5.05×10^{-3} CAL

Temperature (°C)	*Active rate (A)* (ml O_2/g wet wt/h)	*Standard rate (S)* (ml O_2/g wet wt/h)	*Scope* *(A–S)*	*Reduction of energy expenditure with quiescence (A/S)*	*Saving in energy* *(A–S × 0.0051)* (cal/g wet wt/h)
10	0.4	0.12	0.28	× 3.33	1.43×10^{-3}
15	0.5	0.14[1]	0.36	× 3.57	1.84×10^{-3}
20	0.75	0.18	0.57	× 4.17	2.91×10^{-3}
30	1.0	0.30	0.70	× 3.33	3.57×10^{-3}

[1]Interpolated from graphs

Table 1.6 THE METABOLIC COST OF ACTIVITY IN THE AMPHIPOD *GAMMARUS OCEANICUS* (DATA DERIVED FROM HALCROW AND BOYD (1967)). THE ENERGY EQUIVALENT OF OXYGEN CONSUMPTION IS CALCULATED ON THE ASSUMPTION THAT 1 ML O_2 IS EQUIVALENT TO 5.05×10^{-3} CAL

Temperature (°C)	*Routine rate (R)* (ml O_2/g wet wt/h)	*Standard rate (S)* (ml O_2/g wet wt/h)	*Scope* *(R–S)*	*Reduction of energy expenditure with quiescence (R/S)*	*Saving in energy* *(R–S × 0.0051)* (cal/g wet wt/h)
5	0.064	0.044	0.020	× 1.45	0.102×10^{-3}
10	0.124	0.052	0.072	× 2.38	0.367×10^{-3}
15	0.152	0.062	0.090	× 2.45	0.459×10^{-3}
20	0.140	0.106	0.034	× 1.32	0.173×10^{-3}

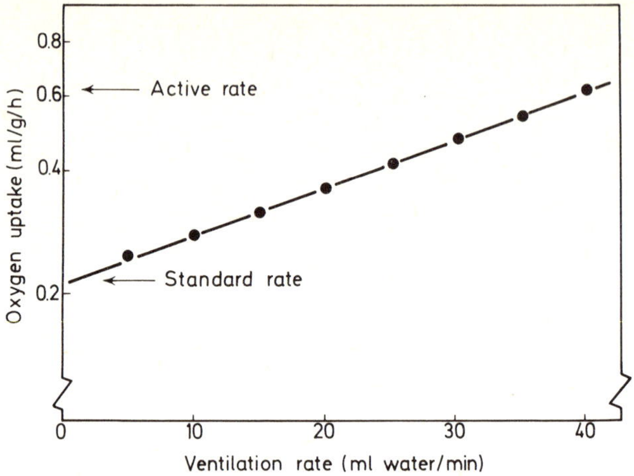

Figure 1.26 Graph showing the relationship between the ventilation rate (ml water/min) and oxygen consumption (ml/g dry weight/h) in a 1.0 g specimen of the mussel Mytilus edulis *at 15°C. (After Newell, and Bayne, 1973; courtesy Editor, Netherlands Journal of Sea Research)*

between oxygen consumption and swimming activity (Halcrow and Boyd, 1967) but in *Mytilus edulis,* as is shown in *Figure 1.26,* the relationship is semi-logarithmic. When measurements are made on mussels at a variety of experimental temperatures it is possible to make similar calculations to those cited above for *Palaemonetes* and *Gammarus.* These are summarised in *Table 1.7* which shows the data not only for active and quiescent animals, but also those for mussels showing routine levels of activity.

Again, *Mytilus edulis* conforms with the general rule that quiescence is associated with approximately a 2-fold reduction of energy expenditure compared with the active rate. This amounts to a saving of as much as 1.8×10^{-3} cal/g dry tissue/h in mussels and a greater saving is achieved at high temperatures much as occurs in *Palaemonetes* and over parts of the range in *Gammarus oceanicus.* Estimates for other animals fall within a similar general range to that cited above. Mangum and Sassaman (1969) found a fall of × 3.45 between the active and standard metabolism of *Diopatra cuprea.* Boyden (1972) estimated a value of ×1.9 for the cockle *Cardium edule* but some seasonal variation in this value has been obtained in other animals. In *Mytilus edulis,* for example, a figure approaching ×6 has been reported for animals collected in the winter (Bayne, Thompson and Widdows, 1973) and this is similar to values cited by Newell (1970) for *Cardium edule* and *Nephtys hombergi.* Comparisons between the metabolic cost of activity in different organisms have, however, little meaning unless we also know the amount of work performed relative to oxygen consumption. A large slow-moving organism, for example, may carry out as much work in movement as a faster moving but smaller animal. Again, irrigatory activities of bivalves can hardly be compared with swimming of crustaceans unless this is calculated per unit of work done. It seems an urgent requirement that the energetic cost of activity be calculated on a more uniform basis so that truly interspecific comparisons can be made.

Table 1.7 THE METABOLIC COST OF ACTIVITY IN THE MUSSEL *MYTILUS EDULIS* (DATA DERIVED FROM BAYNE, THOMPSON AND WIDDOWS (1973)). THE ENERGY EQUIVALENT OF OXYGEN CONSUMPTION IS CALCULATED ON THE ASSUMPTION THAT 1 ML O_2 IS EQUIVALENT TO 5.05×10^{-3} CAL. THE ANIMALS WERE ACCLIMATED TO 15°C AND THE DATA ARE FOR AN ANIMAL OF 1.2 G DRY TISSUE WEIGHT

Temperature (°C)	*Active rate (A)* (ml/g dry wt/h)	*Routine rate (R)* (ml/g dry wt/h)	*Standard rate (S)* (ml/g dry wt/h)	*Scope (A–S)*	*Reduction of energy expenditure with quiescence (A/S)*	*Saving in energy (A–S × 0.0051)* (cal/g/h)
10	0.35	0.2	0.18	0.17	× 1.94	0.87×10^{-3}
15	0.51	0.33	0.22	0.29	× 2.32	1.48×10^{-3}
20	0.68	0.67	0.32	0.36	× 2.13	1.84×10^{-3}

Despite these difficulties, it is possible to say that in any one organism the onset of quiescence may lead to a 2–3 fold reduction in metabolic demand. The widespread occurrence of reduced activity often with bradycardia in limpets (Jones, 1968), winkles (Newell and Pye, 1971c), bivalves (Helm and Trueman, 1967; Trueman and Lowe, 1971; Boyden, 1972) and barnacles (Barnes, Finlayson and Piatigorsky, 1963) may thus not only allow aerial gas exchange to meet the metabolic energy demands (*see* Section 1.3.2) but in itself must lead to a considerable economy of metabolic reserves during the intertidal period.

1.3.3.2 THE INFLUENCE OF TEMPERATURE CHANGE

The influence of temperature on the metabolic energy expenditure of intertidal organisms is directly relevant to the maintenance of energy balance. It is therefore important to know whether a rise in temperature, which often occurs following exposure to air, is accompanied by a passive increase in metabolic energy expenditure despite the fact that energy input is at its minimal level during this phase of the tidal cycle.

Although a great deal is now known about the effects of temperature on living organisms and their component parts (Prosser, 1974; Hochachka and Somero, 1973; Precht *et al.* 1973; Wieser, 1973) it is not always easy to abstract data for the standard or resting metabolism of intertidal animals. This is at least partly because measurements have commonly been made on animals which are showing varying levels of routine activity. It is thus only in comparatively few studies that we can be reasonably sure that the effects of temperature on the standard rate of metabolism are not masked by the much greater metabolic cost of activity. The rate of activity nearly always increases logarithmically with temperature. Instances where this has been recorded include ciliary activity in mussels (Gray, 1923; Schlieper, Kowalski and Erman, 1958), cirral activity in barnacles (Southward, 1964; Ritz and Foster, 1968), radular activity in winkles (Newell, Pye and Ahsanullah, 1971a) and the heart rate of many intertidal animals (Maynard, 1960; Pickens, 1965; Ahsanullah and Newell, 1971). Thus both routine and active rates of oxygen consumption also increase markedly with temperature. Rates of oxygen consumption associated with activity are dependent upon temperature in the amphipod *Gammarus oceanicus* (Halcrow and Boyd, 1967), in the shrimp *Crangon vulgaris* (Hagerman, 1970), in the echinoid *Strongylocentrotus droebachiensis* (Percy, 1972), in the bivalves *Mytilus edulis, Donax vittatus* and *Chlamys opercularis* (Ansell, 1973; Bayne, Thompson and Widdows, 1973; McLusky, 1973) as well as in several polychaetes (Mangum and Sassaman, 1969; Coyer and Mangum, 1973).

In contrast, a variety of different temperature effects have been reported for the oxygen consumption of quiescent intertidal invertebrates. Mangum and Sassaman (1969) showed that in the polychaete *Diopatra cuprea* even the standard rate is temperature-dependent. This animal lives buried in the sediments and probably experiences little variation in environmental temperature during the intertidal period. Again, the subtidal sea-urchin

Strongylocentrotus franciscanus has a respiratory rate which is remarkably dependent upon temperature whereas its intertidal relative *S. purpuratus,* which must experience variable temperatures during the intertidal period, has a rate of oxygen consumption which is essentially independent of temperature between 12 and 21°C (Ulbricht and Pritchard, 1972). On the other hand Davies (1969) showed no marked suppression of the temperature coefficients for the aerial oxygen consumption of *Patella* even though this animal lives on rock surfaces intertidally. Other organisms may show very different temperature effects even though they live in a generally similar intertidal environment. Kennedy and Mihursky (1972) have shown that in the intertidal bivalves *Mya arenaria* and *Mulinia lateralis* the metabolism is strongly affected by temperature change whereas in *Macoma balthica* the metabolism shows little change over the range 10–20°C. Again, Mangum (1972) has shown that in the subtidal polychaete *Hyalinoecia* the oxygen consumption is independent of temperature over a wide range even though the animal does not experience marked temperature changes under natural conditions. It seems then that other factors than merely exposure to fluctuating environmental temperatures may be involved in the occurrence of low temperature coefficients for metabolism.

Without details of the local differences in environmental temperatures which organisms may experience even within the same intertidal habitat, it is difficult to know whether the occurrence of low temperature coefficients, leading to an economy of metabolic reserves as the temperature rises, is related to environmental conditions. However, in addition to those cited above, many intertidal invertebrates (*see* Newell and Northcroft, 1967) including mussels (Read, 1962), limpets (Davies, 1966), littorinids (Newell and Pye, 1970a, b; McMahon and Russell-Hunter, 1973), neogastropods (Huebner, 1969) and rockpool ostracods such as *Hirschmannia viridis* (Hagerman, 1969) each show zones sometimes of as much as 10°C over which the metabolic rate has a low temperature coefficient. Such rate: temperature discontinuities are not confined to intertidal animals and have been reported for Trichoptera larvae (Collardeau, 1961), freshwater gammarids belonging to the *pulex* group (Roux and Roux, 1967), freshwater copepods (Siefken and Armitage, 1968), crayfish (Wiens and Armitage, 1961) and frogs (Dunlap, 1972). These effects have been reviewed by Newell (1969; 1970; 1973a, b) and suggest that discontinuities in the rate: temperature relationships for invertebrate metabolism may be a widespread feature in organisms subjected to major fluctuations in environmental temperature. It is also significant that the temperature range over which metabolism has a reduced temperature sensitivity changes in some intertidal animals such as *Littorina littorea* according to season of the year (Newell and Pye, 1970a; Newell and Roy, 1973) and thermal acclimation (Newell and Pye, 1970b; Pye and Newell, 1973). A similar effect of thermal acclimation has also been reported in some intertidal sea-urchins in which rate: temperature independence was gained at low temperatures following cold acclimation; when the urchins were warm acclimated, the regions of low temperature coefficient occurred at higher temperatures (Ulbricht, 1973).

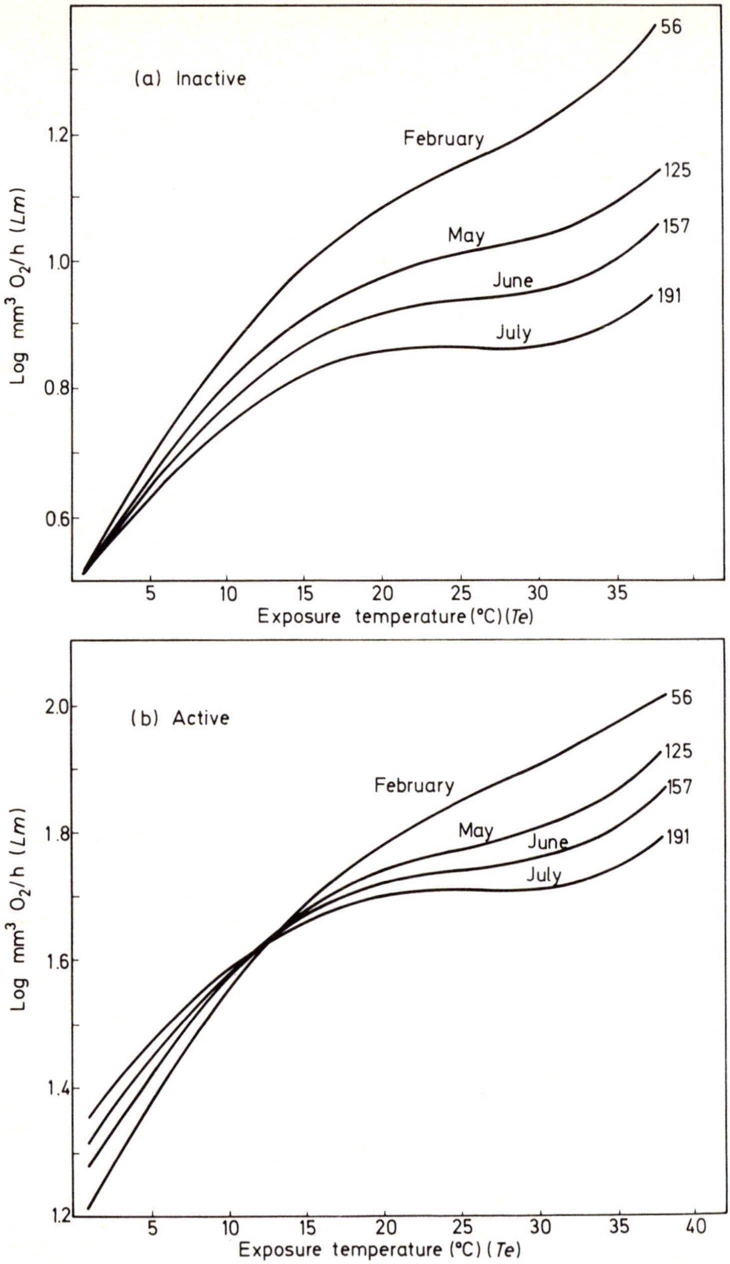

Figure 1.27 Graphs showing the relationship between log metabolism (Lm) *and exposure temperature* (Te) *in a hypothetical specimen of* Littorina littorea *of 40 mg dry tissue weight (a) inactive animals (b) active animals. Curves are for specimens collected in February (day 56), May (day 125), June (day 157) and July (day 191). Generated from a simplified equation where* $Lm = a + x \cdot Te - y \cdot Te^3 + z \cdot Te^4$ *(when* $y = 0.4 \times 10^{-4}$ *and* $z = 0.9 \times 10^{-6}$*). (After Newell and Roy, 1973; courtesy University of Chicago Press)*

One of the problems with the interpretation of these data, and in making comparisons between widely-differing organisms, is that metabolism may be influenced not only by activity level and experimental temperature but also by a wide variety of other factors including photoperiod (Dehnel, 1958; Webb and Brown, 1958; Roberts, 1964, 1967; Unglaub Silverthorn, 1973), body size (Hemmingsen, 1960; Newell, 1970), nutritional state (for review, *see* Marsden, 1973b), whether measurements were made in air or in water (Toulmond, 1967a, b) and various combinations of these and other factors. One way of simplifying the complexity of the data is to make a mathematical model where the direct action of each factor on metabolism is expressed together with their mutual interactions. In the case of the data for *Littorina littorea,* the metabolism of the animals was measured as a function of activity level (*Ac*), date of collection (*Da*), exposure temperature (*Te*) and body size (*D*) expressed as dry weight in mg (Newell and Roy, 1973). Following transformation into a logarithmic scale, metabolism became log metabolism (*Lm*) and body size became log dry weight (*Ld*).

In all, there were four experimentally-determined factors (*Ld, Ac, Te,* and *Da*) plus another nine expressing either curvilinearity or interactions between factors. The number of possible combinations of factors would amount in this case to as many as 8192, so a computer program was used to simplify the multiple regression equation (Quenouille, 1952; Snedecor, 1956; Effroymson, 1960). The independent variables were introduced one by one, tested for significance at the 5% level and either retained, or replaced by another one or removed. The final result produced a shortened multiple regression equation in which all the partial regression coefficients were statistically significant. Of the original thirteen independent variables, eight were retained and the general equation could then be used to predict the effects of season, temperature, body size and activity on metabolism in this animal. The results obtained are of interest insofar as the predicted curves are very similar to those obtained by McFarland and Pickens (1965) for *Palaemonetes vulgaris* and by Bayne, Thompson and Widdows (1973) for *Mytilus edulis.*

Figure 1.27 shows the effect of exposure temperature on the rate of oxygen consumption of a hypothetical specimen of *Littorina littorea* of 40 mg dry weight collected on February 25th (day 56), May 5th (day 125), June 6th (day 157) and July 10th (day 191). It is clear that both inactive and active rates have broadly similar temperature relationships with a marked temperature-dependence early in the year. During the summer, however, the temperature coefficients are progressively suppressed over the range 15–30°C. Both *Palaemonetes varians* and *Mytilus edulis* also have active and standard rates of oxygen consumption which are similar to one another in their temperature relationships and which have a low temperature coefficient. In contrast, the routine rates of both *Littorina littorea* and *Mytilus edulis* are much more strongly dependent upon temperature (Newell and Bayne, 1973). The situation is further complicated in *Littorina* by the fact that large and small specimens do not show a similar response to temperature. The small animals have a much more obvious suppression of their metabolism during the summer than the larger ones

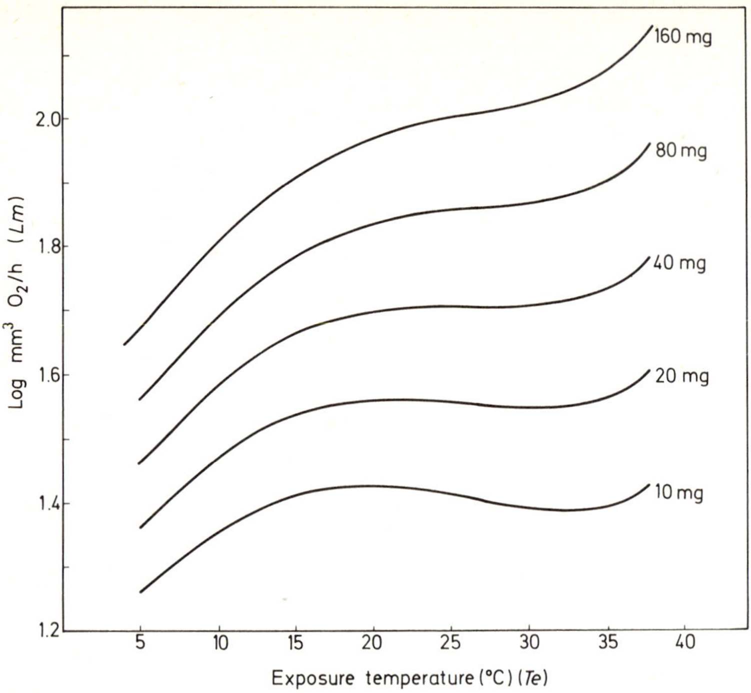

Figure 1.28 Graphs showing the relationship between log metabolism (Lm) *and exposure temperature* (Te) *in active* Littorina littorea *of hypothetical dry tissue weights of 10, 20, 40, 80 and 160 mg. Data for animals collected in July (day 191). See equation in legend to Figure 1.27. (After Newell and Roy, 1973; courtesy University of Chicago Press)*

(*Figure 1.28*). A difference in the effect of temperature on large and small animals is by no means uncommon, although reports in the literature suggest that in some cases the larger sized animals would have a reduced temperature coefficient compared with small ones. Rao and Bullock (1954), for example, cited data for *Talorchestia* from Edwards and Irving (1943a, b) which is essentially similar to that described above for *Littorina.* In *Uca* (Vernberg, 1959), *Arion* (Roy, 1969) and barnacles (Barnes and Barnes, 1969), however, the reverse is the case, with the metabolism of large animals being less sensitive to temperature than small ones.

It follows from this that the temperature coefficient for a particular species may vary according to body size as well as season of the year. The curves for *Littorina littorea* are shown in *Figure 1.29.* It should be emphasised, however, that many other factors which were not measured in this series of experiments may be involved in the control of the metabolic rate of intertidal animals. Roberts (1957), for example, showed that the rate of oxygen consumption of the crab *Pachygrapsus* falls to approximately 60% of the initial rate following starvation at 16°C for 23 days. The most rapid decline occurred within seven days which is a similar time period to that reported by Vernberg (1959) for *Uca.* Davies (1966; 1967) showed that the rate of oxygen consumption of specimens of the limpet *Patella* from high

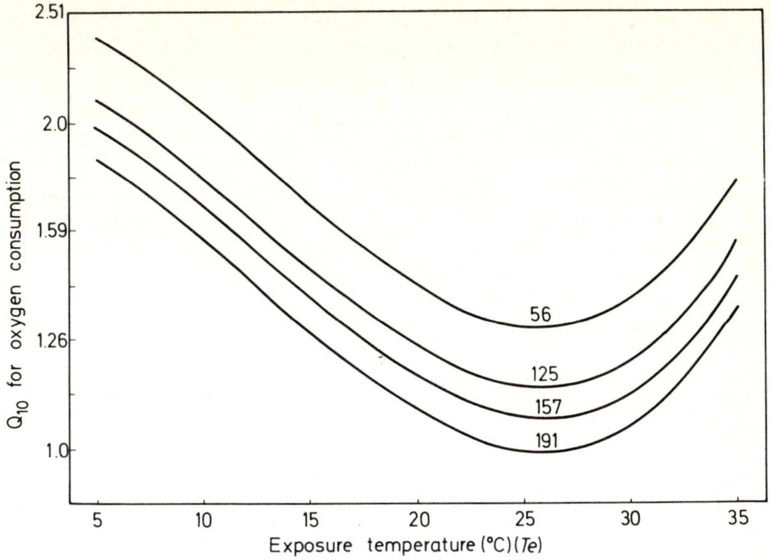

Figure 1.29 Graphs showing the relationship between the temperature coefficient (Q_{10}) for oxygen consumption and exposure temperature (Te) *in February (day 56), May (day 125), June (day 157) and July (day 191). Data for a hypothetical specimen of* Littorina littorea *of 40 mg dry tissue weight. Curves generated from the equation Log Q_{10} = 0.3359 + 0.07743* Ld − *0.0008523* Da − *0.001332* Te^2 + *0.00003415* Te^3 *(for explanation see text). (After Newell and Roy, 1973; courtesy University of Chicago Press)*

shore levels or bare rock surfaces was not only lower but also had a lower temperature coefficient than that of limpets from the lower shore or areas rich in algae. There is also a definite influence of starvation on the level of metabolism and rate : temperature relationships in the shore crab *Carcinus maenas* (Marsden, 1973b; Marsden, Newell and Ahsanullah, 1973; Wallace, 1973b). In this animal both body size and nutritional state are of importance, small specimens showing a more rapid reduction in metabolism and a lower temperature coefficient than large crabs. The evidence suggests, therefore, that intertidal organisms may not be unique in the possession of discontinuous metabolic rate : temperature curves. Where organisms are subjected to a reduced energy supply, whether this is intertidally or subtidally, a reduced rate of metabolism coupled with a low temperature coefficient may represent a principal strategy for the maintenance of energy balance.

Some indication of the mechanisms likely to be involved in these compensatory responses can be gained by a study of the effects of temperature on isolated tissues and subcellular preparations (*see* Troshin, 1967; Vernberg, Schlieper and Schneider, 1963; Newell, 1973a). Rather surprisingly, bearing in mind the drastic treatments involved, there is a good correspondence between the rate of oxygen consumption of the intact organism and that of subcellular preparations of species such as the winkle *Littorina littorea* (Newell and Pye, 1971a, b, c) and the woodlouse *Porcellio scaber* (Newell, Wieser and Pye, 1974) when all rates are expressed in the same units. Studies such as these suggest that in *Littorina* an increase in metabolic rate and in temperature dependence can be induced by increasing substrate concentrations above 1.0 mM pyruvate. At these concentrations the rate of oxygen consumption of subcellular preparations of *Littorina littorea* approach the level and temperature relationships of the active intact winkle. At lower substrate concentrations, the rate of oxygen consumption is reduced and approaches the value for the standard rate of intact quiescent winkles only at approximately 0.01 mM pyruvate (Newell and Pye, 1971a, b; Newell, 1973a) (*see Figure 1.30*). It is of interest to note that, as pointed

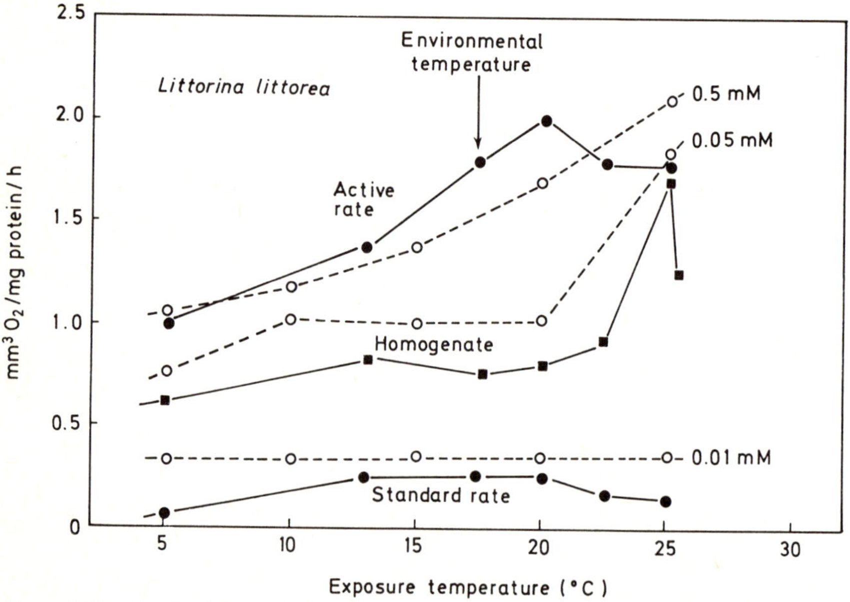

Figure 1.30 Graphs showing the effect of temperature on rate of oxygen consumption of active and inactive winkles (Littorina littorea) *of 30 mg dry protein weight collected in June 1970. Superimposed is the rate for subcellular preparations in the presence of various concentrations of pyruvate. (After Newell and Pye, 1971; courtesy Pergamon Press Ltd)*

out by Somero (1969; *see also* Hochachka and Somero, 1973 and p. 125) at these low substrate concentrations within the physiological range 0.01–1.0 mM, enzyme-substrate affinity may primarily control the reaction rate of many key processes. Positive or negative modulation of enzyme-substrate affinity by temperature itself, pH in the body fluids, or by the induction of repression of different isoenzymes with differing enzyme-substrate affinities may then represent a mechanism by which reaction rates may be controlled and a low temperature coefficient maintained.

We have obtained rather similar results on the isopod *Porcellio scaber* (Newell, Wieser and Pye, 1974) with the sum of the metabolism of subcellular components falling within the range of the metabolic rates of the intact organism. In this case there was little indication of a reduced temperature coefficient in either active or quiescent animals, neither did starvation substantially reduce metabolism below that of the quiescent animals (*Figure 1.31*). It seems, therefore, that some animals such as *Porcellio,* which largely evade temperature stress, do not resemble *Littorina* in their responses to temperature, and in this respect are similar to the subtidal and burrowing organisms referred to on p. 60. Only further investigations aimed at measuring the effects of both combinations of environmental factors on the metabolism of intact organisms, and the responses on their component tissues, will allow us to make more than tentative suggestions on the different patterns of response which might occur in invertebrates from different environmental situations.

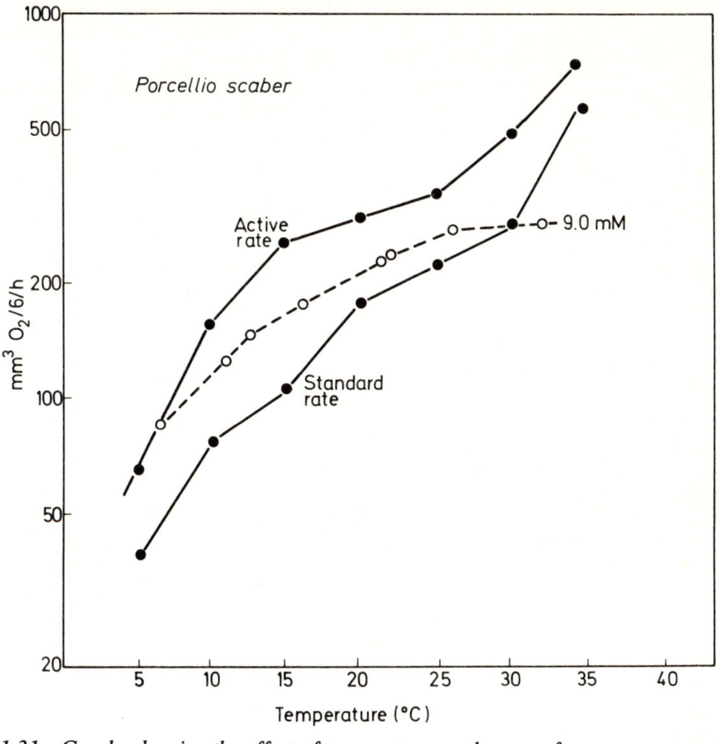

Figure 1.31 Graphs showing the effect of temperature on the rate of oxygen consumption of active and inactive isopods (Porcellio scaber). *Superimposed is the rate obtained for a subcellular preparation in the presence of 9.0 mM succinate. (After Newell, Wieser and Pye, 1974; courtesy Springer-Verlag)*

1.4 CONCLUSION

This survey of the adaptations which intertidal organisms show to life on the sea-shore suggests that the physical limits of tolerance, as well as biological factors principally associated with the maintenance of a positive index of energy balance, play a part in controlling the distribution of animals in the intertidal zone. Lent (1968; 1969) has shown that the intertidal distribution of the mussel *Modiolus demissus* is controlled by several environmental and biological factors depending upon the size of the mussels. Large specimens are less tolerant of heat stress than small ones, whereas small ones are less tolerant of desiccation stress than large mussels. Thus, distribution of this animal on the upper shore is controlled by an interaction between two different environmental factors, both tending to eliminate the extremes of the size range of *Modiolus*. At the lower limits of intertidal distribution, biological, rather than physical factors, limit the occurrence of the mussels. Here again, it seems likely that there is an interaction between two factors each operating maximally on the extremes of the size range of *Modiolus*. Smaller mussels may compete more successfully for food than large ones and so limit the occurrence of large specimens. On the other hand, small mussels have a thin shell so that the smallest specimens are limited by predation. This interaction of physical factors at the upper limit of distribution, and biotic factors at the lower end is illustrated in *Figure 1.32* and may be a common pattern for organisms such as gastropods, bivalves and barnacles which live at the extreme upper limits of the intertidal zone (*see* Connell, 1961; Frank, 1965).

In general, where the distribution of a species borders on an unexploited food resource, there will be a tendency for the new habitat to be exploited to

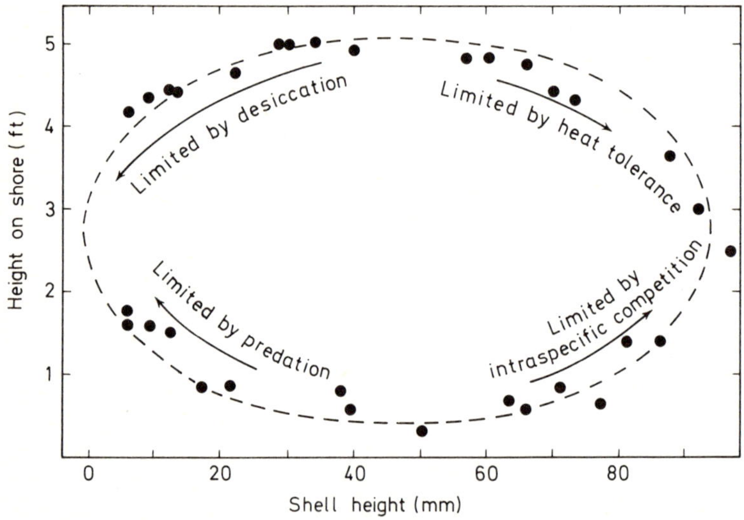

Figure 1.32 Diagrammatic representation of the factors limiting the intertidal distribution of the bivalve Modiolus demissus. *Points show the shell size and intertidal height of the peripheral members of the population at the limits of its distribution. Note that medium-sized individuals survive both higher and lower on the shore than the extremes of the size range. Large individuals tend to be eliminated on the upper shore by their low heat tolerance, and on the lower shore by intraspecific competition with smaller mussels. Small individuals are eliminated on the upper shore by desiccation effects and on the lower shore by predation. (After Lent, 1968; courtesy The Biological Bulletin)*

the limits of the physiological tolerances of the organism concerned. Wolcott (1973), for example, has recently shown that in some intertidal situations the upper shore limpets *Acmaea digitalis* and *A. persona* are flanked by a rich algal carpet near freshwater seepage areas. These animals exploit the food resources to the limits of their hypo-osmotic tolerances. On the other hand, elsewhere *Acmaea digitalis* and *A. scabra* are flanked on the upper shore by an algal film with few other competitors. Under these circumstances the limpets extend their range upshore to the limits of their tolerances of desiccation and thermal stress. Over much of the sea-shore, however, the potential range of distribution of particular organisms overlaps both towards the upper and lower shore with that of competing organisms. Under these circumstances, little extra energy could be gained by an extension in range since the food resources are already utilised by neighbouring species. It is not surprising to find, therefore, that in these cases the distribution range of the organisms is well within the limits of their physiological tolerances. The capacity to survive is then determined by the relative abilities of the organisms to compete with neighbouring species.

This leads us to the general conclusion that studies of the limits of physiological tolerances will have a direct ecological relevance only where

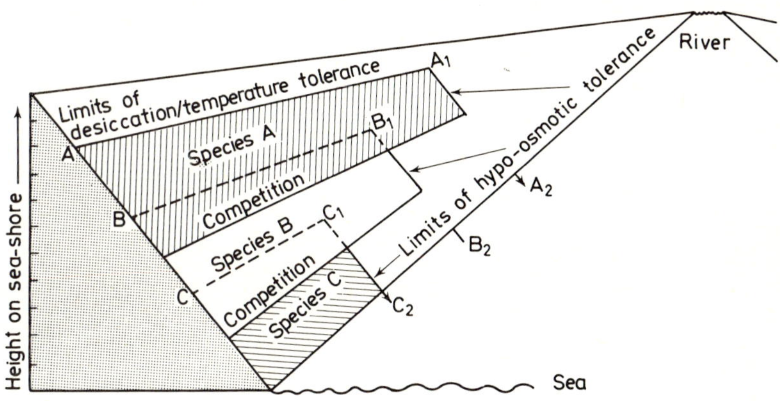

Figure 1.33 Diagram illustrating the factors limiting the distribution of three intertidal species with overlapping limits of physiological tolerance. Note that:
(1) Species A could survive in the whole of the area defined by A A_1 A_2. Because it borders on unexploited food resources, both upshore and towards low salinity its distribution is controlled by (a) its tolerance of desiccation and thermal stress and (b) by its limits of hypo-osmotic tolerance. Its lower limit of distribution is controlled by competition with species B.
(2) The limits of tolerance of species B is defined by area B B_1 B_2, i.e. it overlaps with species A but its distribution on the shore lies well within the limits of its tolerance to desiccation and temperature. Upper and lower limits distributional range are controlled by competition with neighbouring specimens A and C which exploit the available food reserves. In this case species B has adaptations to restrict distribution to a zone where a positive index of energy balance can be maintained. Its upstream distribution is limited by tolerances of hypo-osmotic conditions as in species A.
(3) Finally, the distribution of species C is limited to a zone within its tolerance of temperature and desiccation by competition with species B. However its lower range can spread downshore to the limits of its tolerance of physico-chemical conditions and it can also spread upstream to the limits of its hypo-osmotic tolerances

the distribution of a species borders on an unexploited food resource. Elsewhere in the intertidal zone, behavioural mechanisms to restrict organisms to sites where they can compete advantageously with neighbouring species are of overriding importance. We may thus draw a generalised scheme where there are three species with overlapping zones of tolerance to temperature, desiccation and hypo-osmotic conditions. Under these circumstances, as is shown in *Figure 1.33,* only species (A) will be limited directly towards regions of low salinity by hypo-osmotic tolerances, and towards the upper shore by its tolerance of temperature and desiccation stress. Species (B) will be limited partly by its tolerance of low salinities, but will not extend upshore to the limits of its desiccation and thermal tolerance. On the lower shore, species (C) will be limited upstream by its tolerance of hypo-osmotic conditions, but will extend upshore only until it meets competing species (B). The particular interest of comparative studies on the physiology of intertidal animals is that they give us some insight into the relative abilities of such animals to maintain a positive index of energy balance, and thus compete successfully, under the rigorous conditions which prevail on the sea-shore. It then becomes possible to suggest why one species may replace another in a particular zonational position on the sea-shore, despite the fact that both organisms are capable of survival under the physico-chemical conditions which prevail there.

REFERENCES

ABE, N. (1931). 'Ecological observations on *Acmaea dorsuosa* Gould', *Sci. Rep., Tohoku Imp. Univ. (Sendai),* **6,** 403–427

AHSANULLAH, M. (1969). 'A comparative study of the effects of desiccation and thermal stress on intertidal and sublittoral crabs', Ph.D. Thesis. University of London

AHSANULLAH, M. and NEWELL, R. C. (1971). 'Factors affecting the heart rate of the shore crab *Carcinus maenas* (L.)', *Comp. Biochem. Physiol,* **39A,** 277–287

ALI, R. M. (1970). 'The influence of suspension density and temperature on filtration rate of *Hiatella arctica', Mar. Biol.,* **6,** 291–303

ANSELL, A. D. (1973). 'Oxygen consumption by the bivalve *Donax vittatus* (da Costa)', *J. exp. mar. Biol. Ecol.,* **11,** 311–328

ARNOLD, D. C. (1975). 'The response of the limpet, *Patella vulgata* L., to water of different salinities', *J. mar. biol. Assoc.,* **36,** 121–128

ARNOLD, D. C. (1959). 'The reactions of the limpet, *Patella vulgata* Linnaeus to certain of the ionic constituents of sea water', *J. mar. biol. Assoc. U.K.,* **38,** 569–580

AVENS, A. C. and SLEIGH, M. A. (1965). 'Osmotic balance in gastropod molluscs. I. Some marine and littoral gastropods', *Comp. Biochem. Physiol.,* **16,** 121–141

AYRES, J. C. (1938). 'Relationship of habitat to oxygen consumption by certain estuarine crabs', *Ecology,* **19,** 523–527

BALDWIN, S. (1968). 'Manometric measurements of respiratory activity in *Acmaea digitalis* and *Acmaea scabra', The Veliger,* **11,** 79–82

BALLANTINE, D. and MORTON, J. E. (1956). 'Filtering, feeding and digestion in the lamellibranch *Lasaea rubra', J. mar. biol. Assoc. U.K.,* **35,** 241–274

BARNES, H. and BARNES, M. (1957). 'Resistance to desiccation in intertidal barnacles', *Science,* **126,** 358

BARNES, H. and BARNES, M. (1958). 'Note on the opening response of *Balanus balanoides* (L) in relation to salinity and certain inorganic ions', *Veröff. Inst. f. Meeresforsch. Bremerhaven,* **5,** 160–164

BARNES, H. and BARNES, M. (1969). 'Seasonal changes in the acutely determined oxygen consumption and effect of temperature for three common cirripedes, *Balanus balanoides* (L.), *B. balanus* (L.) and *Chthamalus stellatus* (Poli)', *J. exp. mar. Biol. Ecol.,* **4,** 36–50

BARNES, H., FINLAYSON, D. M. and PIATIGORSKY, J. (1963). 'The effect of desiccation and anaerobic conditions on the behaviour, survival and general metabolism of three common cirripedes', *J. Anim. Ecol.,* **32,** 233–252

BAYNE, B. L., THOMPSON, R. J. and WIDDOWS, J. (1973). 'Some effects of temperature and food on the rate of oxygen consumption by *Mytilus edulis* L.' In: *Effect of temperature on ectothermic organisms,* 181–193. Ed. W. Wieser. Springer-Verlag. Heidelberg

BEAMISH, F. W. H. and MOOKHERJII, P.S. (1964). 'Respiration of fishes with special emphasis on standard metabolism. I. Influence of weight and temperature on respiration of goldfish *Carassius auratus* L.', *Can. J. Zool.,* **42,** 161–175

BLISS, D. E. and MANTEL, L. H. (1968). 'Adaptations of crustaceans to land: A summary and analysis of new findings', *Am. Zool.,* **8,** 673–685

BOCK, C. E. and JOHNSON, R. E. (1967). 'The role of behaviour in determining the intertidal zonation of *Littorina planaxis* Philippi, 1847, and *Littorina scutulata* Gould, 1849', *Veliger,* **10,** 42–54

BOX, G. E. P. (1956). 'The determination of optimum conditions' In: *The design and analysis of industrial experiments,* 495–551. Ed. O. L. Davies. Hafner, New York

BOX, G. E. P. and YOULE, P.V. (1955). 'The exploration and exploitation of response surfaces: an example of the link between the fitted surface and the basic mechanism of the system', *Biometrics,* **11,** 287–323

BOYDEN, C. R. (1972). 'The behaviour, survival and respiration of the cockles *Cerastoderma edule* and *C. glaucum* in air', *J. mar. biol. Assoc. U.K.,* **52,** 661–680

BOYLE, P. R. (1969). 'The survival of osmotic stress by *Sypharochiton pelliserpentis', Biol. Bull.,* **136,** 154–165

BRAFIELD, A. E. and NEWELL, G. E. (1961). 'The behaviour of *Macoma balthica* (L.)', *J. mar. biol. Assoc. U.K.,* **41,** 81–87

BRAND, A. R. and ROBERTS, D. (1973). 'The cardiac responses of the scallop *Pecten maximus* (L.) to respiratory stress', *J. exp. mar. Biol. Ecol.,* **13,** 29–43

BREGAZZI, P. K. and NAYLOR, E. (1972). 'The locomotor activity rhythm of *Talitrus saltator* (Montagu) (Crustacea, Amphipoda)', *J. exp. biol.,* **57,** 375–391

BRETT, J. R. (1971). 'Energetic responses of salmon to temperature. A study of some thermal relations in the physiology and freshwater ecology of sockeye salmon *(Oncorhynchus nerka)', Am. Zool.,* **11,** 99–113

BROEKHUYSEN, C. J. (1940). 'A preliminary investigation of the importance of desiccation, temperature and salinity as factors controlling the vertical distribution of certain marine gastropods in False Bay, South Africa', *Trans. roy. Soc. S. Africa,* **28,** 255–292

BURDON-JONES, C. and CHARLES, G. H. (1958). 'Light reactions of littoral gastropods', *Nature,* **181,** 129–131

BURSELL, E. (1959). 'The water-balance of Tsetse flies', *Trans. Ent. Soc. London.,* **111,** 205–235

CAIN, T. D. (1973). 'The combined effects of temperature and salinity on embryos and larvae of the clam *Rangia cuneata', Mar. Biol.,* **21,** 1–6

CAREFOOT, T. H. (1973). 'Feeding, food preference, and the oxygen uptake of food energy by the supralittoral isopod *Ligia pallasii', Mar. Biol.,* **18,** 228–236

CARRIKER, M. (1955). 'Critical review of biology and control of oyster drills', *Spec. scient. Rep. U.S. Fish. Wildl. Serv.,* **148,** 1–150

CHARLES, G. H. (1961). 'The orientation of *Littorina* species to polarised light', *J. exp. Biol.,* **38,** 189–202

CLARK, M. E. (1968). 'The ecology of supra-littoral rockpools with special reference to the copepod fauna', Ph.D. Thesis, University of Aberdeen, Scotland, 108pp

COLGAN, N. (1910). 'Notes on the adaptability of certain littoral molluscs', *Irish Nat.,* **19,** 127–133

COLLARDEAU, C. (1961). 'Influence de la température sur la consommation d'oxygène de quelques larves Trichopteres', *Hydrobiologia,* **18,** 252–264

COLMAN, N. and TRUEMAN, E. R. (1971). 'The effect of aerial exposure on the activity of the mussels *Mytilus edulis* L. *Modiolus modiolus* (L.)', *J. exp. mar. Biol. Ecol.,* **7,** 295–304

CONNELL, J. H. (1961). 'The influence of interspecific competition and other factors on the distribution of the barnacle *Chthamalus stellatus', Ecology,* **42,** 710–723

COOK, B. A., BAMFORD, O. S., FREEMAN, J. D. B. and TEIDMAN, D. J. (1969). 'A study of the homing habit of the limpet', *Anim. Behav.,* **17,** 330–339

COOK, P. A. and GABBOTT, P. A. (1970). 'Seasonal changes in the free glycerol level in the body parts of the adult barnacle *Balanus balanoides', Mar. Biol.,* **7,** (1), 11–13

COOK, P. A. and LEWIS, A. H. (1971). 'Acquisition and loss of cold-tolerance in adult barnacles *(Balanus balanoides)* kept under laboratory conditions', *Mar. Biol.,* **9** (1), 26–30

COOK, S. B. (1969). 'Experiments on homing in the limpet *Siphonaria normalis', Anim. Behav.,* **17,** 679–682

COOK, S. B. (1971). 'A study of homing behaviour in the limpet *Siphonaria alternata', Biol. Bull.,* **141,** 449–457

CORNELIUS, P. F. S. (1972). 'Thermal acclimation of some intertidal invertebrates', *J. exp. mar. Biol. Ecol.,* **9,** 43–53

COSTLOW, J. D. and BOOKHOUT, C. G. (1968). 'The effect of environmental factors on development of the land-crab *Cardisoma guanhumi* Latreille', *Am. Zool.,* **8,** 399–410

COYER, P. E. and MANGUM, C. P. (1973). 'Effect of temperature on active and resting metabolism in Polychaetes', 173–180. In: *Effects of Temperature on Ectothermic Organisms.* Ed. W. Wieser. Springer-Verlag, Heidelberg

CRISP, D. J. (Ed.) (1969). *Fourth European Marine Biology Symposium.* Cambridge University Press, London. 610pp.

CRISP, D. J. (1971). 'Energy flow measurements', 197–279. In: *Methods for the study of marine benthos.* Eds. N. A. Holme and A. D. McIntyre. Blackwell Scientific Publications

CRISP, D. J. and RITZ, D. A. (1967a). 'Changes in temperature tolerance of *Balanus balanoides* during its life-cycle', *Helgol. wiss Meeresunters.,* **15,** 98–115

CRISP, D. J. and RITZ, D. A. (1967b). Temperature acclimation in barnacles', *J. exp. mar. Biol. Ecol.,* **1,** 236–256

CRISP, M. (1969). 'Studies on the behaviour of *Nassarius obsoletus* (Say) (Mollusca, Gastropoda)', *Biol. Bull.,* **136** (3), 355–373

DALES, R. P. (1963). *Annelids.* Hutchinson, London. 200pp.

DANIEL, M. J. (1971). 'Aspects of the Physiology of the Intertidal Teleost, *Blennius pholis* (L.)', Ph.D. Thesis, University of London

DARWIN, C. (1854). *A Monograph on the Sub-Class Cirripeda with Figures of all the Species.* London

DAVIES, P. S. (1966). 'Physiological ecology of *Patella.* I. The effect of body size and temperature on metabolic rate', *J. mar. biol. Assoc. U.K.,* **46,** 647–658

DAVIES, P. S. (1967). 'Physiological ecology of *Patella.* II. Effect of environmental acclimation on the metabolic rate', *J. mar. biol. Assoc. U.K.,* **47,** 61–74

DAVIES, P. S. (1969). 'Physiological ecology of *Patella.* III. Desiccation effects', *J. mar. biol. Assoc. U.K.,* **49,** 291–304

DAVIES, P. S. (1970). 'Physiological ecology of Patella. IV. Environmental and limpet body temperatures', *J. mar. biol. Assoc. U.K.,* **50,** 1069–1077

DEHNEL, P. A. (1958). 'Effect of photoperiod on the oxygen consumption of two species of intertidal crabs', *Nature Lond.,* **181,** 1415–1417

DENTON, E. J. (1961). 'The buoyancy of fish and Cephalopods', *Prog. Biophys. biophys. Chem.,* **11,** 177–234

DENTON, E. J. and MARSHALL, N. B. (1958). 'The buoyancy of bathypelagic fishes without a gas-filled swimbladder', *J. mar. biol. Assoc. U.K.,* **37,** 753–767

DESHPANDE, R. D. (1957). Ph.D. Thesis, University of Reading (cited by Fretter, V. and A. Graham, 1962)

DUNLAP, D. G. (1972). 'Latitudinal effects on metabolic rates in the cricket frog, *Acris crepitans:* Acutely measured rates in summer frogs', *Biol. Bull.,* **143** (2), 332–343

EDNEY, E. B. (1951). 'The body temperature of woodlice', *J. exp. Biol.,* **28,** 271–280

EDNEY, E. B. (1953). 'The temperature of woodlice in the sun', *J. exp. Biol.,* **30,** 331–349

EDNEY, E. B. (1954). 'Woodlice and the land habitat', *Biol. Rev.,* **29,** 185–219

EDNEY, E. B. (1960). 'Terrestrial adaptations'. In: *The physiology of Crustacea,* **1,** 367–393. Ed. T. H. Waterman. Academic Press, New York and London

EDNEY, E. B. (1961). 'The water and heat relationships of fiddler crabs (*Uca* spp)', *Trans. roy. Soc. S. Africa,* **36** (2), 71–91

EDNEY, E. B. (1962). 'Some aspects of the temperature relations of fiddler crabs (*Uca* spp)', *Biometeorology,* 79–85

EDNEY, E. B. and SPENCER, J. O. (1955). 'Cutaneous respiration in woodlice', *J. exp. Biol.,* **32,** 256–269

EDWARDS, D. C. (1969). 'Zonation by size as an adaptation for intertidal life in *Olivella biplicata*', *Am. Zool.,* **9,** 399–417

EDWARDS, G. A. and IRVING, L. (1943a). 'The influence of temperature and season upon the oxygen consumption of the sand crab, *Emerita talpoida* Say', *J. cell. comp. Physiol.,* **21,** 169–182

EDWARDS, G. A. and IRVING, L. (1943b). 'The influence of season and temperature upon the oxygen consumption of the beach flea, *Talorchestia megalopthalma*', *J. cell. comp. Physiol.,* **21,** 183–189

EFFROYMSON, M. A. (1960). 'Multiple regression analysis', pp. 19–203. In: *Mathematical methods for digital computers,* **1.** Eds. A. Ralston and H. S. Wilf. Wiley, New York

ERCOLINI, A. and SCAPINI, F. (1974). 'Sun compass and shore slope in the orientation of littoral amphipods *Talitrus saltator* Montagu)', *Monitore zool. Ital. (N.S.),* **8,** 85–115

EVANS, F. (1961). 'Responses to disturbance of the periwinkle *Littorina punctata* (Gmelin) on a shore in Ghana', *Proc. zool. Soc. Lond.,* **137,** 393–402

EVANS, F. G. C. (1951). 'An analysis of the behaviour of *Lepidochitona cinereus* in response to certain physical features of the environment', *J. Anim. Ecol.,* **22,** (1), 1–10

EVANS, R. G. (1948). 'The lethal temperatures of some common British littoral molluscs', *J. Anim. Ecol.,* **17** (2), 165–173

FENCHEL, T. and KOFOED, L. H. (1976). 'Evidence for exploitative interspecific competition in mud snails (Hydrobiidae)', *Oikos* (In the press)

FORSMAN, B. (1951). 'Studies on *Gammarus duebeni* Lillj. with notes on some rockpool organisms in Sweden', *Zool. Bidr. Uppsala,* **29,** 215–236

FOSTER, B. A. (1969). 'Tolerance of high temperatures by some intertidal barnacles', *Mar. Biol.* **4,** (4), 326–332

FRAENKEL, G. (1960). 'Lethal temperatures for three marine invertebrates: *Limulus polyphemus, Littorina littorea* and *Pagurus longicarpus*', *Oikos,* **11** (2), 171–182

FRANK, P. W. (1965). 'The biodemography of an intertidal snail population', *Ecology,* **46,** 831–844

FREEMAN, R. F. H. and RIGLER, F. H. (1957). 'The responses of *Scrobicularia plana* da Costa to osmotic pressure change', *J. mar. biol. Assoc.,* **36,** 553–557

FRETTER, V. and GRAHAM, A. (1962). *British Prosobranch Molluscs.* Ray Society London, 755pp.

FRY, F. E. J. (1947). 'Effects of the environment on animal activity', *Univ. Toronto stud. Biol., (55) (Publ. Ontario Fish. Res. Lab.)* **68,** 1–62

FRY, F. E. J. and HART, J. S. (1948). 'The relation of temperature to oxygen consumption in the goldfish', *Biol. Bull.,* **94,** 66–77

FUNKE, W. (1968). 'Heimfindevermogen und Ortstreve bei *Patella* L. (Gastropoda, Prosobranchia)', *Oecologia,* **2,** 19–142

GABBOTT, P. and BAYNE, B. L. (1973). 'Biochemical effects of temperature and nutritive stress in *Mytilus edulis*', *J. mar. biol. Assoc. U. K.,* **53,** 287–298

GALBRAITH, R. T. (1965). 'Homing behaviour in the limpets *Acmaea digitalis* and *Lottia gigantea*', *Am. Midl. Natur.,* **74** (1), 245–246

GANNING, B. (1966). 'Short time fluctuations of the microfauna in a rockpool in the northern Baltic proper', *Veröff. Inst. Meeresforsch. Bremerh. (sonderbd.),* **2,** 149–154

GANNING, B. (1967). 'Laboratory experiments in the ecological work on rockpool animals with special notes on the ostracod *Heterocypris salinus*', *Helgoländer wiss Meeresunters,* **15,** 27–40

GANNING, B. (1970). 'Measurements of community metabolism in some Brackish water rockpools by means of diel oxygen curves', *Oikos,* **21,** 292–298

GANNING, B. (1971a). 'Studies on chemical, physical and biological conditions in Swedish rockpool ecosystems', *Ophelia,* **9** (1), 51–105

GANNING, B. (1971b). 'Studies on Baltic rockpool ecosystems', Ph.D. Thesis, University of Stockholm, Sweden

GANNING, B. and WULFF, F. (1966). 'A chamber for offering alternative conditions to small motile aquatic animals', *Ophelia,* **3,** 151–160

GIBSON, R. N. (1969). 'The biology and behaviour of littoral fish', *Oceanogr. Mar. Biol. Ann. Rev.*, **7,** 367–410

GLYNNE-WILLIAMS, J. and HOBART, J. (1952). 'Studies on the crevice fauna of a selected shore in Anglesey', *Proc. zool. Soc. Lond.*, **122,** 797–824

GOWANLOCH, J. N. and HAYES, F. R. (1926). 'Contributions to the study of marine gastropods. I. The physical factors, behaviour and intertidal life of *Littorina*', *Contr. Canad. Biol. N.S.*, **3,** 133–166

GRAHAME, J. (1973a). 'Assimilation efficiency of *Littorina littorea* (L.) (Gastropoda: Prosobranchiata)', *J. Anim. Ecol.*, **42,** 383–389

GRAHAME, J. (1973b). 'Breeding energetics of *Littorina littorea* (L.) (Gastropoda: Prosobranchiata)', *J. Anim. Ecol.*, **42,** 391–403

GRAINGER, F. and NEWELL, G. E. (1965). 'Aerial respiration in *Balanus balanoides*', *J. mar. biol. Assoc. U.K.*, **45,** 469–479

GRANT, P. T. and MACKIE, A. M. (Eds.) (1974). *Chemoreception in Marine Organisms,* Academic Press, London and New York. 296pp.

GRAY, I. E. (1953). 'Comparative study of gill area in crabs', *Anat. Rec.*, **117,** 567–568

GRAY, J. (1923). 'The mechanism of ciliary movement. III. The effect of temperature', *Proc. roy. Soc. Lond. (B)*, **95,** 6–15

GUNTER, G. (1957). 'Temperature' pp. 159–184. In: *Treatise on Marine Ecology and Paleoecology. (Ecology).* Ed. J. W. Hedgpeth. Mem. (67) Geol. Soc. Amer., **1**

HAEFNER, P. A. (1969). 'Temperature and salinity tolerance of the sand shrimp, *Crangon septemspinosa* Say', *Physiol. Zool.*, **42** (4), 388–397

HAEFNER, P. A. (1970). 'The effect of low dissolved oxygen concentrations on temperature-salinity tolerance of the sand shrimp, *Crangon septemspinosa* Say', *Physiol. Zool.*, **43** (1), 30–37

HAEFNER, P. A. (1971). 'Avoidance of anoxic conditions by the sand shrimp, *Crangon septemspinosa* Say', *Chesapeake Science,* **12** (1), 50–51

HAGERMAN, L. (1969). 'Environmental factors affecting *Hirschmannia viridis* (O. F. Müller) (Ostracoda) in shallow brackish water', *Ophelia,* **7,** 79–99

HAGERMAN, L. (1970). 'The oxygen consumption of *Crangon vulgaris* (Fabricius) (Crustacea, Natantia) in relation to salinity, *Ophelia,* **7,** 283–292

HALCROW, K. and BOYD, C. M. (1967). 'The oxygen consumption and swimming activity of the amphipod *Gammarus oceanicus* at different temperatures', *Comp. Biochem. Physiol.*, **23,** 233–242

HARDIN, D. D. (1968). 'A comparative study of lethal temperatures in the limpets *Acmaea scabra* and *Acmaea digitalis*', *Veliger,* **11,** 83–87

HARVEY, C. E., JONES, M. B. and NAYLOR, E. (1973). 'Some factors affecting the distribution of estuarine isopods (Crustacea)', *Estuarine and Coastal Mar. Sci.*, **1,** 113–124

HELM, M. M. and TRUMAN, E. R. (1967). 'The effect of exposure on the heart rate of the mussel *Mytilus edulis* L.', *Comp. Biochem. Physiol.*, **21,** 171–177

HEMMINGSEN, A. M. (1960). 'Energy metabolism as related to body size and respiratory surfaces and its evolution', *Rep. Steno. Hosp. Copenh.*, **9,** 7-110

HENDERSON, J. T. (1929). 'Lethal temperatures of Lamellibranchiata', *Contr. Can. Biol. and Fish.*, **4** (25), 399–411

HEWATT, W. G. (1940). 'Observations on the homing limpet, *Acmaea scabra* Gould', *Am. Midl. Natur.*, **24,** 205–208

HOCHACHKA, P. W. and MUSTAFA, T. (1972). 'Invertebrate faculative anaerobiosis', *Science,* **178,** 1056–1060

HOCHACHKA, P. W. and SOMERO, G. N. (1973). *Strategies of Biochemical Adaptation.* 358 pp. Saunders, Philadelphia

HODKIN, G. P. (1959). 'Catastrophic destruction of the littoral fauna and flora near Freemantle, January 1959', *W. Aust. Nat.*, **7,** 6–11

HUEBNER, J. D. (1969). 'The effect of body size and temperature on the respiration of *Polinices duplicatus*', *Comp. Biochem. Physiol.*, **44A,** 1185–1197

HUGHES, R. N. (1971). 'Ecological energetics of *Nerita* (Archaeogastropoda, Neritacea) populations on Barbados, West Indies', *Mar. Biol.*, **11** (1), 12–22

HULSCHER, J. B. (1973). 'Burying-depth and trematode infection in *Macoma balthica*', *Neth. J. Sea Res.*, **6,** 141–156

HUNTSMAN, A. G. and SPARKS, M. I. (1924). 'Limiting factors for marine animals. III. Relative resistance to high temperatures', *Contr. Can. Biol. N.S.*, **2** (6), 97–114

HURLEY, D. E. (1968). 'Transition from water to land in amphipod crustaceans', *Am. Zool.* **8,** 327–353

JANSEN, K. P. (1970). 'Effect of temperature and salinity on survival and reproduction in Baltic populations of *Sphaeroma hookeri,* 1814 (Isopoda)', *Ophelia,* **7** (2), 177–184

JANSEN, K. P. (1971). 'Ecological studies on intertidal New Zealand Sphaeromatidae (Isopoda: Flabellifera)', *Mar. Biol.,* **11** (3), 262–285

JANSSON, B. O. (1967). 'Diurnal and annual variations of temperature and salinity of interstitial water in sandy beaches', *Ophelia,* **4,** 173–201

JÄRNEFELT, H. (1940). 'Beobachtungen über die Hydrologie einiger Schärentümpel', *Verh. int. Ver. Limnol.,* **9,** 79–101

JESSEE, W. F. (1968). 'Studies of homing behaviour in the limpet *Acmaea scabra', Veliger,* **11,** 52–55

JONES, H. D. (1968). 'Some aspects of heart function in *Patella vulgata* L.', *Nature, Lond.,* **217** (5134), 1170–1172

JONES, M. B. (1972). 'Effects of salinity on the survival of the *Jaera albifrons* Leach group of species (Crustacea: Isopoda)', *J. exp. mar. Biol. Ecol.,* **9,** 231–237

JØRGENSEN, C. B. (1960). 'Efficiency of particle retention and rate of water transport in undisturbed lamellibranchs', *J. Cons. Int. Explor. Mer.,* **26,** 94–116

JØRGENSEN, C. B. (1966). *The Biology of Suspension Feeding.* Pergamon Press, Oxford. 357pp

KAY, D. G. and BRAFIELD, A. E. (1973). 'The energy relations of the polychaete *Neanthes (=Nereis) virens* (Sars)', *J. Anim. Ecol.,* **42,** 673–692

KENNEDY, V. S. and MIHURSKY, J. A. (1972). 'Effects of temperature on the respiratory metabolism of three Chesapeake Bay bivalves', *Chesapeake Science,* **13** (1), 1–22

KENNEDY, V. S., ROOSENBURG, W. H., ZION, H. H. and CASTAGNA, M. (1974). 'Temperature-time relationships for survival of embryos and larvae of *Mulinia lateralis* (Mollusca: Bivalvia)', *Mar. Biol.,* **24,** 137–145

KENNY, R. (1958). 'Temperature tolerance of the chiton *Clavarizona hirtosa* (Blainville)', *J. roy. Soc. W. Aust.,* **41** (4), 93–101

KENNY, R. (1969a). 'Temperature tolerance of the polychaete worms *Diopatra cuprea* and *Clymenella torquata', Mar. Biol.,* **4** (3), 219–223

KENNY, R. (1969b). 'The effects of temperature, salinity and substrate on distribution of *Clymenella torquata* (Leidy) polychaeta', *Ecology,* **50** (4), 624–631

KENSLER, C. B. (1967). 'Desiccation resistance of intertidal crevice species as a factor in their zonation', *J. Anim. Ecol.,* **36,** 391–406

KENSLER, C. B. and CRISP, D. J. (1965). 'The colonisation of artificial crevices by marine invertebrates', *J. Anim. Ecol.,* **34,** 507–516

KINNE, O. (1963). 'The effects of temperature and salinity on marine and brackish water animals. I. Temperature', *Oceanogr. Mat. Biol. Ann. Rev.,* **1,** 301–340

KINNE, O. (1964). 'The effects of temperature and salinity on marine and brackish water animals. II. Salinity and temperature salinity combinations', *Oceanogr. Mar. Biol. Ann. Rev.,* **2,** 281–339

KINNE, O. (1966). 'Physiological aspects of animal life in estuaries with special reference to salinity', *Neth. J. Sea Res.,* **3,** 222–244

KINNE, O. (1967). 'Physiology of estuarine organisms with special reference to salinity and temperature: general aspects', pp. 525–540. In: *Estuaries.* Ed. G. H. Lauff. *Am. Assoc. Adv. Sci.* (83). Washington D.C.

KLUGH, A. B. (1924). 'Factors controlling the biota of rockpools', *Ecology,* **5,** 192–196

KONTOGIANNIS, J. E. (1973). 'Acquisition and loss of heat resistance in adult tide-pool copepod *Tigriopus californicus', Physiol. Zool.,* **46** (1), 50–54

KROGH, A. (1939). *Osmotic Regulation in Aquatic Animals.* Cambridge University Press, London, 242pp.

KUENZLER, E. J. (1961). 'Structure and energy flow of a mussel population in a Georgia salt marsh', *Limnol. Oceanogr.,* **6,** 191–204

KUSHINS, L. J. and MANGUM, C. P. (1971). 'Responses to low oxygen conditions in two species of the mud snail *Nassarius', Comp. Biochem. Physiol.,* **39A,** 421–435

LANCE, J. (1962). 'Effects of water of reduced salinity on the vertical migration of zooplankton', *J. mar. biol. Assoc. U.K.,* **42,** 131–154

LENT, C. M. (1968). 'Air-gaping by the ribbed mussel, *Modiolus demissus* (Dillwyn): Effects and adaptive significance', *Biol. Bull.,* **134** (1), 60–73

LENT, C. M. (1969). 'Adaptations of the ribbed mussel. *Modiolus demissus* (Dillwyn), to the intertidal habitat', *Amer. Zool.,* **9,** 283–292

LEWIS, J. R. (1954). 'Observations on a high-level population of limpets', *J. Anim. Ecol.,* **23,** 85–100

LEWIS, J. R. (1964). *The Ecology of Rocky Shores.* English Universities Press, London. 323pp.

LINDBERG, H. (1944). 'Ökologisch-Geographische Untersuchungen zur Insektenfauna der Felsentümpel an den Küsten Finnlands', *Acta zool. fenn.,* **41,** 1–178

LOUGH, R. G. and GONOR, J. J. (1973a). 'A response-surface approach to the combined effects of temperature and salinity on the larval development of *Adula californiensis* (Pelecypoda: Mytilidae). I. Survival and growth of three and fifteen-day old larvae', *Mar. Biol.,* **22,** 241–250

LOUGH, R. G. and GONOR, J. J. (1973b). 'A response-surface approach to the combined effects of temperature and salinity on the larval development of *Adula californiensis* (Pelecypoda: Mytilidae). II. Long-term larval survival and growth in relation to respiration', *Mar. Biol.,* **22,** 295–305

MAKINGS, P. (1973). 'Activity of the sea-shore bristle-tail *Petrobius maritimus* (Leach) (Thysanura) at low temperatures', *J. Anim. Ecol.,* **42,** 585–598

MANGUM, C. P. (1972). 'Temperature sensitivity of metabolism in offshore and intertidal onophid polychaetes', *Mar. Biol.,* **17,** 108–114

MANGUM, C. P. and SASSAMAN, C. (1969). 'Temperature sensitivity of active and resting metabolism in a polychaetous annelid', *Comp. Biochem. Physiol.,* **30,** 111–116

MANGUM, C. P. and WINKLE, W. VAN. (1973). 'Responses of aquatic invertebrates to declining oxygen conditions', *Am. Zool.,* **13,** 529–541

MARSDEN, I. D. (1973a). 'The influence of salinity and temperature on the survival and behaviour of the isopod *Sphaeroma rugicauda* from a salt-marsh habitat', *Mar. Biol.,* **21,** 75–85

MARSDEN, I. D. (1973b). 'The influence of starvation on temperature relationships of metabolism in ectotherms', pp. 165–172. In: *Effects of Temperature on Ectothermic Organisms.* Ed. W. Wieser. Springer-Verlag, Heidelberg

MARSDEN, I. D. (1975). 'Adaptations of *Sphaeroma rugicauda* (Leach) from a salt marsh habitat', Ph.D. Thesis, University of London

MARSDEN, I. D., NEWELL, R. C. and AHSANULLAH, M. (1973). 'The effect of starvation on the metabolism of the shore crab, *Carcinus maenas', Comp. Biochem. Physiol.,* **45A,** 195–213

MARSHALL, N. B. (1965). *The Life of Fishes.* Weidenfeld and Nicolson, London. 402pp.

MAYES, P. A. (1962). 'Comparative investigations of the euryhaline character of *Littorina* and the possible relationship to intertidal zonation', *Nature,* **195,** 1269–1270

MAYNARD, D. M. (1960). 'Circulation and heart function', pp. 161–226. In: *The Physiology of Crustacea,* **1.** Ed. T. H. Waterman. Academic Press, New York

McALISTER, R. O. and FISHER, F. M. (1968). 'Responses of the false limpet, *Siphonaria pectinata* Linnaeus (Gastropoda, Pulmonata) to osmotic stress', *Biol. Bull.,* **134** (1), 96–117

McFARLAND, W. N. and PICKENS, P. E. (1965). 'The effects of season, temperature, and salinity on standard and active oxygen consumption of the grass shrimp, *Palaemonetes vulgaris* (Say)', *Can. J. Zool.,* **43,** 571–585

McLUSKY, D. S. (1973). 'The effect of temperature on the oxygen consumption and filtration rate of *Chlamys (Aequipecten) opercularis* (L.) (Bivalvia)', *Ophelia,* **10,** 141–154

McMAHON, R. F. and RUSSELL-HUNTER, W. D. (1973). 'Respiratory adaptability in relation to vertical zonation in littoral and sublittoral snails', *Biol. Bull.,* **145** (2), 447

MICALLEF, H. (1966). 'The ecology and behaviour of selected intertidal gastropods', Ph.D. Thesis, University of London

MICALLEF, H. (1968). 'The activity of *Monodonta lineata* in relation to temperature as studied by means of an aktograph', *J. Zool. Lond.,* **154** (2), 155–159

MICALLEF, H. (1969). 'Zonation of certain trochids under an artificial tidal regime', *Neth. J. Sea Res.,* **4** (3), 380–393

MICALLEF, H. and BANNISTER, W. H. (1967). 'Aerial and aquatic oxygen consumption of *Monodonta turbinata* (Mollusca: Gastropoda)', *J. Zool. Lond.,* **151,** 479–482

MILLER, R. J. and MANN, K. H. (1973). 'Ecological energetics of the seaweed zone in a marine bay on the Atlantic coast of Canada. III. Energy transformations by Sea-urchins', *Mar. Biol.*, **18,** 99–114

MILNE, A. (1940). 'Some ecological aspects of the intertidal area of the estuary of the Aberdeenshire Dee', *Trans. roy. Soc. Edinburgh,* **60,** 107–140

MONTEROSSO, B. (1930). 'Studi cirrepedologici. VI. Sul comportamento di *"Chthamalus stellatus"* in diverse condizione sperimentale', *R.C. Accad. Lincei (Ser 6)* **11,** 501–505

MOON, T. W. and PRITCHARD, A. W. (1970). 'Metabolic adaptations in vertically-separated populations of *Mytilus californianus* Conrad', *J. exp. mar. Biol. Ecol.,* **5,** 35–46

MORTON, J. E. (1954). 'The crevice faunas of the upper intertidal zone at Wemburg', *J. mar. biol. Assoc. U.K.,* **33,** 187–224

MORTON, J. E. (1960). 'The responses and orientation of the bivalve *Lasaea rubra* Montagu', *J. mar. biol. Assoc. U.K.,* **39,** 5–26

MORTON, J. E., BONEY, A. D. and CORNER, E. DS. (1957). 'The adaptations of *Lasaea rubra* (Montagu), a small intertidal lamellibranch', *J. mar. biol. Assoc. U.K.,* **36,** 383–405

MOULTON, J. M. (1962). 'Intertidal clustering of an Australian gastropod', *Biol. Bull.,* **123,** 170–178

MUIR, B. S., NELSON, G. J. and BRIDGES, K. W. (1965). 'A method for measuring swimming speed in oxygen consumption studies on the aholehole, *Kuhlia sandvicensis', Trans. Am. Fish. Soc.,* **90,** 323–327

MUIR, B. S. and NIIMI, A. J. (1972). 'Oxygen consumption of the euryhaline fish aholehole *(Kuhlia sandvicensis)* with reference to salinity, swimming and food consumption', *J. Fish. Res. Bd. Can.,* **29,** 67–77

NAYLOR, E. and SLINN, D. J. (1958). 'Observations on the ecology of some brackish water organisms in pools at Scarlett Point, Isle of Man', *J. Anim. Ecol.,* **27,** 15–25

NEWELL, G. E. (1958a). 'The behaviour of *Littorina littorea* (L) under natural conditions and its relation to position on the shore', *J. mar. biol. Assoc. U.K.,* **37,** 229–239

NEWELL, G. E. (1958b). 'An experimental analysis of the behaviour of *Littorina littorea* (L) under natural conditions and in the laboratory', *J. mar. biol. Assoc. U.K.,* **37,** 241–266

NEWELL, R. C. (1962). 'Behavioural aspects of the ecology of *Peringia (=Hydrobia) ulvae* (Pennant) (Gastropoda, Prosobranchia)', *Proc. zool. Soc. Lond.,* **138,** 49–75

NEWELL, R. C. (1965). 'The role of detritus in the nutrition of two marine deposit feeders, the prosobranch *Hydrobia ulvae* and the bivalve *Macoma balthica', Proc. zool. Soc. Lond.,* **114,** 25–45

NEWELL, R. C. (1969). 'Effects of fluctuations in temperature on the metabolism of intertidal invertebrates', *Am. Zool.,* **9,** 293–307

NEWELL, R. C. (1970). *Biology of Intertidal Animals.* Elek Books, London. 555pp

NEWELL, R. C. (1973a). 'Environmental factors affecting the acclimatory responses of ectotherms', pp. 151–164. In: *Effects of Temperature on Ectothermic Organisms.* Ed. W. Wieser. Springer-Verlag, Heidelberg

NEWELL, R. C. (1973b). 'Factors affecting the respiration of intertidal invertebrates', *Am. Zool.,* **13,** 513–528

NEWELL, R. C., AHSANULLAH, M. and PYE, V. I. (1972). 'Aerial and aquatic respiration in the shore crab *Carcinus maenas* (L.)', *Comp. Biochem. Physiol.,* **43A,** 239–252

NEWELL, R. C. and BAYNE, B. L. (1973). 'A review on temperature and metabolic acclimation in intertidal marine invertebrates', *Neth. J. Sea. Res.,* **7,** 421–433

NEWELL, R. C. and NORTHCROFT, H. R. (1967). 'A re-interpretation of the effect of temperature on the metabolism of certain marine invertebrates', *J. Zool. London.,* **151,** 277–298

NEWELL, R. C. and PYE, V. I. (1970a). 'Seasonal changes in the effect of temperature on the oxygen consumption of the winkle *Littorina littorea* (L) and the mussel *Mytilus edulis* L.', *Comp. Biochem. Physiol.,* **34,** 367–383

NEWELL, R. C. and PYE, V. I. (1970b). 'The influence of thermal acclimation on the relation between oxygen consumption and temperature in *Littorina littorea* (L) and *Mytilus edulis* L. *Comp. Biochem. Physiol,'* **34,** 385–397

NEWELL, R. C. and PYE, V. I. (1971a). 'Quantitative aspects of the relationship between metabolism and temperature in the winkle *Littorina littorea* (L).', *Comp. Biochem. Physiol.,* **38B,** 635–650

NEWELL, R. C. and PYE, V. I. (1971b). 'Temperature induced variations in the respiration of mitochondria from the winkle *Littorina littorea* (L)', *Comp. Biochem. Physiol.*, **40B,** 249–261

NEWELL, R. C. and PYE, V. I. (1971c). 'Variations in the relationship between oxygen consumption, body size and summated tissue metabolism in the winkle, *Littorina littorea', J. mar. biol. Assoc. U.K.,* **51,** 315–338

NEWELL, R. C., PYE, V. I. and AHSANULLAH, M. (1971a). 'Factors affecting the feeding rate of the winkle *Littorina littorea', Mar. Biol.,* **9** (2), 138–144

NEWELL, R. C., PYE., V. I. and AHSANULLAH, M. (1971b). 'The effect of thermal acclimation on the heat tolerance of the intertidal prosobranchs *Littorina littorea* (L) and *Monodonta lineata* (Da Costa)', *J. Exp. Biol.,* **54,** 525–533

NEWELL, R. C. and ROY, A. (1973). 'A statistical model relating the oxygen consumption of a mollusc *(Littorina littorea)* to activity, body size, and environmental conditions', *Physiol. Zool.,* **46** (4), 253–275

NEWELL, R. C., WIESER, W. and PYE, V. I. (1974). 'Factors affecting oxygen consumption in the woodlouse *Porcellio scaber* Latr.' *Oecologia,* **16,** 31–51

NEWMAN, W. A. (1967). 'On the physiology and behaviour of estuarine barnacles', *Proc. Symp. Crustacea,* **3:** *Mar. Biol. Assoc. India,* 1038–1066

ODUM, H. T. and SMALLEY, A. E. (1959). 'Comparison of population energy flow of a herbivorous and a deposit-feeding invertebrate in a salt marsh ecosystem', *Proc. natn. Acad. Sci. U.S.A.,* **45,** 617–622

OHGUSHI, R. (1954). 'Ethological studies on the intertidal limpets. I. On the rhythmic activities of two species of limpets', *Jap. J. Ecol.,* **4,** 120 (Japanese with English summary)

ORR, P. R. (1955). 'Heat death. I. Time-temperature relationships in marine animals', *Physiol. Zool.,* **28,** 290–294

ORTON, J. H. (1929). 'Observations on *Patella vulgata.* III. Habitats and habits', *J. mar. biol. Assoc. U.K.,* **16,** 277–288

ORTON, J. H. (1933). 'Some limiting factors in the environment of the common limpet, *Patella vulgata', Nature Lond.,* **131,** 693–694

PAJUNEN, V. I. and JANSSON, A. (1969). 'Dispersal of the rockpool corixids *Arctocorisa carinata* (Sahlb) and *Callicorixa producta* (Reut.) (Heterogtera, Corixidae)', *Ann. zool. Fennici.,* **6,** 391–427

PAPI, F. and PARDI, L. (1953). 'Ricerche sull'orientamento di *Talitrus saltator* Montagu (Crustacea-Amphipoda). II. Sui fattori che regolano la variazione dell angolo di orientamento nel corso del giorno. L'orientamento di notte. L'orientamento diurno di altre popolazioni', *Z. vergl. Physiol.,* **35,** 490–518

PAPI, F. and PARDI, L. (1959). 'Nuovi reperti sull'orientamento lunare di *Talitrus saltator* Montagu (Crustacea, Amphipoda)', *Z. vergl. Physiol.,* **41,** 583–596

PARDI, L. (1960). 'Innate components in the solar orientation of littoral Amphipods', *Cold Spring Harb. Symp. Quant. Biol.,* **25,** 395–401

PARDI, L. and PAPI, F. (1952). 'Die Sonne als Kompass bei *Talitrus saltator* (Montagu) (Amphipoda, Talitridae)', *Naturwiss,* **39,** 262–263

PARDI, L. and PAPI, F. (1953). 'Ricerche sull'orientamento di *Talitrus saltator* (Montagu) (Crustacea-Amphipoda). I. L'orientamento durante il giorno in una popolazione del litorale tirrenico', *Z. vergl. Physiol.,* **35,** 459–489

PARDI, L. and PAPI, F. (1961). 'Kinetic and tactic responses.' In: *The Physiology of Crustacea,* **2,** 365–399. Ed. T. H. Waterman. Academic Press, New York and London

PARRY, D. A. (1951). 'Factors determining the temperature of terrestrial arthropods in sunlight', *J. Exp. Biol.,* **28,** 445–462

PATANÉ, L. (1933). 'Sul compartamento di *Littorina neritoides* (L) mantenuta in ambiente subaero ed in altre condizione sperimentale', *R.C. Accad. Lincei (Ser. 6),* **17,** 961–967

PEARSE, A. S. (1929). 'Observations on certain littoral and terrestrial animals at Tortugas, Florida, with special reference to migrations from marine to terrestrial habitats', *Papers Tortugas Lab.,* **26,** 205–223

PERCY, J. A. (1972). 'Thermal adaptations in the boreo-arctic echinoid *Strongylocentrotus droebachiensis* (O. F. Müller, 1776). I. Seasonal acclimation of respiration', *Physiol. Zool.,* **45** (4), 277–289

PERTUNEN, V. (1963). 'Effect of desiccation on the light reactions of some terrestrial arthropods', *Ergeb. Biol.,* **26,** 90–97

PETERSEN, J. A. and JOHANSEN, K. (1973). 'Gas exchange in the giant sea cradle *Cryptochiton stelleri* (Middendorff), *J. exp. mar. Biol. Ecol.*, **12,** 27–43

PETRUSEWICZ, K. and MACFADYEN, A. (1970). 'Productivity of terrestrial animals, principles and methods'. In: *International Biological Programme Handbook* (13). Blackwell, Oxford. 190pp.

PICKENS, P. E. (1965). 'Heart rates of mussels as a function of latitude, intertidal height and acclimation temperature', *Physiol. Zool.*, **38,** 390–405

PORTER, W. P. and GATES, D. M. (1969). 'Thermodynamic equilibria of animals with the environment', *Ecol. Monogr.*, **39,** 227–244

PRECHT, H., CHRISTOPHERSEN, J., HENSEL, H. and LARCHER, W. (1973). *Temperature and Life.* Springer-Verlag, Heidelberg. 760pp

PROSSER, C. L. (1974). *Comparative Animal Physiology.* W. B. Saunders, Philadelphia

PYE, V. I. and NEWELL, R. C. (1973). 'Factors affecting thermal compensation in the oxidative metabolism of the winkle *Littorina littorea', Neth. J. Sea. Res.*, **7,** 411–419

PYEFINCH, K. A. (1943). 'The intertidal ecology of Bardsey Island, North Wales, with special reference to the recolonisation of rock surfaces, and the rock-pool environment', *J. Anim. Ecol.*, **12,** 82–108

QUENOUILLE, M. H. (1952). *Associated measurements.* Academic Press, New York

RALSTON, A. and WILF, H. S. (Eds). (1960). *Mathematical methods for digital computers.* John Wiley & Sons, New York. 293pp

RAO, K. P. and BULLOCK, T. H. (1954). 'Q_{10} as a function of size and habitat temperature in poikilotherms', *Am. Nat.*, **87** (838), 33–43

READ, K. R. H. (1962). 'Respiration of the bivalved molluscs *Mytilus edulis* L. and *Brachidontes demissus plicatulus* Lamark as a function of size and temperature', *Comp. Biochem. Physiol.*, **7,** 89–101

REESE, E. S. (1969). 'Behavioural adaptations of intertidal hermit crabs', *Am. Zool.*, **9** (2), 343–355

REGIS, M. B. (1969). 'Écologie et aspects quantitatifs de la croissance de quelques monodontes et gibbules de la Mediterranée', *Recl. Trav. Stn. mar. Endoume,* **45,** 199–304

RITZ, D. A. (1968). 'The effect of temperature on the activity and survival of barnacles', Ph.D. Thesis, University College of North Wales

RITZ, D. A. and FOSTER, B. A. (1968). 'Comparison of the temperature responses of barnacles from Britain, South Africa and New Zealand, with special reference to temperature acclimation in *Elminius modestus', J. mar. biol. Assoc. U.K.*, **48,** 545–599

ROBERTS, J. L. (1957). 'Thermal acclimation of metabolism in the crab *Pachygrapsus crassipes* Randall. I. The influence of body size, starvation and molting', *Physiol. Zool.*, **30,** 232–242

ROBERTS, J. L. (1964). 'Metabolic responses of freshwater sunfish to seasonal photoperiods and temperatures', *Helgol. wiss. Meeresunters,* **9,** 459–473

ROBERTS, J. L. (1967). 'Metabolic compensations for temperature in sunfish', 245–262. In: *Molecular Mechanisms of Temperature Adaptation.* Ed. C. L. Prosser. *Am. Assoc. Adv. Sci. Symp.*, (84), Washington D.C.

ROBERTS, M. H. (1971a). 'Larval development of *Pagurus longicarpus* Say reared in the laboratory. II. Effects of reduced salinity on larval development', *Biol. Bull.*, **140** (1), 104–116

ROBERTS, M. H. (1971b). 'Larval development of *Pagurus longicarpus* Say reared in the laboratory. III. Behavioural responses to salinity discontinuities', *Biol. Bull.*, **140,** 489–501

ROSENBERG, R. and ROSENBERG, K. (1973). 'Salinity tolerance in three Scandinavian populations of *Littorina littorea* (L.) (Gastropoda)', *Ophelia,* **10** (2), 129–139

ROUX, C. and ROUX, A. L. (1967). 'Température et métabolisme respiratoire d'espèces sympatriques de gammares du groupe *pulex* (Crustacés Amphipodes)', *Ann. Limnol,* **3,** 3–16

ROY, A. (1969). 'Analyse des facteurs du taux de métabolisme chez la limace *Arion circumscriptus', Rev. Can. Biol.*, **28,** 33–43

SANDISON, E. E. (1966). 'The oxygen consumption of some intertidal gastropods in relation to zonation', *J. Zool. Lond.*, **149,** 163–173

SANDISON, E. E. (1967). 'Respiratory response to temperature and temperature tolerance of some intertidal gastropods', *J. exp. mar. Biol. Ecol.*, **1,** 271–281

SASSAMAN, C. and MANGUM, C. P. (1970). 'Patterns of temperature adaptation in North American Atlantic coastal actinians', *Mar. Biol.*, **7,** 123–130

SCARRATT, D. J. and RAINE, G. E. (1967). 'Avoidance of low salinity by newly hatched lobster larvae', *J. Fish Res. Board Can.*, **24,** 1403–1406

SCHLIEPER, C. R., KOWALSKI, R. and ERMAN, P. (1958). 'Beitrag zur ökologisch-zellphysiologischen Characterisierung des borealen Lamellibranchiers *Modiolus modiolus* L.', *Kieler Meeresforsch,* **14,** 3–10

SEELEMANN, U. (1968). 'Zur Überwindung der biologischen Grenze Meer-Land durch Mollusken. II. Untersuchungen an *Limapontia capitata, Limapontia depressa* und *Assiminea grayana', Oecologia,* **1,** 356–368

SEGAL, E. (1956). 'Adaptive differences in water-holding capacity in an intertidal gastropod', *Ecology,* **37,** 174–178

SEGAL, E. and DEHNEL, P. A. (1962). 'Osmotic behaviour in an intertidal limpet, *Acmaea limatula', Biol. Bull.,* **122,** 417–430

SEGAL, E., RAO, K. P. and JAMES, T. W. (1953). 'Rate of activity as a function of intertidal height within populations of some littoral molluscs', *Nature Lond.,* **172,** 1108–1109

SHOTWELL, J. A. (1950). 'Distribution of volume and relative linear measurement changes in *Acmaea,* the limpet', *Ecology,* **31,** 51–61

SIEFKEN, M. and ARMITAGE, K. B. (1968). 'Seasonal variations in metabolism and organic nutrients in three *Diaptomus* (Crustacea: Copepoda)', *Comp. Biochem. Physiol.,* **24,** 591–609

SJOBERG, B. (1967). 'On the ecology of the *Jaera albifrons* group (Isopoda'), *Sarsia,* **29,** 321–348

SMITH, J. E. and NEWELL, G. E. (1955). 'The dynamics of the zonation of the common periwinkle *(Littorina littorea* (L.)), on a stony beach', *J. Anim. Ecol.,* **24** (1), 35–56

SMITH, W. K. and MILLER, P. C. (1973). 'The thermal ecology of two South Florida fiddler crabs: *Uca rapax* Smith and *U. pugilator', Physiol. Zool.,* **46** (3), 186–207

SNEDECOR, G. W. (1956). *Statistical Methods Applied to Experiments in Agriculture and Biology.* Iowa State University Press, USA

SOMERO, G. N. (1969). 'Enzymic mechanisms of temperature compensation: immediate and evolutionary effects of temperature on enzymes of aquatic poikilotherms', *Am. Nat.,* **103,** 517–529

SOURIE, R. (1954). 'Contribution a l'étude ecologique des côtes rocheuse du Sènègal', *Mem. Inst. fr. Afr. noire,* **38,** 7–342

SOUTHWARD, A. J. (1958). 'Note on the temperature tolerance of some intertidal animals in relation to environmental temperatures and geographical distribution', *J. mar. biol. Assoc. U.K.,* **37,** 49–66

SOUTHWARD, A. J. (1964). 'The relationship between temperature and rhythmic cirral activity in some cirripedia considered in connection with their geographical distribution', *Helgol. wiss. Meeresunters.,* **10,** 391–403

SPOOR, W. A. (1946). 'A quantitative study of the relationship between the activity and oxygen consumption of goldfish, and its application to the measurement of respiratory metabolism in fishes', *Biol. Bull.,* **91,** 312–325

STEPHENSON, T. A., ZOOND, A. and EYRE, J. (1934). 'The liberation and utilisation of oxygen by the population of rock pools', *J. Exp. biol.* **11,** 162–172

SUTHERLAND, J. P. (1970). 'Dynamics of high and low populations of the limpet, *Acmaea scabra', Ecol. Monogr.,* **40,** 169–188

SVERDRUP, H. U., JOHNSON, M. W. and FLEMING, R. H. (1946). *The Oceans, their Physics, Chemistry and General Biology.* Prentice-Hall, New York. 1087pp

SWENNEN, C. (1969). 'Crawling tracks of trematode infected *Macoma balthica* (L.)', *Neth. J. Sea Res.,* **4** (3), 376–379

TENORE, K. R. and DUNSTAN, W. M. (1973). 'Comparison of feeding and biodeposition of three bivalves at different food levels', *Mar. Biol.,* **21,** 190–195

THOMPSON, R. J. and BAYNE, B. L. (1972). 'Active metabolism associated with feeding in the mussel *Mytilus edulis* L.', *J. exp. mar. Biol. Ecol.,* **9,** 111–124

THOMPSON, R. J., RATCLIFFE, N. A. and BAYNE, B. L. (1974). 'Effects of starvation on structure and function in the digestive gland of the mussel *(Mytilus edulis* L.)', *J. mar. biol. Assoc. U.K.,* **54,** 699–712

THORSON, T. B. and SVIHLA, A. (1943). 'Correlation of the habitats of amphibians with their ability to survive the loss of body water', *Ecology,* **24,** 374–381

TOULMOND, A. (1967a). 'Étude de la consommation d'oxygène en fonction du poids, dans l'air et dan l'eau, chez quatre espèces de genre *Littorina* (Gastropoda, Prosobranchiata)', *C.R. Acad. Sci. Paris,* **264,** 636–638

TOULMOND, A. (1967b). 'Consommation d'oxygène dans l'air et dans l'eau chez quatre Gastropodes du genre *Littorina', J. Physiol. (Paris),* **59,** 303–304

TROSHIN, A. S. (Ed) (1967). *The cell and environmental temperature. Int. Ser. Pure and Appl. Biol. Zool. Div.* **34:** 463pp. Pergamon Press, London

TRUEMAN, E. R. and ANSELL, A. D. (1969). 'The mechanisms of burrowing into soft substrata by marine animals', *Oceanogr. Mar. Biol. Ann. Rev.,* **7,** 315–366

TRUEMAN, E. R. and LOWE, G. A. (1971). 'The effect of temperature and littoral exposure on the heart rate of a bivalve mollusc, *Isognomon alatus,* in tropical conditions,' *Comp. Biochem. Physiol.,* **38A,** 555–564

TURNER, M. J. and GEORGE, C. J. (1955). 'Some aspects of the behaviour of the quahaug *Venus mercenaria* during the early stages', *8th Rep. Invest. Shellf. Mass. Dept. Nat. Res. Div. Mar. Fish., Commonwealth Mass.,* **8,** 5–14

ULBRICHT, R. J. (1973). 'Effect of temperature acclimation on the metabolic rate of sea urchins', *Mar. Biol.,* **19,** 273–277

ULBRICHT, R. J. and PRITCHARD, A. W. (1972). 'Effect of temperature on the metabolic rate of sea-urchins', *Biol. Bull.,* **142,** 178–185

UNGLAUB SIVERTHORN, S. (1973). 'Respiration in eyestalkless *Uca* (Crustacea: Decapoda) acclimated to two temperatures', *Comp. Biochem. Physiol.,* **45A,** 417–420

UTINOMI, H., YAMIZI, I. and IKERI, M. (1950). 'The ecology of tide pools. I. Topographical and tidal conditions as environmental factors. II. Meteorological and hydrological conditions as environmental factors. III. Biota of tide pools, their composition and fluctuation', *Results from Physiol-Ecol. Lab. Kyoto Univ.,* **66-68,** 1–23 (Japanese with English Summary)

VAHL, O. (1972a). 'Efficiency of particle retention in *Mytilus edulis* L.', *Ophelia,* **10,** 17–24

VAHL, O. (1972b). 'Particle retention and relation between water transport and oxygen uptake in *Chlamys opercularis* (L.)', *Ophelia,* **10,** 67–74

VAHL, O. (1973a). 'Porosity of the gill, oxygen consumption and pumping rate in *Cardium edule* (L.) (Bivalvia)', *Ophelia,* **10** (2), 109–118

VAHL, O. (1973b). 'Pumping and oxygen consumption rates of *Mytilus edulis* L. of different sizes', *Ophelia,* **12,** 45–52

VAHL, O. (1973c). 'Efficiency of particle retention in *Chlamys islandica* (O. F. Müller)', *Astarte. J. Arctic. Biol.,* **6** (1), 21–25

VERMEIJ, G. J. (1971a). 'Temperature relationships of some tropical Pacific intertidal gastropods', *Mar. Biol.,* **10,** 308–314

VERMEIJ, G. J. (1971b). 'Substratum relationships of some tropical Pacific intertidal gastropods', *Mar. Biol.,* **10** (4), 315–320

VERMEIJ, G. J. (1972). 'Intraspecific shore-level size gradients in intertidal molluscs', *Ecology,* **53,** 693–700

VERMEIJ, G. J. (1973). 'Morphological patterns in high-intertidal gastropods: Adaptive strategies and their limitations', *Mar. Biol.,* **20,** 319–346

VERNBERG, F. J. (1959). 'Studies on the physiological variation between tropical and temperate zone fiddler crabs of the genus *Uca.* II. Oxygen consumption of whole organisms', *Biol. Bull.,* **117,** 163–184

VERNBERG, F. J. and VERNBERG, W. B. (1970). 'Lethal limits and the zoogeography of the faunal assemblages of coastal Carolina waters', *Mar. Biol.,* **6** (1), 26–32

VERNBERG, F. J., SCHLIEPER, C. and SCHNEIDER, D. E. (1963). 'The influence of temperature and salinity on ciliary activity of excised gill tissue of molluscs from North Carolina', *Comp. Biochem. Physiol.,* **8,** 271–285

VOVELLE, J. (1969a). 'Complexity of the opercular materials in *Astralium rugosum* (Linné) (Gastropoda Prosobranchia, Turbinidae)', *Proc. malac. Soc. Lond.,* **38** (6), 557

VOVELLE, J. (1969b). 'Elaboration de la matière operculaire chez *Tricolia pullus* (L.), Gastropoda, Prosobranchia', *Malacologia,* **9** (1), 293–294

VOVELLE, J. (1970). 'Étude embryologique, histologique et histochimique de l'opercule et du disque operculigere de *Neptunea antiqua* L., *Buccinum undatum* L. et *Nucella lapillus* (L.)', *Proc. Congr. Soc. Fr. de Malac.,* (Abstract)

VOVELLE, J. (1973). 'Transfert du calcium a travers l'epithelium du repli operculaire chez *Astrea rugosa* L. (Turbinidae)', *Malacologia,* **14,** 47–51

WALLACE, J. C. (1972). 'Activity and metabolic rate in the shore crab, *Carcinus maenas* (L.)', *Comp. Biochem. Physiol.*, **41A,** 523–533

WALLACE, J. C. (1973a). 'Observations on the relationship between the food consumption and metabolic rate of *Blennius pholis* L.', *Comp. Biochem. Physiol.*, **45A,** 293–306

WALLACE, J. C. (1973b). 'Feeding, starvation and metabolic rate in the shore crab, *Carcinus maenas*', *Mar. Biol.*, **20,** 277–281

WALNE, P. R. (1972). 'The influence of current speed, body size and water temperature on the filtration of five species of bivalves', *J. mar. biol. Assoc. U.K.*, **52,** 345–374

WARBURG, M. R. (1968). 'Behavioural adaptations of terrestrial isopods', *Am. Zool.*, **8,** 545–559

WARBURTON, K. (1973). 'Solar orientation in the snail *Nerita plicata* (Prosobranchia: Neritacea) on a beach near Watamu, Kenya', *Mar. Biol.*, **23,** 93–100

WARREN, C. E. and DAVIS, G. E. (1967). 'Laboratory studies on the feeding, bioenergetics and growth of fish', pp. 175–214. In: *The biological basis of freshwater fish production.* Ed. S. D. Gerking. Blackwell Scientific Publication

WATERMAN, T. H. (1961). 'Light sensitivity and vision', pp 1–64 In: *The Physiology of Crustacea,* **2,** Ed. T. H. Waterman. Academic Press, New York and London

WEBB, H. M. and BROWN, F. A. (1958). 'The repetition of pattern in the respiration of *Uca pugnax*', *Biol. Bull.*, **115,** 303–318

WELLS, G. P. (1949). 'Respiratory movements of *Arenicola marina* L.', *J. mar. biol. Assoc. U.K.*, **28,** 447–464

WELLS, M. J. and BUCKLEY, S. K. L. (1972). 'Snails and trails', *Anim. Behav.*, **20,** 345–355

WIDDOWS, J. (1973). 'The effects of temperature on the metabolism and activity of *Mytilus edulis*', *Neth. J. Sea Res.*, **7,** 387–398

WIENS, A. W. and ARMITAGE, K. B. (1961). 'The oxygen consumption of the crayfish *Orconectes immunis* and *Orconectes nais* in response to temperature and oxygen saturation', *Physiol. Zool.*, **34,** 39–54

WIESEPAPE, L. M., ADRICH, D. V. and STRAWN, K. (1972). 'Effects of temperature and salinity on thermal death in postlarval brown shrimp, *Penaeus aztecus*', *Physiol. Zool.*, **45** (1), 22–33

WIESER, W. (1973). *Effects of Temperature on Ectothermic Organisms.* Springer-Verlag, Heidelberg. 298pp

WILKENS, J. L. and FINGERMAN, M. (1965). 'Heat tolerance and temperature relationships of the fiddler crab *Uca pugilator,* with reference to body coloration', *Biol. Bull.*, **128** (1), 133–141

WILLIAMS, G. B. (1964). 'The effects of extracts of *Fucus serratus* in promoting the settlement of larvae of *Spirorbis borealis* (Polychaeta)', *J. mar. biol. Assoc. U.K.*, **44,** 397–414

WILLIAMSON, D. I. (1953). 'Landward and seaward movement of the sandhopper *Talitrus saltator*', *Rep. Brit. Assoc.*, D, 71–73

WINBERG, G. G. (1956). 'Rate of metabolism and food requirements of fishes', *Fish Res. Bd. Can. Transl. Ser.*, (194), 1960

WINTER, J. E. (1969). 'Über den Einfluss der Nahrungskonzentration und anderer Factoren auf Filtrierleistung und Nahrungsausnutzung der Muscheln *Arctica islandica* und *Modiolus modiolus*', *Mar. Biol.*, **4,** 87–135

WOLCOTT, T. G. (1973). 'Physiological ecology and intertidal zonation in limpets *(Acmaea):* A critical look at "limiting factors" ', *Biol. Bull.*, **145,** 389–422

WULFF, F. (1972). 'Experimental studies on physiological and behavioural response mechanisms of *Nitocra spinipes* (Crustacea: Harpacticoidea) from brackish water rock pools', *Mar. Biol.*, **13** (4), 325–329

Two

Settlement responses in marine organisms

D. J. CRISP
Marine Science Laboratories, University College of North Wales, Anglesey

2.1 INTRODUCTION

Marine organisms are essentially opportunists, their pelagic larvae being produced in large numbers, each with only a remote expectation of survival. In this respect larvae of marine organisms resemble seeds of plants. Indeed it was at one time generally believed that pelagic invertebrate larvae, like seeds, fell indiscriminately on stony ground and on good ground and therefore had only a single chance of reaching a suitable habitat (Nelson, 1928; Coleman, 1933) but a few biologists, notably Matthews (1917), Wilson (1932) and Cole (1938) believed that pelagic larvae might be able to exercise discrimination between favourable and unfavourable habitats if their development were not rigidly scheduled. They believed that larvae might be able to delay metamorphosis if they encountered an unsuitable site. The patient work of Wilson (1932, 1937) on the influence of the character of deposits on the settlement of the larvae of a number of polychaetes, and similar studies by Jägersten (1940) on *Protodrilus rubropharyngeus* larvae, together with the investigations of Knight-Jones on gregariousness in the larvae of oysters, serpulids and barnacles, eventually proved the latter view to be right, at least in a large number of cases. Since then a great many more examples of settlement selection by invertebrate larvae have been recorded so that random settlement must now be regarded as unusual if indeed it occurs at all.

The evolution of habitat selection by the larvae of marine animals offers them a much greater potential to exploit highly specialised and sparse habitats than is possible for plants. More important still is the possibility which this reproductive strategy offers to sessile animals of successfully occupying ephemeral habitats, notably the surfaces of other species of animals and plants. All sites are to some degree transient, even a rocky shore may become so densely crowded with sessile organisms that the young must search for vacant spaces at a considerable distance from their parents. I have shown that pelagic transfer from site to site by larvae may be essential to the survival of species whose habitat may from time to time disappear or become unsuitable (Crisp, 1976).

The way in which larvae find their way back to their original habitat, the clues by which they recognise suitable sites, and the sensory mechanisms involved is the subject of this chapter.

2.2 BEHAVIOUR PRIOR TO SETTLEMENT

During the free-swimming period prior to settlement the larva drifts in the direction of the prevailing current system. In coastal and estuarine areas the oscillatory tidal currents generally reach greater velocities than the non-tidal (residual) currents and are therefore likely to be the chief influence on larval transport in the short term. A purely sinusoidally varying current system would, on average, carry the larva furthest if the length of larval life was a half, one, one and a half etc. times the period of a complete tidal cycle (12.6 h). Hence any extension of the period beyond 6 h would not increase dispersal unless the larval life was sufficiently prolonged to be able to take advantage of non-tidal currents. Any extension of larval life in non-feeding larvae beyond a few hours would therefore use up some of the energy required for metamorphosis and growth without any compensating advantage.

It is therefore significant that larvae should be fairly sharply divided between those that are short-lived, usually settling after about 2 to 6 h and which do not feed, and those which remain in the water and feed for periods of about a week to several months. Extremely long-lived larvae (teleplanic larvae) have been shown by Scheltema (1971) to be not uncommon in tropical and warm temperate waters and to be capable of transoceanic passages.

The view that larvae drift entirely at random is probably as fallacious as the view that they settle at random. Evidence is growing to show that the swimming behaviour helps to bring them into the vicinity of their natural habitat, after which the settlement behaviour enables them to select a favourable site. Dispersal and habitat searching should be seen, therefore, as part of an integrated pattern of behaviour rather than two separate processes.

The first step in habitat selection is found in the response to light and gravity during the pelagic stage. The great majority of larvae are strongly photopositive at first but their behaviour may change subsequently. *Figure 2.1* taken from Ryland's (1960) work on the larvae of Polyzoa, illustrates the changes in response to light in four species over periods of a few hours after release. The width of the kite diagram shows the proportion of larvae occupying a defined section of a horizontal tube with the light source marked at +. The larvae of *Celleporella hyalina,* which settle at and below low water spring tide level, rapidly reversed their sign of phototaxis, almost all individuals swimming away from the light after 4½ h (*Figure 2.1*). The larvae of *Alcyonidium hirsutum,* a low intertidal species settling on fucoid algae, showed a slower change which did not extend to all individuals, so that the population as a whole changed its response to light from positive to variable (*Figure 2.1(b)*). A second intertidal species, *Flustrellidra hispida,*

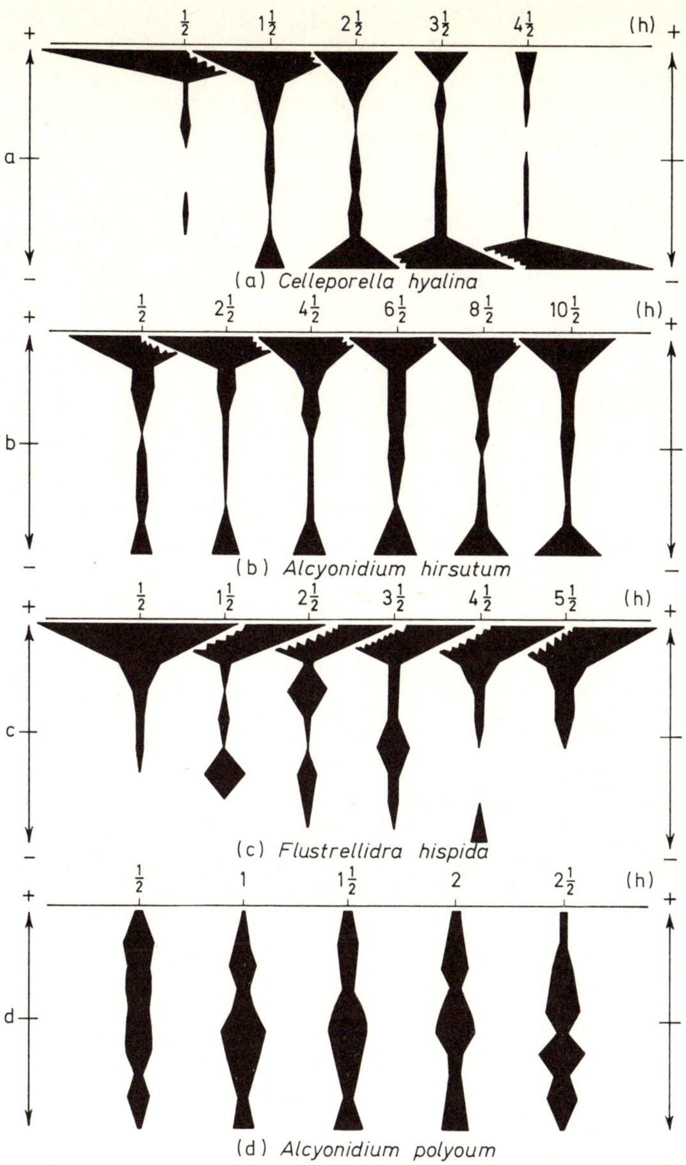

Figure 2.1 Responses of polyzoan larvae to directional illumination. The kite diagrams show the behaviour of four species in horizontal troughs illuminated from one end (+). The troughs were marked into divisions and the distribution of larvae noted at the time intervals given. Four types of behaviour shown: (a) Celleporella hyalina, *photopositive becoming photonegative (b)* Alcyonidium hirsutum, *photopositive becoming variable (c)* Flustrellida hispida, *photopositive throughout (d)* Alcyonidium polyoum, *indifferent throughout. (After Ryland, 1960; courtesy R. J. Skaer)*

which is found rather higher upshore, also on fucoids, remained strongly photopositive (*Figure 2.1(c)*) while the last species, *Alcyonidium polyoum,* was apparently insensitive to light throughout its larval life. Responses to gravity are also shown by free swimming larvae, though these are less well documented because they are not immediately obvious as are the responses to light. Generally, responses to gravity reinforce responses to light.

Thorson (1964) critically reviewed what was then known of these responses and showed that there was some degree of correlation between the level occupied by the adult and the behaviour of the larva. The larvae of intertidal species displayed any one of the three types of response illustrated in the *Figures 2.1 (a), (b),* and *(c).* After an initial period of upward swimming they might continue to swim upwards, they might become variable and indifferent, swimming either up or down, or they might reverse their behaviour and swim downwards. However, the larvae of invertebrates living in the sublittoral zone gave only the third type of behaviour, invariably swimming away from the light prior to settlement. It is obviously essential to species living below the tide marks for their larvae eventually to leave the surface waters, but it is somewhat surprising to find no unanimity among the larvae of intertidal animals to remain near the surface. But provided the latter are shortlived, so that the majority do not drift far offshore, a number of different responses may help to partition the habitat efficiently among the great diversity of species which occupy the intertidal zone.

Of even clearer adaptive value is the behaviour of the pelagic larvae of some estuarine species. If allowed to drift passively near the sea surface, the downstream residual flow would carry them out to sea and if they remained in the surface they would be unlikely to return to the estuary. Early stage larvae of the estuarine barnacle, *Balanus improvisus,* swim to the surface and must be carried downstream. But Bousfield (1955) found that the later stage larvae, unlike those of the coastal species *Balanus balanoides,* sank to the bottom. In all stratified estuaries there is an upstream flow of seawater at deeper levels which compensates for the surface drift of seawater entrained in the downstream flow of fresh water. Thus by descending to deeper levels the late stage larvae of *Balanus improvisus* would be carried up the estuary to regions of low salinity. In a similar way large concentrations of the older larvae of the estuarine oyster, *Crassostrea virginica,* are found near the bottom whereas the early stages were more uniformly distributed throughout the water column (Haskin, 1964). Furthermore an old observation of Nelson and Perkins (1930) that the larvae of *Crassostrea* sink when the salinity falls on the ebb and swim when it rises on the flood, provides a further method of navigating upstream in a tidal estuary. Wood and Hargis (1971) tested this theory under natural conditions in the James river (*see also* Chapters 6 and 7). They compared the distribution of larvae with particles of coal of similar size and found that, whereas the inert particles were brought into suspension at half ebb and half flood, the maximum number of larvae was encountered only towards the end of the flood tide when the salinity had risen appreciably. It is of course possible for an estuarine species to survive without means of upstream navigation by relying on the retention of a proportion of its larvae within the estuary. Nelson and Perkins (1930) believed that many molluscan larvae tended to concentrate close to the discontinuity layer of a stratified estuary, thereby minimising their net transport. Retention would clearly be more likely if the estuary were large and had a small proportion of its water exchanging with the open sea and if the species possessed high fecundity and a short pelagic life. Carriker (1967) tentatively suggested that the length of larval pelagic life may generally be less in estuarine than in marine species but a sufficiently wide ranging survey has not been carried out to be sure that this is so.

It is clear that by maintaining itself at a certain depth the pelagic larva can increase its chances of being carried in a favourable direction and that light and gravity give the larva a reference orientation. It is not clear exactly how the larva determines its depth and what stimulates it to swim up or down. Light intensity is a poor clue since it is so variable. Nevertheless, larvae do have the capacity to respond to the light gradient even on moonlit nights if they remain within a few metres of the surface (Crisp and Ritz, 1973) so that photopositive larvae would be capable of maintaining themselves continuously within the vicinity of the sea surface. However, it is not generally realised that a clean water surface is a very dangerous place for a larva. Small arthropod larvae with hydrofuge cuticles, such as newly moulted cyprids, can become stranded on the surface and unable to re-enter the sea. Unprotected ciliated larvae face an even crueller fate; they can be torn apart by the surface forces and their protoplasm spread as a monomolecular film on the water surface. Therefore it seems likely that most larvae would require a depth regulating mechanism.

Pressure is theoretically the most consistent and reliable indicator of depth. The majority of larvae that have been examined are pressure sensitive (Rice, 1964; Knight-Jones and Morgan, 1966), though there is no accepted theory to explain the mechanism of pressure sense, nor any known pressure deformable structures through which it could be mediated.

2.3 SETTLEMENT BEHAVIOUR

When the pelagic larva has reached the stage of development at which settlement is possible it may come into contact with a solid surface. The process of settlement from this time on may usually be divided into 3 steps — attachment, exploration and fixation. Attachment is not necessarily permanent, but allows the larva to test the nature of the substratum. If it elicits the full settlement response the larva will ultimately become permanently cemented, often with a preferred orientation, and proceed to metamorphose. If the substratum proves to be unsatisfactory, metamorphosis can usually be delayed, the larva swimming off to locate and test other surfaces. Larvae are therefore able to make repeated and active attempts to find a suitable place for development and growth. In this respect they have a great advantage over seeds, for though the latter may be able to delay germination and thereby take advantage of the possibility that the habitat may improve, they lack the motility and sensory refinements of invertebrate larvae.

2.3.1 The cyprid of *Balanus balanoides*

Settlement behaviour has been studied most fully in the last larval stage, or cyprid, of the barnacle. The barnacle represents the peak of evolution of sessile animals and its larvae therefore provide the best illustration of the sensory adaptations and pattern of behaviour during settlement. An important factor which has made exhaustive experimental analysis of the larvae of *Balanus balanoides* possible is the great prevalence of its cyprids in the spring plankton of European coastal waters, particularly almost land-locked areas such as the Menai Straits and Firth of Clyde. In late April and early May they can be obtained in thousands by a few casts with a plankton net, thus obviating the tedium of artificially rearing this fairly long-lived larva.

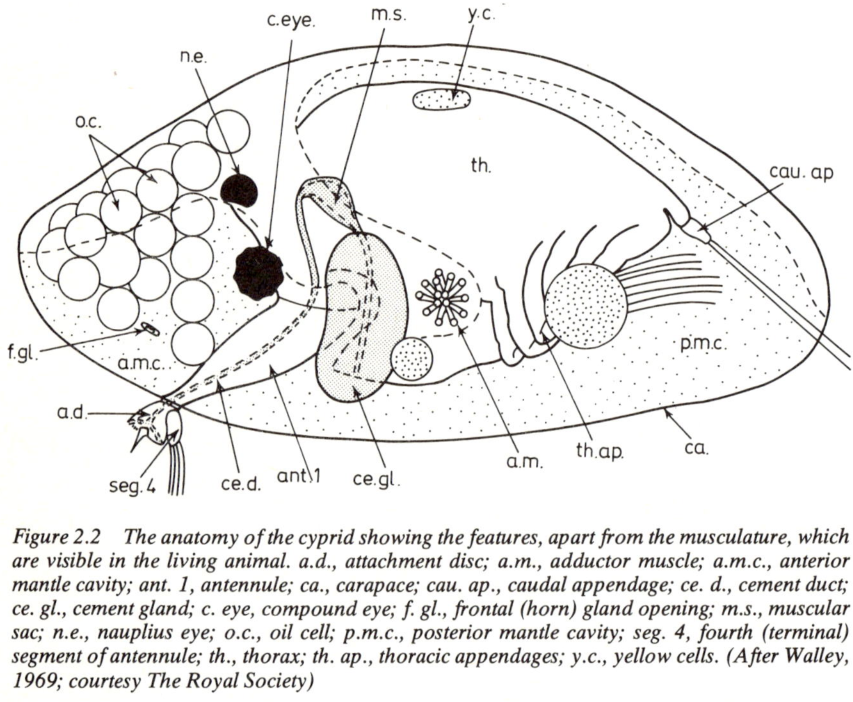

Figure 2.2 The anatomy of the cyprid showing the features, apart from the musculature, which are visible in the living animal. a.d., attachment disc; a.m., adductor muscle; a.m.c., anterior mantle cavity; ant. 1, antennule; ca., carapace; cau. ap., caudal appendage; ce. d., cement duct; ce. gl., cement gland; c. eye, compound eye; f. gl., frontal (horn) gland opening; m.s., muscular sac; n.e., nauplius eye; o.c., oil cell; p.m.c., posterior mantle cavity; seg. 4, fourth (terminal) segment of antennule; th., thorax; th. ap., thoracic appendages; y.c., yellow cells. (After Walley, 1969; courtesy The Royal Society)

The cyprid (*Figure 2.2*) is a unique larval stage, its sole function being to select a site for settlement. It has no functional gut but can survive for several weeks on reserves of triglyceride contained in oil cells (o.c. *Figure 2.2*) which accumulate during the preceding nauplius stages (Holland and Walker, 1975). The cyprid has a bivalve carapace with an anterior and posterior mantle cavity. The anterior encloses the prominent antennules (ant. 1) with their attachment discs (a.d.) which are used in walking, while the posterior encloses the thoracic appendages which are used in swimming and are later modified to form the adult feeding organs — the cirri.

The cyprid, like most final stage larvae, is more richly endowed with sense organs than any other stage in the life history. The persistent nauplius eye, which is involved in the phototactic response of the nauplius stages and in the shading response of the adult (Forbes, Seward and Crisp, 1971), is augmented in the cypris stage by two compound eyes which are later

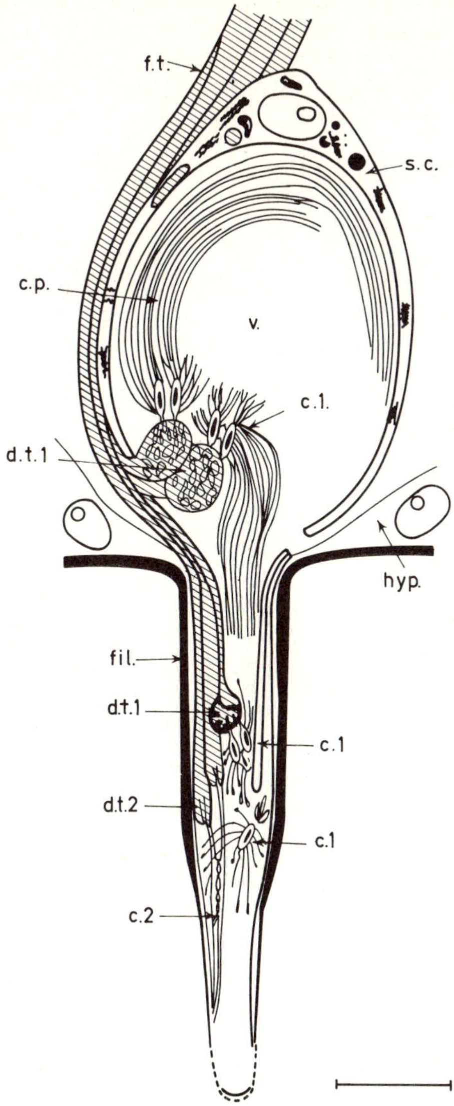

Figure 2.3 Diagram of the frontal filament complex based on ultrastructural observations of stage II B. hameri *nauplii. c.1., branched cilia; c. 2., simple cilia; c.p., ciliary projections; d.t.1., swollen dendritic terminations; d.t.2., non-swollen dendritic terminations; fil., external filament; f.t., filament tract; hyp., hypodermal cell; s.c., supporting cell; v, vesicle. Scale is 10 μm. (After Walker, 1974; courtesy Springer-Verlag)*

discarded during metamorphosis. Close to the compound eyes are the vesicles of the frontal filaments with nerve tracts connecting branched sensory cilia of the vesicles to filament centres in the brain adjacent to the optic centres. Simple cilia arising from dendritic terminations of the filament tracts enter and connect with the filaments. The whole frontal filament complex (*Figure 2.3*) recently described by Walker (1974) is clearly sensory. It persists throughout the nauplius and cypris stages but, like the compound eyes, is lost at metamorphosis. Its function is not known but circumstantial and structural evidence suggests that it is probably either for orientation or pressure reception or perhaps both.

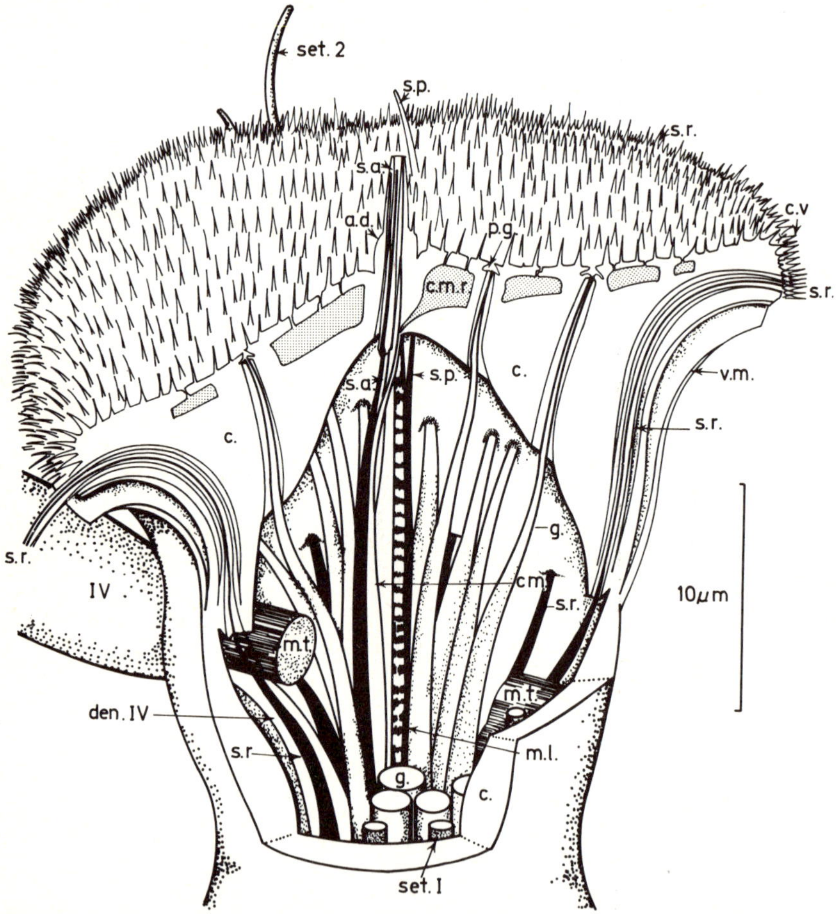

Figure 2.4 The attachment organ of the antennule of the cyprid of Balanus balanoides *reconstructed from sections. The internal structures are seen by cutting away the pre-axial side. Sensory organs shown black. a.d., axial dome; c., cuticle; cm., cement gland duct; cm.r., radial canals of cement gland duct; c.v., cuticular villi; den. IV, dendrites going to fourth segment; IV, fourth segment; g., antennular glands and ducts (some severed by cut-away); m.l., longitudinal muscle; m.t., transverse muscle; p.g., pore of antennular gland; s.a., axial sense organ; s.p., post axial sense organ; s.r., radial sense organ; set. 1, pre axial seta; set. 2, post axial seta; v.m., velum. (After Nott and Foster, 1969; courtesy The Royal Society)*

Each attachment disc of the cyprid (a.d.), an enlargement of the third segment of the antennule, is a pad covered by cuticular villi (Nott, 1969; Nott and Foster, 1969) with pores through which it is thought a sticky secretion may exude. Certainly the antennules can adhere extremely firmly so that the larva is not readily dislodged even by a powerful jet of water. Nevertheless, when the larva voluntarily releases itself it swims off readily (Crisp, 1955). The cyprid walks over the substratum using the antennules one after the other, planting one deliberately forward and then, after a short pause, as though to test the adhesion, withdraws the other. Each step is laboriously taken in a space of five or six seconds, the movements of the cyprid comically resembling those of an old man uncertain of his footing. The attachment disc is a highly complex and important organ with a 'singularly uniform structure' throughout the Cirripedia (Darwin, 1854). Its fine structure has been described by Nott and Foster (1969). Distributed over its surface and around its rim are numerous sense organs of the form of arthropod scolopidia (*Figure 2.4*). Most of these probably serve as proprioceptors, having their sensory processes ensheathed in a supporting tube which does not open to the exterior, responding to changes in the shape of the attachment organ as it is pushed on to and withdrawn from a substratum. A few are apparently open to the exterior and may be chemoreceptors. There are two other areas where batteries of sensory setae, almost certainly functioning as mechanoreceptors, are concentrated. One is on the terminal segment of the antennule (Gibson and Nott, 1971) and the other is at the hind end of the cyprid where a pair of long caudal setae, each associated with a complex of four shorter setae, project beyond the carapace and make contact with the substratum (Walker, private communication). As the cyprid explores the surface, the cirri of the terminal antennular segment are continuously swept across it while, during pauses between steps, the animal may swing round on the antennules so that the caudal setae describe arcs. These movements no doubt enable the larva to appreciate the texture and contour of the surface and to locate obstacles. Some of the sensory setae may also detect water currents. There are numerous small sensory setae projecting all over the carapace which may have the same function (Walker, private communication). The 'acoustic organs' of Darwin however are in fact the openings of the frontal glands and are not sensory structures (Walker and Lee, 1975).

The sequence of events described below indicates the need for such a varied repertoire of sense organs.

2.3.1.1 ATTACHMENT

It is not known whether cyprids are brought into the vicinity of the substratum by chance or by some stimulus causing them to descend through the water column or approach a shaded object. Crisp and Meadows (1963) thought that cyprids of *Balanus balanoides* might have transitory phases of photonegative or photokinetic behaviour which would cause them to attach to shaded surfaces. Crisp and Ritz (1973) have shown that the cyprids of this species settle in the shade but require a somewhat higher light intensity for this response than for normal phototaxis. No definite mechanism has been established, largely because of the difficulty of observing in detail the movements of freely swimming cyprids.

As soon as the cyprid brushes against the surface it attempts to attach by the antennules. The 'clinging response' is stimulated by the movement of water over the surface, as will immediately be apparent to anyone who tries to transfer cyprids with a Pasteur pipette. As long as the water is being steadily drawn up or expelled they cling firmly to the walls of the pipette. In order to remove them the water must be left motionless for a short time; they then release their hold and swim. At this moment a quick press may expel them with a sudden jet of water.

Although the relationship between water flow and settlement of barnacles and other fouling organisms is of great importance to the fouling of ships and pipelines, very little useful data exists. Biologists have apparently been overawed by the hydrodynamical problems and engineers inhibited by their ignorance of larval behaviour. As a result most of the investigations have tried to provide an answer to the question, 'At what current speed can larvae settle?' meaning by current speed the velocity of water at such a distance from the settlement surface that the flow is not affected by it. A moment's reflection will reveal that this question is futile. What would determine whether the larva can settle is the relative velocity between the larva and the surface at the moment it comes into contact. In general, larvae are small compared with the dimensions of the hydrodynamic boundary layer around a visible object. Hence at the moment of contact the rate of flow of water around the larva will be reduced to a value much less than that of the normally measured external current because of the drag of the solid surface. Furthermore, the normally measurable flow can be related to the flow which the larva would experience at settlement only under rather precise and simple experimental conditions. To make observations on settlement under other conditions where the flow over different parts of the surface is variable and unpredictable is therefore useless.

The simplest system for examining the relationship between water movement and settlement is the flow through a long uniform tube. The velocity, v, of the water relative to the surface is zero at the solid boundary and increases with the distance, r, along the radius according to the formula

$$\left[\frac{dv}{dr}\right]_0 = \frac{4q}{\pi r^3}$$

where r is the radius and q the flow per unit time. The quantity dv/dr is known as the velocity gradient and is measured in reciprocal seconds. In the above formula the subscript 0 refers to the value of dv/dr at the vessel wall.

Using tubes 1.5 metres in length, the percentage of cyprids which settled was related to the applied velocity gradient (Crisp, 1955). With the two species *Balanus balanoides* and *Elminius modestus* attachment was not possible at velocity gradients greater than 500 s^{-1}. When the gradient was reduced an increasing proportion were able to attach, but at rather lower velocity gradients, for example 70 s^{-1} for the cyprids of *Balanus balanoides*, there was a change in behaviour. Instead of attempting to attach, the cyprids were trundled passively down the tube and a much smaller proportion actually settled. The threshold velocity gradient to stimulate *Elminius modestus* cyprids was rather lower than that for the cyprids of *Balanus balanoides*. It was evident therefore that the maximum rate of attachment was when the gradient was sufficient to produce a stimulus but not so great as to prevent the cyprid from making contact with the wall of the tube.

A criticism of these experiments is that they related the percentage which attached in a single transit through the tube rather than the number that attached in unit time. Thus, at the higher velocity gradients the chances of successful attachments grew less, not only because the cyprids were carried faster but also because they would have had less time in the tube in which to attach. Making allowance for the time of stay in the tube the results indicate that the cyprids of *Balanus balanoides* attach most readily at about 150 s^{-1} and those of *Elminius modestus* at about 300 s^{-1}. Observations suggest that, in order to attach, the cyprids swim strongly against the direction of the current. Since the cyprids of both species swim at approximately the same speed, namely 4 to 5 cm/s, they would be brought to rest at distances of approximately 300 μm for *Balanus balanoides* and 150 μm for *Elminius modestus*. This is approximately half the height of the cyprids of each species (Crisp, 1955). It therefore seems most probable that the cyprids respond to being brushed against the surface by swimming upstream and if they are able to maintain station against the flow of water they can attach by means of the antennule. Light evidently plays no part in rheotaxis, the cyprids being able to attach equally well in light or dark and being quite unaffected by the presence of light and dark stripes painted on the tube. The appreciation of current and contact with the surface must therefore by mediated by mechanoreceptors.

2.3.1.2 EXPLORATION

The cyprid begins to 'walk' as soon as it attaches. The first steps taken are generally in a straight path, interrupted by turns when it meets obstacles or irregularities in the surface contour. It is not difficult to record the track by means of the camera lucida. A few typical tracks made by cyprids settling on a flat sheet of phenolformaldehyde plastic are shown in *Figure 2.5*. The circles represent the point of attachment, each small dot the position of the animal at each step, and the arrow the point from which the cyprid swims off again. The great majority of cyprids obviously swam off this surface, only the one where a large black dot is shown in the bottom left corner succeeded in settling.

The surface was crossed by parallel grooves 5 mm apart which are shaded in the figure. It will be seen that although the cypris larva is known eventually to settle in grooves and hollows, during its exploration it moved freely over the surface, climbing down into the grooves and out

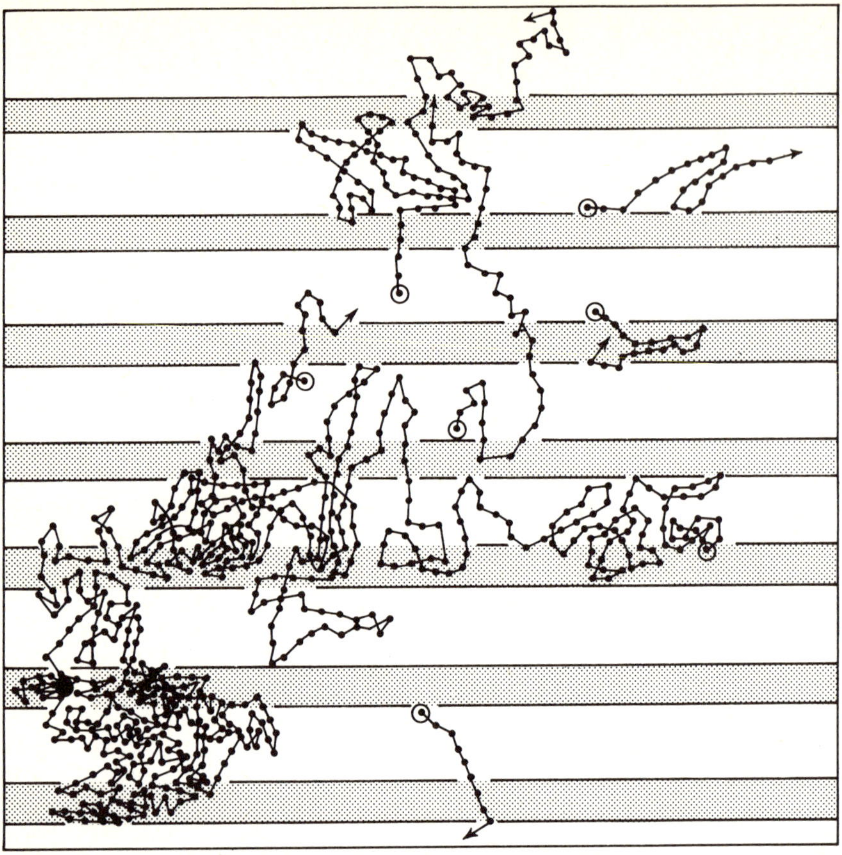

Figure 2.5 Paths traced by means of camera lucida, of seven cypris larvae exploring a grooved non-toxic panel. The grooves are shaded and approximately 5 mm apart. The point of initial attachment is shown by an open circle, the point of swimming off by an arrow. One cyprid, which explored for 30 or 40 min, eventually settled and metamorphosed in the groove at the point marked with a full circle. (After Crisp and Austen, 1960; courtesy Association of Applied Biologists)

again. Indeed there was little evidence at first of the ultimate pattern of settlement. One noticeable feature of the exploratory behaviour was the greater tendency for cyprids to become detached when they were on the surface of convexities, such as the external edges of grooves or high points on the surface. Convexities were not the only deterrents to continued exploration. By watching the cyprids on a variety of surfaces I have observed that when loose objects such as algal filaments, silt particles or air bubbles are tested with the antennulary disc the cyprid often swims off soon afterwards. A simple explanation of these facts might be that the stimulus for continued exploration is the strength of adhesion between the antennule and the surface.

The exploratory behaviour of barnacle cyprids of various species has been described by a number of authors (e.g. Visscher, 1928; Doochin, 1951; Knight-Jones and Crisp, 1953; Barnes, 1955) and all are in substantial agreement. The most significant feature, the change in behaviour as exploration is prolonged, is clearly seen in *Figure 2.5*. Initially the cyprid walks in a more or less steady path with few changes in direction or pauses if uninterrupted. 'Wide searching' behaviour is a suitable designation for the first element in the exploratory behaviour pattern. It allows the cyprid quickly to assess the likelihood of the surface having favourable areas and if none are encountered or if an unfavourable stimulus is received the cyprid swims off. Detachment is in fact the most frequent termination of such behaviour on inert and particularly on smooth surfaces. However if the cyprid receives a favourable stimulus or even if it remains for a sufficient time on the surface, its behaviour changes. The rate of stepping slows down, not because the movements are made more slowly, but because the cyprid pauses, apparently testing the substratum more closely. At each halt it may remain pivoted by one antennule and swing the body in an arc, taking the next step in a quite different direction. As a result the steady path is transformed into a random walk with short links. The immediate area is therefore explored much more thoroughly at the expense of translation. This change in behaviour from wide to close searching is not abrupt but its effect can be clearly seen by comparing the initial paths in *Figure 2.5* with most of the paths of the one cyprid that eventually settled. When pivoting on the antennules the cyprid may sweep the caudal appendages in an arc, evidently testing the contour of the surface.

The change from wide to close searching behaviour should thus indicate the kind of stimulus which leads to settlement. Observations have never been published in quantifiable form but the evidence is that the cyprids are stimulated (a) by concavities in the surface (Crisp and Barnes, 1954) and (b) by contact with their own species (Knight-Jones and Crisp, 1953). Towards the end of the period of exploration the cyprid displays a third element of its behaviour pattern which may be called 'inspection'. By this time the translatory movements have virtually ceased, the cyprid stepping to and fro around a single point swinging the body repeatedly in arcs. With the extended caudal appendages it establishes there is no nearby object protruding from the surface. In this way previously settled spat are avoided and the unoccupied area thus marked out around each settled cyprid is an arc with a radius slightly greater than its length. The individuals are therefore separated from one another by at least this distance and so their behaviour in this final stage can be described as territorial (Crisp, 1961).

The cyprids display certain other activities during the period of inspection which can be interpreted as adaptive. Not only do the antennules appear to test the surface, but periodically the cyprid can be seen to flick the thoracic appendages violently several times, even to the extent of dislodging loose particles from the surface. At intervals the antennules can be seen to pull the cyprid down on to the surface and then to rotate the body slowly so that the anterior end rubs against the substratum. These movements may be interpreted as preparing the surface so that the cement will make a good bond.

2.3.1.3 HABITAT SELECTION

The most usual source of evidence from which selective behaviour can be inferred is the positions in which recently settled juveniles are found. It is extremely tedious to watch the actual movements of the larvae at settlement and observe the process of selection. On the other hand, it is relatively easy either to record the pattern of settlement on various habitats in the field or to set up choice experiments in the laboratory.

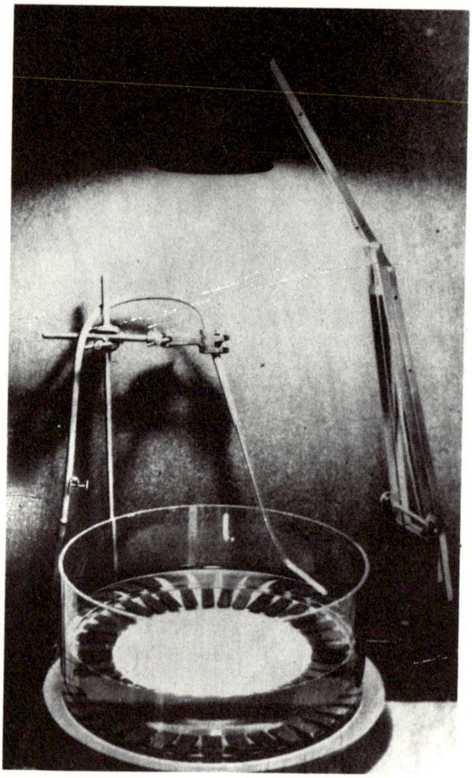

Figure 2.6 Apparatus for testing larval preference. About forty slate panels, 5 × 2 cm, each with ten 1½ mm diameter pits drilled in them, with surfaces treated in different ways, are arranged at the periphery of a rotating cylindrical dish with overhead illumination. An air jet circulates the water gently in the opposite direction to that of the rotation of the dish. Other test objects can be substituted for slate panels (see also Figure 2.14)

A widely applicable method is shown in *Figure 2.6*. At the periphery of a circular dish rotated slowly on a turntable are placed a series of test objects between which the larvae are allowed to choose. The dish is filled with seawater and air jets blowing across the surface in a direction opposing that of the rotation of the dish produce a current of water and aerate the dish. The effect of the rotation of the water is to cause debris, dead larvae and other unwanted material to accumulate in the centre of the dish away from the test objects. When everything is ready the larvae are introduced and left to settle. Panels of plastic, slate or glass, the surfaces of which are treated in different ways, are generally used but pieces of weed, shell, small piles of sand or other objects can equally well be set out according to the particular larva being investigated. Despite the greatest care taken in equalising the shape and surface texture of each test object and in evening up the variation in the light field by rotating the dish, considerable differences are always obtained in the numbers settling on each apparently identical replicate. It is therefore necessary to use large numbers of replicates for each treatment. Furthermore, each batch of larvae used in an experiment may differ not only in numbers but also in its intrinsic rate of settlement. Therefore all treatments should, if possible, be tested together. These two requirements underline the need for large shallow cylindrical dishes accommodating 30–50 test panels at least. If for any reason enough panels cannot be accommodated, a series of experiments of incomplete block-design (Ryland, 1959) can be substituted for a single experiment. In all cases however a carefully prepared experimental design with a view to the subsequent statistical analysis is essential.

Field observations and experiments on barnacles (Knight-Jones and Stephenson, 1950) as well as laboratory choice experiments (Knight-Jones, 1953b) showed that barnacle cyprids are strongly gregarious, settling preferentially in the vicinity of living or dead individuals of their own species. Cyprids of *Balanus balanoides* also prefer rough to smooth surfaces (Barnes, 1956), settle more densely in pits and grooves (Crisp and Barnes, 1954; *Figure 2.14*) and in the shade (Crisp and Ritz, 1973).

Superficially, it might be thought that once a cyprid encounters an appropriate stimulus or group of stimuli it responds automatically and inevitably by settling. However, casual observations suggest that this is not so. When pitted panels are colonised, the cyprids occupy the pits singly until almost all the pits have one cyprid apiece, and only then does multiple occupation begin. When the pits have accumulated several individuals in each the cyprids begin to colonise the plane surface. Clearly the cyprids appear to have the ability to exercise real choice, rejecting the less favourable sites in the order: plane surface, occupied pit, unoccupied pit, whenever a more favourable position is available. An experiment to test this question more rigorously was designed. A panel was prepared with nine well spaced out pits of a size and shape strongly favoured by cyprids. Three pits were solitary, three pits were surrounded by a single, and three by a pair of concentric shallow grooves known to be less favourable for settlement, (*Figure 2.7*). In reaching the central pits the cyprid's pattern of exploration would inevitably include excursions across the surrounding grooves. Thus any cyprid moving towards a pit surrounded by a groove would be trapped in the groove whereas those moving towards an unprotected pit would be free to enter. Therefore, if settlement were an automatic process the pits surrounded by grooves ought to be less rapidly colonised than the others. When the panels were exposed in the sea, however, all the pits were occupied with equal facility and well before any cyprids settled in the surrounding grooves.

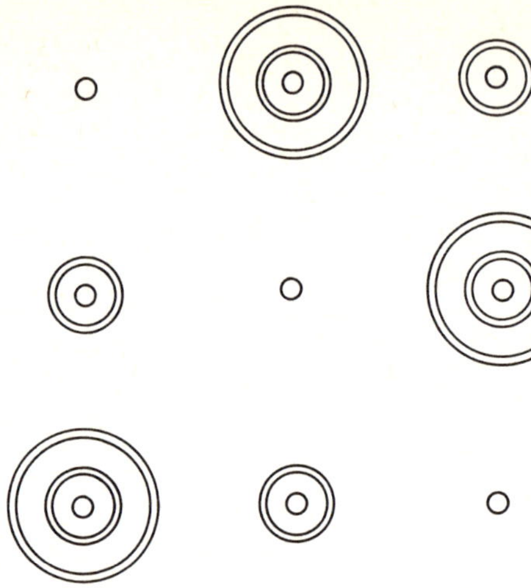

Figure 2.7 Diagram of test for larval preference. When offered to cypris larvae, the centre pits, which were the most attractive shape, were occupied first. The surrounding grooves were occupied next, and the plane surfaces last. 3 × 3 Latin square design. (See text)

To explain the power of choice by cyprids, Crisp and Meadows (1963) put forward the classical pattern of instinctive behaviour in which close searching and inspection were to be regarded as steps in the pattern leading to the consummatory act of settlement. An encounter with the specific stimulus would lead to settlement only if the threshold for releasing the act of settlement had been lowered by a period of exploration with several previous encounters with suitable stimuli. Furthermore, it was shown that the rate of settlement, when tested against a standard stimulus, increased the longer the period that the cyprids were denied access to an appropriate releaser. This implies, therefore, that the threshold is lowered with increasing age.

During the exploratory phase therefore, the larvae will be stimulated at first to settle only in the most favourable sites, but as exploration continues and the threshold stimulus falls, less attractive sites will eventually release the settlement response. The result of this process would give the appearance of individual memory and choice. It is in reality a purely statistical effect resulting from the distribution of settlement thresholds in the natural population combined with a drop in the response threshold with time.

2.3.1.4 ORIENTATION

During these final movements the cyprid determines its orientation. It will already have identified a shaded concavity during its close searching behaviour but it will not have accommodated to the particular shape of the cavity until the last moment, nor will it have determined its orientation to light or to the prevailing current. By observing the orientation of cyprids settled under controlled conditions it can be shown that all these three factors are important in determining the direction in which they settle. Briefly, the cyprid orientates primarily to contour, aligning itself to the long axis of any groove along the surface (Crisp and Barnes, 1954). Secondly it orientates to light, directing its anterior end towards the prevailing light source (Barnes, Crisp and Powell, 1951) and, thirdly, it may orientate to the water flow, settling with its posterior end awkwardly pointing to the current source (Crisp, 1955). There is a clear hierarchy among these three stimuli, contour having the greatest influence, light the next, and current direction the least. Consequently a strong orientation to light can be demonstrated only on a smooth surface or on one where the rugosities run parallel to the direction of the light (Crisp and Barnes, 1954). To demonstrate orientation to current is even more difficult. It is necessary to conduct the experiments not only on uniformly contoured surfaces but also in the dark or under uniform illumination. Furthermore, if the barnacle is not correctly aligned to the current it can reorientate during its growth. It does so by torsion about its vertical axis, and so in species with a calcareous base, leaves a spiral pattern in the canals. Torsion is most rapid in early growth and may quickly account for so much more of the ultimate orientation that the weak component brought about by the behaviour of the cyprid at settlement might be left in doubt (Crisp and Stubbings, 1957). However, subsequent unpublished laboratory observations made jointly with P. S. Meadows leaves in no doubt that if other stimuli are effectively removed the cyprids will settle predominantly orientated so that the cirral net of the juvenile barnacle fishes into the current.

The hierarchy of orientational responses — contour, light and current — is in the same order as the consistency of operation of the stimulus. Grooves on the surface are absolutely constant, the direction of light somewhat variable and the current direction the most capricious of the three factors. The adaptive significance of the response to current is clear; barnacles which are correctly orientated grow somewhat faster than the average (Crisp, 1960). Similarly the delicate juvenile barnacles which have settled neatly in grooves are protected against damage from stones, scouring by sand and browsing by molluscs. Orientation to light is less easy to explain. It results in the adult eye being turned to the least illuminated part of the visual field, and thus tends to increase the sensitivity of the barnacles in those sectors which would otherwise be least likely to evoke the shading response (Forbes, Seward and Crisp, 1971).

It is necessary for the above stimuli to operate just before the cyprid pours out its store of permanent cement. At this moment the cyprid can be seen to nestle into a pit or groove, pulling itself down and rolling slowly from side to side adjusting to secure maximum contact with the sides of the pit. As a result, in a hemispherical pit of about 1 mm radius the first cyprid usually settles at the bottom but later settlers, driven by their territorial behaviour to avoid the first, arrange in a circlet just below the rim. In grooves they become spaced out in a linear series. If the section is cylindrical each settles in the middle of the groove but in a groove of square section they attach at the angles along either side. In all cases they appear to obtain the maximum protection even at the expense of a diminished growth rate (Crisp, 1960). The reaction to light takes place almost at the last moment and indeed if the direction of the incident light is changed during cementation the cyprid attempts to turn towards it. It is evident therefore that the sensory equipment of the cyprid is functional up to the last moment before metamorphosis.

2.3.1.5 CEMENTATION

Figure 2.8(a) illustrates the cement apparatus of the cyprid. The paired cement glands (c.g.) are large structures occupying a considerable part of the body of the cyprid. Each is connected through a muscular sac (m.s.) to a duct (c.d.) which traverses the antennule and opens on the attachment disc through a series of canals and pores. Each cement gland (*Figure 2.8(b)*) has

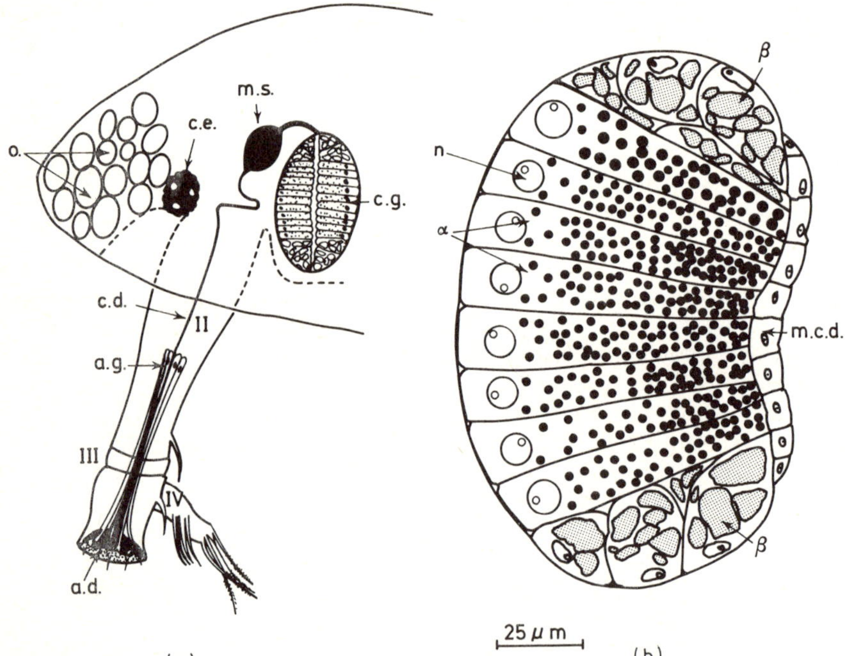

Figure 2.8 Cyprid cementing apparatus. (a) Arrangement for manufacturing and discharge of cement. The antennulary glands (a.g.) are believed to produce a temporary adhesive used in exploring, but there is as yet no proof that this is their function. The cement gland c.g. produces the permanent cement (After Walker, 1971). (b) Cytological detail of the cement gland as seen in section. (After Walker, 1971). a.d., attachment disc; a.g., antennulary glands; c.d., cement duct; c.e., compound eye; m.s., muscular sac; m.c.d., cells of median collecting duct of cement gland; n., nucleus of α cell; o., oil globules; II, III, IV, segments of antennule; α, α cell type; β, β cell type. (Courtesy Springer-Verlag)

two kinds of cells, a central mass of α cells making up most of the gland and peripheral groups of β cells. The granules of the α cells, like the cement itself, (Saroyan, Lindner, Dooley and Bleile, 1970) contain protein and give cytochemical reactions for tyrosine, tryptophan, sulphhydryl and disulphide as well as for phenol and polyphenol oxidase but contain no appreciable carbohydrate or lipid (Walker, 1971). The β cells contain protein but give no other reaction. When the cyprid cements itself to the substratum both components are discharged together, though some α cell material remains in the gland. The antennules become wholly embedded in a mass of cement. Curiously, after discharge is complete there is no trace of cement left in the duct system although secretory material remains in the glands.

The double character of the gland and the composition of the α cells suggest strongly a degree of polyphenol tanning of the α cell protein. The tanning reaction is probably set in motion by some component of the β cells. Although the cement is probably tanned, it does not become hard and brittle but remains plastic. The adult cement, which is produced by different generations of cells (Walker, 1973) also retains a sticky, glue-like character, probably holding the animal down by 'Stefan adhesion' rather than by chemical union with the substratum (Crisp, 1973a). A glue-like adhesive is probably better suited than a brittle cement for the adhesion of a small growing animal particularly as the forces of adhesion become progressively more important with decrease in the size of the animal.

2.3.1.6 METAMORPHOSIS

An excellent study has been published by Walley (1969) which describes in detail the processes taking place during development through the six nauplius stages, during the transformation of the sixth stage nauplius into the cypris larva and during metamorphosis of the cypris larva into the young barnacle. Walley traced the relationship between the larval and the adult organs and demonstrated how few of the organ systems of the larva persisted into the adult (*Figure 2.9*). With the important exception of the nauplius eye, all the sense organs and their centres in the nervous system, the three main nauplius appendages and their associated musculature, the antennules of the cyprid, the larval mouth and the larval excretory system are lost. Haemocytes, which become especially abundant during metamorphosis, act as phagocytes ingesting fragments of hystolysing organs. They also cluster around regions of rapid synthesis and may be responsible for transporting raw materials needed for the growth of new structures. She also showed that the new organ systems were developed well in advance of the time at which they would need to become functional, so that the transition from one stage to the next could take place smoothly and quickly.

Hystolysis and phagocytosis are characteristic of dramatic morphological change where disposal of redundant tissue and recycling of the material is urgent. An alternative procedure, adopted by some polychaete (Wilson, 1932), nemertean (Cantell, 1966), gastropod and echinoderm larvae is to eat and digest the discarded larval tissue.

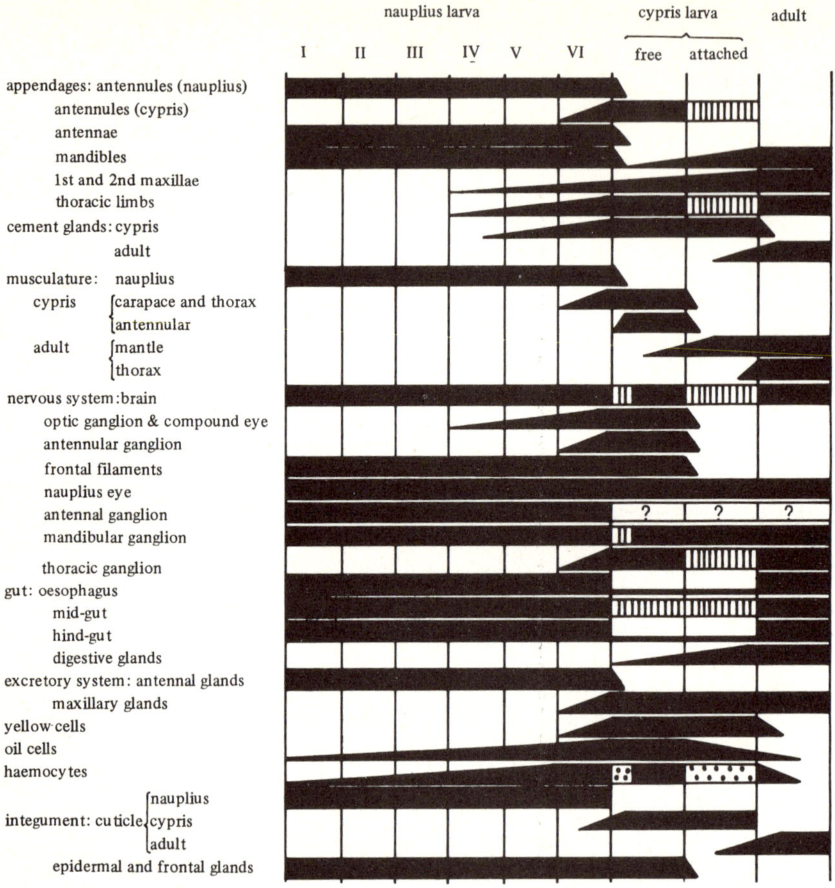

Figure 2.9 Table summarising the anatomical changes that take place during the larval development and metamorphosis of B. balanoides. *The development, persistence and/or loss of each organ system and set of appendages is represented by the solid black areas.* [|||] *indicates histolysis,* [∵] *indicates a phase of phagocytic activity,* [?] *indicates that the fate of that structure is not known. (After Walley, 1969; courtesy The Royal Society)*

Often, as for example in insect pupae the active physiological functions of feeding and locomotion are suspended during metamorphosis. The cyprid, although an active swimmer, is unable to feed, so that Darwin's epithet (1854) 'locomotive pupa' is very apt. After the cyprid has become permanently cemented to the substratum it remains entirely quiescent while the crucial metamorphic changes to the adult take place.

In bivalve larvae and in other invertebrates where metamorphosis is less radical the change may take place rather more gradually, the stage intervening between larva and adult being able to alternate between a pelagic and benthic existence. Carriker refers to such a swimming and crawling stage as the 'pediveliger'.

2.3.2 Behaviour of other invertebrate larvae

The essential similarity of the role of almost all invertebrate larvae has led to a remarkable convergence in sensory equipment and behaviour patterns despite the wide differences in the morphology of the various larval types. It is, therefore, necessary only to re-emphasise these common features and to show how they have become modified in particular instances where there may be unusual circumstances.

The three elements of exploratory behaviour in the cyprid, namely wide searching, close searching and inspection have their counterparts in *Spirorbis borealis* and *Ostrea edulis,* two species where the tracks of the larvae have been individually recorded (Wisely, 1960; Cranfield, 1973). Whereas the cyprid walks freely on the attachment discs, *Spirorbis* and *Ostrea* spin fine sticky threads which attach to the substratum and may serve to anchor the larva as it glides over the surface or, more probably, enable it to regain the surface if it should be accidentally washed off. Cranfield (1973) describes how the behaviour of the oyster larva changes quite abruptly from a fast straight gliding path on the pedal cilia to a slow deliberate looping action of the larval foot which attaches alternately by glands at the tip and on the sole, secreting a complex thread as it moves over the surface. After a period of inspection when it remains virtually in one spot it attaches permanently by the byssus. Gruffydd and Lane (1975) have recently compared the morphology of the foot in three contrasting bivalves — the oyster, which is permanently cemented, the mussel which is mobile when juvenile but becomes more or less sedentary as an adult, and the scallop which, though initially attached by the byssus, lives freely after a short juvenile period. They describe the homologies of the complex series of glands present in the larval foot and show the relationship between the development of these glands and the behaviour of the larva. It is probably quite usual for bivalves to form threads at settlement and polyzoa, such as *Bugula* (Lynch, 1947), polychaete and planula larvae are also retained by fine threads.

One type of invertebrate larva which does not appear to explore the surface before settling is the ascidian tadpole. These tadpoles are strongly influenced by light, being stimulated to swim upwards by any reduction in the light intensity. This response will naturally bring them on to the underside of overhangs and other dark objects. On approaching a surface they seek out the darkest areas which they can locate with an accuracy of a millimetre or less. Although they do not possess the rugophilic response, the larvae of *Diplosoma* can often settle in grooves as a result of their seeking out the shade formed by the furrow (Crisp and Ghobashy, 1971). There are usually three adhesive papillae by which the tadpoles attach at the anterior end. Each papilla consists of a hollow, cup-shaped organ with a central mass of cells containing predominantly proteinaceous granules (Lane, 1973). This material can pass through a small hole at the apex of the papilla in the form of small droplets which coalesce to form a sticky adhesive. Small quantities of this material are probably exuded while the larva is still free-swimming (*Figure 2.10*) so that the larva sticks immediately on contact

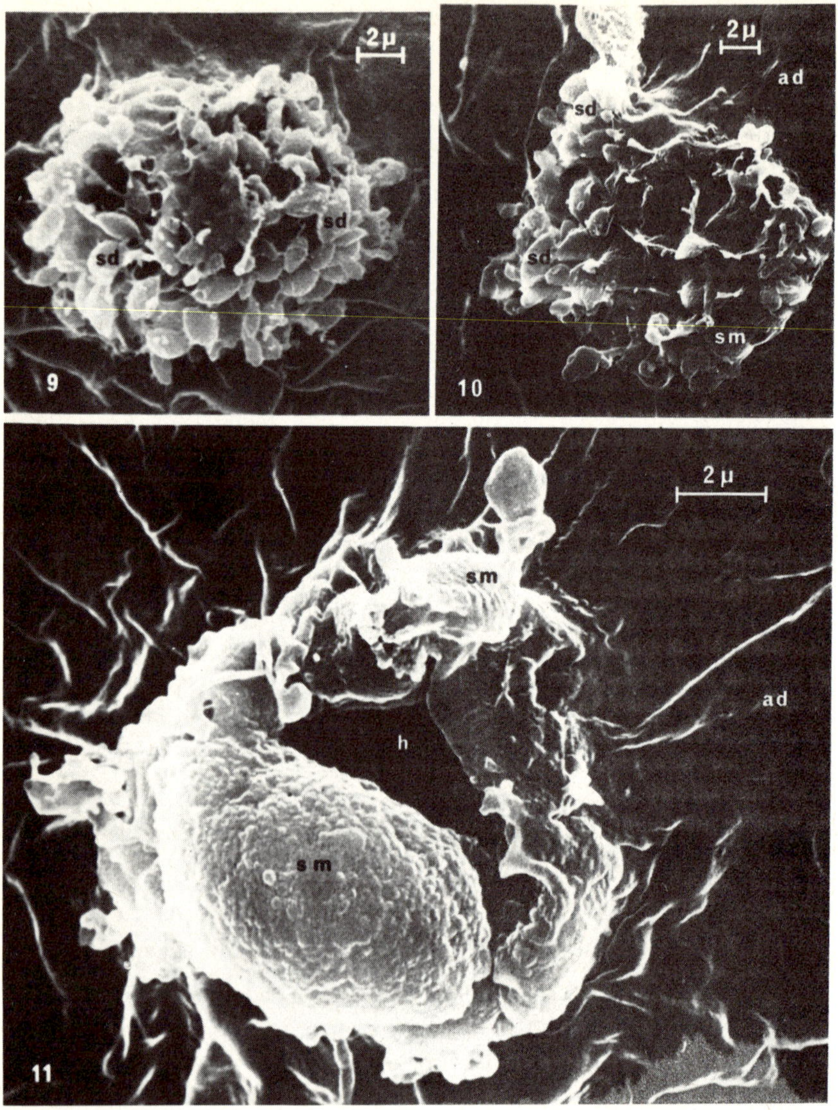

Figure 2:10 Scanning electron micrograph of the adhesive disc (ad) of a free-swimming larva showing billowy masses of secretion (sm) formed from droplets, emerging through the central hole (h) in the tunic covering the disc. (After Lane, 1973; courtesy Springer-Verlag)

with an object. After this larger quantities pour out, binding the animal more firmly to the surface. The cement does not become solid, since if the larva is pulled off it can stick again to another object. Some coelenterate larvae, such as those of *Tubularia larynx* and *Hydractinia echinatum* which adhere by nematocysts to a surface may also be exceptional in lacking decisive exploratory patterns of behaviour. However, according to Williams

(1965) the planulae of *Clava squamata* explore and, by means of their reaction to light and chemical stimuli, locate the dark regions of the axils of *Ascophyllum* where they congregate.

2.3.2.1 RESPONSES TO WATER MOVEMENT

We have seen in barnacle cyprids that while water current has little effect on the exploring larva, other than possibly to dislodge it, it may be critical in the early stage of the settlement process in stimulating or permitting attachment to take place and important at the end in controlling orientation.

Little is known of the velocity gradients under which other types of larva can settle, though it is usually assumed that there will be periods of calm slack water or sanctuaries remote from the effects of waves where settlement of the more sensitive forms will always be possible. However, no one has yet attempted to relate the behaviour of larvae to water currents to the tolerance of the adult to wave exposure.

Larval size must be an important factor since the smaller the larva the greater the protection it will receive from the reduced flow in the boundary layer adjacent to the surface. Wood (1965), in tests on natural settlement on rotating discs in Sydney Harbour, found that the minute spores of *Enteromorpha,* which measure only 10–15μm, settle on the more rapidly moving parts whereas the spat of *Balanus amphitrite* and *Hydroides norvegica* were confined to the slower moving parts. Houghton, Peerman and Tierney (1973) studied the settlement of *Enteromorpha* spores in a flume and concluded similarly that settlement would be possible on surfaces moving at speed in the water, even on ships' hulls 'steaming at a relatively high speed'. However, because the hydrodynamic situation was not defined, this important conclusion has still to be confirmed using more rigorous techniques.

The larvae of several groups of organisms, notably of serpulids, bivalves and bryozoans, are known to orientate at settlement, probably in response to water current, but there have not yet been sufficient well-controlled experiments to rule out the possibility that other factors are involved, notably light and gravity. Nor has the adaptive value of orientation to current, which is quite clear in cirripedes, been clearly demonstrated among other groups.

2.3.2.2 RESPONSES TO LIGHT AND GRAVITY

Responses to light and gravity during exploration are less evident than responses in swimming larvae and there is a lack of well founded data on which to base general conclusions. The results of settlement experiments in which, for example, larvae are observed to settle on the shaded side of test objects may have one of several possible explanations. In ascidian tadpoles such as those of *Diplosoma listerianum,* which do not explore the surface, settlement away from the direction of incident light must imply photonegative behaviour at the end of the pelagic stage (Crisp and Ghobashy, 1971). On the other hand, shaded areas might be chosen as a result of negative phototaxis during the exploratory phase as is claimed by Williams (1965) for the planulae of *Clava squamata.* Thirdly, larvae might accumulate in the shade as a result of low photokinesis.

The majority of larvae of the Porifera, Coelenterata, Bryozoa and Tunicata settle away from the light in shaded places, often on the underside of objects. They also tend to sink and therefore settle at the bottom of containers in which they are placed. For some of the larvae of economically important bivalves quite detailed accounts have been given of their behaviour. The larva of *Mytilus edulis,* after a somewhat labile response to light and gravity in the free-swimming stages, becomes photonegative and either geonegative or indifferent to gravity at the time of settlement. It usually orientates with its anterior end away from the light. The larva of *Ostrea* and *Crassostrea* behave rather similarly to each other, being indifferent to light but negative to gravity, and settling more frequently on the underside of shells etc. (Cole and Knight-Jones, 1939, 1949; Crisp, 1967; Hopkins, 1935, 1937). During their exploratory phase the larvae of *Ostrea* tend to work their way up a slope and then to orientate with the hinge uppermost, perhaps an adaptation to prevent the young oyster from becoming occluded with silt. *Teredo* larvae are photopositive when swimming but become photonegative when about to settle, showing low photokinesis in a strong light. As a result they drop on to the surface below them where they explore without reference to the light field (Isham *et al.,* 1951).

Few species appear to choose strong illumination. The larvae of *Hydroides* sp. and *Pomatoceros* appear to be photopositive or geonegative at settlement; at all events they form a band close to the water line when allowed to settle in glass finger bowls or beakers. But other serpulids, notably *Spirorbis spirorbis* larvae, become photonegative at settlement (Knight-Jones, 1951, 1953). The larvae of *Salmacina dysteri* behave similarly (Giard, 1876) and retain their aversion to light into the adult stage. Among the few other animal species reputed to settle in brightly illuminated places or on the upper surfaces of substrata are *Sabellaria vulgaris* (McDougal, 1943), *Elminius modestus* (Crisp and Ritz, 1973). Grave and McCash (1923) claimed that the ascidian *Perophora veridis* settled in bright light, but McDougal found colonies predominantly on the underside of collectors. Obviously, larvae which distinguish between light and shade can only do so if there is sufficient light to allow them to discriminate.

There have been several experiments to ascertain the influence of colour of surface on settlement (e.g. Neu, 1933). These investigations are generally aimed at answering the question 'Can a particular colour help to prevent fouling?' Unfortunately they have not tested whether colour, as distinct from subjective reflectance, is a factor in the settlement of larvae, nor therefore is it known whether larvae possess colour discrimination.

2.3.2.3 RESPONSES TO SURFACE TEXTURE

Whereas it is easy to define a smooth surface, biologists have not considered the exact meaning of a rough surface, preferring to leave the judgment subjective, or to quote the grade of abrasive used to produce the surface. Roughness is in fact a complex property which is not amenable to definition by a single index. It is probably best understood in terms of the amplitude of component waves in the surface and illustrated as a spectrogram. Because of this difficulty it is scarcely profitable to attempt comparisons between the results of various authors on surfaces of undefined roughness except insofar as they have shown differences in the larval response between a rough and a smooth surface or between surfaces of subjectively increasing roughness in the same experiment. There are two further difficulties. First, any increase in surface roughness must be accompanied by a change in the reflectance of light. The greater scattering of light from a dark surface as a result of roughening may therefore influence the photic as much as the rugophilic behaviour of the larva. Secondly, a roughened surface gives a better key for the cementation process which takes place at settlement. Hence there is a greater chance that a larva will be washed off a smooth than off a rough surface. Although the confusion between initial choice and ultimate survival may be unlikely in laboratory experiments, such a possibility must be considered when the result of the experiment is based on the distribution of the spat which had settled some time previously on surfaces exposed in the sea. It is perhaps because of better adhesion as much as a recognition of the general preference for rough surfaces on the part of settling larvae (Pomerat and Weiss, 1946) that in fouling studies test panels made from smooth material are generally abraded before being exposed to settlement. However there are a number of larvae that settle preferentially on relatively smooth surfaces. *Crassostrea virginica* (Crisp, 1967) and *Spirorbis spirorbis* (Crisp and Ryland, 1960) are two examples, while other larvae, such as those of *Tubularia larynx* (Pyefinch and Downing, 1949) and *Bugula flabellata* (Crisp and Ryland, 1960) appear to be indifferent.

2.3.2.4 SURFACE CONTOUR

When the scale of roughness is larger than the larva itself one speaks of the contour of the surface. The strong tendency shown by cyprids to congregate at settlement into pits and grooves and to avoid convex surfaces has its parallel in larval behaviour throughout the animal kingdom. It is understandable that boring organisms, such as *Xylotrya* and *Teredo,* should seek out depressions as likely sites where they can enter the substratum, but evidently the initial protection afforded by concavities is of such great importance even to the larvae of epibenthic filter feeders that they settle in protected hollows despite their eventual need to extend their feeding organs as far as possible into the surrounding water. The ability of ciliated larvae to distinguish surface textures is surprising but even more remarkable is their recognition of concavities which are very large in comparison with the larva itself. A good example illustrated in *Figure 2.11* is the settlement of the larvae of *Celleporella hyalina,* a bryozoan, on *Laminaria saccharina.* The frond of this kelp bulges out on either side of the centre line giving a succession of mounds and hollows. The colonies of *Celleporella* are concentrated mainly in the concave regions. It would be tempting to think that the distribution might result from abrasion, only the colonies which were fortunate in settling in the hollows being able to survive the frequent wafting of the frond over the sandy bed of the sea. However, experiments on pieces of frond containing plain, concave and convex areas showed that there was a genuine selection of the concavities (Ryland, 1959).

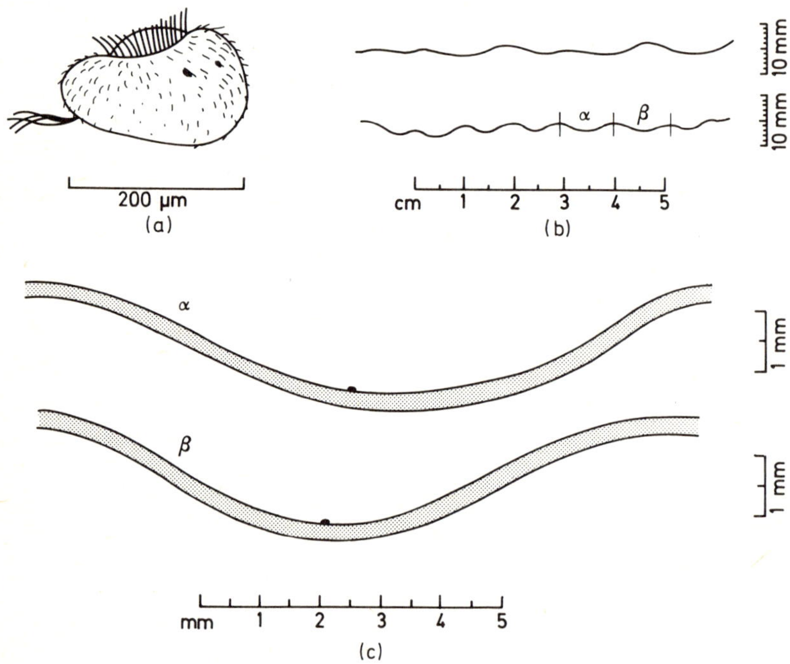

Figure 2.11 Diagram to show the larva of Celleporella hyalina *(a) sections across the wrinkled area of the fronds of* Laminaria saccharina *(b) and an enlarged section to illustrate the position selected and the scale of the larva relative to the concavity (c). (After Ryland, 1959; courtesy R. J. Skaer)*

Concavities were recognised quite independently of their position so that the larva did not just fall in to the centre under gravity. Furthermore, larvae settled in concavities, not only in the fronds of *Laminaria* but also in other species of algae, including those not present in the larval habitat. The disparity between the very large size of the concavity and the small size of the larva is demonstrated in *Figure 2.11(c).* Evidently the larvae, during their meandering spiral path just before settlement, must build up a primitive three-dimensional image and thus be able to detect quite small variations in height above or below the plane of the surface.

2.3.2.5 TERRITORIAL BEHAVIOUR

Surface projections seem to be detected in a similar way, but as they often rise abruptly from the plane of the surface there is not the same difficulty in understanding how they are appreciated by the wandering larva. Wisely (1960) described the movements of *Spirorbis spirorbis* when about to settle. *Figure 2.12* shows the typical wide searching and close searching behaviour of this larva. If during its path it collides with a protruding object, for example, with a sand particle or another individual, it turns away and tries to complete the pattern again in another area close by. If the surface is densely packed with settled individuals and the path is therefore frequently interrupted the larva may swim off. As a result each larva eventually locates a small vacant territory before committing itself to settle. The use of the term 'territorial behaviour' (Crisp, 1961) has been criticised on the grounds that the larvae do not defend their territory (de Wolf, 1973). There seems no

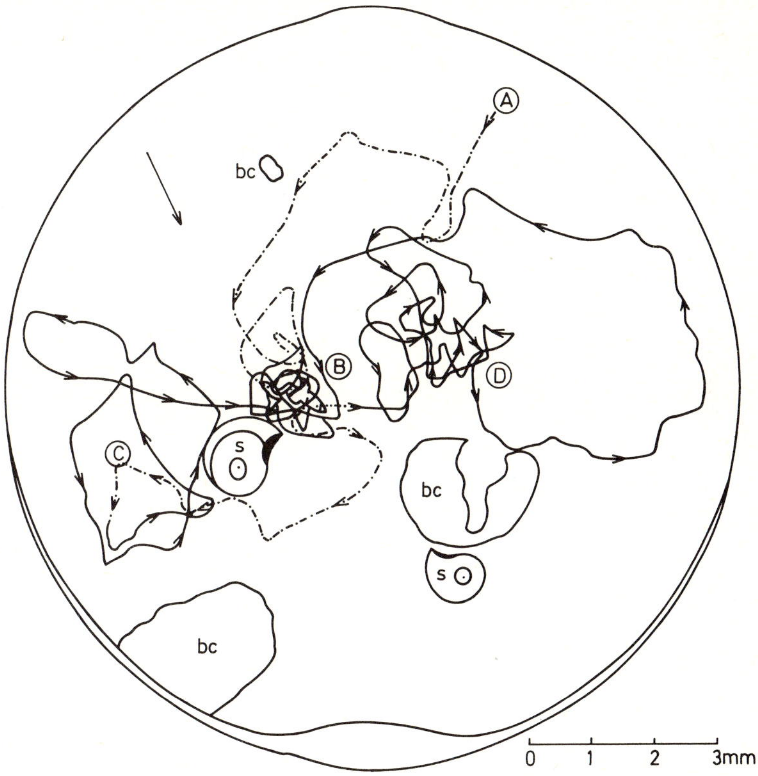

(a)

Figure 2.12 (a) Path of the larve of Spirorbis spirorbis *settling on a piece of* Fucus serratus *already populated by* Spirorbis *(s) and bryozoa (bc). The larva alighted at A, crawled past B, circled twice at C fairly rapidly, slowed down at D, searched closely without settling, returned to wide searching, but finally searched closely and settled at B. (After Wisely, 1960; courtesy CSIRO)*

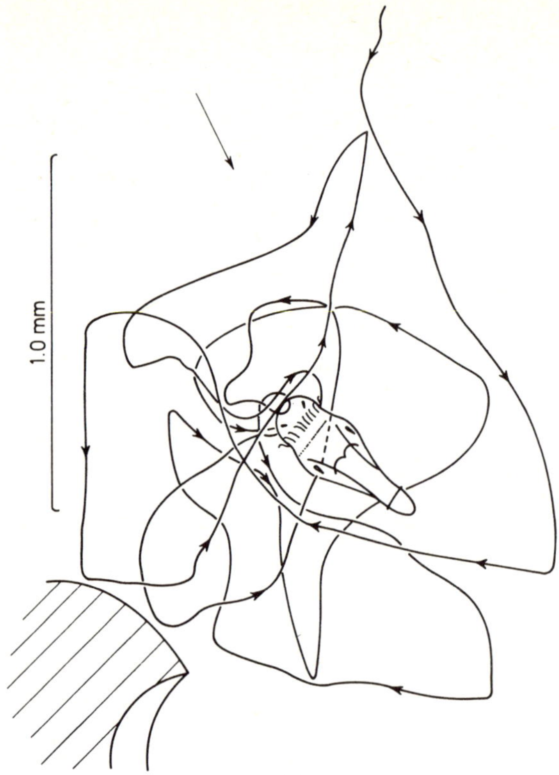

Figure 2.12 (b) Details of final close searching and inspection. Arrow, direction of light, time taken 3½ min. Note avoidance of obstacle at lower left corner (After Wisely, 1960; courtesy CSIRO)

good reason why the term territory should be restricted to space acquired or retained by aggressive activity, and my use of the word is in the ordinary sense of individual spatial possession, however established.

Territorial behaviour can readily be surmised from the pattern of settlement since individuals will be spaced out from each other or 'under-dispersed' — a confusing term implying that the statistical dispersion of variation in quadrat frequencies is too low. There are several procedures that can be adopted to establish spacing out, the simplest being to find whether in quadrats of a scale corresponding to that of the territory the variance is significantly less than the mean (Knight-Jones and Moyse, 1961; Crisp, 1961). Another method is nearest-neighbour analysis (Clarke and Evans, 1954) for one- or two-dimensional systems (Crisp, 1961; Wisely, 1960). However it is much more informative, though rather more laborious, to determine the distribution of population density as a function of distance from a reference individual. This can be done by taking each individual in turn and counting the numbers of spat settled within successive annuli and expressing the result as numbers per unit area. When these are averaged over all individuals they produce a figure such as that illustrated below (*Figure 2.13*). From such a figure the size of the territory can be

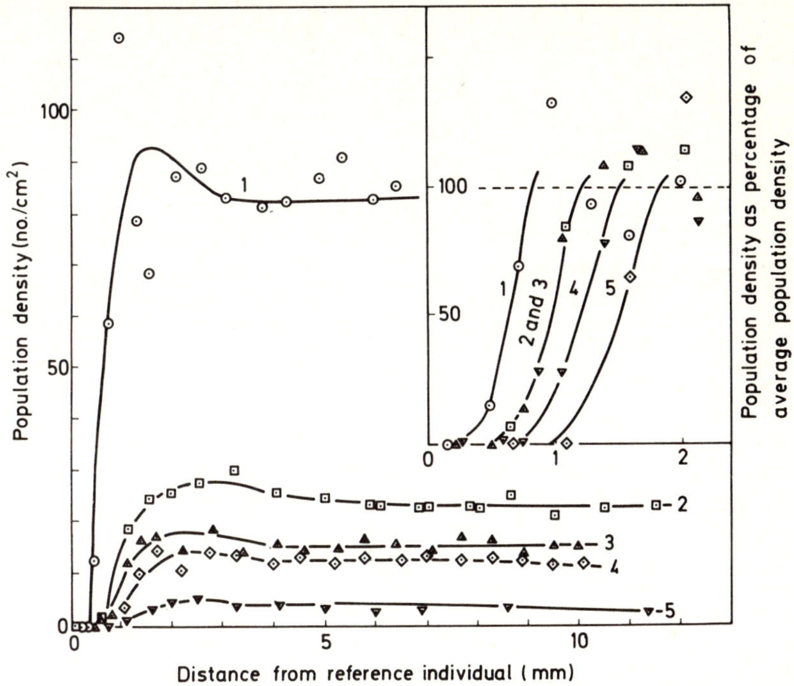

Figure 2.13 Results obtained by counting the numbers of barnacles present in successive annuli at increasing distance (shown on the abscissa) from each individual taken in turn as a reference point. The ordinate shows the radially dependent population density (at distance r to $r + \Delta r$) obtained by dividing average count by annulus area ($2\pi r\Delta r$). Five populations of decreasing density were analysed, the mean densities being: Curve 1, 85 cm^{-2}; Curve 2, 22.5 cm^{-2}; Curve 3, 15cm^{-2}; Curve 4, 12.5 cm^{-2}; Curve 5, 3.5 cm^{-2}. The fall in density on approaching the reference point represents territory from which individuals tend to be excluded. At distances of <0.4 mm, which represent an overlap, the density is likely to approach zero in any case. Inset figure represents the radially dependent density expressed as a percentage of the average density. As the average density of population pressure increases the territory diminishes in area. (After Crisp, 1961; courtesy R. J. Skaer)

measured. The distance both in barnacles and in *Spirorbis* which separates individual territories does not appear to be the area which the spat will require to reach adulthood; it is much smaller and relates to the behaviour pattern and dimensions of the larva. Both in *Spirorbis* (Wisely, 1960) and in barnacles (Crisp, 1961) the territory became smaller as the settlement pressure was increased and more individuals were forced to settle (*Figure 2.13* inset). Wisely found that the territories diminished because the pre-settlement behaviour became abbreviated by the omission of the wide searching movements. It is most important in analysing territorial behaviour to ensure that the settlement intensity is sensibly constant throughout the area investigated, otherwise any of the above tests may be vitiated.

Whereas Wisely and Crisp believed that territorial behaviour was essentially an avoidance reaction to objects projecting from the surface, including settled spat, Knight-Jones and Moyse (1961) considered that in barnacles there was a specific element. They noticed that cyprids in the field avoided settling on barnacles of their own, but not on those of a different species. Recently however experiments on the simultaneous settlements of cyprids of *Elminius modestus* and *Balanus balanoides* in small pits gave no such evidence of specific avoidance of their own species. On the contrary, although cyprids avoided entering occupied pits whenever possible, those which did so favoured pits in which their own species had been established.

Surfaces with a fibrous texture present the greatest possible concentration of convex surfaces. Not surprisingly therefore they are avoided by the majority of larvae; Barnes and Powell (1950) for example found that staple cloths with filaments of glass fibre 8 μm in diameter were avoided by barnacle and tubeworm larvae. Fibrous collectors, though unsuitable for the settlement of most marine animals, are commonly used to encourage the settlement of *Pecten* larvae which evidently search for substrata of this shape. The pediveliger of *Mytilus edulis* behaves in precisely the same manner towards algal filaments of about 180 μm diameter (Bayne, 1965). The foot can curl round the filament and thereby secure the juvenile mussel in a position where the water is frequently renewed and where it is likely to be free from competition by other filter feeders. After a period of rapid growth, the young mussel leaves the algal filaments and eventually finds its way to the adult mussel bed (Bayne, 1964).

2.3.2.6 SETTLEMENT OF LARVAE IN BOTTOM DEPOSITS

Most of the species living in deposits of mud, sand and gravel have pelagic larvae which need to locate the right kind of substratum at the end of their free-swimming stage. A few, however, like *Scoloplos armiger,* lay their eggs in gelatinous capsules which are anchored to the sand by a narrow tube. The photonegative larvae crawl directly down the neck of the capsule and into the sand.

A few of the early investigators including Mortensen (1921) noticed that the presence of deposits was important in encouraging larvae to settle. It was however Wilson's pioneering studies of polychaete larvae, extending over two decades, that drew together various strands of evidence which gave us the understanding of substrate selection that is widely accepted today. The most fundamental property distinguishing different kinds of deposits is the particle size since it controls so many of the characteristics that determine whether it will be suitable for a particular species. Particle size is the main influence on such physical properties as permeability, thixotropy and dilatency, and the capacity for adsorption. These properties in turn influence the composition of the microflora on which deposit feeding animals live.

Wilson's early work soon established that the kind of deposit, whether mud, sand or gravel could be distinguished by the various species of larvae. Thus the larvae of *Notomastus latericeus* and *Scolecolepis fuliginosa,* two worms normally found in mud or muddy sand, metamorphosed more readily in such a deposit than in clean sand or shell gravel (Day and Wilson, 1934; Wilson, 1937). *Owenia fusiformis* on the other hand, a worm which builds tubes in clean, fine sand, metamorphosed in response to a sprinkling of sand grains, though a somewhat thicker layer was more conducive (Wilson, 1932). Wilson (1948) next turned his attention to the larvae of *Ophelia bicornis*. This worm was found to be restricted to a particular type of sand and the larvae metamorphosed readily and healthily only if this type of sand was present. Wilson (1952; 1954) offered the larvae sands of varying grain size and found that they favoured those in which the grain size corresponded with that of their natural habitat. Similar results could be obtained by using artificial sands made from glass beads. Further experiments, however, showed that particle size was not the only, nor indeed the most important, factor inducing metamorphosis. If the sand was heated to redness, or if other highly destructive agents were used to destroy any organic matter on its surface, then although the shape of the sand grains was unaffected Wilson found that the suitability of the natural sand was considerably diminished. However it was possible to restore the metamorphosis-inducing property to the sand by allowing it to stand in seawater for a period of time. Wilson (1955) concluded that the surface of the sand grains required to be covered with microflora of a specific type and density before it could induce *Ophelia* larvae to settle. Jägersten (1940) had found that the larvae of an archiannelid, *Protodrilus rubropharyngeus,* similarly required shell gravels to induce metamorphosis and that the property associated with shell gravel could be transferred to other deposits or small stones to which the larvae had previously shown no response. Jägersten's experiments could, therefore, for the most part be interpreted in terms of the transfer of a microflora which the larvae could recognise. Gray (1967) carried out similar experiments on adults and larvae of *Protodrilus rubropharyngeus* and on the adults of *P. symbiotica* and *P. hypoleucus* (Gray, 1966; 1967b) and found not only that destructive agents would remove the attractiveness of the natural sand but also that bacterial cultures from naturally occurring sand were the most effective in restoring it to its original condition. Other bacteria capable of improving the attractiveness of the sands were usually those which grew attached to surfaces, non-sessile bacteria being less effective. Gray also showed that the density of the bacterial cells on the surface of the sand was not necessarily the operative factor, since natural sands with quite small numbers of bacteria were usually more attractive than artificially restored sands which were much more heavily coated. Gray therefore believed that the larvae responded to an adherent organic film produced by the bacteria which served as a habitat indicator. The mechanism by which the larvae distinguish the organic covered surface from a clean surface is not understood but it is clear from the observations of almost all observers that the larvae are neither attracted to the sand nor influenced at a distance. It is only after they have made actual contact that they respond by remaining in the sand and undergoing metamorphosis. Evidently therefore the mechanism involves close range physical forces rather than any diffusing chemical substance.

2.3.2.7 RESPONSE TO SURFACE FILMS

As soon as a chemically clean solid is placed in seawater any dissolved molecules of high molecular weight will begin to adsorb on to its surface. Most widespread among such substances in seawater are humic compounds which consist of the more refractory breakdown products of organic origin. Following this initial 'molecular fouling' the surface gradually accumulates bacteria, sessile diatoms and algal spores, soon followed by motile and sessile Protozoa (Zobell and Allen, 1935; Zobell, 1939). All these micro-organisms secrete colloidal materials, mainly polysaccharides or mucopolysaccharides, which contribute towards the formation of a 'slime film'. Slime films, together with their attached micro-organisms, may become sufficiently thick to be clearly noticeable to the naked eye after a period of a day or two.

Invertebrate larvae do not usually settle in quantity during the first few days and consequently appear after the slime film has formed. This fact had led to the erroneous belief that the primary film was necessary for settlement. It is true that the majority of larvae of invertebrates — serpulid, barnacle, oyster and bryozoan larvae — settle more readily on filmed than on clean surfaces. However, this is a preference not a precondition. Furthermore, there are several well-authenticated examples of larvae which avoid filmed surfaces in favour of unfilmed ones. Films of some micro-organisms may encourage while those of others may discourage the settlement of the same invertebrate larvae (Meadows and Williams, 1963), while the metabolic activity of the micro-organisms may also influence the settlement. It seems unlikely, therefore, that the response of the larva depends on the physical properties of the film alone. As with the films on the surfaces of the particles forming bottom deposits, it seems probable that larvae can appreciate both physical and chemical differences.

2.3.2.8 SETTLEMENT IN RESPONSE TO CHEMICAL SUBSTANCES

The reaction of marine invertebrate larvae to bacterial films and diatom slimes raises the important question whether chemical substances diffusing from the surfaces of living organisms or the chemical constitution of the surface itself plays any part in habitat selection. If a recognition of complex chemical substances could reinforce the appreciation of the physical attributes of the substratum and of its environment then a very much more precise and definite choice could be made.

The first real evidence of such specificity came from the work of Knight-Jones on gregarious settlement. He realised that strong circumstantial evidence already existed. The gregarious distribution of sessile marine organisms in nature (Burton, 1949), the close association between epiphytic animals and their host plants, and the importance of the proximity for sexual reproduction all indicated that an element of specific recognition might be incorporated in the settlement process. Cole and Knight-Jones (1949) and Knight-Jones (1952) first demonstrated gregariousness in the flat oyster

Ostrea edulis while Knight-Jones and Stephenson (1950), again by means of field experiments, observed that *Elminius modestus* settled in much greater density on surfaces already bearing spat of its own species. The really crucial demonstration, however, was made in the laboratory. First Knight-Jones showed that two species of *Spirorbis, S. borealis* and *S. pagenstecheri* as they were then called, chose specifically the fronds of *Fucus* on which their own species had already settled. Secondly, barnacle cyprids settled on surfaces populated by other barnacles rather than on bare surfaces, preferring surfaces bearing their own species to those bearing barnacles of other species (Knight-Jones, 1953b; 1955).

The gregarious response is stronger in barnacles than in other groups and may well be stronger in *Balanus balanoides* than in many other barnacle species (Larman and Gabbott, 1975). Moreover its cyprids are very readily obtained from the spring plankton. It was not surprising, therefore, that research was concentrated on this species and demonstrated not only the mechanism and significance of gregarious settlement but also a hitherto unsuspected chemical sense. Through a series of elegantly simple experiments Knight-Jones was able to locate the settlement promoting factor in the cuticle of the barnacle (Knight-Jones, 1953b). He found that, despite its specificity, it was extremely robust chemically, withstanding high temperatures, strong solvents, years of immersion in water and attack by destructive chemicals. Only the tanned protein of the cuticle — assumed to be like that of other arthropods — appeared to meet these criteria. As a large complex molecule it would probably possess minor differences from species to species and, being chemically bound and relatively inert, it would possess the refractory properties needed and would be insoluble in water. The problem therefore remained, how could the cyprid appreciate its presence?

The next step was taken by Crisp and Meadows (1962; 1963) who found, in apparent contradiction to the conclusions reached by Knight-Jones, that material could be extracted from the barnacle and from other arthropod integuments which, if transferred to previously unattractive surfaces, would cause the cyprids to settle abundantly on them (*Figure 2.14*). It soon became evident that the extractable settlement factor was a heat stable integumental protein of the kind previously referred to by earlier workers as 'arthropodin'.

As so often happens, the contradiction between the two approaches led to a fuller and an entirely compatible understanding. Crisp and Meadows were able to show that arthropodin was ineffective in promoting settlement when in solution and presumably was not appreciated by the chemical sense of the cyprid as normally understood. Only when the arthropodin was adsorbed on to a surface would the cyprid respond to it. The only hypothesis consistent with observation was that when extractable arthropodin was applied to a surface it was held by the physico-chemical forces of adsorption in the same orientation as it would normally occupy on the surface of the cuticle. Thus in Knight-Jones' investigations, the protein was held at the surface of the natural cuticle by chemical bonds resulting from quinone tanning and was therefore insoluble. Crisp and Meadows' methods removed untanned protein of the same kind and allowed it to adsorb on the surface of a clean piece of slate

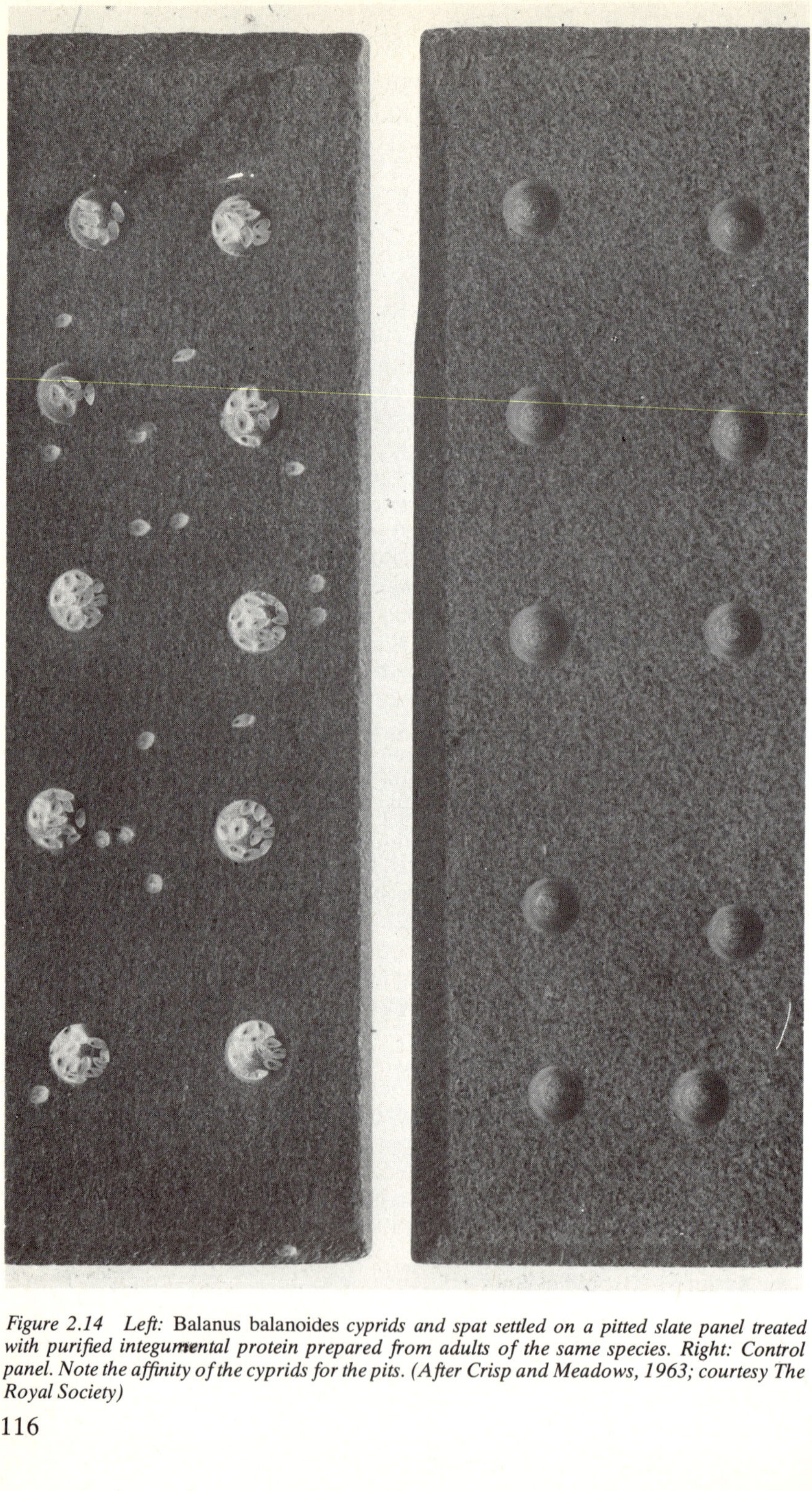

Figure 2.14 Left: Balanus balanoides *cyprids and spat settled on a pitted slate panel treated with purified integumental protein prepared from adults of the same species. Right: Control panel. Note the affinity of the cyprids for the pits. (After Crisp and Meadows, 1963; courtesy The Royal Society)*

so that the cyprid was presented with the same or with a similar molecular configuration.

As a result of these experiments the concept of a 'tactile chemical sense' was postulated by which the molecular nature of a surface could be recognised in the way that a blind man reads braille. Perhaps an even closer analogy would be the reading of a molecular structure in the same way that a protein recognises its antigen (Crisp, 1975).

The receptor through which this remarkable ability is mediated is generally believed to be the attachment disc of the antennule, simply because this is the organ by which the cyprid makes close contact with the substratum. The detailed studies of its structure by Nott and Foster (1969) and in particular the arrangement of its sense organs make this a probable interpretation. If the molecular force field of the disc complements that of the surface of the cuticle, specific recognition could be achieved by registering the force of adhesion. Since adhesive forces are proportional to area, whereas mass and inertial forces increase with volume, adhesion plays an extremely important part in the behaviour of very small animals particularly in a buoyant medium. Hence contact between two solid surfaces under water might be sufficient to generate an appreciable species specific force.

The sensory mechanism responding to the surface structure of a tough, insoluble material is probably not confined to barnacle cyprids. Settling larvae of oysters appear to respond to the periostracum of oyster shells in the same way that barnacle larvae do towards arthropodin, though with less discrimination (Crisp, 1967; 1974). Wilson (1968; 1970) found that *Sabellaria* larvae needed to make contact with the tube-forming cement of the adult colony to induce settlement. The response was also specific. Mussel larvae, however, are not gregarious, even though the adults live in colonies which exclude nearly all other sessile animals (Scheer, 1945). Perhaps the very success of the adult mussel as a competitor makes gregarious larval settlement too hazardous for the larva.

'Gregarious settlement', in which the larva responds to the presence of its own species, has its counterpart in what I have called 'associative settlement', in which the larva responds to an unrelated species. Generally the association is between a sessile invertebrate and its living substratum. An example would be the association of certain Bryozoa and hydroids with fucoid algae (Ryland, 1962; Crisp and Williams, 1960; Williams, 1965) or the association of various species of *Spirorbis* with a variety of organic substrata (Crisp, 1974). The relation between barnacles on the one hand and turtles, whales, sponges and corals may well fall into this class though the settlement mechanism has not yet been fully demonstrated.

A different kind of association exists between polychaetes and archiannelids and the specific microflora of the gravels, sands and muds which form their habitat. Here the second species is not the substratum itself but serves as an indicator of an appropriate type of habitat. This second kind of association is likely to be extended in future to a larger assemblage of benthic forms including gastropods, bivalves and echinoderms. Possibly the response of the larva of the mud snail *Nassarius obsoletus* to extracts of the mud in which it lives is to be regarded as an indirect recognition of the habitat mediated through microbial byproducts (Scheltema, 1961). *Teredo* larvae similarly respond to diffusates from wood (Harington, 1921).

A third kind of associative settlement response was observed by Thompson (1958), who found that larvae of nudibranch *Adalaria proxima* required a stimulus from its food organism *Electra pilosa* before it would settle. A number of similar interactions between nudibranchs and their food have been reported (Thompson, 1964; Crisp, 1974).

Both gregarious and associative settlement will have the same two advantageous results for the organisms which practise it. First, the adults will be ultimately congregated into small groups instead of being scattered at random. This is an obvious aid in reproductive efficiency. Secondly, the clusters of individuals will become centred on suitable habitats thereby promoting their longer survival. Gregarious settlement emphasises the former objective and incidentally entails the latter since settling near an established individual is some guarantee that the habitat will be suitable. Associative settlement emphasises the attainment of a suitable habitat but since suitable habitats form only a small fraction of the environment the net result is that the larvae are brought into proximity with each other. Since the larvae settling in any one group are likely to be derived from a wide circle of origins both mechanisms will encourage genetic exchange without unduly reducing the prospects of individual survival.

Not a great deal is yet known about the chemical structure of settlement-inducing substances, nor is there any reason *a priori* that a chemical structure which stimulates one type of larva need in any way be similar to that which stimulates another. The only necessity is that they should be symbolic and reasonably specific. Of course, they need not be entirely specific and perhaps in any event this would be an unattainable objective. Indeed settlement-inducing substances need only permit the larva to be able to improve its chances of settlement on a suitable substratum above random for their recognition by the larva to have selective advantage. Thus we have seen, for example, that the degree of specificity displayed by cyprids at settlement is by no means complete. Substances capable of stimulating barnacle settlement can be derived not only from barnacles themselves but also from all species of arthropod so far tried. The evolution of barnacle genera such as *Chelonibia* and *Octolasmis* which settle on decapod Crustacea is therefore not at all remarkable. But cyprids will settle also in response to extracts of sponge, vertebrate and even molluscan tissue when the heat stable protein fraction is suitably concentrated. Recently Larman and Gabbott (1975) examined a number of such proteins and found them to have several properties in common. However, we are still a long way from understanding in molecular terms what constitutes a settlement-inducing substance, even for the most thoroughly studied larva, the cyprid.

2.4 PREVENTION OF SETTLEMENT

The settlement of marine organisms on ships' hulls greatly increases the drag on the moving ship, 80% of which is caused by skin friction. Various types of seawater installation can also become fouled with serious economic losses, particularly since engineers rarely make provision for the eventuality. Research on marine invertebrate larvae can be justified economically as well as scientifically because any measures for the prevention of fouling must interrupt the larval settlement process at some point. The measures must also be one hundred per cent successful, not only because the resistance even of a lightly fouled surface is much greater than that of a smooth one, but also because any organism that settles gregariously will quickly spread its effects over the whole area (Knight-Jones and Crisp, 1953).

At present the standard method of preventing ship fouling is by the application of a toxic paint, classically one based on cuprous oxide but more recently one employing organo-tin derivatives. The latter are more effective against a wide range of animals and plants and are more easily incorporated into the paint. Various additional toxins have been used, for example mercury, arsenicals, DDT etc., to spice the main course. However, the primary aim of the formulator must be to control, as economically as possible, the rate of diffusion (or leaching) of the toxic ingredient above a certain limiting level. In one of the older types of paint, the vehicle itself slowly wore down, releasing the reserves of toxin from below its original surface. Unfortunately such materials created their own roughness in the course of defoliation. After a period of development of smoother paints based on insoluble polymers, the more modern trend has reverted to the basically sound idea of a slowly dissolving medium. The newest developments achieve the property of self-polishing, the only practical way of actually reducing skin friction after the paint has been applied.

All paints, therefore, have in the past depended on killing the larva after it had settled. There is no evidence that barnacles, or for that matter other organisms, are deterred from settling by the toxins present in paints (Crisp and Austin, 1960). There is a growing demand for controlling fouling more elegantly and the protection of the health of dock operators and the supposed danger to the natural environment may eventually force new toxins or more novel measures on the market. However, the problem is an intractable one requiring a heavy research investment and is therefore not assisted by the present fragmented nature of the industry (Crisp, 1973b).

An obvious ploy would be to attempt to interrupt the settling behaviour during the exploratory phase. Small obstacles or fibres might be effective but would naturally be ruled out on account of the increase in friction. Very smooth surfaces, which are clearly desirable from the ship owners' standpoint if they can be maintained, would deter but are not entirely capable of preventing settlement. The fact that settlement-inducing substances are known has suggested the possibility of settlement-arresting substances, but the outlook is not encouraging. The whole background of larval behaviour shows that there is a natural tendency to defer settlement in the absence of a specific chemical stimulus. Hence there is no reason why larvae would need to distinguish between an inert and a positively discouraging surface, and therefore no need for them to possess a receptor system to respond to particular substances which would prevent settlement.

Generally a very clean surface is the least attractive that can be devised.

Another attack might be directed at the point of secretion of the primary cement. A smooth surface of low energy would reduce the forces of adhesion, possibly to the point where waves or the current produced by the motion of the ship would strip off the fouling. However, low energy paints do not adhere well and might therefore involve a complex system of priming coats. Other suggestions that have been made from time to time and which can be found extensively in the patent literature include radioactive paints, loudspeakers, ultrasonics, air bubbles, 'balano-toxin' derived from decomposing cyprids, moulting and sterilising hormones. All these remedies suffer from at least the one drawback: they do not work.

The problem of occlusion of pipes, which involves mainly the prevention of mussel fouling, cannot be so readily solved by the application of paints. However, since the seawater in the system is somewhat more limited in volume than that surrounding a ship, a continuous injection of low concentrations of cheap toxin, almost invariably chlorine, is often feasible. The introduction of the halogen, though usually effective, has its environmental drawbacks (Hoare and Hiscock, 1974). Nevertheless, since industrial installations using seawater are usually located in heavily polluted estuaries the environmental objections under these circumstances seem unreal, if not churlish. In estuaries where mariculture is practised, chlorination might be objectionable.

REFERENCES

BARNES, H. (1955). 'Further observations on rugophilic behaviour in *Balanus balanoides* (L.)', *Vidensk. Meddr dansk naturh. Foren. for 1955,* **117,** 341–348

BARNES, H. (1956). 'Surface roughness and the settlement of *Balanus balanoides* (L)', *Arch. Soc. Zoo. bot. fenn. Vanamo,* **10,** 2

BARNES, H., CRISP, D. J. and POWELL, H. T. (1951). 'Observations on the orientation of some species of barnacles', *J. Anim. Ecol.,* **20,** 227–241

BARNES, H. and POWELL, H. T. (1950). 'Some observations on the effect of fibrous glass surfaces upon the settlement of certain sedentary marine organisms', *J. mar. biol. Assoc. U.K.,* **29,** 299–302

BAYNE, B. L. (1964). 'Primary and Secondary settlement in *Mytilus edulis* L.', *J. Anim. Ecol.,* **33,** 513–523

BAYNE, B. L. (1965). 'Growth and the delay of metamorphosis of the larvae of *Mytilus edulis* (L.)', *Ophelia,* **2,** 1–47

BOUSFIELD, E. L. (1955). 'Ecological control of the occurrence of barnacles in the Miramichi Estuary', *Bull. natn. Mus. Can.,* **137,** 69pp

BURTON, M. (1949). 'Observations on littoral sponges including the supposed swarming of larvae, movement and coalescence in mature individuals, longevity and death', *Proc. zool. Soc. Lond.,* **118,** 893–915

CANTELL, C. E. (1966). 'The devouring of the larval tissues during metamorphosis of pilidium larvae', *Ark. Zool.,* **18,** 489–492

CARRIKER, M. R. (1967). 'Ecology of estuarine benthic invertebrates', In: *Estuaries.* Ed. G. H. Lauff. *Am. Assoc. Adv. Sci. Publ. No. 83.* Washington D.C. 442–457

CLARKE, P. J. and EVANS, F. C. (1954). 'Distance to nearest neighbour as a measure of spatial relationships in populations', *Ecology,* **35,** 445–453

COLE, H. A. (1938). 'The fate of the larval organs in the metamorphosis of *Ostrea edulis', J. mar. biol. Assoc. U.K.,* **22,** 469–84

COLE, H. A. and KNIGHT-JONES, E. W. (1939). 'Some observations and experiments on the settling behaviour of *Ostrea edulis', J. Cons. perm. int. Explor. Mer.,* **14,** 86–105

COLE, H. A. and KNIGHT-JONES, E. W. (1949). 'The settling behaviour of larvae of the European oyster *Ostrea edulis* L., and its influence on methods of cultivation and spat collection', *Fishery Invest. Lond. Ser. II,* **17** (3), 39pp

COLEMAN, J. S. (1933). 'The nature of the intertidal zonation of plants and animals', *J. mar. biol. Assoc. U.K.,* **18,** 435–476

CRANFIELD, H. J. (1973). 'Observations on the behaviour of the pediveliger of *Ostrea edulis* L. during attachment and cementing', *Mar. Biol.* **22,** 203–209

CRISP, D. J. (1955). 'The behaviour of barnacle cyprids in relation to water movement over a surface', *J. exp. Biol.,* **32,** 569–590

CRISP, D. J. (1960). 'Factors influencing growth rate in *Balanus balanoides', J. Anim. Ecol.,* **29,** 95–116

CRISP, D. J. (1961). 'Territorial behaviour in barnacle settlement', *J. Exp. Biol.,* **38,** 429–446

CRISP, D. J. (1967). 'Chemical factors inducing settlement in *Crassostrea virginica* Gmelin', *J. Anim. Ecol.,* **36,** 329–335

CRISP, D. J. (1973a). 'Mechanisms of adhesion of fouling organisms'. In: *3rd Int. Congress on marine corrosion and fouling in the sea—Gaithersburg, Maryland, U.S.A.,* Oct. 1972, 691–709. Ed. B. Floyd Brown

CRISP, D. J. (1973b). 'The role of the biologist in anti-fouling research'. In: *3rd Int. Congress on marine corrosion and fouling in the sea—Gaithersburg, Maryland, U.S.A.,* Oct. 1972, 88–93. (Ed. B. Floyd Brown)

CRISP, D. J. (1974). 'Factors influencing the settlement of marine invertebrate larvae', In: *Chemoreception in Marine Organisms.* Ed. P. T. Grant and A. N. Mackie. pp. 177–265

CRISP, D. J. (1975). 'Surface chemistry and life in the sea (The Sir Eric Rideal Lecture 1974)', *Chem. Ind.* **5,** 187–193

CRISP, D. J. (1976). 'The role of the pelagic larva', In *Perspectives in Experimental Biology,* **1,** 145–155. Ed. P. Spencer Davis. SEB 50th Anniversary Meeting. Pergamon Press

CRISP, D. J. and AUSTEN, A. P. (1960). 'The action of copper in anti-fouling paints', *Ann. appl. Biol.,* **48,** 787–799

CRISP, D. J. and BARNES, H. (1954). 'The orientation and distribution of barnacles at settlement with particular reference to surface contour', *J. Anim. Ecol.,* **23,** 142–162

CRISP, D. J. and GHOBASHY, A. F. A. A. (1971). 'Responses of the larvae of *Diplosoma listerianum* to light and gravity'. In: *Proc. 4th European Marine Biology Symposium.* Ed. D. J. Crisp. Cambridge University Press. 443–465

CRISP, D. J. and MEADOWS, P. S. (1962). 'The chemical basis of gregariousness in cirripedes', *Proc. roy. Soc. B.,* **156,** 500–520

CRISP, D. J. and MEADOWS, P. S. (1963). 'Adsorbed layers: the stimulus to settlement in barnacles', *Proc. roy. Soc. B,* **158,** 364–387

CRISP, D. J. and RITZ, D. A. (1973). 'Responses of cirripede larvae to light. I. Experiments with white light', *Mar. Biol.,* **23,** 327–335

CRISP, D. J. and RYLAND, J. S. (1960). 'Influence of filming and of surface texture on the settlement of marine organisms', *Nature, Lond.,* **185,** 119

CRISP, D. J. and STUBBINGS, H. G. (1957). 'The orientation of barnacles to water currents', *J. Anim. Ecol.,* **26,** 179–196

CRISP, D. J. and WILLIAMS, G. B. (1960). 'Effect of extracts from Fucoids in promoting settlement of epiphytic polyzoa', *Nature Lond.,* **188,** 1206–1207

DARWIN, C. (1854). *A Monograph of the Sub-class Cirripedia,* **II,** *The Balanidae, the Verrucidae.* Ray Society London, 684pp

DAY, J. H. and WILSON, D. P. (1934). 'On the relation of the substratum to the metamorphosis of *Scolecolepis fuliginosa* (Claparede)', *J. mar. biol. Assoc. U.K.,* **19,** 655–662

DE WOLF, P. (1973). 'Ecological observations on the mechanism of dispersal of barnacle larvae during planktonic life and settlement', *Netherlands J. of Sea Res.,* **6,** 1–129

DOOCHIN, H. D. (1951). 'The morphology of *Balanus improvisus* Darwin and *Balanus amphitrite niveus* Darwin during initial attachment and metamorphosis', *Bull. mar. Sci. Gulf Caribb.,* **1,** 15–39

FORBES, L., SEWARD, M. J. B. and CRISP, D. J. (1971). 'Orientation to light and the shading response in barnacles', In: *Proc. 4th Marine Biology Symposium,* 539–558. Ed. D. J. Crisp; Cambridge University Press

GIARD, A. (1876). 'Note sur l'embryogénie de la *Salmacina dysteri* Huxley', *C.r. hebd. Séanc. Acad. Sci. Paris,* **82,** 233–235 and 285–288

GIBSON, P. H. and NOTT, J. A. (1971). 'Concerning the fourth antennula segment of the cypris larva of *Balanus balanoides*', In: *Proc. 4th European Marine Biology Symp.*, 227–236. Ed. D. J. Crisp

GRAVE, C. and McCASH, G. K. (1923). '*Perophora viridis:* The activities and structure of the free-swimming larvae', *Wash. Univ. Stud. scient. Ser.*, **11,** 89–116

GRAY, J. S. (1966). 'The attractive factor of intertidal sands to *Protodrilus symbioticus*', *J. mar. biol. Assoc. U.K.*, **46** (3), 627–645

GRAY, J. S. (1967a). 'Substrate selection by the archiannelid *Protodrilus rubropharyngeus* Jägersten', *Helgoländer wiss. Meeresunters,* **15,** 253–269

GRAY, J. S. (1967b). 'Substrate selection by the archiannelid *Protodrilus hypoleucus* Armarante', *J. exp. mar. Biol. Ecol.*, **1,** 47–54

GRUFFYDD Ll. D. and LANE, D. J. W. (1975). 'The glands of the larval foot in *Pecten maximus* and possible homologues in other bivalves', *J. mar. biol. Assoc. U.K.*, (in the press)

HARINGTON, C. R. (1921). 'A note on the physiology of the ship-worm, *(Teredo norvegica)*', *Biochem. J.*, **15,** 736–741

HASKIN, H. H. (1964). 'The distribution of oyster larvae'. In: *Symp. Exp. Marine Ecol. Occasional Pub.*, **2,** 76–80, Narrasangett Marine Laboratory

HOARE, R. and HISCOCK, K. (1974). 'An ecological survey of the rocky coast adjacent to a bromine extraction works', *Estuarine and Coastal Mar. Sci.*, **2,** 329–348

HOLLAND, D. L. and WALKER, G. (1975). 'The biochemical composition of the cypris larva of the barnacle *Balanus balanoides*', *J. cons. int. Explor. Mer.* **36,** 162–165

HOPKINS, A. E. (1935). 'Attachment of larvae of the Olympia oyster, *Ostrea lurida,* to plane surfaces', *Ecology,* **16,** 82–86

HOPKINS, A. E. (1937). 'Experimental observations on spawning, larval development and setting in the Olympia oyster, *Ostrea lurida*', *Bull. Bur. Fish. Wash.*, **48,** No. 23

HOUGHTON, D. R., PEERMAN, I. and TIERNEY, D. (1973). 'The effect of water velocity on the settlement of swarms of *Enteromorpha* spp.', In: *Proc. 3rd Int. Congress on marine corrosion and fouling, Gaithersburg, Maryland,* 1972, 682–690. Ed. B. Floyd Brown

ISHAM, L. B., WALTON SMITH, F. G. and SPRINGER, V. (1951). 'Marine borer attack in relation to conditions of illumination', *Bull mar. Sci. Gulf Caribb.*, **1,** 46–63

JÄGERSTEN, G. (1940). 'Die Abhängigkeit der Metamorphose vom Substrat des Biotops bei *Protodrilus*', *Ark. Zool.*, (Stockholm), **32A** (17), 1–12

KNIGHT-JONES, E. W. (1951). 'Gregariousness and some other aspects of the setting behaviour of *Spirorbis*', *J. mar. biol. Assoc. U.K.*, **30,** 201–222

KNIGHT-JONES, E. W. (1952). 'Reproduction of oysters in the Rivers Crouch and Roach, Essex, during 1947 and 1949', *Fishery Invest. Lond.*, Ser. II, (2)

KNIGHT-JONES, E. W. (1953a). 'Decreased discrimination during settling after prolonged planktonic life in larvae of *Spirorbis borealis* (Serpulidae)', *J. mar. biol. Assoc. U.K.*, **32,** 337–345

KNIGHT-JONES, E. W. (1953b). 'Laboratory experiments on gregariousness during setting in *Balanus balanoides* and other barnacles', *J. Exp. Biol.*, **30,** 584–598

KNIGHT-JONES, E. W. (1955). 'The gregarious setting reaction of barnacles as a measure of systematic affinity', *Nature, Lond.*, **174,** 266

KNIGHT-JONES, E. W. and CRISP, D. J. (1953). 'Gregariousness in barnacles in relation to the fouling of ships and to anti-fouling research', *Nature, Lond.*, **171,** 1109

KNIGHT-JONES, E. W. and MORGAN, E. (1966). 'Responses of marine animals to changes in hydrostatic pressure', *Oceanogr. mar. Biol. ann. Rev.*, **4,** 267–299

KNIGHT-JONES, E. W. and MOYSE, J. (1961). 'Intra specific competition in sedentary marine animals', *Symp. Soc. exp. Biol.*, **15,** 72–95

KNIGHT-JONES, E. W. and STEVENSON, J. P. (1950). 'Gregariousness during settlement in the barnacle *Elminius modestus* Darwin', *J. mar. biol. Ass. U.K.*, **29,** 281–297

LANE, D. J. W. (1973). 'Attachment of the larva of the ascidian *Diplosoma listerianum*', *Mar. Biol.*, **21,** 47–58

LARMAN, V. N. and GABBOTT, P. A. (1975). 'Settlement of cyprid larvae of *Balanus balanoides* and *Elminius modestus* induced by extracts of adult barnacles and other marine animals', *J. mar. biol. Assoc., U.K.*, **55,** 183–190

LYNCH, W. F. (1947). 'The behaviour and metamorphosis of the larva of *Bugula neretina* (Linnaeus): Experimental modification of the length of the free-swimming period and the responses to light and gravity', *Biol. Bull.*, **92,** 115–150

McDOUGAL, K. D. (1943). 'Sessile marine invertebrates of Beaufort, N. Carolina', *Ecol. Monogr.*, **13**, 323–374

MATTHEWS, A. (1917). 'The development of *Alcyonium digitatum* with some notes on early colony formation', *Q. J. microsc. Sci.*, **62**, 43–94

MEADOWS, P. S. and WILLIAMS, G. B. (1963). 'Settlement of *Spirorbis borealis* Daudin larvae on surfaces bearing films of micro-organisms', *Nature, Lond.*, **198**, 610–611

MORTENSEN, T. (1921). *Studies of the development and larval forms of echinoderms*. G.E.C. Gad. Copenhagen, 266 pp

NELSON, T. C. (1928). 'Pelagic dissoconchs of the common mussel, *Mytilus edulis*, with observations on the behaviour of the larvae of allied genera', *Biol. Bull.*, **55**, 180–192

NELSON, T. C. and PERKINS, E. B. (1930). 'The reactions of oyster larvae to currents and to salinity gradients', *Anat. Rec.*, **47**, 288

NEU, W. (1933). 'Der Einfluss des Farbtons der Unterlage auf die Besiedlung mit *Balanus* da Costa und *Spirorbis* Mont.', *Internat. Rev. Ges. Hydrobiol. u. Hydrograph.*, **28**, 228–246

NOTT, J. A. (1969). 'Settlement of barnacle larvae: surface of the antennular attachment disc by scanning electron microscopy', *Mar. Biol.*, **2**, 248–251

NOTT, J. A. and FOSTER, B. A. (1969). 'On the structure of the antennular attachment organ of the cypris larva of *Balanus balanoides* (L.)', *Phil. Trans. roy. Soc. B.*, **256**, 115–134

POMERAT, C. M. and WEISS, C. M. (1946). 'The influence of texture and composition of surface on the attachment of barnacles and of other sedentary organisms', *Biol. Bull.*, **91**, 57–65

PYEFINCH, K. A. and DOWNING, F. S. (1949). 'Notes on the general biology of *Tubularia larynx* Ellis and Solander', *J. mar. biol. Assoc. U.K.*, **28**, 21–43

RICE, A. L. (1964). 'Observations on the effects of changes of hydrostatic pressure on the behaviour of some marine animals', *J. mar. biol. Assoc. U.K.*, **44**, 163–175

RYLAND, J. S. (1959). 'Experiments on the selection of algal substrates by polyzoan larvae', *J. Exp. Biol.*, **36**, 613–631

RYLAND, J. S. (1960). 'Experiments on the influence of light on the behaviour of polyzoan larvae', *J. Exp. Biol.*, **37**, 783–800

RYLAND, J. S. (1962). 'The association between Polyzoa and algal substrata', *J. Anim. Ecol.*, **31**, 331–338

SAROYAN, J. R., LINDNER, E., DOOLEY, C. A. and BLEILE, H. R. (1970). 'Barnacle cement—Key to second generation anti-fouling coatings', *Ind. Eng. Chem. Prod. Res. Develop.*, **9**, 122–133

SCHEER, B. T. (1945). 'The development of marine fouling communities', *Biol. Bull.*, **89**, 103–121

SCHELTEMA, R. S. (1961). 'Metamorphosis of the veliger larvae of *Nassarius obsoletus* (Gastropoda) in response to bottom sediment', *Biol. Bull.*, **120**, 92–109

SCHELTEMA, R. S. (1971). 'The dispersal of the larvae of shoal-water benthic invertebrate species over long distances by ocean currents', In: *Proc. 4th European Marine Biological Symposium*, 7–28. Ed. D. J. Crisp. Cambridge University Press

THOMPSON, T. E. (1958). 'The natural history, embryology, larval biology and post larval development of *Adaleria proxima* (Alder and Hancock) Gastropoda Opisthobranchia)', *Phil. Trans. roy. Soc. Lond. B.*, **242**, 1–58

THOMPSON, T. E. (1964). 'Grazing and the life cycles of British Nudibranchs'. In: *Grazing in Terrestial and Marine Environments. Brit Ecol. Soc. Symp. No. 4*, 275–297. Ed. D. J. Crisp. Oxford, Blackwell

THORSON, G. (1964). 'Light as an ecological factor in the dispersal and settlement of larvae of marine bottom invertebrates', *Ophelia*, **1**, 167–208

VISSCHER, J. P. (1928). 'Reactions of the cyprid larva of barnacles at the time of attachment', *Biol. Bull.*, **54**, 327–335

WALKER, G. (1971). 'A study of the cement apparatus of the cypris larva of the barnacle *Balanus balanoides*', *Mar. Biol.*, **9**, 205–212

WALKER, G. (1973). 'The early development of the cement apparatus in the barnacle *Balanus balanoides* (L.) (Crustacea: Cirripedia)', *J. exp. mar. Biol. Ecol.*, **12**, 305–314

WALKER, G. (1974). 'The fine structure of the frontal filament complex of barnacle larvae (Crustacea: Cirripedia)', *Cell. Tiss. Res.*, **152**, 449–465

WALKER, G. and LEE, V. E. (1975). 'Surface structures and sense organs of *Balanus balanoides* (L.) as seen by scanning and transmission electron microscopy', *J. Zool. (Lond.)*, **178**, 161–172

WALLEY, L. J. (1969). 'Studies on the larval structure and metamorphosis of *Balanus balanoides*', *Phil. Trans. roy. Soc. B.*, **256,** 237–280

WILSON, D. P. (1948). 'The relation of the substratum to the metamorphosis of *Ophelia* larvae', *J. mar. biol. Assoc. U.K.*, **27,** 723–760

WILSON, D. P. (1952). 'The influence of the nature of the substratum on the metamorphosis of the larvae of marine animals, especially the larvae of *Ophelia bicornis Savigny*', *Annls. Inst. Oceanogr. Monaco,* **27,** 49–156

WILSON, D. P. (1954). 'The attractive factor in the settlement of *Ophelia bicornis* Savigny', *J. mar. biol. Assoc. U.K.,* **33,** 361–380

WILSON, D. P. (1955). 'The role of micro-organisms in the settlement of *Ophelia bicornis* Savigny', *J. mar. biol. Assoc. U.K.,* **34,** 531–543

WILSON, D. P. (1968). 'The settlement behaviour of the larvae of *Sabellaria alveolata*', *J. mar. biol. Assoc. U.K.,* **48,** 387–435

WILSON, D. P. (1970). 'The larvae of *Sabellaria spinulosa* and their settlement behaviour', *J. mar. biol. Assoc. U.K.,* **50,** 33–52

WISELY, B. (1960). 'Observations on the settling behaviour of larvae of the tubeworm *Spirorbis borealis* Daudin (Polychaete)', *Aust. J. mar. Freshwat. Res.,* **11,** 55

WOOD, E. J. F. (1955). 'Effect of temperature and rate of flow on some marine fouling organisms', *Aust. J. Sci.,* **18,** 34–37

WOOD, L. and HARGIS, W. J. (1971). 'Transport of bivalve larvae in a tidal estuary'. In: *Proc. 4th European Marine Biology Symposium,* 29–44. Ed. D. J. Crisp. Cambridge University Press

ZOBELL, C. E. (1939). 'The role of bacteria in the fouling of submerged surfaces', *Biol. Bull.,* **77,** 302

ZOBELL, C. E. and ALLEN, E. C. (1935). 'The significance of marine bacteria in the fouling of submerged surfaces', *J. Bact.,* **29** (3), 239–251

Three

Biochemical adaptations to temperature

G. N. SOMERO
Scripps Institution of Oceanography, La Jolla, California

P. W. HOCHACHKA
Department of Zoology, University of British Columbia, Vancouver

3.1 INTRODUCTION

Of all factors in the marine environment, temperature has the most pervasive effects on the functions and distribution patterns of organisms. To appreciate the complexities and the magnitudes of thermal effects on the physiology and biochemistry of marine organisms, and to understand the basic mechanisms of biochemical adaptation which are utilised to deal with temperature effects, one must have a detailed appreciation of the primary interactions which occur between changes in temperature and the cellular chemistry. We have, therefore, organised this chapter around two major questions. First, we shall deal in some detail with the basic effects of temperature changes on the molecular structures and functions of the cell. Second, we shall outline certain of the major adaptive patterns or 'strategies' which appear most important in tailoring the biochemistry of the organism to function well under the particular thermal conditions it experiences.

In writing this chapter we wish to do more than to review existing information concerning temperature effects and temperature adaptations. In almost no case are there sufficient data to permit anything resembling 'final words' on a particular topic. We therefore hope that the phenomena we discuss will arouse in the readers' minds new and exciting questions which may lead to profitable new approaches to the study of the biochemistry of environmental adaptation.

3.2 THE BASIC EFFECTS OF TEMPERATURE ON MARINE ORGANISMS

3.2.1 The critical element of time

The element of time plays a critical role in determining the magnitude of stress imposed by a temperature change and the avenues of adaptive response open to an organism. The intensity of the stress arising from a change in temperature is basically proportional to the product of two terms: (a) the magnitude of the temperature change, and (b) the rapidity with which the change occurs. Temperature changes of sufficient speed may prevent even the simplest behavioural adaptations to the thermal stress, e.g. rapid migration to an area where temperature conditions are more favourable (*see* Chapter 1). At the physiological and biochemical levels as well, the speed of a temperature change will be instrumental in determining what types of adaptive mechanism can be brought into play. As a general (and obvious) rule, the longer the time available to the organism to accomplish its physiological and biochemical reactions to temperature stress, the more thoroughly can the organism 'rebuild' its cellular chemistry to facilitate survival and enhance success in its new thermal regime.

When we examine the time component in the thermal stress equation in some detail, we find that three more or less distinct time courses of temperature stress confront marine organisms. Most rapid are the temperature changes which accompany the tide cycle and sudden changes in weather, e.g. cloud cover. In intertidal and estuarine habitats, these short-term temperature changes may exceed 15-20°C. Whereas motile organisms usually are able to stabilise their body temperatures by behavioural means, many sessile organisms manage to endure these large and rapid changes in body temperature.

A second time course of temperature stress is due to seasonal temperature changes. Again, as has been discussed in Chapter 1, the shallow intertidal regions and temperate zone estuaries are especially apt to confront organisms with extremes of thermal stress. Changes of several degrees Celsius may occur in the open seas as well, above the thermocline. As in the case of short-term temperature changes, seasonal variations in temperature frequently are adapted to through migration. In fact, in spite of the emphasis placed here on biochemical adaptations to temperature, it is only fair to point out that adaptations at this level of biological organisation often appear to be a 'last resort' type of response which is made if and only if the organism lacks behavioural means for reducing or eliminating thermal stress.

A third and final time course of temperature stress is associated with the very long-term changes in temperature which are experienced, for example, by populations of organisms colonising a new habitat with a different thermal regime from that known by the species during its past evolutionary history. Colonisation of high latitude waters and the deep-sea no doubt demanded extensive changes in the physiology and biochemistry of marine organisms as they developed capacities to cope with relatively low temperatures. These adaptations in most cases required new genetic information, e.g. genes coding for new enzyme variants which were able to function well at low temperatures. Adaptations which occur over many generations thus add a significant new potential for success in a different environment, for unlike adaptation processes which occur only during the lifespan of the individual, evolutionary adaptations alter the genetic repertoire and allow more fundamental responses to an environmental change.

One additional aspect of evolutionary adaptation to a new thermal habitat must be emphasised. These adaptations may involve not only a tolerance for new absolute temperatures, but also an ability to cope with a different range of temperatures. Thus a species which colonises an estuarine environment probably must become increasingly tolerant of a wide range of temperatures, i.e. it must become 'eurythermal'. In contrast, a species which colonises an environment which is highly thermally stable can 'afford' to lose some of its ability to withstand temperature fluctuations, as evidenced by the stenothermality of Antarctic fishes, for example (Somero and DeVries, 1967).

This brief discussion of the role of time in thermal stress and adaptation raises many of the major questions to be discussed in this chapter. For example, do the biochemical mechanisms of temperature adaptation utilised during seasonal acclimatisation processes resemble those characteristic of evolutionary adaptation to new temperatures? What are the primary biochemical mechanisms for enhancing eurythermality? Does a eurythermal organism benefit from possessing a wider array of variants on each enzyme 'theme', i.e. do eurythermal species have more complex allozyme and isozyme systems than stenothermal species? Is a variable thermal regime necessarily stressful, or does a regular (predictable) change in habitat (body) temperature offer favourable potentials for a marine organism? What biochemical factors are most instrumental in extending or altering the tolerance to extremes of temperature?

To approach these and related questions about temperature adaptation by marine organisms, we must first examine in some detail the ways in which temperature changes impinge on and perturb the structures and functions of the cell, especially its macromolecular constituents. This brief discourse on biophysics and biochemistry of temperature effects will allow us, first, to appreciate how vulnerable ectothermic organisms in particular are to thermal stress and, second, to gain some insight into the molecular properties which are most apt to be adaptively modifiable and thus serve as the 'raw material' for fabricating biochemical adaptations to temperature.

3.2.2 The effects of temperature on biochemical structures and processes

3.2.2.1 TEMPERATURE EFFECTS ON REACTION RATES

When heat energy is added to or removed from the cell, the resulting changes in molecular kinetic energies (*Figure 3.1*) can lead to a multitude of biologically important effects. To a physical chemist, all of these diverse effects could be grouped under two headings: (a) temperature effects on reaction equilibria, and (b) temperature effects on reaction rates. Most biologists interested in the interactions between temperature and living processes are far more familiar with the second class of effects, and we shall examine these 'rate effects' of temperature before considering the biologically crucial influences temperature can have on equilibria involving, in particular, non-covalently ('weak') bonded systems.

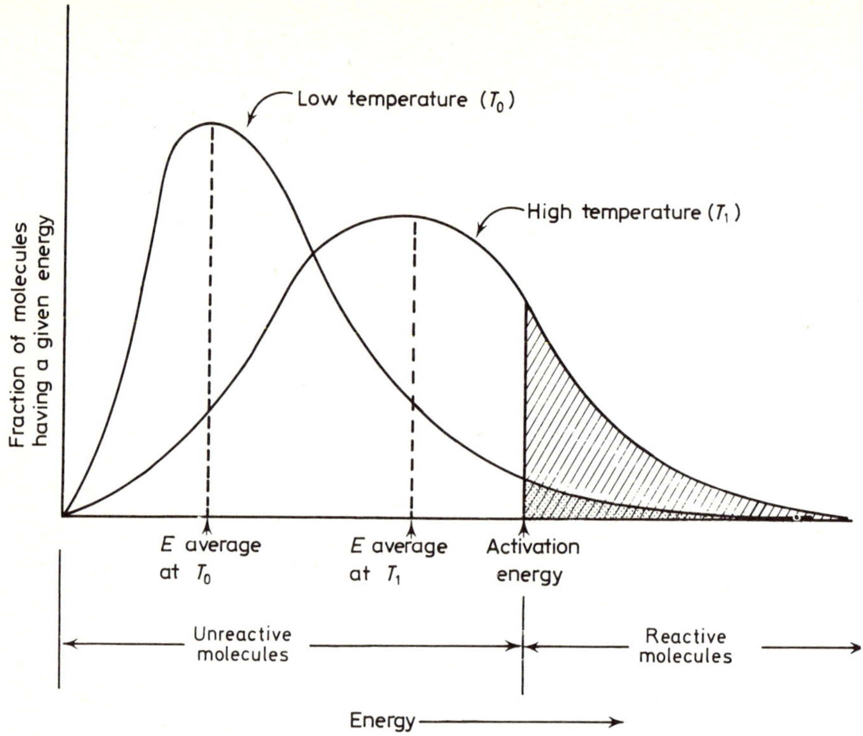

Figure 3.1 Energy distribution curves for a population of molecules at two different temperatures, T_0 and T_1. Only the molecules which possess energy equal to or greater than the activation energy are reactive (as indicated by stippling at T_0 and shading at T_1). (After Hochachka and Somero, 1973; courtesy W. B. Saunders & Co.)

The rate effects of temperature changes derive from the dependence of reaction velocities on the fraction of molecules in a given population which contain at least the minimal amount of kinetic energy to be reactive (*Figure 3.1*). A small percentage change in absolute temperature leads to a very much larger percentage change in the fraction of molecules which can react. For example, a 10°C change in absolute temperature represents only about a 3 per cent change in the *average* kinetic energy of a population of molecules held near 25°C (298°K). However, the fraction of the population of molecules which now possesses energy equal to or greater than the minimal activation energy may double or triple due to this 3 per cent change in average kinetic energy (*Figure 3.1*).

This basic physical-chemical relationship is one of the fundamental ground rules which biological processes must obey. It is nonetheless clear, however, that under many circumstances organisms would benefit from being able to free their metabolic reactions from a strict dependence on this relationship. We will observe, in fact, that many of the most innovative biochemical adaptations to temperature are what Barcroft (1934) would term means for freeing the cell from the 'tyranny of the Arrhenius equation'.

For well over a century biologists have been aware of the sharp dependence of biological processes on temperature, especially in the case of such gross manifestations of life as oxygen consumption. Recently biologists have come to appreciate more subtle manifestations of the rate effects of temperature changes. Not only can temperature changes alter the overall metabolic rate of an organism, but in addition temperature can lead to sharply differential effects on different components of metabolism. These differential effects are perhaps most obvious in the case of comparisons of temperature influences on rates of thermochemical, photochemical and diffusional processes. Photochemical reactions are essentially temperature-independent, and most diffusional processes are less temperature-dependent than chemical reactions which involve the formation or rupture of chemical bonds. However, it is among reactions of the latter category that we find the most diverse effects of temperature. Activation enthalpies differ among metabolic reactions, so a given change in temperature will accelerate (or retard) different reactions to different extents. Temperature effects on substrate binding also differ among enzymes, as discussed below. It is therefore important to keep in mind that the task which an organism must accomplish as it attempts to control its metabolic processes in the face of temperature changes includes (a) some regulation of the overall rate of metabolic activity, and (b) close coordination of a large array of enzymic processes which may be affected by temperature changes in highly diverse manners.

3.2.2.2 TEMPERATURE EFFECTS ON WEAK-BONDED SYSTEMS

In addition to affecting the rates at which equilibria are attained, changes in temperature can influence the equilibrium position of chemical reactions. In the cell, the equilibria which are most temperature-sensitive are those which involve the formation or rupture of non-covalent ('weak') chemical bonds such as hydrogen bonds, electrostatic interactions, van der Waals' forces and hydrophobic interactions. Covalent bonds are generally stable at biological temperatures, as evidenced by the fact that catalysis is required to facilitate rapid synthesis or rupture of these strong chemical bonds.

The enthalpy changes which occur during weak bond formation (*Table 3.1*) reveal why these types of chemical bonds are termed 'weak'. At

Table 3.1 'WEAK' CHEMICAL BONDS AND THEIR ENTHALPIES OF FORMATION (AFTER HOCHACHKA AND SOMERO, 1973)

Class of 'weak' bond	*Approximate enthalpy of formation* (kcal/mole)
van der Waals' forces	−1
Hydrogen bonds	−(3–7)
Ionic (electrostatic) interactions	−5
Hydrophobic interactions	+(1–3)

biological temperatures, weak bonds are continuously breaking and reforming as a result of the thermal energy present in the cell. The extreme lability of all types of weak bond might lead one to ask if it 'makes sense' to rely so heavily on these fragile interactions for supporting the integrities of the crucial structures and processes listed in *Table 3.2*. The answer to such a

Table 3.2 BIOCHEMICAL STRUCTURES AND PROCESSES WHICH ARE DEPENDENT ON 'WEAK' CHEMICAL BONDS

1. Higher orders of protein structure: helical structures, tertiary conformation, and quaternary structure.
2. Enzyme-ligand interactions.
3. Membrane structure: lipid-lipid and lipid-protein interactions.
4. Nucleic acid-nucleic acid interactions.
5. Nucleic acid-protein interactions.
6. Protein-protein interactions, e.g. microtubule and muscle contractile elements.
7. Hormone-receptor protein interactions.
8. Water structure.

question has come into sharp focus during the past decade or two: the specificities, the accuracies, the sensitivities and the efficiencies of all the structures/processes listed in *Table 3.2* are intimately dependent on a fine balance between structural rigidity and structural flexibility. For example, enzymic catalysis and regulation are frequently, perhaps always, accompanied by conformational changes in the enzyme. These critical changes in enzyme conformation are possible because the tertiary structures of proteins are stabilised largely by weak bonds which can be broken or formed under the effects of energy released or taken up during substrate and modulator binding, the splitting of substrates to products etc. Another familiar example of the importance of weak bonds is in the case of double-stranded nucleic acids. The ability of double-stranded DNA to unwind during replication results from the fact that the inter-chain stabilisation energy is due to weak bonds which can rapidly and easily be broken at cell temperatures. Strong covalent bonds do, of course, provide a much greater degree of structural stability. However, biological molecules must also possess the flexibility of structure which only weak bonds are able to provide.

The threats imposed by temperature changes on weak-bond-dependent structures and processes are of two general sorts. First, because the enthalpies of weak bond formation (rupture) are so small (*Table 3.1*) minor changes in cell temperature may be sufficient to disrupt large numbers of important weak bonds. Increases and decreases in temperature may have adverse effects on weak-bond-dependent structures and processes in the sense that the formation of too many additional weak bonds, e.g. at low temperatures for hydrogen-bonded systems, may make the system too rigid for effective function.

The second mode of thermal perturbation of weak-bonded systems stems from the fact that the sign of the enthalpy change for bond formation differs among the various classes of weak bonds. Hydrogen-bond formation and the establishment of electrostatic interactions generally are exothermic processes (*Table 3.1*). Thus removing heat energy from the cell will stabilise these classes of weak bonds. Hydrophobic interactions form endothermically, so at reduced temperatures those structures and processes which rely heavily on hydrophobic interactions may be weakened (Brandts, 1967). The basis of this temperature dependence of hydrophobic interactions lies in the role played by changes in water structure during bond formation. When a hydrophobic group, e.g. an isoleucine side-chain, protrudes into water at the surface of a protein molecule, water molecules are thought to form a dense, highly-ordered 'iceberg' around the hydrophobic group (Brandts, 1967; Lewin, 1974). The water organised around the hydrophobic group has a lower entropy than the surrounding 'bulk' water, i.e. the accommodation of the hydrophobic group in water is energetically unfavourable on entropy grounds, and this entropy decrease serves as the driving force tending to lead to 'burial' of the hydrophobic group within the non-polar interior of the protein. The movement of the hydrophobic group from the exterior to the interior of the protein requires an enthalpy input, however, since the 'iceberg' of water molecules around the group must be melted before the group can move into the interior of the protein. Thus the net free energy change in this transfer process is the algebraic sum of a positive enthalpy change and a negative entropy term ($T\Delta S$). Note that as temperature is reduced, the $T\Delta S$ term becomes smaller, i.e. the favourable (negative) transfer free energy is reduced in absolute value.

Our reasons for dwelling in some detail on the thermodynamics of weak bond-temperature interactions are two-fold. First, it is obvious that a change in cell temperature will affect different weak-bond-dependent structures and processes in quite diverse manners. Systems which are largely reliant on hydrogen bonds, van der Waals' forces and electrostatic interactions will be disrupted at high temperatures and stabilised at low temperatures. Hydrophobic interactions will confer the opposite temperature sensitivities on a system.

A second important outcome of this analysis concerns a potential mechanism for temperature adaptation of weak-bond-dependent systems. If an organism must adapt to a decrease in cell temperature, there may be a selective advantage in replacing some hydrophobic interactions with, say, hydrogen bonds or electrostatic interactions. Warm adaptation might involve the opposite changes. Thus the availability of weak bonds with enthalpies of formation which differ in sign may provide organisms with an important source of adaptational raw material for effecting temperature-related changes in their cellular chemistry.

3.3 ENDOTHERMY IN THE MARINE ENVIRONMENT: PHYSIOLOGICAL AND ANATOMICAL AVENUES OF ESCAPE FROM THERMAL STRESS

3.3.1 Basic problems of endothermy in an aqueous environment

In view of the magnitudes and complexities of effects which result from changes in cell temperature, one would predict that organisms will benefit in general from keeping their cell temperatures relatively stable. Temperature regulation can be accomplished by several means and the simplest of these is behavioural. Many marine species undergo diurnal and/or seasonal migrations which greatly reduce the range of cell temperatures the organisms experience. However, the benefits which accrue from this strategy of thermal regulation must be balanced against a host of other environmental considerations. Thus, a habitat which offers a favourable thermal regime may lack the proper types and amounts of food required for optimal rates of growth and reproduction. An agreeable thermal habitat may not provide satisfactory breeding conditions. The density of predators may exceed that which can be tolerated. Because of the need to balance temperature considerations against these other environmental parameters, one can easily rationalise the selective advantages of anatomical and physiological adaptations which enable an organism to regulate its own body temperature and thus gain it the freedom to select its habitat on the basis of criteria other than temperature.

The ability to rely on one's own metabolically-generated heat for body temperature regulation is termed 'endothermy'. For non-mammalian aquatic organisms, the acquisition of an endothermic capability faces stiff obstacles since most aquatic species respire via gills or other membraneous surfaces which are bathed by large volumes of water. The exchange of gases across respiratory surfaces is several-fold slower than the rate of thermal equilibration, and since gas exchange must be given precedence over heat retention, virtually all of the heat gained by the circulatory fluids in rapidly metabolising tissues is exhausted to the surrounding water during gas exchange. Thus for marine ectotherms (poikilotherms, 'cold-blooded' organisms), the development of endothermic capabilities requires two distinct types of adaptation: (a) an ability to generate sufficient metabolic heat to keep the body temperature above ambient when necessary; and (b) a means for retaining this heat, or at least a major share of it, within the body when low ambient temperatures dictate a need for thermal regulation.

3.3.2 Mechanisms of heat generation

3.3.2.1 BASIC CONSIDERATIONS OF HEAT SOURCES IN METABOLISM

Since all organisms generate heat during metabolism, even unicellular species are potentially endothermic. However, considerations of surface-volume relationships, insulation abilities (which must be paired with a need for surfaces through which gases and solutes are exchanged with the surrounding water), and absolute rates of metabolic heat production all argue against the occurrence of endothermic abilities in all but large and/or rapidly metabolising organisms. In fact, in most endotherms we find that the heat produced during normal metabolic function must be supplemented by additional heat generated specifically for thermoregulatory purposes when cold stress is present.

In considering the likely sources for the generation of heat in thermogenic processes, we might at first predict that virtually any metabolic reaction which is exothermic could serve as a source of heat for thermal regulation. However, we find that the biochemical processes which have been harnessed specifically for thermogenic purposes are largely restricted to reactions involving the synthesis and degradation of ATP, reactions in which the enthalpy changes are very large. ATP-associated reactions of two fundamental sorts have become important in thermogenic processes. First, when the ATP synthesis reactions occurring during electron transport are uncoupled, the energy released by the electrons flowing towards oxygen is given off to the cell as heat. Second, we will see that other important thermogenic reactions utilise the energy released when large quantities of ATP are split to ADP and inorganic phosphate (P_i). These basic heat generating schemes have been reviewed by Prusiner and Poe (1968) and Hochachka (1974b).

The general adaptive strategy which is followed in thermogenic processes can be summarised thus: to liberate large quantities of heat when cold stress is present, the organism has learned to utilise metabolic reactions which are strongly exothermic and which, under ordinary circumstances, perform a metabolic role distinct from heat production. The development of all thermoregulatory schemes (*see Table 3.3*) thus appears to be based on the

Table 3.3 MECHANISMS OF THERMOGENESIS

I. *Enhanced splitting of ATP:*
   1. Shivering.
   2. Non-shivering thermogenesis (thyroid stimulated).
   3. 'Warming-up' exercises, e.g. wing movements by insects prior to flight.
   4. Metabolic 'short-circuits': the PFK/FDPase 'short circuit'.
   5. Activity *per se* in the course of normal activity.

II. *Uncoupled or loosely coupled respiration:* releasing energy as heat prior to ATP synthesis.
   1. Brown fat metabolism.

acquisition of the necessary regulatory mechanisms to enable pre-existing catalytic reactions to be selectively utilised for a new function, thermogenesis, when low temperatures dictate that heat production is of more critical importance than the normal function of the reactions.

In the following discussion of heat generation mechanisms, it will become apparent that most of the examples given are based on studies of terrestrial organisms. Such an approach may seem inappropriate in a volume which is concerned with marine organisms. However, aside from marine mammals and a small number of fish species (Carey *et al.*, 1971), mechanisms for heat production/retention have not received attention in marine species. Our intent is thus one of acquainting the reader with many of the fascinating 'tricks' used by terrestrial species to produce heat, hoping that the interested reader might consider examining certain marine species which, we feel, might be potential users of similar or identical metabolic adaptations.

3.3.2.2 BROWN ADIPOSE TISSUE

The only animal tissue known which is specialised for conducting the sole function of heat generation is brown adipose tissue (BAT). Found in hibernants and neonatal mammals, BAT serves as a highly important source of heat under such conditions as arousal from hibernation.

BAT consists largely of a supply of lipid fuel and the mitochondrial machinery required for lipid oxidation. It has been suggested that the generation of heat in BAT derives from two mechanisms. First, as shown in *Figure 3.2(a),* free fatty acids formed by lipase-catalysed breakdown of triglycerides may uncouple ATP synthesis from electron transport. The energy released during fatty oxidation is thus released as heat instead of being used to 'drive' ATP synthesis. Alternatively, hormonal effects on the plasma membrane of BAT may lead to a large-scale activation of ion pumping enzymes and, hence, to a major increase in ATP splitting *(Figure 3.2(b)).* Elevated ATP synthesis for 'driving' ion transport will also lead to a large increase in cellular heat production, since only a fraction of the energy released during fatty acid degradation will be trapped in ATP, even under

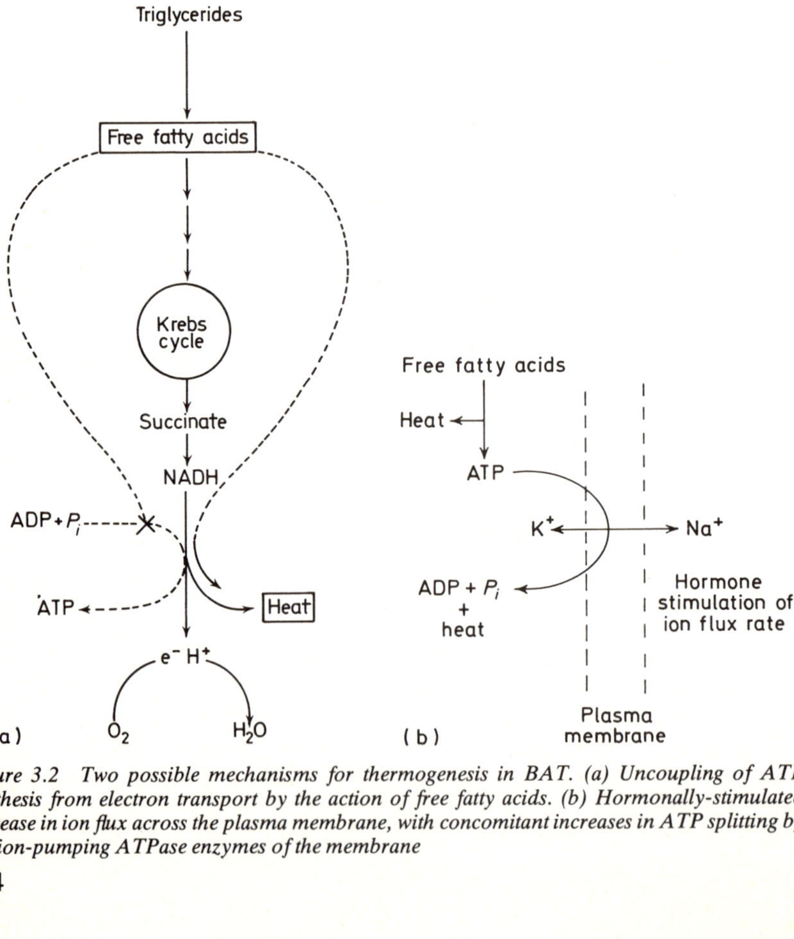

Figure 3.2 Two possible mechanisms for thermogenesis in BAT. (a) Uncoupling of ATP synthesis from electron transport by the action of free fatty acids. (b) Hormonally-stimulated increase in ion flux across the plasma membrane, with concomitant increases in ATP splitting by the ion-pumping ATPase enzymes of the membrane

conditions of tight coupling between electron transport and ATP synthesis. The contributions made by these two heat generation mechanisms in BAT are still under active investigation.

The occurrence of BAT in marine organisms other than mammals has not been investigated. Study of warm-bodied fishes would seem an especially relevant area of investigation, for the abilities of certain tuna fishes to maintain retinal and brain temperatures above ambient (Stevens and Fry, 1971) may indicate that localised sources of heat generation are present to warm these small, relatively inactive tissues. It would be intriguing to find that a non-mammalian organism had evolutionally converged on a BAT-like mechanism for heat generation. Such an achievement does not appear extraordinarily difficult in a basic 'engineering' sense, for the major advance required for the development of a BAT type of metabolism is the provision of a regulatory mechanism to uncouple electron transport from ATP synthesis — a feat which in mammals is accomplished with apparent simplicity by free fatty acids.

3.3.2.3 METABOLIC SHORT-CIRCUITS

The utilisation of an exothermic reaction for work under some circumstances and for thermogenesis under cold-stress conditions is not limited to the electron transport system. As stated above, any reaction or reaction sequence in which large amounts of heat can be released can serve as a potential thermogenic site, provided that the organism is able to use the reaction(s) for heat generation when, and only when, additional heat is required. An example of such an adaptation involving a pair of reactions normally associated with glycolytic and gluconeogenic processes has recently been discovered: the metabolic 'short-circuit' in fructosediphosphate (FDP) metabolism in bumblebees (genus *Bombus*) (Newsholme *et al.*, 1972; Clark *et al.*, 1973).

The metabolism of FDP involves different enzymes for synthesis and breakdown of this metabolite. FDP synthesis from fructose-6-phosphate occurs via the strongly exergonic phosphofructokinase (PFK) reaction:

$$\text{F6P} + \text{ATP} \rightleftharpoons \text{FDP} + \text{ADP}$$

Because the equilibrium position of this reaction is strongly to the right, reversal of the PFK reaction is largely precluded under cellular conditions. A second enzyme is required to reform F6P, namely FDPase, which catalyses the reaction:

$$\text{FDP} + H_2O \rightleftharpoons \text{F6P} + P_i$$

If PFK and FDPase are both working simultaneously in a tissue, their net achievement is the breakdown of ATP to ADP, i.e. a metabolic 'short-circuit' at this point in metabolism. Thus, in strongly glycolytic tissues, FDPase levels usually are very low, whereas in gluconeogenic tissues such as liver and kidney cortex, FDPase levels are high.

It was very surprising, therefore, to find that bumblebees contained high concentrations of PFK and FDPase in their flight musculature (Newsholme *et al.*, 1972). The high levels of FDPase in this glycolysing muscle seemed to establish a situation in which the glycolytic activity needed to support flight movements could be short-circuited. However, the joint presence of FDPase and PFK also creates a favourable thermogenic potential for this tissue, assuming that the bee can turn-on FDPase only when additional heat is required, e.g. during a warm-up period prior to flight at low ambient temperatures.

Clark *et al.* (1973) have elucidated the mechanism which is involved in the regulation of FDPase activity in bumblebee flight muscle. When the bee is stationary and muscle temperatures are below the levels which permit flight, FDPase and PFK are highly active. Under these conditions the muscle is splitting large amounts of ATP and thereby generating significant quantities of heat. As the muscle warms to flight temperature and muscular activity commences, calcium ions are released from the sarcoplasmic reticulum. Ca^{2+} strongly inhibits bumblebee FDPase, and this single regulatory effect appears sufficient to turn-on and turn-off FDPase function according to the thermal needs of the insect.

We do not know if this type of thermogenic mechanism is present in marine organisms. However, as in the case of BAT, the raw material for developing the thermogenic system is already largely present in most organisms. Have marine mammals or warm-bodied fishes 'discovered' the required regulatory switches to put this mechanism to use?

3.3.2.4 ATPase heat generators: thermogenesis via the sodium pump

An alternative means for releasing large amounts of heat via ATP splitting is to increase the rate of a physiological process in which large amounts of ATP are normally utilised. The largest single use of ATP in metabolism is in the maintenance of ion disequilibria, e.g. the concentration gradients of sodium and potassium ions between the extra- and intracellular fluids. In mammals, maintaining these disequilibria may require as much as 45 per cent of the energy generated under basal metabolic conditions (Prosser, 1973). Thus, a potential for increasing the activities of the ion pump ATPases during thermogenesis would seem to confer a significant selective advantage to an organism. In particular, this mechanism for heat production is one that is present in *all* cells, so unlike BAT, for example, ion ATPase heat generation mechanisms could directly warm each region of the body.

Ismail-Beigi and Edelman (1970) have presented evidence that ion ATPase generated heat is of major importance in what is termed 'non-shivering thermogenesis'. When a mammal is exposed to low ambient temperatures, piloerection and shivering are the first responses geared to increasing heat production and retention. After a number of days at reduced temperatures, shivering ceases, and heat production shifts to non-shivering types of mechanism. Non-shivering thermogenesis has been known for many years to be dependent on the release of thyroid hormones (thyroxine and triiodothyronine). However, the mechanism(s) of action of these hormones has remained a mystery until recently. It now appears that the action of thyroid hormones in non-shivering thermogenesis is the stimulation of membrane-bound Na–K ATPase enzymes. The thermogenic effects of these hormones can be blocked by the Na–K ATPase inhibitor ouabain. Additional evidence that thyroid hormone-mediated non-shivering thermogenesis involves Na–K ATPases is the finding that transmembrane K^+ and Na^+ gradients are increased in thyroid hormone treated tissues (Ismail-Beigi and Edelman, 1970). A further effect of these changes in ion concentration might involve direct ion activation of enzymes involved in energy metabolism. K^+ is a key activator, and Na^+ is an inhibitor, of the glycolytic enzyme, pyruvate kinase (Somero and Hochachka, 1968). Thus, the observed changes in intracellular ion concentrations could lead to stimulation of glycolysis and further heat production.

As in the case of BAT metabolism and metabolic 'short-circuits', the catalytic machinery for generating heat via ion pumps is a trait present in all marine organisms. The utilisation of this potential is known only in mammals, of course.

The phylogeny of endothermy has recently been discussed in a speculative fashion by Stevens (1973), who proposes that the present day mammalian thermogenic systems using ion ATPase-derived heat have arisen from hormonal and osmoregulatory 'raw material' already present in fishes. His article can be consulted for a good review of these topics.

3.3.3 Heat retention mechanisms

Even if an organism possesses the ability to generate large quantities of heat via metabolic schemes like those discussed above, regulation of body temperature will still not be possible unless the flow of heat to the environment is closely regulated. This statement of course applies to warm- and cold-blooded organisms, whether terrestrial or aquatic.

The most familiar mechanism for regulating heat flow between the body and the environment is superficial insulation. Mammals, birds, and certain insects (Heinrich, 1974), exhibit excellent abilities to contain metabolic heat within their bodies through creation of dead-air-spaces around much of the body surface. However, for aquatic species this means of reducing heat flow is virtually eliminated, for obvious physical reasons. Marine mammals, therefore, have shifted their superficial insulative layer within the body, employing a thick layer of fat (blubber) in place of a deep layer of dry hair.

Marine ecotherms such as fishes encounter much more difficult problems in regulating heat flow. Superficial insulation, in itself, could not be an adequate mechanism for heat retention since the major site of heat exchange with the environment is at the gills. Thus, for a marine fish the critical problem to solve involves the prevention of heat flow from the rapidly metabolising tissues such as the swimming musculature to the respiratory surfaces.

The means by which this control of heat flow is accomplished in warm-bodied fishes such as tuna species (Carey *et al.*, 1971) are illustrated in *Figure 3.3*. Counter-current heat exchangers, which of course are also present in birds and mammals, all have a common anatomy: warmed blood passing from actively metabolising tissues is brought into close contact with cooled blood arriving from the gills (or, in the case of birds and mammals, from the cooler extremities such as the legs and feet). The bed of fine, closely intertwined capillaries, the rete mirabile, of the heat exchanger permits a rapid and nearly quantitative transfer of heat from the venous circulation to the arterial circulation.

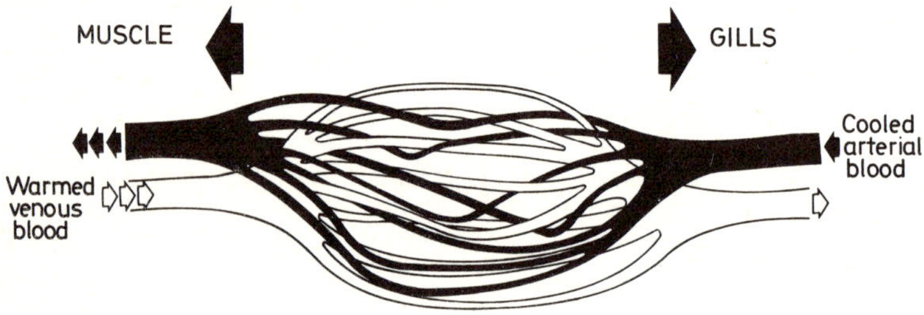

Figure 3.3 The anatomy of a counter-current heat exchanger. Warmed venous blood passes into intimate contact with cooled arterial blood arriving from the gills, in the case of a fish system. Thermal equilibration occurs in the rete mirabile, the fine capillary bed where venous and arterial systems come into contact. (After Hochachka and Somero, 1973; courtesy W. B. Saunders & Co.)

Several large and rapidly swimming tuna and shark species are now known to be capable of holding their deep-body temperatures several degree Celsius above ambient temperatures through use of such heat exchangers (Carey *et al.,* 1971; Stevens and Fry, 1973). Furthermore, the large bluefin tuna is not only endothermic, but in addition is impressively homeothermic, i.e. it can not only generate enough heat and control its release to maintain body temperatures above ambient, but it can also hold its body temperature at a relatively stable level. This finding implies that the flow of blood through the heat exchanger can be regulated to allow only a needed amount of heat to be retained within the organism. The major advantage of homeothermy for this species has been suggested earlier in this chapter: through the acquisition of homeothermy, an organism gains the ability to select its habitat on the basis of other than thermal criteria. Thus, the bluefin tuna can breed in the tropics, where warm temperatures may prove advantageous for the non-homeothermic young, and yet journey into high latitude waters during non-breeding periods to feed in these food-rich environs.

Less well understood are the mechanisms which help to enable tuna species to maintain their brain and retinal temperatures at levels above ambient (Stevens and Fry, 1971). As we have suggested above, these organs may offer us examples of heat generation mechanisms similar to those found in endothermic insects and mammals.

We now turn our attention to marine species which are unable to regulate their body temperatures through anatomical and physiological means. True ectotherms, which represent the vast majority of marine species and individuals, illustrate the magnitudes and complexities of biochemical adaptations which are required when the chemistry of the cell cannot be shielded against the effects of changes in ambient temperature.

3.4 ECTOTHERMY

3.4.1 Temperature compensation of metabolic rates

Ectothermic organisms which are unable to control their cell temperatures often exhibit considerable degrees of temperature-independence in their metabolic rates. Whereas one would predict that each 10°C change in cell temperature would lead to an approximately two-fold change in metabolic rate, this expectation often is not realised, i.e. many ectotherms exhibit good abilities to compensate their metabolic rates for changes in temperature (Prosser, 1974).

Typical patterns of metabolic temperature compensation are illustrated in *Figure 3.4*. Observe that metabolic compensation may occur over three time courses. Species evolutionally adapted to different temperatures are often much more similar in their rates of whole organism and *in vitro* tissue respiration (Peiss and Field, 1950; Scholander *et al.,* 1953; Wohlschlag, 1964; Somero, Giese and Wohlschlag, 1968; Prosser, 1974) and growth (Dehnel. 1955) than would be expected on the basis of simple Q_{10} relationships. Similar compensatory patterns have been observed for shorter-term, phenotypic acclimation processes.

A note of caution must be sounded in making interspecific and interpopulation comparisons of metabolic rates, however. In the case of whole organism oxygen consumption, the observed metabolic rate will be strongly influenced by the physiological, e.g. nutritional, and behavioural states of the organisms. Since resting metabolism may be only 10% of active metabolism, as measured by oxygen consumption rates, the activity level of the specimens is an especially critical variable. Holeton (1974) has criticised past attempts to perform broad, interspecific comparisons of fish respiration, basing his criticisms on the points made above. His review should be consulted for a succinct resumé of the uncertainty principles inherent in such studies. What these criticisms suggest in terms of the correct experimental procedures for comparing true differences in metabolic levels among species is that tissue respiration studies may provide a more valid index of interspecific differences in metabolic rates than whole organism studies. Excised tissues obviously will not be prone to generate artifacts resulting from behavioural disturbances.

Lastly, some organisms have been found to exhibit complete, or nearly complete, temperature-independence in certain rate processes (*Figure 3.4 (b)*; Gordon, 1968; Newell, 1969; Newell and Pye, 1970a, 1970b, 1971). This pattern of 'immediate' or 'instantaneous' temperature compensation

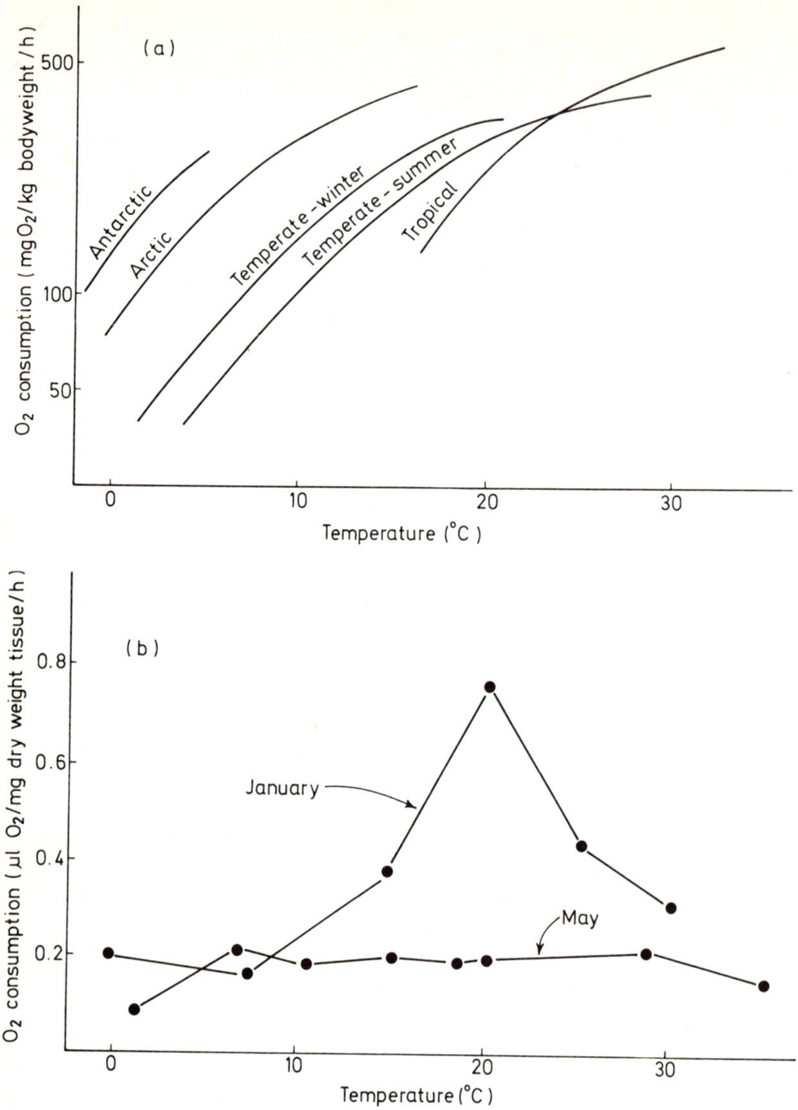

Figure 3.4 (a) Metabolic compensation to temperature. The relationship between temperature and rate of oxygen consumption (standard metabolism) for fishes adapted or acclimated to different temperatures (from Hochachka and Somero, 1973; modified after Brett, 1971). Temperature compensation in rates of oxygen consumption is found for whole organism respiration and tissue respiration (see text). (b) The effect of temperature on the standard (non-active) rate of oxygen consumption of the winkle, Littorina littorea, *acclimatised to temperatures of approximately 4°C (January) and 15°C (May). Note that the rate of oxygen consumption is essentially independent of temperature over the range of temperatures the animal is apt to experience at each season. (Data from Newell and Pye, 1970; figure from Hochachka and Somero, 1973; courtesy W. B. Saunders & Co.)*

seems most characteristic of ectotherms which experience very rapid and often quite large changes in cell temperature, e.g. intertidal invertebrates which are exposed to air during low tide (e.g. *see* Newell, 1969 and Chapter 1).

3.4.1.1 POTENTIAL BIOCHEMICAL MECHANISMS OF RATE COMPENSATION

Since the regulation of metabolic rates must of necessity involve control of the velocities of many enzymic reactions, it is logical to begin our analysis with a discussion of the manners by which the activities of enzymes can be turned-up and turned-down in response to needs for different amounts of metabolism. There would appear to be four distinct ways of achieving these ends:

1. Changes in enzyme concentration. For temperature compensation purposes this would involve decreasing enzyme concentrations during warm adaptation and increasing concentrations during cold adaptation.
2. Changes in substrate and cofactor concentration. Increased availability of substrates and cofactors could boost metabolic rates at low temperatures, for example.
3. Modulation of enzyme activities.
4. Formation of new enzyme variants with different catalytic efficiencies. Low temperature compensation could be achieved through synthesis of new enzyme forms which exhibit enhanced abilities to catalyse reactions on a per enzyme molecule basis.

3.4.1.1.1 Metabolic compensation via changes in enzyme concentration

Our familiarity with enzyme induction phenomena in bacteria and eukaryotic organisms might lead us to predict that the major, if not sole, way of adjusting metabolic rates in temperature compensatory manners is through changes in enzyme concentration. In terms of the demands placed on enzyme systems, a change in cell temperature is analogous to a change in, for example, metabolite availability. Both alterations in the cellular chemistry call for changes in the amounts of enzymic activity present in the cell.

Before discussing the available data concerning temperature-dependent changes in enzyme concentration, we wish to consider briefly some of the limitations of this strategy of adaptation. First, changing enzyme concentrations to adjust metabolism in temperature compensatory manners seems unlikely in the case of short-term temperature compensations as might occur, for example, on a diurnal basis. The 'immediate' compensation found in certain organisms (*Figure 3.4(b)*) almost certainly cannot result from a rapid change in enzyme concentration.

Changing enzyme concentrations also seems a sub-optimal strategy for evolutionary temperature adaptation. If an organism can develop new enzyme variants over many generations which function better at its new thermal regime, it seemingly could avoid having to synthesise relatively large quantities of enzymes during cold adaptation. Thus, given evolutionary time spans to effect temperature compensation, it would seem advantageous for an organism to develop 'better' enzymes, rather than rely on increasing enzyme concentrations. [The antithesis of this argument, namely the 'advantage' of developing 'poorer' catalysts during warm adaptation may seem absurd at first sight. However, as we discuss below and elsewhere (Low and Somero, 1974; Somero, 1975a), such a seemingly absurd type of adaptation does appear reasonable when considered in the context of the overall stresses on both structure and function which high temperature imposes on an enzyme.]

Another questionable aspect of temperature compensation via changing enzyme concentrations derives from the fact that a particular enzyme may function well over only a part of the temperature range experienced by an organism. For example, if an enzyme loses a great deal of its catalytic and/or regulatory abilities at high or low extremes of temperature, mere adjustment of enzyme concentration does not appear an optimal mechanism of adaptation. This consideration seems especially relevant in the case of evolutionary processes.

One can also question the feasibility of adjusting *all* enzyme concentrations during temperature adaptation. On the one hand, the solvent capacity of the cell is finite (Atkinson, 1969), and there are only so many enzyme binding sites on membranes and other cellular structures to which enzymes are attached. Secondly, increased enzyme synthesis at low temperatures would have to occur under conditions of reduced metabolic rates, so compensation via increased enzyme concentrations would probably take a great deal of time, e.g. several days to a few weeks. These, in fact, are the typical time courses observed for cold acclimation of enzymic activities (Sidell *et al.,* 1973).

Although temperature compensation via changes in enzyme concentration appears to have limitations, there are many data which suggest that the process of temperature acclimation does involve major alterations in the amounts of enzymes present in the cells (Hazel and Prosser, 1974). Our qualification, 'suggests', is used since in virtually all studies to be discussed, enzymic activities, not enzyme concentrations, have been estimated. The reason for this experimental approach no doubt lies in the difficulties inherent in measuring enzyme concentrations in the cell (*see* Schimke, 1969). Thus, most workers have been content to use the activities of enzymes (usually measured using supernatant fractions of tissue homogenates) as indicators of changing concentrations during acclimation. However, one must remember that an observed change in enzymic activity can result from any of the four factors listed above, at the beginning of this section.

The many studies of enzymic activity changes as a function of thermal acclimation which have been performed are excellently reviewed by Hazel and Prosser (1974), so in this chapter we shall attempt to provide only a general view of these studies. A first point worth stressing is that there are virtually no data bearing on the question of whether enzyme concentration changes are important in evolutionary temperature compensation or short-term 'immediate' compensation. One recent study (Wilson, Somero and Prosser, 1974) has shown that for two closely related species of the genus *Sebastes,* the species which lives in cool waters below the thermocline (*S. miniatus*) exhibits 70% higher cytochrome oxidase activities than a shallow water species, *S. auriculatus,* which is subject to higher cell temperatures. However, there has been no systematic study of enzyme activity or concentration levels in marine ectotherms from different latitudes. Likewise, there have been no studies of possible diurnal changes in enzyme concentrations in organisms exposed to daily changes in temperature. As we argued above, however, changes in enzyme concentration seem a sub-optimal means for temperature adaptation to both evolutionary and short-term changes in temperature.

One broad generalisation which seems possible on the basis of available data on enzymic activities in differently-acclimated ectotherms is that the enzymes involved in the primary pathways of energy metabolism, notably the glycolytic sequence and the Krebs citric acid cycle and electron transport system, tend to display at least partial compensation to changes in temperature (Hazel and Prosser, 1974). In view of the observed compensations in whole organism and tissue-level oxygen consumption rates, this finding is not surprising.

Although temperature compensation in rates of oxygen consumption and ATP generating enzymic pathways is significant, in most cases compensation to reduced temperatures is not complete, i.e. at their respective acclimation temperatures, cold-acclimated individuals frequently have lower metabolic and enzymic rates than warm-acclimated individuals (e.g. *see Figure 3.4(a)*). We shall discuss the implications of this finding later in this chapter.

Another common observation recorded in studies of enzymic activity changes during temperature acclimation is that the relative activities of different metabolic pathways change during acclimation. Adjusting to a new habitat temperature thus may involve changes in the extents to which different pathways contribute to metabolism as well as changes in total metabolic flow through these pathways. These qualitative changes have been termed 'metabolic reorganisations' (Hochachka, 1967).

One of the most characteristic metabolic reorganisations involves the metabolism of glucose-6-phosphate (Hochachka, 1967). G-6-P metabolism is complex, since this metabolite exists at a critical metabolic branchpoint. Catabolism of G-6-P may occur via the glycolytic series or via the hexose monophosphate pathway (the pentose shunt). Alternatively, G-6-P may be split to free glucose and P_i by the enzyme glucose-6-phosphatase. Free glucose may then be transported out of the cell, e.g. from the liver to the blood. Lastly, glucose-phosphate may be channelled towards glycogen synthesis. Because of the likelihood that a change in temperature may shift the relative needs of the organism for these different patterns of glucose-6-phosphate metabolism, one might predict that the relative abilities of these different pathways to compete for G-6-P will vary with acclimation temperature.

The major shift in G-6-P metabolism during cold acclimation is an increased channelling of this metabolite into the hexose monophosphate pathway, away from glycolysis. Even though the activities of both pathways may be increased in cold-acclimated ectotherms (Hazel and Prosser, 1974), hexose monophosphate pathway enzymes are frequently observed to display the greater increase in activity. What does the observed increase (Hochachka and Hayes, 1962) in glucose-6-phosphate metabolism via the hexose monophosphate pathway mean in terms of temperature adaptation? An answer to this question can be proposed on the basis of the differing roles played by the glycolytic sequence and the hexose monophosphate pathway. Glycolysis has the primary function of generating ATP and substrates for the oxidative reactions of the Krebs cycle. The hexose monophosphate pathway, in contrast, is not a system for supplying ATP, but instead is a major source of important intermediates and reducing power (NADPH) for biosynthetic processes. The pentose sugars produced by this pathway are important in nucleotide synthesis, and the NADPH is of course the primary source of hydrogen for reductive steps in biosynthesis, e.g. reduction of fatty acids. The reorganisation of G-6-P metabolism during temperature acclimation therefore may reflect an important shift towards biosynthetic reactions at low temperatures. This enhanced biosynthetic ability may be directed towards the synthesis of increased amounts of enzymes for temperature compensatory purposes. At least this function could be important during the initial phases of temperature compensation. Prolonged reorganisation of this type could indicate that, at reduced temperatures, an organism can afford to direct more of its energy into processes such as growth than at higher temperatures. Indeed, there are many excellent studies which indicate that growth of fishes is faster at intermediate-to-low temperatures than at high temperatures (Brett, 1971). It is not possible currently to state why this is the case, but reductions in activity levels and, perhaps, in the need for energy to maintain ion disequilibria (Maetz and Evans, 1972; Motais and Isaia, 1972), may free additional energy for biosynthetic reactions such as those involved in protein and lipid synthesis.

A final interpretation of the biosynthetically-directed metabolic reorganisation which occurs during cold acclimation does not involve temperature compensation *per se,* but instead is phrased in terms of season-specific changes in metabolism. Thus, a shift towards hexose monophosphate pathway activity would seem an appropriate response for an organism which undergoes gametogenesis, especially egg production, during the cold season. In this context, metabolic reorganisation in response to changing temperature can be viewed as a process which is triggered by temperature but not directed primarily towards overcoming adverse effects of reduced temperature (Somero *et al.,* 1968).

Metabolic reorganisation also involves the 'inverse' compensation of certain enzymic activities (Hazel and Prosser, 1974), i.e. for some enzymes activities are greater in warm- than in cold-acclimated individuals. According to Hazel and Prosser (1974), this pattern of compensation is characteristic of enzymes that are involved in detoxification processes. Increased activities of peroxidases and esterases in warm-acclimated individuals is viewed as adaptive owing to the fact that the higher metabolic rates evident in warm-acclimated organisms (at their higher acclimation temperature) are apt to lead to the production of higher amounts of toxic end-products. It would appear, using this line of reasoning, that the acceleration in velocities of these detoxification reactions as temperature rises is not sufficient to cope with the increased rate of production of toxic end-products at higher temperatures. Whatever the correct biological interpretation of 'inverse' compensation is, it has become abundantly clear that temperature compensation is not effected by uni-vectorial adjustment of all enzymic reaction velocities. Different cell temperatures impose quantitative and qualitative changes in metabolic demands.

If we are willing to accept the interpretation that enzymic activity changes are the result of changes in enzyme concentration, we can then consider the question as to how an ectothermic organism can vary its enzyme concentrations in response to alterations in cell temperature. Two mechanisms are possible. First, rates of enzyme synthesis can be adaptively varied in response to temperature change. Second, rates of protein degradation can be adaptively altered. This second mechanism would seem to offer the cold-acclimating ectotherm the possibility of a 'free ride'. Thus, if the activities of proteolytic enzymes are reduced by a fall in cell temperature, rates of protein degradation may be reduced as well. This state of affairs could be of considerable help in promoting increased concentrations of enzymes, even if low temperature also reduced rates of protein synthesis.

On closer analysis, this simplified mechanism for enzymic temperature compensation is found to be lacking in important characteristics. One of its failures is its lack of specificity. A non-specific, general reduction in protein degradation rates could not lead to the reorganisation of enzymic activities discussed above. Thus, at least some control via synthetic reactions is mandatory for effecting the observed patterns of metabolic compensation (unless we are willing to make the questionable assumption that the enzymes whose activities are relatively low in cold-acclimated individuals are especially susceptible to degradation at low temperatures).

An even stronger objection to the hypothesis that decreased rates of protein degradation could play a role in cold acclimation is based on current theories of the mechanisms involved in the control of protein catabolism (Schimke, 1969). The rates at which proteins are degraded are not determined primarily by the activities of proteolytic enzymes, i.e. the half-life of a protein does not depend on the concentration of proteolytic enzymes in its immediate vicinity in any simple way. Instead, the rate of protein degradation appears to be established primarily by the rate at which proteins are *rendered susceptible* to the action of proteolytic enzymes. Factors in the environment of the enzyme which reduce its susceptibility to degradation will prolong its half-life. For example, the presence of substrate is known to stabilise the higher orders of structure of an enzyme, e.g. its conformation, and to extend its half-life (Schimke, 1969). Enzymes bound to other cellular structures may be more stable than when they are free in solution. The presence of modulators, cofactors and inorganic ions which can alter protein structure may influence the half-life of an enzyme. All of these considerations argue against the notion that decreased temperatures will uniformly reduce rates of protein degradation. Furthermore, the finding that many enzymes are cold labile (Beyer, 1972) indicates that reduced temperature may increase the rates of degradation of many proteins, especially multimeric ones. Temperature-dependent changes in protein stability could also result from temperature-dependent changes in the ligand binding ability of an enzyme (*see below*). Enhanced substrate binding at low temperatures might stabilise the structure of an enzyme, for example.

Experimental data are consistent with the view that rates of protein degradation are not a strict function of temperature. In a study of protein degradation rates in the eurythermal estuarine fish *Gillichthys mirabilis* (Somero and Doyle, 1973), only the proteins of gill tissue were degraded more rapidly at increasing temperatures. No temperature effects on degradation rates were observed in liver and brain, and in muscle degradation rates were higher at low temperatures. These findings indicate that rates of protein degradation do not follow simple Q_{10} relationships, but instead are determined by a complex, interacting set of factors, including protein structural parameters and physiological considerations (Somero and Doyle, 1973).

We therefore conclude that the apparent changes which occur in enzyme concentration during temperature acclimation are largely a manifestation of highly specific changes in protein synthetic and gene regulatory activities. This conclusion is supported by several studies which have shown that during cold acclimation the nucleic acid metabolism (Das, 1967) and the protein synthetic processes (Haschemeyer, 1968, 1969a, 1969b; Smith, Colombo and Munn, 1968) of ectotherms change in manners consistent with the view that rates of enzyme synthesis vary inversely with acclimation temperature. These studies are reviewed in detail by Hazel and Prosser (1974).

To conclude this discussion of enzyme concentration changes as a mechanism of temperature compensation, we can offer the following brief summary of the current state of knowledge. Changes in enzyme concentration, as opposed to activity changes, have been unequivocally demonstrated in only one multicellular organism during cold acclimation (Wilson, 1973). All other activity data cannot be unambiguously interpreted. Where alterations in enzymic activity are noted, one finds a diversity of responses to changing temperature. We argue that this 'reorganisation' of metabolism may reflect altered metabolic demands, in a qualitative sense as well as a quantitative sense, when temperature changes. Furthermore, the specificity displayed in enzymic activity changes suggests that precise gene activation mechanisms are critical in temperature acclimation.

We must now consider an alternative means for adapting to different temperatures, an adaptive process which will be shown to be critically important when the effect of temperature on the functional and structural properties of an enzyme are so great as to preclude adaptation via simple upwards or downwards adjustments of enzyme concentrations.

3.4.1.1.2 Temperature-related changes in catalytic efficiency

The alternative mechanisms for adjusting rates of enzymic activity to compensate for changes in temperature all involve adjustments in the rates at which single enzyme molecules catalyse their reactions. These changes in rate on a per enzyme molecule basis can be achieved by altering the inherent catalytic efficiency of an enzyme, or by changing the substrate binding ability of the enzyme. These two mechanisms will be seen to play important roles in both evolutionary and short-term ('immediate') temperature compensation processes.

The inherent catalytic efficiency of an enzyme can be measured in two ways. First, one can determine the *substrate turnover number* of the enzyme, the number of substrate molecules converted to product per unit time per mole of enzyme. This is a direct measure of how well an enzyme conducts its given catalytic role. A second means for estimating catalytic efficiency involves measurement of the thermodynamic activation parameters of an enzymic reaction. Since the free energy of activation ($\Delta G^{\ddagger}$) of an enzymic process indicates how extensively an enzyme has reduced the 'energy barrier' to a metabolic reaction, $\Delta G^{\ddagger}$ will be inversely proportional to the substrate turnover number of the catalyst (*Figure 3.5*).

For many years biologists have speculated about the possibility that organisms with low cell temperatures might possess enzymes with greater abilities to reduce the energy barriers to a given reaction than the homologous enzymes of organisms such as mammals which have relatively high cell temperatures (Hochachka and Somero, 1972, 1973). These speculations generally were phrased in terms of the Arrhenius activation energy (Ea), an enthalpy-derived parameter. Inverse correlations between the magnitudes of Ea and the cell temperatures of organisms have been observed in many cases (Hochachka and Somero, 1972; Low, Bada and Somero, 1973). However, since the true measure of the ability of an enzyme to drive a reaction is the free energy of activation, which equals the activation enthalpy ($\Delta H^{\ddagger}$) minus the absolute temperature times the activation entropy ($\Delta S^{\ddagger}$), it is obvious that Ea (or $\Delta H^{\ddagger}$) cannot provide a quantitative measure of enzymic efficiency unless the magnitude of $\Delta S^{\ddagger}$ is also known.

Because measurement of $\Delta S^{\ddagger}$ values necessitates knowledge of the number of enzyme molecules present in the assay system (Low *et al.*, 1973), information which in turn is dependent on prior purification and characterisation (e.g. molecular weight) of an enzyme, there have been few studies in which the effort has been taken to determine all three activation parameters for different homologues of a single enzymic reaction. Most of the available data are given in *Table 3.4*. One conclusion is obvious: the enzymes of low cell temperature species, e.g. marine fishes and invertebrates, are more efficient catalysts than the homologous enzymes of birds and mammals. For example, the M_4-LDH reaction of a tuna species proceeds three times as rapidly at 5°C as the homologous reaction of birds and mammals.

Differences in catalytic efficiency appear related to the adaptation temperatures of the organisms, not merely to phylogenetic status. This is most clearly shown in the case of pyruvate kinases (*Table 3.4*; Low and

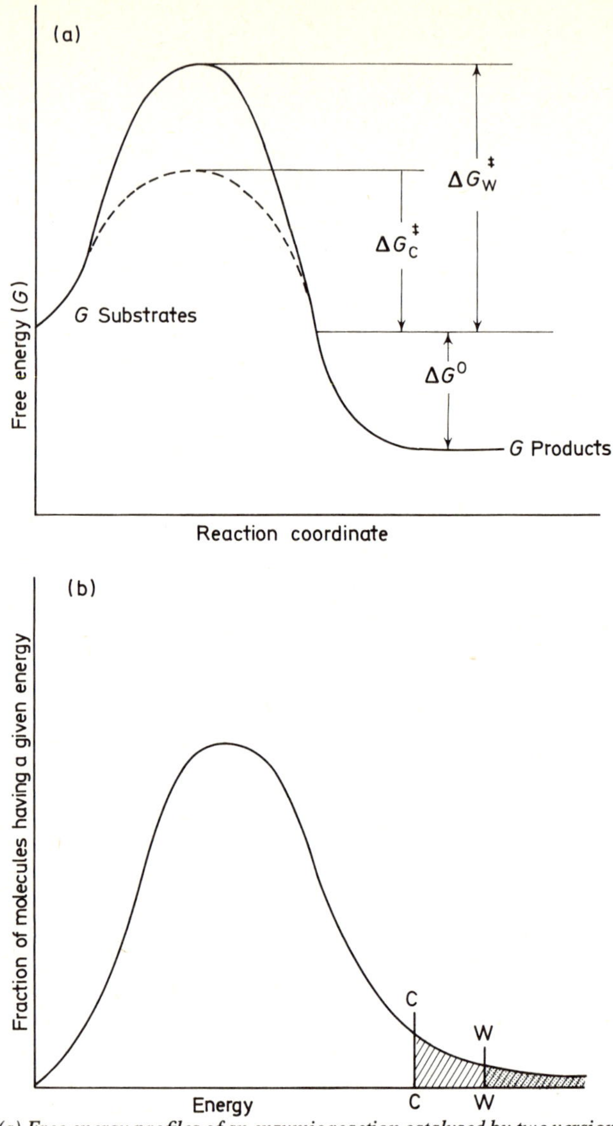

Figure 3.5 (a) Free energy profiles of an enzymic reaction catalysed by two versions of the same enzyme which differ in their abilities to reduce the free energy of activation ($\Delta G^{\ddagger}$) of the reaction, i.e. the energy which must be added to raise the ground-state enzyme-substrate complex to the activated (transition) state. Whereas the chemistry of the substrates and products determines the standard free energy change (ΔG^0) of the reaction, i.e. the equilibrium state of the system, enzyme C($\Delta G_C{}^{\ddagger}$) drives the reaction at a much faster rate than enzyme W ($\Delta G_W{}^{\ddagger}$), indicating that the rate of approach to equilibrium is faster with the more efficient enzyme. (b) An energy distribution (see Figure 3.1) illustrating the effect which reductions in activation free energy have on the velocity of a reaction at a constant temperature. The less efficient enzyme lowers the energy barrier to the reaction to the value indicated by line W—W; with this enzyme only molecules under the stippled portion of the curve are reactive. Enzyme C (activation energy indicated by line C—C) reduces the energy barrier to the extent that all molecules (enzyme-substrate complexes) with energies in the shaded region of the curve are reactive. (After Hochachka and Somero, 1973; courtesy W. B. Saunders & Co.)

Table 3.4 CATALYTIC ACTIVATION PARAMETERS (ACTIVATION FREE ENERGIES, $\Delta G^{\ddagger}$; ENTHALPIES, $\Delta H^{\ddagger}$; AND ENTROPIES, $\Delta S^{\ddagger}$) FOR HOMOLOGOUS ENZYMIC REACTIONS OF SPECIES ADAPTED TO DIFFERENT TEMPERATURES

	Cell temperature range	V_{max}[2]	$\Delta H^{\ddagger}$[3] (cal/mole)	$\Delta S^{\ddagger}$[3] (entropy units)	$\Delta G^{\ddagger}$[3] (cal/mole)
PYRUVATE KINASES[1]					
Chicken	39°	205			
5°			17 450	13.4	13 720
30°			11 100	−8.0	13 520
Rabbit	37°	200			
5°			15 000	5.3	13 640
30°			11 500	−6.7	13 530
Bufo marinus (toad)	25–32°	225			
5°			14 450	3.5	13 490
30°			11 350	−7.0	13 460
Mugil cephalus (mullet fish)	18–30°	245			
5°			13 200	−0.5	13 330
30°			10 950	−8.1	13 410
Scorpaena gutatta (fish)	8–17°	305			
5°			13 150	−0.6	13 320
30°			11 150	−7.0	13 280
Trematomus borchgrevinki (Antarctic fish)	−2°				
5°			11 700		
30°			11 700		

Table 3.4 *continued*

	Assay temperature	V_{max}[2]	$\Delta H^{\ddagger}$ (cal/mole)	$\Delta S^{\ddagger}$ (entropy units)	$\Delta G^{\ddagger}$ (cal/mole)
M_4-LACTATE DEHYDROGENASES[4]					
Rabbit	5°	95	12 525	−2.5	13 230
	35°	958	12 525	−2.5	13 310
Chicken	5°	168	10 500	−8.7	12 920
	30°	1184	10 500	−8.7	13 180
Tuna	5	355	8 775	−13.4	12 500
	35°	1846	8 775	−13.4	12 900
Halibut	5°	355	8 700	−13.7	12 500
	35°	1826	8 700	−13.7	12 910
D-GLYCERALDEHYDE-3-PHOSPHATE DEHYDROGENASES[4]					
Rabbit	5°	6.1	15 300	11.4	18 450
	35°	180	14 900	11.3	18 400
Lobster	5°	22.7	14 550	−2.2	13 950
	35°	220	14 800	−2.9	13 900
Cod	5°	18.5	14 700	−2.6	13 950
	35°	225	14 800	−2.9	13 900
MUSCLE GLYCOGEN PHOSPHORYLASE-b[4]					
Rabbit	0°	0.8	15 950	17.2	20 650
	30°	60	15 200	17.8	20 600
Lobster	0°	4.5	15.050	1.1	15 350
	30°	70.8	15 100	0.8	15 300

[1] Data from Low and Somero (1976)
[2] μmoles substrate converted to product/mg enzyme/min at an assay temperature of 25°C
[3] Except for the PK of the Antarctic fish, *Trematomus borchgrevinki,* the PK's existed in two temperature-dependent conformational states. The transition temperatures ranged between 20 and 26°C, depending on the species (5°C values are for the low temperature conformation of PK; 30°C values are for the high temperature conformer)
[4] Data from Low and Somero (1974)

Somero, 1976). Much as a cold-water fish's enzyme differs from the homologous enzyme of a bird or a mammal, so does the cold-adapted enzyme differ from the homologous enzyme in a warm-adapted ectotherm. Thus we observe a regular variation in catalytic efficiency with adaptation temperature which cuts across taxonomic lines and suggests that temperature-adaptive modification of enzymic properties has continued subsequent to the divergence of the major animal groups.

If we interpret these differences in catalytic efficiency from the standpoint of cold adaptation, the reductions in size of $\Delta G^{\ddagger}$ and the increases in substrate turnover number we observe as we examine species with lower and lower cell temperatures appear perfectly reasonable. However, if we instead try to interpret these differences in terms of the probable time sequence of their evolutionary origin, we run into some perplexing problems. Let us make the reasonable assumption that a fish-type enzyme, i.e. one with relatively high catalytic efficiency, was ancestral to the enzymes found in modern birds and mammals. If we accept this assumption we must then rationalise an apparent loss of enzymic efficiency during the process of biological evolution, i.e. we must attempt to account for the appearance of a seemingly poorer catalyst during the evolution of higher organisms.

To approach an answer to this question we must consider the additional selective pressures which changes in cell temperature imposed on enzymes. Whereas we have restricted our discussion on this point entirely to questions of rates of catalysis, a second important temperature effect must be considered to make our treatment biologically reasonable: the influence of temperature changes on enzyme structural stability. In adapting to temperature, an enzyme must not only satisfy the criterion of catalytic efficiency, but in addition it must achieve the correct structural properties to insure satisfactory regulation and stability of higher orders of structure (Somero, 1975a).

Interpreting the observed interspecific differences in catalytic efficiency in this holistic context, we find reasons for believing that an 'adaptational compromise' may have to be reached between the demands for high catalytic efficiency, on the one hand, and correct regulatory and structural traits, on the other (Somero, 1975). The basis of this compromise is the role which changes in enzyme conformation play in catalysis. It is well known that rapid, reversible changes in enzyme conformation occur during the rate-limiting, activation event in catalysis (Koshland and Neet, 1968; Low and Somero, 1974, 1975a, b). In an admittedly overly simplified sense, one can propose that an enzyme with a relatively flexible structure will be capable of undergoing these conformational changes with less input of energy. In other words, an enzyme with a relatively flexible conformation may be able to change its conformation more easily and, as a result, be a more efficient catalyst. Certain of these catalytic conformational changes will lead to exergonic reactions, for example, the exposure of buried charged groups to the surrounding water (Low and Somero, 1975b). The more readily these exposures can occur, the more efficient will the enzyme be as a catalyst.

The relationship between enzyme thermal stability and catalytic efficiency can now be better understood. For a low temperature-adapted ectotherm, a different compromise can be reached between these two factors than in the case of a tropical ectotherm or a bird or mammal. In the high cell temperature species, increased structural stability may become more and more important, and some sacrifice of catalytic efficiency may be selectively advantageous if the gain in structural stability is great enough. It should be realised that structural stability refers to more than just resistance to denaturation. We must also recall that correct regulatory abilities demand proper structural characteristics, e.g. correct modulator binding site geometries and proper abilities to alter conformation as a result of modulator binding. Thus, at least three factors will be critically important in enzymic temperature adaptation, and no one factor can be optimised if this optimisation leads to adverse effects on one or more other crucial enzymic traits.

An example of such a balance between the thermal stability of an enzyme and its catalytic efficiency is given by Thompson, Militzer and Georgi, (1958) for FDP aldolase of a thermophilic bacterium. This enzyme, which functions at temperatures above 80°C *in situ,* has its conformation stabilised in part by disulphide bridges. When these bridges are broken by reducing agents, the enzyme displays (a) a great increase in thermal lability, and (b) an enhanced catalytic activity. Here, then, rigidity of structure is shown to be inversely correlated with catalytic efficiency.

A final question about the importance of activation free energy values in temperature compensation concerns the possibility that changes in cell temperature may directly alter the catalytic efficiency of an enzyme, i.e. a single enzyme may display lower $\Delta G^{\ddagger}$ values at low temperatures than at higher temperatures. (Here we are not considering solely the decreases in $\Delta G^{\ddagger}$ values at low temperatures due to the $-T\Delta S^{\ddagger}$ term; *see Table 3.4.)* This type of enzymic adaptation would seem especially advantageous to intertidal species which must cope with large and sudden temperature changes.

The available data (Hochachka and Somero, 1973; Low and Somero, 1976) suggest that activation free energies are not subject to regular variation in any adaptive way as the cell temperature of an organism varies. The only cases in which the activation free energies of a reaction display apparently adaptive differences as temperature varies are found with membrane-associated enzymes (*see below*). In these cases, changes in the activation parameters of the reaction may derive from temperature-induced changes in the physical state of the lipids of the system. These adaptations will be discussed later in this chapter.

Whereas activation free energies do not appear to play a role in short-term temperature compensation processes, interspecific differences in activation enthalpies may be interpreted as temperature-adaptive, at least to a certain degree. Notice that the activation enthalpies of the low-cell-temperature enzymes (*Table 3.4*) are invariably lower than those of avian and mammalian enzymes.This difference is apparently adaptive in that the ectothermic species' enzymes will have lower Q_{10} values than the enzymes (reactions) of birds and mammals (assuming no differences exist in terms of temperature effects on substrate binding; *see below*). One can inquire further if enzymes of highly eurythermal ectotherms are characterised by lower activation enthalpies than the homologous enzymes of stenothermal ectotherms. Here we find no adaptive differences (*Table 3.4;* Low and Somero, 1976; Somero and Low, 1976): the activation enthalpy (like the activation free energy and entropy) correlates with the absolute

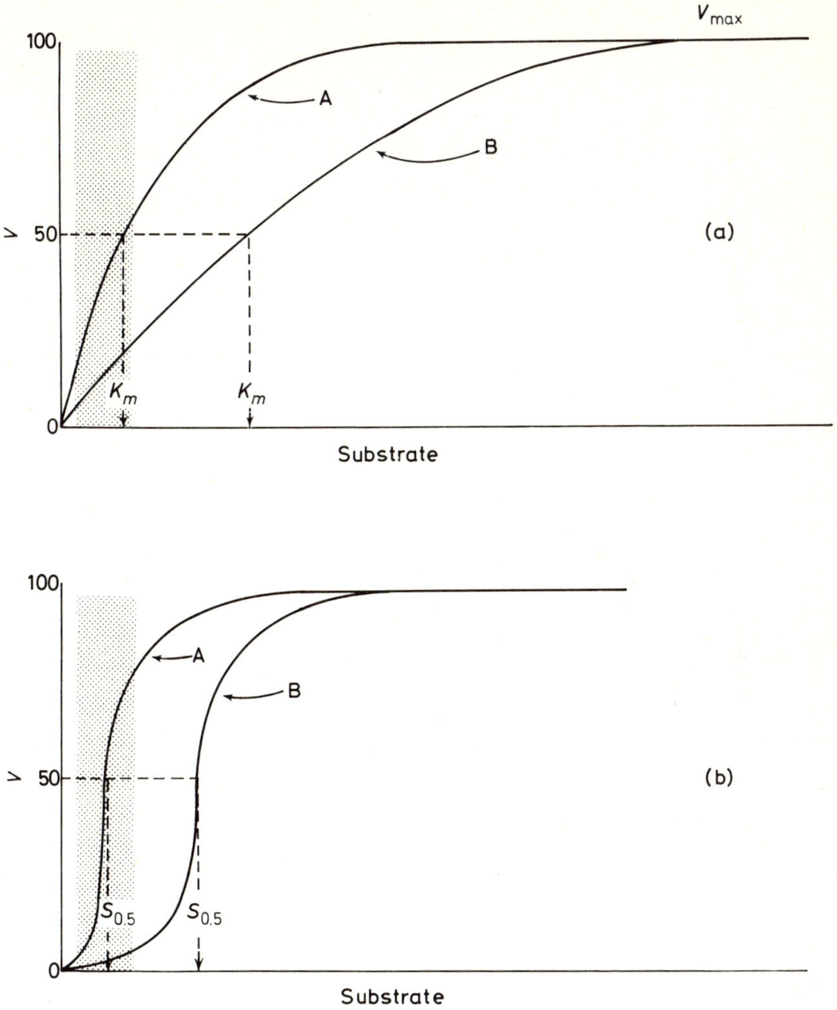

Figure 3.6 Substrate saturation curves for enzymes having (a) hyperbolic and (b) sigmoidal kinetics. The substrate concentration at which the reaction velocity equals half of the maximal velocity (V_{max}) equals the apparent Michaelis constant (K_m) for hyperbolic enzymes and the $S_{0.5}$ value for sigmoidal enzymes. Physiological substrate concentrations are indicated by shading. For each type of enzyme, two variants with different apparent K_m ($S_{0.5}$) values are shown to illustrate the interplay between the ability of the enzyme to bind substrate under non-saturating substrate concentrations and the reaction velocity. (After Hochachka and Somero, 1973; courtesy W. B. Saunders & Co.)

temperature to which the organism is adapted, not the range of temperatures the organism faces. This finding suggests that short-term compensation of enzymic activity to temperature changes must be achieved by mechanisms different from those involved in adjusting activation parameters. We now turn our attention to these other mechanisms.

3.4.1.1.3 Temperature effects on enzyme-substrate interactions

Mechanisms for adjusting the activities of enzymes are not, of course, limited to effects which involve the generation of activated complexes. While it is customary to think that the primary catalytic function of enzymes is to reduce the free energy barriers to reactions, the actual extent to which the catalytic potential of an enzyme is put to use in the cell is found to be highly dependent on the concentration of substrate available to the enzyme (*Figure 3.6*). Only when the enzyme is fully saturated with substrate, i.e. when the reaction rate reaches its maximal velocity (V_{max}), does the cell extract the full catalytic potential of the enzyme.

To one unfamiliar with mechanisms of enzyme activity regulation, it might seem advantageous for enzymes to function at maximal velocities all of the time, for under these circumstances each enzyme molecule is being put to maximal use as a catalyst. However, demands for precise metabolic regulation, i.e. for the turning-on and turning-off of metabolic reactions according to the needs of the cell for different metabolic products, outweigh the possible benefits of continuous V_{max} activities. The regulation of enzymic activity is most commonly effected by altering the position or the shape of the substrate saturation curve (*Figure 3.7*). Positive modulators (activators) increase the substrate binding ability of the enzyme, as measured by the

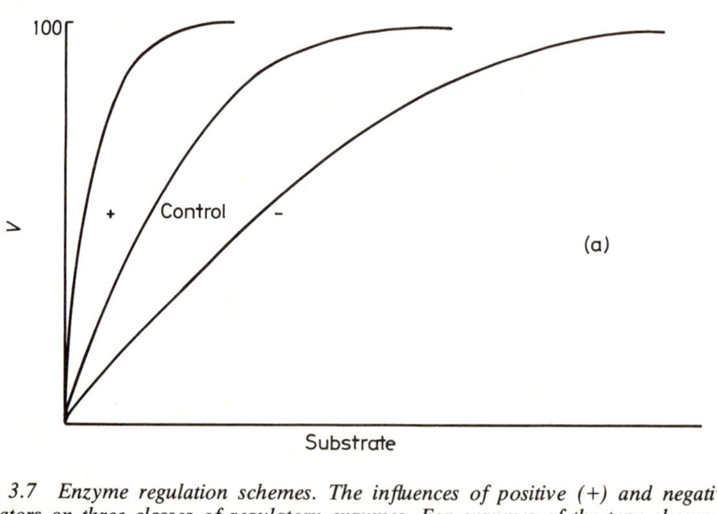

Figure 3.7 Enzyme regulation schemes. The influences of positive (+) and negative (−) modulators on three classes of regulatory enzymes. For enzymes of the type shown in (a), modulators affect only the apparent K_m of substrate. Positive modulators lower K_m (enhance substrate binding); negative modulators raise K_m.

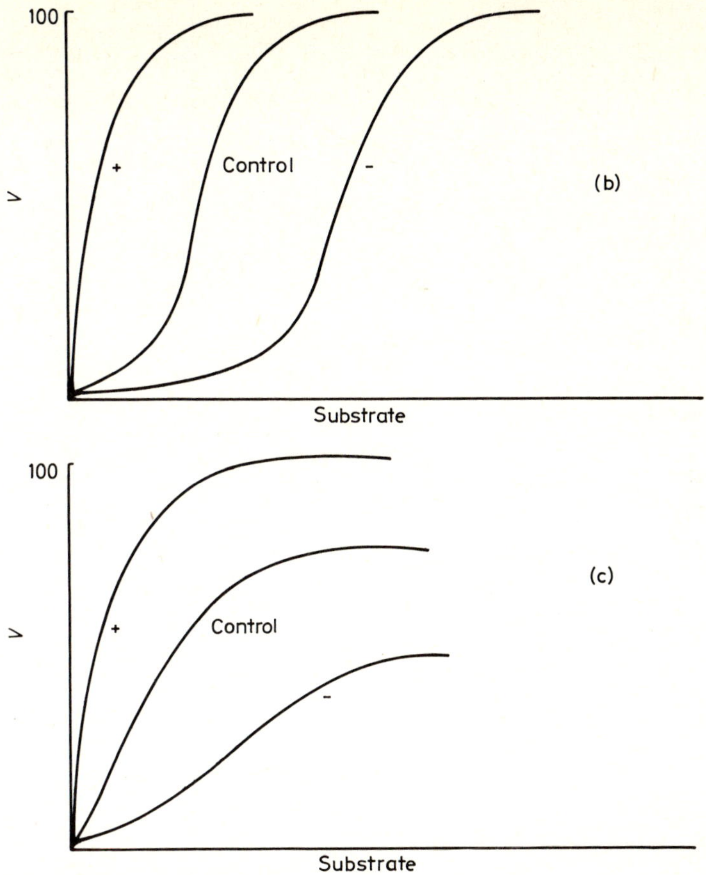

Figure 3.7 Enzymes of type (b) again display the same type of kinetics, sigmoidal, under different modulator conditions, and vary only the $S_{0.5}$ *value of substrate. Also positive modulators can change the shape of sigmoidal saturation curves to hyperbolas.*
Enzymes of type (c) display a more complex response to modulators. Positive modulators reduce the sigmoidicity (cooperativity) of the saturation curve. For some enzymes, albeit a minority, modulators also affect the V_{max} *of the reaction, as shown here. Shifts between sigmoidal and hyperbolic kinetics can occur without* V_{max} *effects, however. (After Hochachka and Somero, 1973; courtesy W. B. Saunders & Co.)*

apparent Michaelis constant (K_m), and/or change the shape of the substrate saturation curve from sigmoidal to hyperbolic. Negative modulators exert the opposite effects. For positive and negative modulators to exert their influences, the enzyme cannot be operating under fully saturated conditions. Thus, we observe that substrate concentrations in the cell are almost invariably much lower than the levels needed for V_{max} activity. In general, intracellular substrate concentrations are of the order of the apparent K_m of the enzyme or lower.

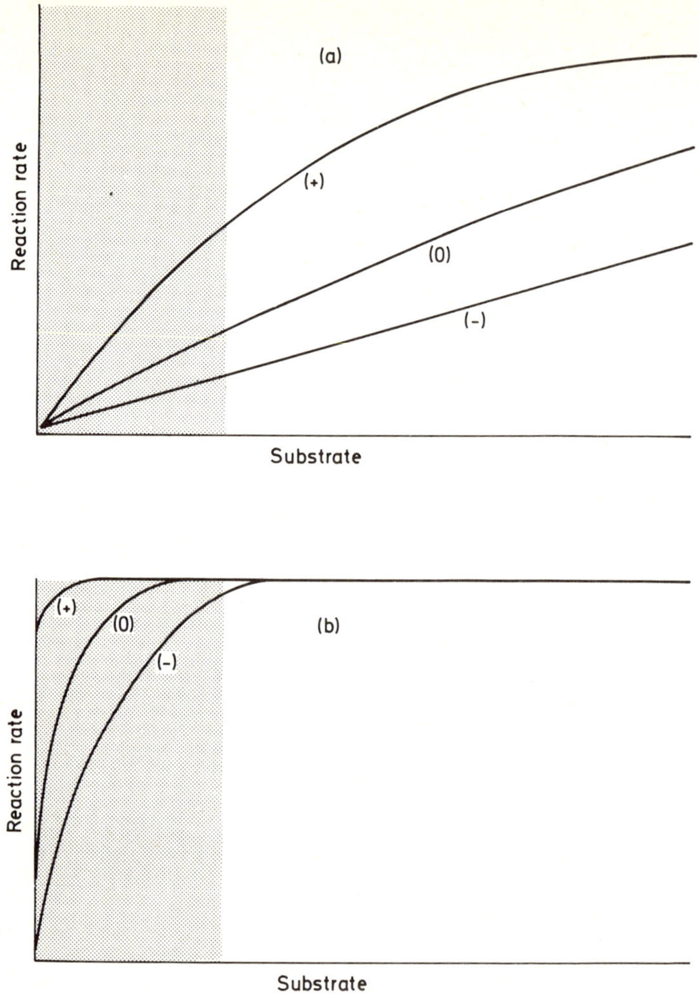

Figure 3.8 *Substrate saturation curves for enzymes which have apparent K_m values which are either too high (a) or too low (b) to permit satisfactory catalysis and regulation. In case (a), the enzyme never attains a significant fraction of its catalytic potential, even in the presence of a positive modulator (+). In such a case the signal for increased rate of function might not lead to an adequate elevation in the rate of the reaction. When a negative modulator (−) binds to the enzyme, activity is grossly low. In this case, a signal for a slow-down of metabolism might lead to a virtual cessation of the activity of the enzyme.*
In case (b), the enzyme binds substrate so strongly that under conditions of no modulation (O) or positive modulation (+) the enzyme is operating at V_{max}, a dangerous situation (see text). A negative modulator (−) will have little effect in reducing the activity of the enzyme. This case illustrates clearly why temperature compensation during evolutionary adaptation and acclimation is not effected by large decreases in apparent K_m values in cold-adapted (acclimated) organisms. Also, these curves show why temperature-dependent K_m changes must be held within strict limits in the process of 'immediate' temperature compensation (see text). (After Hochachka and Somero, 1973; courtesy W. B. Saunders & Co)

Owing to the requirement that enzyme-substrate affinity, as measured by the reciprocal of the apparent K_m value, be of a magnitude that enables modulators to exert their effects on rates of catalysis, the absolute value of the apparent K_m (or $S_{0.5}$) is subject to intense selective pressure. Substrate binding ability must be great enough to insure adequate rates of catalysis, yet not be so high that the enzyme will become saturated with substrate if a positive modulator increases substrate binding ability, i.e. reduces the apparent K_m (*Figure 3.8*). Whenever an enzyme becomes substrate-saturated, the concentration of substrate can build-up exponentially. If this occurs, the further transformations of the substrate can proceed according to mass action relationships rather than according to the rules established by enzyme regulatory schemes. It is clear that this type of uncontrolled chemical reaction is intolerable for the cell (Atkinson, 1969), especially in the case of substrates which are highly reactive, highly acidic or otherwise capable of reacting with a wide variety of cellular metabolites and structures. Thus, the requirement for apparent K_m and $S_{0.5}$ values which permit effective regulation and prevent possible saturation of enzymes will be seen to act as a major shaping force in enzyme evolution (Somero, 1969a; Somero, 1975a; Hochachka and Somero, 1973).

Let us now consider how temperature can affect enzyme-substrate interactions and how organisms can adapt to these effects. On the basis of our earlier discussion of weak chemical bonds, which are important for stabilising enzyme-substrate and enzyme-modulator complexes, it should be clear that changes in temperature will have significant effects on enzyme-substrate and enzyme-modulator complex formation. Temperature changes will not only enhance or disrupt these complexes, but in addition will have differential influences depending on whether the complex in question is stabilised primarily by hydrophobic interactions (low temperature labile) or hydrogen bonds, electrostatic interactions or van der Waals' forces (high temperature labile). Further effects of temperature on enzyme-ligand interactions will arise from temperature dependent changes in protein structure, e.g. in the geometry of ligand binding sites, since protein structures are also stabilised to a great extent by weak bonds (*Table 3.1*).

As a model system for examining temperature effects on enzyme-ligand interactions we will consider the well-studied substrate (acetylcholine; ACh) binding site of acetylcholinesterase (AChE) (*Figure 3.9*).The catalytic site of the enzyme has two distinct regions. The binding of ACh, with concomitant positioning of the substrate in the correct position for catalysis, is largely the responsibility of the anionic site which consists of a hydrophobic pocket (a depression in the enzyme surface lined largely with hydrophobic amino acid side-chains) and a dissociated carboxylate group (COO^-). The splitting of the ACh molecule occurs at the esteratic site (*Figure 3.9*).

Stabilisation of the ACh-AChE complex is seen to involve two types of weak bond. Hydrophobic interactions between the non-polar amino acid side-chains lining the hydrophobic pocket and the methyl groups bound to the nitrogen atom of ACh provide a major share of the stabilisation free energy. The electrostatic interaction between the carboxylate group and the

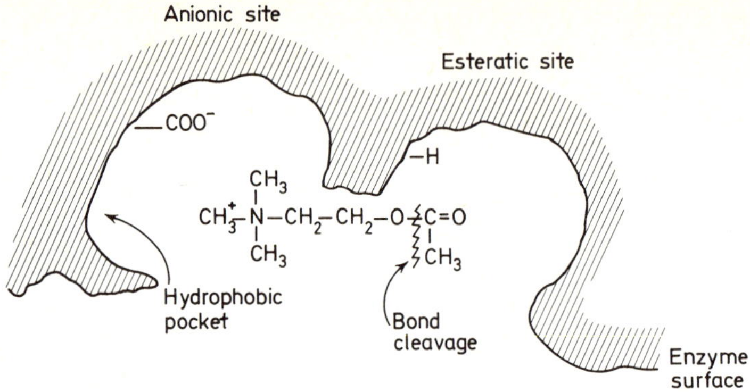

Figure 3.9 The substrate-binding site of acetylcholinesterase. (After Hochachka and Somero, 1973; courtesy W. B. Saunders & Co.)

positively charged quaternary ammonium group further contributes to stabilisation of the ACh–AChE complex. Since these two classes of weak bonds have opposite temperature dependencies, it is interesting to inquire as to whether the AChE's of species adapted to different temperatures differ in terms of the relative roles played by the hydrophobic and electrostatic contributions to ACh–AChE stabilisation. That such differences could be of critical importance in temperature adaptation is implicit in the recent finding that the binding of ACh analogues, relying largely either on the hydrophobic or the electrostatic contribution to enzyme-ligand complex stabilisation, displays major differences in thermal responses (Hochachka, 1974a). The effect of temperature on the hydrophobic contribution to ACh–AChE complex stabilisation can be deduced from experiments in which the substrate analogue, 3,3-dimethylbutylacetate, is used. Binding of this compound would involve hydrophobic interactions almost exclusively, since the quanternary nitrogen (with positive charge) is absent. Using the purified AChE of the electric eel, it was found that the apparent K_m for this analogue was approximately ten-fold higher than the apparent K_m of ACh at 35°C, and this difference between analogue and substrate K_m values was accentuated at reduced temperatures (*Figure 3.10*). If the apparent K_m for the carbon analogue is a valid estimate of the true dissociation constant, then the binding reaction occurs with a free energy change of –3.4 kcal/mole, an enthalpy change of +12.8 kcal/mole, and an entropy change of 54.3 kcal/mole/degree (Hochachka, 1974a).

Estimates of the effects of temperature on the electrostatic interactions between the quanternary ammonium nitrogen and the carboxylate group of the anionic site can be obtained from studies using specific inhibitors of the AChE reaction (Hochachka, 1974a). For a simple inhibitor such as dimethylammonium ion, binding to AChE is almost exclusively due to electrostatic interactions (Froede and Wilson, 1972). As one would predict (*Table 3.2*), the binding of this inhibitor is exothermic, and the binding constant (K_I) is directly proportional to temperature (*Figure 3.11*).

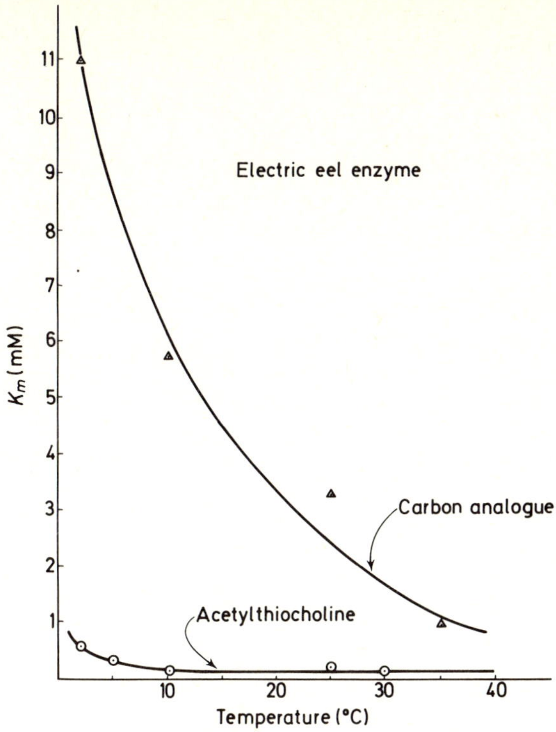

Figure 3.10 The effects of assay temperature on the apparent Km values for acetylcholine and the synthetic substrate, 3,3-1dimethylbutyl acetate, for electric eel acetylcholinesterase. (After Hochachka, 1974a; courtesy Biochemical Journal)

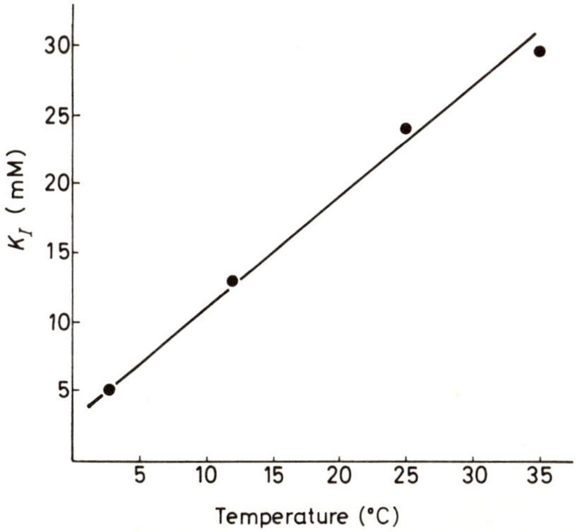

Figure 3.11 The effect of temperature on the KI for dimethylammonium ion of electric eel acetylcholinesterase. (After Hochachka, 1974a; courtesy Biochemical Journal)

The data shown in *Figures 3.10* and *3.11* demonstrate that the net effect of temperature on AChE–ACh binding will depend on the relative importance of two classes of weak interactions. In the absence of any changes in enzyme binding site conformation due to temperature, an AChE variant which relies heavily on hydrophobic interactions for substrate binding should display an inverse relationship between temperature and the apparent K_m of ACh, i.e. substrate binding affinity will decrease as temperature falls. Conversely, an

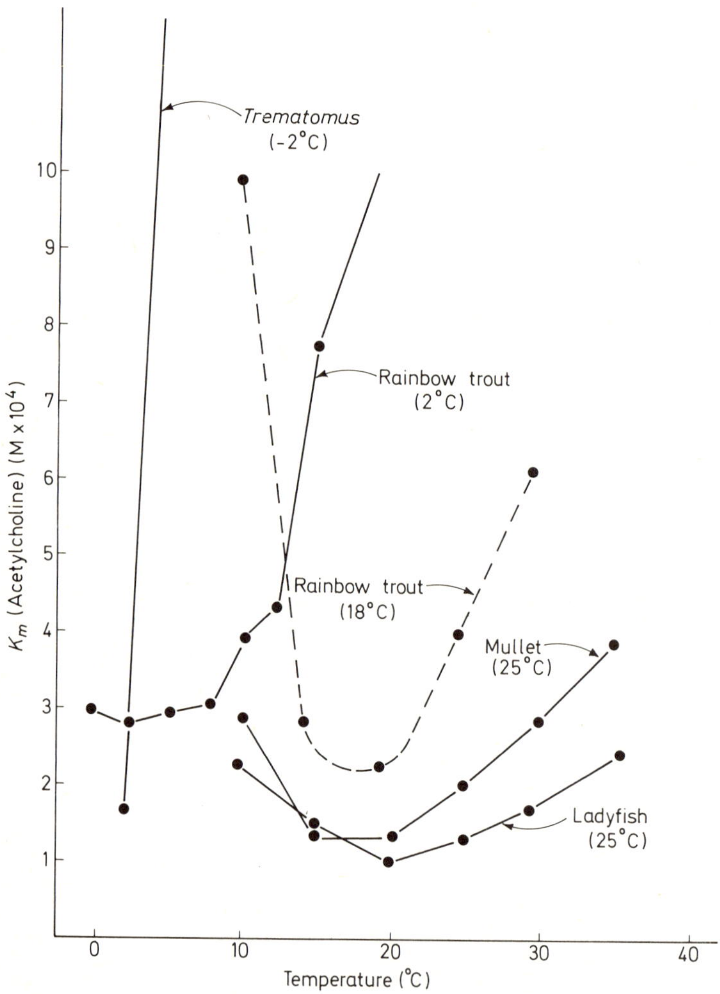

Figure 3.12 The effect of temperature on the apparent K_m of acetylcholine for acetylcholinesterases of four fish species: rainbow trout (Salmo gairdneri) *acclimated to 2 and 18°C; an Antarctic species,* Trematomus borchgrevinki; *the stripped mullet* (Mugil cephalus); *and the ladyfish* (Elops hawaiensis). *The approximate adaptation or acclimation temperature of the fish is given in parentheses. (Data from Baldwin, 1971, and Baldwin and Hochachka, 1970; figure from Hochachka and Somero, 1973; courtesy W. B. Saunders & Co.)*

AChE which relies most heavily on electrostatic interactions should display a positive correlation between temperature and apparent K_m of AChE. If both types of interaction are about equally important, the enzyme might exhibit very complex apparent K_m-versus-temperature responses.

Available data show that major inter-specific differences exist in the effect of temperature on ACh binding by AChE (Baldwin and Hochachka, 1970; Baldwin, 1971; *Figure 3.12*). For AChE of the Antarctic fish, *Trematomus borchgrevinki,* the electrostatic contribution to binding would seem dominant. For most other AChE's, both classes of weak interaction appear to play a role in substrate binding, and the relative importance of hydrophobic and electrostatic interactions may vary with temperature. Thus, over the higher range of temperatures for an enzyme, the apparent K_m of ACh is directly proportional to temperature, suggesting that the high temperature lability of electrostatic interactions is of measurable importance. However, at lower temperatures the apparent K_m of ACh begins to rise as temperature is lowered. This finding is consistent with the hypothesis that low temperature disruption of hydrophobic interactions is now a significant factor in stabilising the ACh–AChE complex. Of course, these conclusions cannot be definite since in no case is it known whether changes in enzyme conformation with temperature are contributing to the observed temperature-dependencies in substrate binding. Nonetheless, species-specific temperature responses seem readily accountable, at least in part, on the basis of amino acid substitutions at the anionic pocket. For example, increased concentrations of hydrophobic groups within the pocket could enhance hydrophobic interactions and reduce the electrostatic interaction [increased numbers of hydrophobic groups might reduce water activity in the pocket which, in turn, could hamper dissociation of the carboxylic acid group (*Figure 3.9*)]. Enhanced electrostatic binding could be achieved by reducing the hydrophobicity of the pocket and by facilitating the dissociation of the carboxylic acid group.

Let us now analyse the observed interspecific differences in temperature effects on substrate binding for AChE and pyruvate kinase (PK) (*Figure 3.13*), and attempt to deduce the major evolutionary goals involved in adapting substrate binding abilities to a specific thermal regime. The first general conclusion we suggest is that for all enzymes the substrate binding ability, as measured by the apparent K_m of $S_{0.5}$ value, is not allowed to vary widely over the range of temperatures experienced by the cell. At non-biological temperatures for the cell (enzyme), apparent K_m values may exhibit extremely great sensitivities to temperature (*Figures 3.12* and *3.13*). We believe that the relative stability in apparent K_m and $S_{0.5}$ values seen over the biological temperature range of an organism reflects the critical importance of preserving the regulatory capacity of an enzyme at all temperatures (*see Figure 3.8*).

A second general finding is that when enzyme-substrate affinity varies with temperature, it does so in a manner which leads to rate stabilisation, i.e. over the normal temperature range of the organism, when the apparent K_m varies with temperature, the trend is for enhanced binding ability at lower temperatures. This increased capability to bind substrate at lower

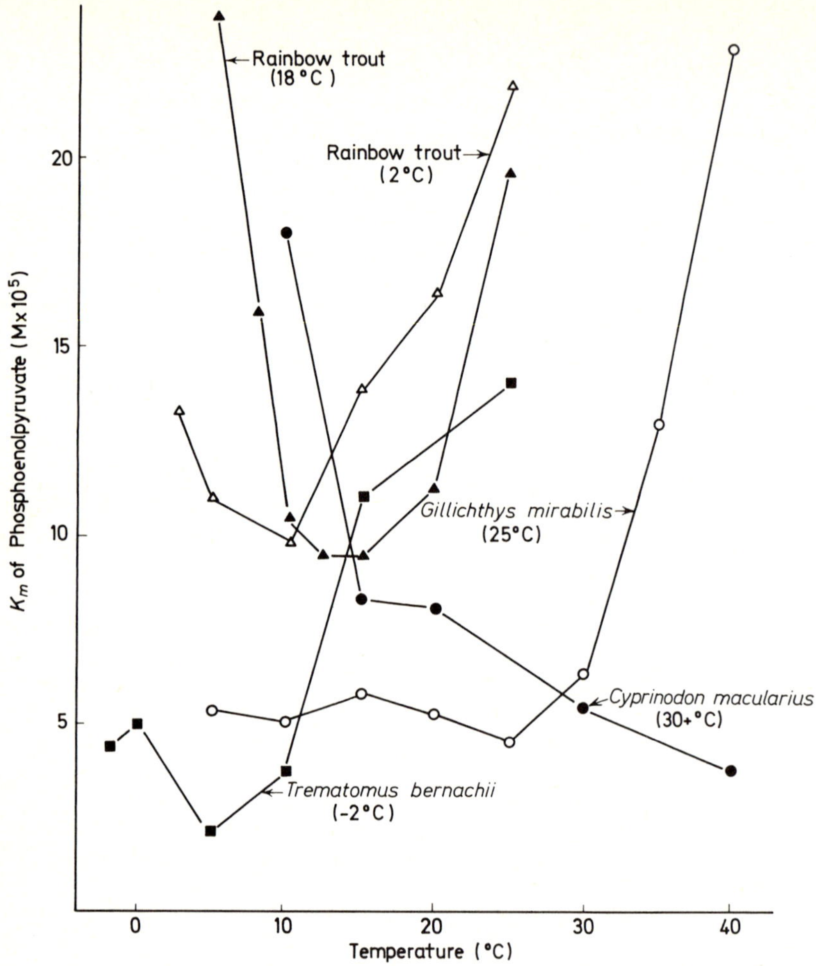

Figure 3.13 The effect of temperature on the apparent K_m of phosphoenolpyruvate (PEP) for pyruvate kinases of four fish species: rainbow trout, acclimated to 2 and 18°C; the Antarctic fish, Trematomus bernacchii*; the estuarine species,* Gillichthys mirabilis *(longjaw mudsucker); and the desert pupfish,* Cyprinodon macularius. *(Data from Hochachka and Somero, 1973; Somero, 1975b)*

temperatures helps to offset the reduced thermal energy in the cell, and leads to lower Q_{10} values at non-saturating substrate concentrations than at V_{max} substrate levels (Somero, 1969a; Hochachka and Somero, 1973). In this situation a decrease in temperature affects the enzyme analogously to a positive modulator. This 'positive thermal modulation' may be an important mechanism in immediate temperature compensation (*Figure 3.4(b)*).

A third common attribute of temperature-apparent K_m interactions is that when very rapid changes in apparent K_m occur, these are almost invariably at temperatures near the lethal limits of the species. These extremely rapid and large changes in apparent K_m values with temperature, e.g. for AChE of the Antarctic fish (*Figure 3.12*) at temperatures only a few degrees Celsius above 0°C, may be instrumental in establishing the temperature tolerance of an organism (Somero, 1969a). At low temperatures, the simultaneous reductions in substrate binding ability and thermal energy can lead to enormous Q_{10} values at physiological substrate concentrations (Somero and Hochachka, 1971); e.g. for PK of the rainbow trout, the Q_{10} for the reaction catalysed by the enzyme from warm-acclimated individuals is about 25 at physiological PEP concentrations over the temperature range 3–7°C. Such a rapid change in enzymic reaction rate with temperature could (a) be lethal in and of itself by slowing down the rate of glycolytic function, and (b) be of major stress in terms of metabolic imbalance, since other reactions of glycolysis could display very different Q_{10} values. At higher temperatures, where apparent K_m values may rise extremely quickly, the ability of the enzyme to bind substrate may fall to such a low level that the reaction may be blocked even though ample thermal energy is available to activate the enzyme-substrate complex. It is interesting in this connection that the upper lethal temperature of Antarctic *Trematomus* fishes adapted to –1.86°C is approximately 7°C (Somero and DeVries, 1967), a temperature at which the ability of the important brain enzyme, AChE, to bind substrate is already vastly less than at physiological temperatures.

Another general observation in studies of temperature effects on enzyme-substrate affinity is that neither cold acclimation nor evolutionary cold adaptation appears to involve selection for enzymes with lower apparent K_m values than those of homologues in warm-acclimated or warm-adapted organisms (*Figures 3.12* and *3.13*). As we have argued above, the advantages which such a change would confer on the catalytic potential of an enzyme probably would be more than offset by reductions in the regulatory properties of the enzyme, i.e. its abilities to vary its rate of function when substrate concentrations change and when modulators interact with the enzyme (*Figure 3.8(b)*).

One might ask, however, if the apparent primacy of regulatory function over catalytic function is also noted for enzymes which are unlikely to have a regulatory role. In the above discussion we have considered only enzymes which are incorporated into tightly regulated multi-enzyme pathways. Might different adaptive strategies exist for enzymes such as those involved in digestion in the gut where the sole function of the enzyme is to break down rapidly ingested materials? For trypsins of a variety of vertebrate species, the absolute value of the apparent K_m of substrate (an artificial peptide analogue, benzoyl-DL-arginine-p-nitroanilide) was directly proportional to the preferred temperatures of the species (Hofer *et al.,* 1975), an observation which suggests that enzymes that are not constrained by regulatory demands may alter their catalytic functions more freely during thermal adaptation. Additional studies of enzymes involved in multi-enzyme sequences and of enzymes which function independently of any other enzymes will be needed before we can fully appreciate differences in adaptive strategies among classes of enzymes.

The major role played by temperature-dependent changes in apparent K_m

values likely is in the case of short-term or immediate temperature compensation (*Figure 3.4 (b)*). When the apparent K_m value is directly proportional to temperature, rates of catalysis are less temperature sensitive than under conditions in which the apparent K_m is either temperature-independent or varies inversely with temperature. However, in spite of the potential raw material for effecting temperature-insensitive rates of enzymic function offered by this mechanism, a biologically convincing demonstration that this raw material is actually utilised must be achieved using systems more complex than *in vitro* enzyme assays. Let us consider what types of experiments must be done to examine the roles played by temperature-dependent apparent K_m values in true living systems.

At the very least, such experiments must demonstrate (a) that the influence of temperature on the apparent substrate affinities of the key regulatory enzymes governing the rates and directions of metabolic flow are in agreement with, for example, observed temperature effects on oxygen consumption, and (b) the substrate concentrations available to the regulatory enzymes are such that binding phenomena can control rates of catalysis. While to date there have been no studies in which both of these requirements have been met, there are data which are at least consistent with the hypothesis that increased substrate binding ability at reduced temperatures can lead to reductions in metabolic Q_{10} values. For example, Newell and co-workers (e.g. Newell and Pye, 1971) have 'dissected' the respiratory machinery of an intertidal mollusc (*Littorina littorea*) to determine if the temperature-independent respiratory metabolism of the organism under inactive conditions is reflected in the oxygen uptake of isolated mitochondria. They in fact observed that oxygen consumption of mitochondria was virtually temperature-independent at low (i.e. physiological) concentrations of substrate (pyruvate), but that at high substrate concentrations the rate of oxygen consumption exhibited a significant temperature dependence. One interpretation of their data is as follows: under conditions of low pyruvate concentration the enzymes of the Krebs citric acid cycle were operating well below saturating (V_{max}) conditions, and temperature-dependent changes in enzyme-substrate affinity, e.g. of the enzymes of the pyruvate dehydrogenase complex, were sufficient to stabilise rates of catalysis in the face of varying temperature. When higher concentrations of pyruvate were used in these *in vitro* preparations, the enzymes approached or reached saturation, and the respiratory Q_{10} of the mitochondria was then a function of the activation enthalpies of the enzymic reactions.

Results from other studies of temperature effects on the metabolism of tissue slices and tissue homogenates *in vitro* are consistent with the mechanism just outlined. Dean (1969) observed high degrees of temperature-independence in rates of lipid oxidation in isolated trout tissues when physiological substrate concentrations were used. Hochachka (1968) observed similar effects using fish liver homogenates supplied with physiological concentrations of a variety of metabolites. In this latter study, the observed Q_{10} values for different metabolites varied considerably, suggesting that a sudden change in cell temperature will lead to a qualitative rechannelling of metabolic flow, much in the way that thermal acclimation over a period of several days or weeks leads to a reorganisation of intermediary metabolism. An especially clear example of the influence of temperature on the relative activities of metabolic pathways has been provided by the work of van Handel (1966) who found that changes in temperature led to significant differences in the relative amounts of carbon channelled into the two major classes of depot energy stores, glycogen and lipids, in mosquitoes. These immediate changes in the relative activities of metabolic pathways are consistent with the hypothesis that differential effects of temperature on the substrate-binding abilities of branch-point enzymes can lead to immediate redirections of metabolic flow when the cell temperature of an ectotherm changes. These findings also imply that to speak of a Q_{10} value for 'metabolism' is to ignore the complexity of effects engendered by changes in temperature at the level of metabolic pathways.

3.4.2 The roles of multiple enzyme forms in temperature adaptation

3.4.2.1 STATEMENT OF THE PROBLEM

If we accept the thesis that critical structural and functional traits of enzymes which are highly temperature sensitive (*Table 3.2*) must be preserved over the entire range of temperatures experienced by an organism in its native habitat, we must consider the potential mechanisms which might serve to enhance the eurythermality of enzymes. These mechanisms would appear to fall into two general categories. First, the structure and function of a single enzyme may develop the necessary eurythermality to insure satisfactory catalysis and regulation over the entire thermal range of the organism. Adaptations of this type might involve such changes as reductions in the binding enthalpies for substrate and modulator interactions. For example, if the binding of substrate was strongly endothermic, a concomitant exothermic reaction elsewhere on the enzyme surface (or within the enzyme) during substrate binding could 'titrate' the effects of the enthalpy change occurring as the substrate is bound (Somero, 1975a).

Second, if a single enzyme species is unable to acquire sufficient eurythermality to enable it to function over the entire habitat temperature range, the eurythermality of the particular enzymic *reaction* may yet be achieved if two or more forms of the enzyme catalysing the reaction are present in the cell, and these multiple variants on the single enzyme theme have different thermal optima (*Figure 3.14*). Let us consider the benefits and the disadvantages of these two mechanisms for eurythermality.

3.4.2.2 MULTIPLE ALLELIC ISOZYMES (ALLOZYMES)

There are two genetic mechanisms available for increasing the number of variants of an enzyme (functionally defined). Multiple allelic forms of an enzyme, allozymes, may be coded at a single gene locus. Alternatively,

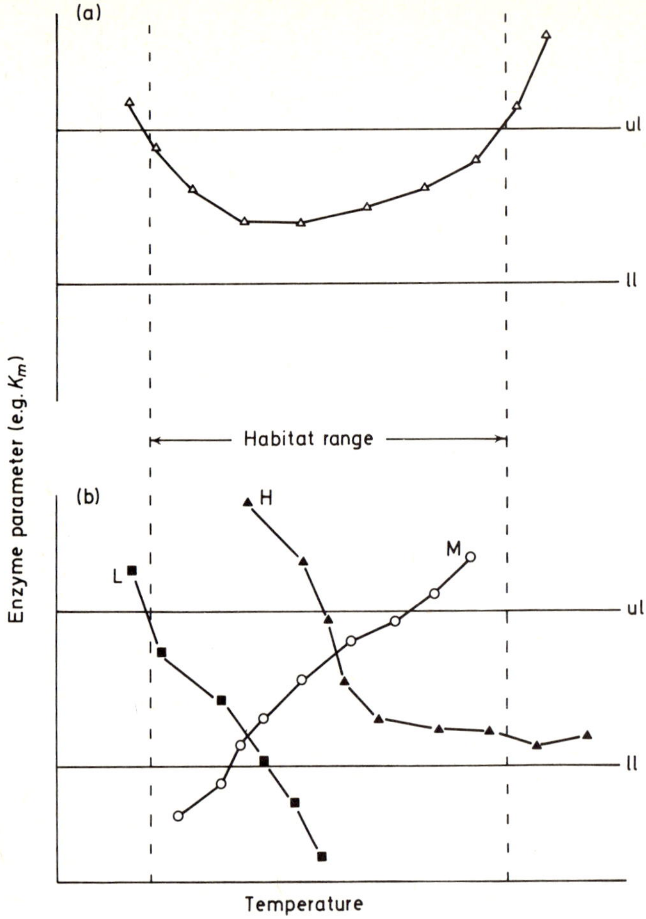

Figure 3.14 A schematic representation of two mechanisms for maintaining enzymic function over the full range of habitat temperatures experienced by a eurythermal organism. (a) The 'Eurytolerant Protein' Strategy: In this case a single enzyme species in terms of primary structure is able to maintain the necessary kinetic and structural traits within the acceptable limits (upper limit designated 'ul'; lower limit designated 'll') over the entire temperature range experienced by the organism. (b) The 'Multiple Variant' Strategy: In this case the vital enzymic parameters are maintained within acceptable limits by the joint functionings of three enzymes (allozymes or multiple locus isozymes), designated 'L', a low temperature optimum variant; 'M', a mid-range optimum variant; and 'H', a high temperature optimum variant. All three variants must be present in the cell if the full range of habitat temperatures is to be tolerated

additional gene loci may code for a particular type of enzyme. We shall refer to multiple locus isozymes simply as 'isozymes'.

The role of allozymes in adaptation to variable environments is currently a topic of active study and debate among population biologists (*see* Levins, 1968; Wills, 1973; Somero and Soulé, 1974; Somero, 1975b; for references). Many workers argue that the presence of multiple allelic forms of enzymes confers a significant advantage on organisms which experience environments that vary in time and space. The molecular basis of this advantage is indicated by the scheme shown in *Figure 3.14,* wherein the presence of two or more variants on each enzyme theme which have different thermal optima and tolerance ranges, greatly extends the habitat range of the organism. If an enzyme cannot acquire the pattern of eurythermality illustrated in *Figure 3.14(a),* then successful adaptation to a varying environment, e.g. thermal regime, may be contingent on the development of multiple allelic forms of an enzyme (or multiple isozymes, as discussed below).

These arguments form the basis for the following hypothesis: if adaptation to varying thermal environments depends, in part, on the acquisition of increased numbers of allelic variants on different protein themes, then ectothermic species which inhabit very stable thermal regimes would be expected to display lower levels of allelic polymorphism than phylogenetically and ecologically similar species living in highly variable thermal conditions. Recently this particular statement of the 'niche-variation hypothesis' has been tested by examining thirteen species of marine teleosts from widely different thermal regimes (Somero and Soulé, 1974). Contrary to the predictions of the niche-variation hypothesis (Levins, 1968; Selander and Kaufman, 1973), there was no correlation between the annual temperature range experienced by a species in its native habitat(s) and the amount of allelic polymorphism in the sampled populations. The highest levels of polymorphism were found in tropical and deep-sea fishes which, of course, live under relatively stable temperature conditions compared to, say, temperate zone estuarine and intertidal species. Workers who have examined levels of genetic polymorphism in marine invertebrates (Ayala *et al.,* 1973; Gooch and Schopf, 1972) also have reported fairly high levels of allelic polymorphism in tropical and deep-sea species, albeit there are so few data on marine invertebrates that meaningful comparisons probably are difficult at best.

Available data on fishes, while also limited in number, permit the following tentative conclusions about the importance of allozymes in temperature adaptation. First, at least on a gross, inter-family basis, fishes which live in stable habitats such as the Antarctic Ocean are not significantly less polymorphic than ecologically similar species living in such highly variable temperature regimes as those of temperate zone estuaries and intertidal zones. Whether more fine-level analysis, e.g. of different populations of a single species, will reveal positive correlations between water temperature variation and allozymic polymorphism, is at present an open question meriting immediate study. Certainly the data available from studies of terrestrial and freshwater species do not seem adequate to permit a clear decision on the correctness of the niche-variation hypothesis as it pertains to temperature adaptation.

A second conclusion is that the evolutionary history of a species may play a major role in establishing the level of genetic polymorphism characteristic of the species. For example, the 'time divergence' model of evolution (Soulé, 1973) predicts highest levels of genetic polymorphism in species which inhabit environments which have changed relatively little over long spans of time. Interestingly, both the deep-sea and tropical reefs have been subject to relatively little perturbation in climate, latitude and species composition compared to most other marine habitats, and the fishes from tropical reefs and the deep-sea display the highest observed levels of allelic polymorphism (Somero and Soulé, 1974).

In conclusion, it appears simplistic to predict simple positive correlations between environmental and genetic variabilities, especially in the case of phylogenetically diverse species living in habitats with markedly different evolutionary histories. Also, on purely genetic grounds, one can fault the niche-variation hypothesis. Thus, the reliance on multiple allozymes would create significant genetic 'problems' in terms of segregational mechanics. If survival depended on heterozygosity at, say, ten loci, it would be exceedingly unlikely that any offspring would be heterozygous at all loci and thus able to cope with the full environmental spectrum it is likely to encounter.

3.4.2.3 MULTIPLE LOCUS ISOZYMES AND TEMPERATURE ACCLIMATION

Although multiple allelic variants have not been found to be of broad importance in adapting fishes to variable thermal regimes, there is evidence showing that multiple locus isozymes may play such a role. As shown in *Figures 3.12* and *3.13*, rainbow trout (*Salmo gairdneri*) possess kinetically distinct 'warm' and 'cold' isozymes of AChE and PK. The kinetic properties of the AChE and PK isozymes present in warm (17–18°C) and cold (2–4°C) acclimated trout are distinct and apparently adaptive. Each single isozyme species displays a characteristic U-shaped apparent K_m-versus-temperature curve, with a minimal value of the apparent K_m near the acclimation temperature. Note that the minimal K_m values for the 'warm' and 'cold' isozymes are approximately the same, supporting the view stated earlier to the effect that cold adaptation over seasonal and evolutionary time-courses is not effected by increases in the absolute substrate binding ability of an enzyme.

The advantages which accrue from the two isozyme systems found with trout AChE and PK would seem to be as follows. First, throughout the year the substrate binding ability of each class of enzyme is maintained at a relatively stable value. Second, rapid upswings in apparent K_m values at extremes of temperature are avoided. For example, the synthesis of a 'cold' isozyme at winter temperatures eliminates the sharp Q_{10} effects which would result from the functioning of the 'warm' isozyme form at winter temperatures. As stated earlier, simultaneous reductions in thermal energy and substrate binding ability can lead to Q_{10} values greater than 20 at physiological substrate concentrations (Somero and Hochachka, 1971). Another advantage of a multiple locus isozyme system, compared to a multiple allelic system, is that the cell need contain only the enzyme variants which are capable of efficient functioning under the thermal conditions experienced by the cell at that particular season. If the cell contained two allozymes, one similar to the 'cold' trout AChE and PK isozyme and one similar to the 'warm' isozymes, then at high and low temperature ranges a major fraction of the enzymes being synthesised and held within the cell would be non-functional. A multiple locus isozyme system thus possesses a regulatory efficiency not found with multiple allelic systems. Segregational problems (*see above*) would also be absent in a multiple locus isozyme system.

Quantitative, but usually not qualitative, isozyme changes in response to altered temperature were first observed in tissues of the rainbow trout (Baldwin and Hochachka, 1970; Hochachka and Lewis, 1970; Moon and Hochachka, 1971; Hochachka and Somero, 1973). The apparent significance of temperature-specific isozymes in this species prompted examination of other freshwater and marine teleosts to determine how general this mechanism of temperature adaptation is. The results of these latter studies suggest that the rainbow trout, if not unique, is at least highly atypical in having a potential for synthesising temperature-specific isozymes. In most other fishes studied, including such eurythermal species as the goldfish (Wilson, 1975), the longjaw mudsucker (*Gillichthys mirabilis*), an estuarine species, the brown bullhead, *Ictalurus nebulosus,* (Somero, 1975b) and three species of the intertidal genus *Gibbonsia* (Davis and Somero, unpublished), identical isozyme patterns were observed in warm-and cold-acclimated specimens. For the *Gibbonsia* species, populations sampled throughout the year, i.e. naturally acclimatised individuals, also revealed no changes in isozyme patterns.

In two other species of fish, kinetic evidence has been presented which is consistent with the occurrence of distinct isozymes in differently acclimated individuals: brain choline acetyltransferase in the goldfish (Hebb, Stephens and Smith, 1972) and L-alanine: 2-oxoglutarate aminotransferase in the pond loach, *Misgurnus fossilis* L. (Mester, Iordachescu and Niculescu, 1973). However, in the absence of electrophoretic data, it cannot be concluded that different isozyme forms were responsible for the kinetic differences observed (*see below*).

In view of the fact that only in the case of the rainbow trout are both kinetic and genetic (electrophoretic) data available showing that multiple locus isozymes play a role in temperature acclimation, we might consider certain of the genetic bases for the uniqueness of this species. One of the distinguishing attributes of the rainbow trout, and other Salmonid fishes, is their high content of DNA per nucleus (Ohno, 1970). The Salmonid fishes are tetraploid organisms, i.e. they possess at least twice as many copies of each type of gene (or did at the time of the origin of the tetraploid state) as a so-called 'normal' species of fish. Thus, the rainbow trout may have sufficient genetic raw material to fabricate season-specific isozymes, much as the normal diploid organism has enough information for cell- and tissue-specific isozymes (Moon, 1975; Somero, 1975b). The latest increase in ploidy in the Salmonid fishes probably occurred after the organisms had already developed the necessary cell- and tissue-specific isozymes, so this newest genetic information could be utilised for generating isozymes for specific environmental conditions. It would be interesting to examine other tetraploid fishes for seasonal changes in isozyme patterns. The observation that the tetraploid goldfish (*Carassius auratus*) does not exhibit different isozymes in differently-acclimated specimens (Wilson, Whitt and Prosser, 1973; Wilson *et al.,* 1975) indicates that there may be diversity in adaptational strategies even among the tetraploid fishes.

A final example of environmentally-related isozyme changes bears mentioning at this juncture, even though the isozyme effects do not appear necessarily related to temperature adaptation. Massaro and Brooke (1971) examined the effects of temperature and photoperiod on lactate dehydrogenase (LDH) isozyme patterns in *Fundulus heteroclitus.* Although they found no temperature-induced changes in LDH patterns, change in photoperiod did lead to isozyme changes. Whether these isozyme changes were temperature-adaptive is not known, since kinetic studies were not performed. What is especially important about these findings is that they raise an important point concerning experimental design in acclimation studies. What may trigger a temperature-adaptive change is not temperature variation itself, but rather another environmental cue which, in the case of photoperiod, is a more reliable indicator of season. Acclimation experiments which have failed to find changes, e.g. in isozyme patterns, may have failed to induce the changes the organisms are capable of making, if the laboratory experimental regime involved variation in temperature but not in photoperiod. Indeed, Duman and DeVries (1974a) observed that the disappearance of organic 'antifreeze' compounds from the blood of an Arctic fish required experimental lengthening of the photoperiod as well as an increase in holding temperature. This type of environmental regulation of freezing resistance is of obvious value as a 'fail-safe' mechanism which insures that unseasonably warm temperatures will not induce the loss of freezing resistance which may yet be required later in the year (*see below*).

3.4.2.4 CONFORMATIONAL VARIANTS OF ENZYMES AND TEMPERATURE ADAPTATION

Because the higher orders of enzyme structure are stabilised by various types of weak bonds which are highly temperature sensitive (*Table 3.1*), it is not unreasonable to suggest that the conformation of a protein may be quite different at different temperatures. If the new conformation assumed by an enzyme alters its kinetic properties, the possibility arises that a single enzyme, in terms of primary structure, might be able to function as both a 'warm' and 'cold' isozyme (*see Figures 3.12* and *3.13*). A temperature-induced change in conformation could lead to adaptive changes in, for example, the thermal stability and substrate binding ability of the enzyme.

The hypothesis that an enzyme can exist in two or more conformations which give the enzyme two or more distinct sets of kinetic properties has been clearly stated and well-developed by Nickerson and Day (1969) and Nickerson (1973). Their basic concepts of the roles of 'metastable' and 'multistable' proteins in biological processes are essentially identical with the example given above, namely a change in the environmental (e.g. temperature) conditions surrounding a protein can induce the molecule to adopt a new conformation which leads to improved capabilities to deal with the new environment. The mechanistic basis of these changes in structure and function deserves some discussion, for it illustrates what we regard as a new and exciting way of approaching questions of environmental adaptation of proteins.

In the model of 'metastable' protein function (*Figure 3.15*), an energy barrier exists between conformational states A and B. Thus, even though state B is thermodynamically the preferred state due to its lower free energy, the conversion of A to B could be very slow due to the need for an input of energy to 'climb' the energy barrier between A and the activated (transition) state species, $A^{\ddagger}$. Thus at low temperatures there could be significant amounts of conformation A in the cell if this conformation occurs first in the sequence of folding events leading to the final, most stable conformation, B.

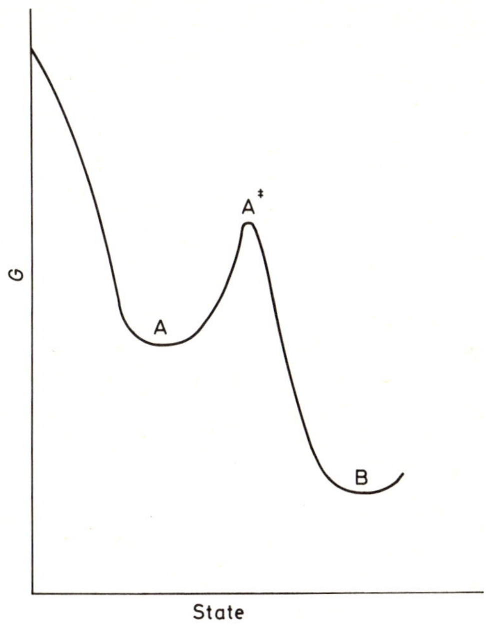

Figure 3.15 The 'metastable' protein model. Following completion of the synthesis of the primary amino acid sequence, a protein undergoes a series of folding reactions leading to the final, thermodynamically most stable, conformation (B). However, if conformation A precedes conformation B in the folding sequence, as shown, and if the energy barrier between A and B is large, then at low temperatures a substantial amount of the protein may remain in conformation A

The 'multistable' model of protein conformation is a thermodynamic, as opposed to kinetic, model. As shown in *Figure 3.16,* a single primary structure has different thermodynamically favourable states at high and low temperatures. State A has the lower free energy at low temperatures; conformation B has the lower free energy at high temperatures. If the energy

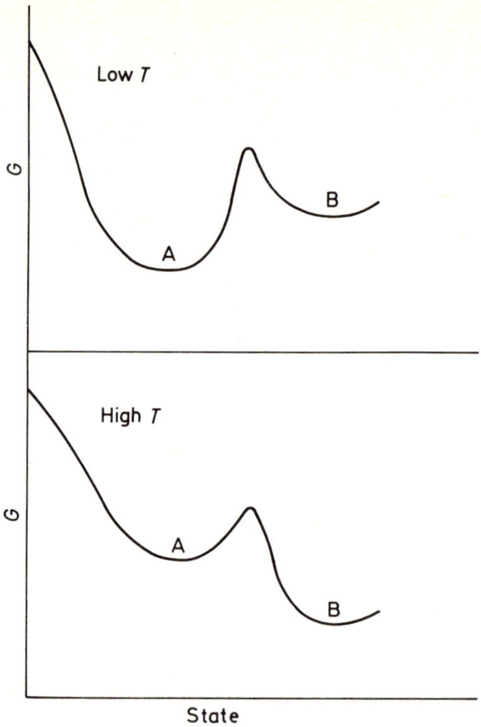

Figure 3.16 The 'multistable' protein model. In this system the thermodynamically most stable conformation varies with temperature. At low temperatures, conformation A is more stable. At high temperatures, conformation B is more stable. If conformation A has a low temperature optimum and conformation B a high temperature optimum, then a single amino acid sequence can, in effect, generate two functionally distinct and adaptively different enzyme variants. This type of system may be responsible for the kinetic properties of king crab pyruvate kinase (Figures 3.17 and 3.18). (Model after Nickerson, 1973)

barrier between the states is not so large as to prevent fairly rapid interconversion between the two states, then a change in cell temperature could lead to a rapid conversion of A to B, or vice-versa. [The interested reader should consult the original papers by Nickerson and Day (1969) and Nickerson (1973) for additional examples of environmental and physiological effects which may be involved in the interconversion of multistable and metastable proteins.]

We believe that there is strong evidence in support of the role of multistable proteins in temperature adaptation processes. For instance, the observation that a single enzyme can continue to bind substrate well over a wide range of temperatures, whereas other, inter-specific variants of the same enzyme do not (compare the different AChE patterns in *Figure 3.12*), is at least consistent with the hypothesis that temperature-induced changes in enzyme conformation lead to adaptive adjustments in substrate binding ability. An alternative mechanism to account for these interspecific differences, one invoking amino acid substitutions at the substrate binding site, has been discussed earlier.

Another finding which is consistent with the existence of temperature-dependent multistable states of proteins is shown in *Figure 3.17*. Pyruvate kinase of the Alaskan king crab (*Paralithodes camtschatica*) displays complex saturation kinetics, as illustrated. At low temperatures, e.g. 2°C, the substrate saturation curve is basically hyperbolic, and only at the highest concentrations of substrate is a 'bump' obvious. As the assay temperature is raised, the anomalous 'bump' in the saturation curve comes to assume a greater and greater role in the activity of the enzyme. At temperatures above 15°C, the saturation curve is sigmoidal, indicating that the form of the enzyme responsible for the 'bump' at lower temperatures is now responsible for virtually all of the enzymic activity at all PEP concentrations.

These kinetic patterns were interpreted to mean that this enzyme is capable of existing in two conformational states, one exhibiting classical Michaelis Menten kinetics and one displaying sigmoidal kinetics (Somero, 1969b). The hyperbolic state is favoured at low temperatures, the sigmoidal state is favoured at high temperatures. This hypothesis is identical with Nickerson's (1973) suggested two-state 'multistable' protein (*Figure 3.16*), wherein the hyperbolic form of the enzyme is represented by state A, and the sigmoidal form by state B. The observation that prolonged incubation of the king crab enzyme at an intermediate temperature such as 10°C at which both forms are kinetically apparent did not lead to complete conversion to one state or the other argues strongly against a 'metastable' model (*Figure 3.15*) for this system.

The biologically important effects of this apparent temperature-

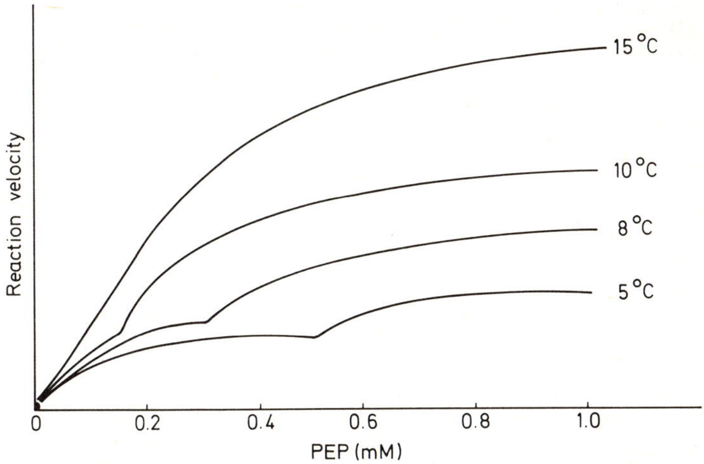

Figure 3.17 The effect of temperature and varying PEP concentrations on the activity of Alaskan king crab (Paralithodes camtschatica) *pyruvate kinase. Notice how the 'bump' contribution to activity increases as temperature rises. (Data from Somero, 1969b; figure from Hochachka and Somero, 1973; courtesy W. B. Saunders & Co.)*

dependent interconversion between two conformational states of the enzyme are suggested by the apparent K_m (or $S_{0.5}$)-versus-temperature profiles of *Figure 3.18*. Note the striking similarity between these two curves and those found for the rainbow trout 'warm' and 'cold' isozymes. In both the trout and king crab enzyme systems, the presence of two forms of an enzyme leads to stabilisation of substrate binding ability over the full range of habitat temperatures of the species. Multiple locus isozymes and multistable forms of a single primary structure thus seem capable of effecting an identical adaptive response.

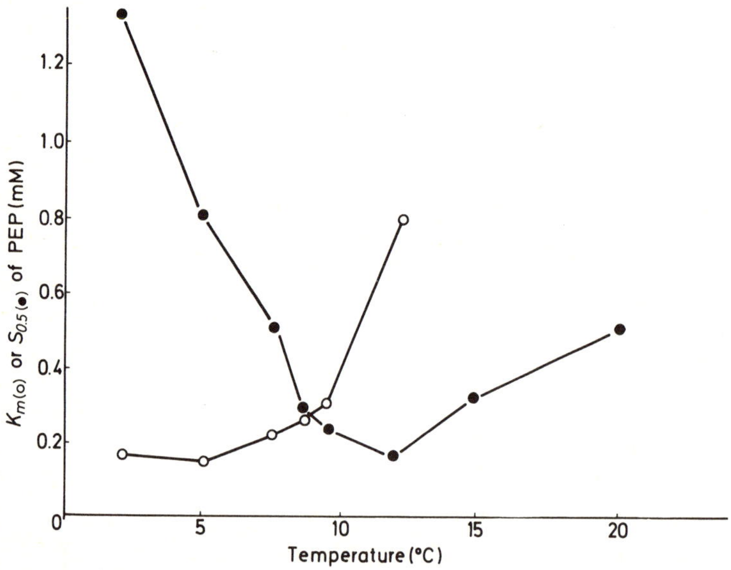

Figure 3.18 The effect of assay temperature on the apparent K_m or $S_{0.5}$ value for the two conformational variants postulated to exist in the pyruvate kinase system of the Alaskan king crab. The hyperbolic form of the enzyme (open circles) has highest substrate affinity at low temperatures. The sigmoidal form of the enzyme (closed circles) has highest substrate affinity over the upper portion of the thermal range experienced by the organism. (Data from Somero, 1969b; figure from Hochachka and Somero, 1973; courtesy W. B. Saunders & Co.)

The observation that conformational variants of a single primary structure can exhibit kinetic properties akin to those resulting from the activities of two multiple locus isozymes leads us to sound a note of caution when interpreting published kinetic data. Reports of kinetically distinct forms of enzymes, e.g. in differently acclimated individuals, should not be taken as a sufficient basis for concluding that different allozymes or multiple locus isozymes are present in the organisms. Perhaps in many cases in which kinetic differences have been observed between the enzymes of warm- and cold-acclimated specimens, whereas no electrophoretic differences were apparent (Somero and Hochachka, 1971; Hochachka and Clayton-Hochachka, 1973; Mester, Iordachescu and Niculescu, 1973), the 'new' enzyme form appearing during acclimation is different only in terms of tertiary structure (conformation), not in primary structure.

Lastly, the pyruvate kinase data presented in *Table 3.4* show that temperature-dependent conformational states of an enzyme may lead to differences in the catalytic activation parameters of the reaction, as well as to changes in apparent substrate affinity (*Figure 3.18*). Thus below a certain temperature (approximately 20–26°C depending on the species) the activation enthalpy, free energy and entropy exhibit increases for all PK's studied except the enzyme of *Trematomus* (*Pagothenia*) *borchgrevinki,* an Antarctic fish. Interestingly, only the low temperature conformer of PK exhibits apparently temperature-adaptive differences in activation parameters (*Table 3.4*; Low and Somero, 1976).

3.4.2.5 COUNTERACTING ENTHALPY CHANGES AS A MECHANISM FOR LESSENING THE TEMPERATURE SENSITIVITIES OF ENZYME-LIGAND BINDING EVENTS

We have already discussed two mechanisms for reducing the temperature-dependence of enzyme-ligand binding events. First, changes in the amino acid composition of the ligand binding site(s) of an enzyme could alter the binding enthalpies in temperature-adaptive manners (*see* the discussion of the AChE binding site above). Second, temperature-induced conformational changes in an enzyme could lead to temperature-adaptive changes in ligand binding, as has been suggested to occur, for example, with king crab pyruvate kinase (*Figures 3.17* and *3.18*).

A third mechanism for reducing the temperature sensitivities of substrate and modulator binding events has been alluded to only briefly and will now be discussed in some detail. This is the mechanism involving a pairing of two reactions which occur with enthalpy changes of approximately equal absolute value, but opposing signs. Consider, for example, a substrate binding reaction in which the interaction between enzyme and substrate involves two hydrogen bonds. Excluding the effects of water-protein and water-substrate interactions, which of course could contribute significantly to the energetics of the binding event (*see* Low and Somero, 1975b), we would predict a binding enthalpy of approximately –8 kcal/mole (*Table 3.1*). The formation of the enzyme-substrate complex would therefore have a significant dependence on temperature. To reduce this temperature effect, a chemical reaction with an approximately equal enthalpy change in terms of absolute value, but with opposite sign, could be triggered elsewhere on the enzyme (or within the enzyme). Since thermodynamic quantities are additive, the net enthalpy change could approximate zero, i.e. the binding event would be temperature-independent.

An example of this type of paired, opposing enthalpy changes which lead to temperature-independence in ligand binding is found in the case of mammalian haemoglobin (Hb) (Benesch, Benesch and Yu, 1969). The binding of oxygen to Hb is temperature-dependent, and the temperature effect observed in purified Hb preparations is much greater than in whole blood. This observation indicates that some component in the erythrocyte may modify the temperature-dependence of the oxygenation reaction. The compound responsible has been shown to be the important organophosphate modulator of Hb, 2,3-diphosphoglycerate (2,3-DPG). The binding of this ligand to Hb is weakly exothermic, as is the binding of oxygen. Since 2,3-DPG must be removed from Hb for oxygen to bind, we find a situation in which the potential for counteracting enthalpy changes like those discussed above can occur. Thus, some of the heat released during oxygen binding can be used to 'pay' for the removal of 2,3-DPG from Hb. It has been shown that the heat of the oxygenation reaction is −7.3 kcal/mole in the presence of 2,3-DPG, and −10.7 kcal/mole in the absence of this modulator.

The possible importance of this type of mechanism for reducing reaction enthalpies in ectotherms has not been investigated. Interestingly, for the Hb of the bluefin tuna, which displays an extreme degree of temperature-independence in oxygen binding (Rossi-Fanelli and Antonini, 1960), the opposed effects of modulator- and oxygen-binding events do not appear important in this regard. Purified tuna Hb is capable of binding oxygen in a virtually temperature-independent fashion. We suggest that paired and opposing enthalpy changes could still be important, however. Rather than invoking enthalpy changes arising from ligand binding or release, we propose that changes in the Hb molecule itself, e.g. the formation or rupture of a weak bond between amino acid side-chains, or between amino acid side-chains or peptide backbone linkages and the surrounding water could provide the energy changes required to adaptively titrate ligand binding enthalpies (Low and Somero, 1975b; Somero, 1975a). In fact, the energy changes which result from altered protein group hydration are both large enough and of frequent enough occurrence to serve as a vast reservoir of raw material for adjusting binding energetics.

3.4.3 Temperature-membrane interactions

3.4.3.1 FUNDAMENTALS OF MEMBRANE STRUCTURE

The importance of temperature-induced changes in the structure/function of cellular membranes has been appreciated for many years (Brock, 1967; Tansey and Brock, 1972; Bowler *et al.*, 1973). As discussed below, changes in membrane structure caused by high or low extremes of temperature may be of primary importance in establishing the thermal tolerance limits of organisms (Tansey and Brock, 1972).

The basis of the extreme temperature-sensitivity of membrane structure derives from the fact that the stability of membrane organisation and the physical state of the cell membrane are dependent on weak chemical bonds. The alignment of the fatty acid chains of phospholipids (*Figure 3.19*) involves van der Waals' interactions. The stabilisation of lipid-protein complexes involves at least two types of weak bonds. The proteins which occur on the surface of the membrane, the so-called 'extrinsic' or 'peripheral' (Singer and Nicolson, 1972) proteins, are electrostatically bound to the charged ends of the phospholipids. The proteins which occur partly or entirely within the membrane ('intrinsic' or 'integral' proteins) tend to have non-polar surfaces (Singer and Nicolson, 1972) and are held within the fatty acid layer by hydrophobic interactions.

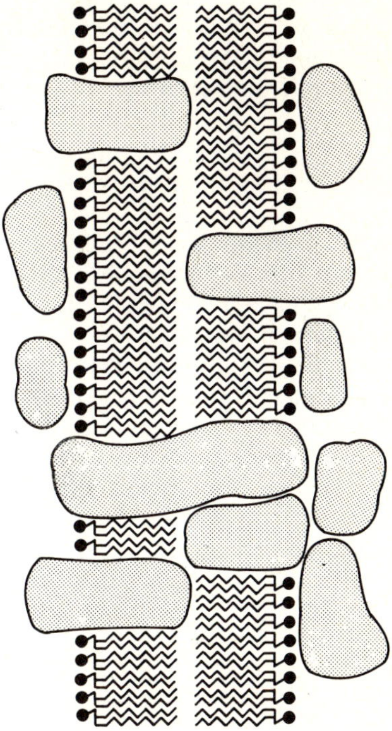

Figure 3.19 A schematic diagram of the structure of a functional biological membrane, e.g. a plasma membrane. The basic framework of the membrane is a phospholipid bilayer within which and on which protein molecules are bound by 'weak' bonds (see text). (Figure after Fox, 1972; from Hochachka and Somero, 1973; courtesy W. B. Saunders & Co.)

Changes in cell temperature can therefore be expected to have several potentially damaging effects on membrane structure and function. The viscosity of a membrane is determined by the degree of structure in the fatty acid side-chain bilayer. Reductions in temperature will stabilise the van der Waals' interactions among the non-polar aliphatic chains, leading to large increases in membrane viscosity. If the membrane becomes too viscous, many of its essential functions will be impaired (*see below*).

Changes in temperature can also be expected to affect the structures of membrane proteins and their interactions with membrane lipids. For example, the binding of 'extrinsic' ('peripheral') membrane proteins might be disrupted at elevated temperatures. Since the release of an enzyme from the surface of a membrane can lead to major changes in the kinetic properties of an enzyme (Karpatkin, 1967), a temperature effect of this type could severely disrupt metabolism. To date, temperature effects on enzyme binding to membrane surfaces have not been systematically investigated.

Lastly, for proteins which function more or less within the non-polar interior of the membrane, changes in the viscosity of the membrane could exert major effects on the functional properties of the proteins. For example, a highly viscous, rigid membrane structure might preclude the proper movements or conformational changes by 'integral' ('intrinsic') proteins. Functions such as transport could be blocked under these circumstances.

Let us now examine some of the available information concerning temperature effects on membrane structure and function and the types of membrane restructurings which seem important in adapting membranes to different temperatures.

3.4.3.2 TEMPERATURE EFFECTS ON MEMBRANE-ASSOCIATED ENZYMES

There have been several recent reviews of temperature effects on the kinetics of membrane-associated enzymes (*see* Hazel and Prosser, 1974; Hochachka and Somero, 1973), so we need consider only a small number of examples to illustrate the salient aspects of these phenomena. The most characteristic effect of temperature on membrane-associated enzymes is illustrated in *Figure 3.20.* An Arrhenius plot (log V_{max}-versus-the reciprocal of the absolute temperature) with two slopes, above and below the 'break' temperature, has been reported for several membrane-associated enzymes from tissues of mammals and chilling-sensitive plants (Lyons and Raison, 1970a, 1970b; Inesi, Millman and Eletr, 1973; McMurchie, Raison and Cairncross, 1973).

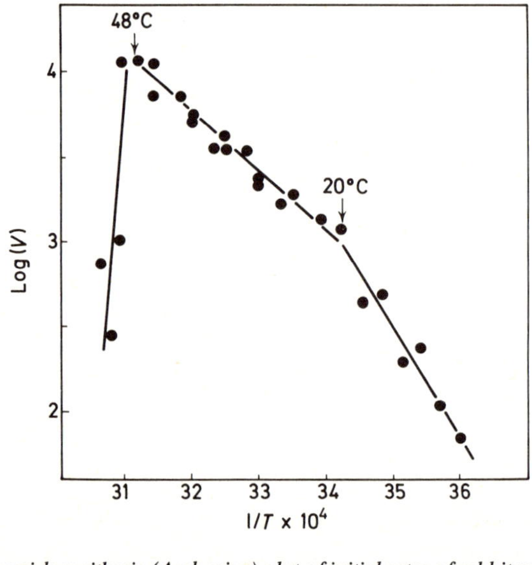

Figure 3.20 A semi-logarithmic (Arrhenius) plot of initial rates of rabbit muscle sarcoplasmic reticulum Ca-dependent ATPase activity. Note the 'break' in the slope of the plot at 20°C, a temperature at which the lipid phase of the membrane (Figure 3.19) undergoes a major change in viscosity (see text). (After Inesi et al., 1973; courtesy Academic Press)

Table 3.5 THERMODYNAMIC ACTIVATION PARAMETERS FOR ATPASE ACTIVITY ABOVE AND BELOW THE 'BREAK' TEMPERATURE IN THE ARRHENIUS PLOT (AFTER INESI, MILLMAN AND ELETR, 1973)

Temperature range (°C)	$\Delta H^{\ddagger}$ (kcal/mol)	$\Delta G^{\ddagger}$ (kcal/mol)	$\Delta S^{\ddagger}$ (entropy units)
5–20	28–30	17–19	+38–+40
20–35	15–17	14–17	0–+ 3

The most thorough analysis of this temperature effect has been made by Inesi, Millman and Eletr (1973) who examined the effect of temperature on a Ca^{2+} dependent ATPase found in sarcoplasmic reticulum vesicles of rabbit skeletal muscle. These workers determined the activation thermodynamic parameters for the ATPase reaction above and below the break temperature of approximately 20°C (*Table 3.5*). These data show that large changes in activation enthalpy and activation entropy occur at the break temperature. Inesi, Millman and Eletr (1973) interpret these findings as follows: below 20°C the fatty acid side-chains of the phospholipids exist in a tightly organised, semi-crystalline state. This rigid or viscous environment limits the potential for movement (conformational, translational, rotational) of the ATPase enzyme. The large activation enthalpy required at temperatures below 20°C stems from a need to disrupt the ordered lipid molecules in order for the ATPase enzyme to undergo the changes in shape or position which accompany catalysis. Disruption of the lipid organisation will of course lead to a large activation entropy. This interpretation of the kinetic data is strongly supported by spin label studies which revealed that the motion of the fatty acid chains greatly increased, and their organisation decreased, as the experimental temperature was raised above 20°C. In addition, spin labels attached to the reactive sites on the ATPase molecules behaved differently above and below the break temperature; the motion of the protein side-chains also increased above 20°C. These findings support the view that decreases in temperature can lead to marked disruptions of enzymic activities in membranes owing to a primary change in the viscosity of the hydrophobic regions in which the 'intrinsic' proteins are embedded which leads to impairment in the abilities of the enzymes to undergo the necessary structural and/or positional changes involved in catalysis.

3.4.3.3 TEMPERATURE-ADAPTIVE ALTERATIONS IN MEMBRANE LIPID COMPOSITION: 'HOMEOVISCOUS' ADAPTATION

Since 'intrinsic' membrane proteins require an environment which is sufficiently fluid to permit the structural and positional changes involved in catalysis, the adjustment of membrane viscosity is apt to be a critical component of the temperature adaptation response. Viscosity adjustment in a temperature compensatory manner, termed 'homeoviscous adaptation' by Sinensky (1974), has in fact been studied for several decades in both warm- and cold-blooded organisms (*see* Prosser, 1974).

The major adaptive change observed in all species studied is an adjustment in the degree of saturation of the fatty acid chains of the membrane phospholipids (Johnston and Roots, 1964; Roots, 1968; Caldwell and Vernberg, 1970; Smith and Kemp, 1971; Hazel, 1972a, 1972b; Sinensky, 1974). An increase in the number of double bonds in a fatty acid, i.e. a decrease in saturation, enhances the fluidity of a fatty acid since double bonds cause bends in the carbon chain and thereby make it difficult for close alignment, and strong van der Waals' contacts, to occur among fatty acid chains. Decreased saturation of membrane lipids from brain (Roots, 1968), mitochondria (Caldwell and Vernberg, 1970; Hazel, 1972a, 1972b) and intestine (Smith and Kemp, 1971) of cold-acclimated fish show the generality of this type of adaptation.

Further evidence that the viscosity of membrane lipids can affect enzymic function is given by the data of Hazel (1972a, 1972b). He found that lipids purified from mitochondria of warm- and cold-acclimated goldfish had different activating abilities on purified succinic dehydrogenase (SDH) from the fish. The less saturated lipids from cold-acclimated specimens displayed the greater activating ability. The molecular basis of this effect may be the same as that suggested by Inesi, Millman and Eletr (1973) for the observed influence of lipid viscosity on membrane-bound ATPase function.

The changes observed in membrane lipid composition during thermal acclimation parallel the differences seen among species adapted to different temperatures. Although data are quite sparse, available information on fishes (Patton, 1975) and bacteria (Ray, White and Brock, 1971) is all consistent with the view that 'homeoviscous' adaptation of cellular and intracellular membranes is an important component of the temperature adaptation response.

3.4.3.4 TEMPERATURE AND RATES OF ION AND WATER FLUX THROUGH MEMBRANES: NON-ACTIVE TRANSPORT PROCESSES

Temperature-dependent changes in membrane viscosity could also affect membrane-based processes which are not dependent on enzymic activity. For example, if the rate of non-active transport of water and solutes through a membrane is partly dependent on the structure of the membrane, changes in temperature might alter rates of these non-enzyme-mediated processes. Thus, if decreases in temperature led to more viscous membranes, rates of non-active transport might fall rapidly as temperature is reduced. Conversely, a looser membrane structure at higher temperatures might enhance the passive flux of water and solutes through membranes, thereby increasing the demands on the energy supply of the cell for active transport processes needed to restore ion and water balance.

The effects of temperature on the passage of water and sodium through the gill epithelia of the eel, *Anguilla anguilla,* have been measured by Motais and Isaia (1972). The percentage of body water exchanged with the environment in eels maintained at 25, 15 and 5°C was 56%, 35%, and 14%, respectively. The diffusional permeability of sodium was affected in a highly similar manner. Whether these temperature-dependent changes in water and ion permeabilities are due entirely to temperature effects on gill epithelial structure is not clear, since temperature-dependent changes in gill circulatory patterns (reduced circulation through the filaments at low temperature, for example) could lead to the same type of effect. However, these observations do carry an important implication for temperature compensation processes, regardless of the mechanistic basis of the permeability changes. Thus, the observation that metabolic compensation is seldom complete may find partial explanation in the fact that the energy demands for ionic and osmotic regulation are reduced at low temperatures.

A relevant observation in this connection is the finding by Maetz and Evans (1972) that the activity of the sodium pump enzyme responsible for sodium extrusion in the seawater-adapted flounder, *Platichthys flesus* L., exhibits 'inverse' temperature compensation, ATPase activity was higher in 16°C-acclimated fish than in 6°C-acclimated specimens. As Hazel and Prosser (1970) argue, enzymes which exhibit 'inverse' compensation to temperature generally are involved in processes that lead to removal of harmful substances from the cell. This explanation could account for the observed pattern of flounder ATPase activities as well if elevated temperatures promoted increased permeability to sodium ion.

3.4.4 Freezing avoidance mechanisms in marine teleosts

3.4.4.1 THE NATURE OF THE PROBLEM

All marine teleosts are hypotonic to seawater* (Dobbs and DeVries, 1975). For most species of marine teleosts blood freezing points are approximately −0.5 to −0.8°C. The fact that these values are at least 1°C higher than the freezing point of seawater indicates that teleosts living in high latitude waters and coming into contact with ice must find mechanisms to prevent ice formation in their cellular and extracellular fluids.

As in the case of many environmental adaptations, the apparently simplest strategy for avoiding freezing involves migration to regions where waters are not cold enough to permit ice formation or, if the water temperature is below the freezing point of the body fluids of the fish, there are no ice crystals present to seed ice formation within the organism. Many marine teleosts from high latitudes do in fact behaviourally avoid ice formation by remaining at depths where the absence of ice crystals enables

*It has been reported (Potts and Morris, 1968) that certain Antarctic fishes of the genus *Trematomus* are hypertonic to seawater. This conclusion is based on data gathered with a Fiske osmometer, which measures the freezing point of a solution. If the solutes present are ideal, the solute concentration can be determined directly from the freezing point depression observed. In the case of these Antarctic fishes, however, there is a difference of several tenths of a degree Celsius between the freezing and melting points of the body fluids owing to the presence of glycoprotein 'antifreeze' molecules (DeVries, 1971). The correct measure of solute concentration is the melting point of a solution containing these 'antifreezes'. Thus, as Dobbs and DeVries (1975) have shown, even these freezing-resistant Antarctic species are hypotonic to seawater.

the fishes to remain in a super-cooled state (Gordon, Amdur and Scholander, 1962). The obvious drawback of this mode of adaptation is that the organism is ecologically restricted, i.e. its choice of habitat cannot be made on the basis of other than the single criterion of ice presence or absence. It would therefore seem to be advantageous for marine teleosts to develop freezing resistance mechanisms which will allow them to remain in the presence of ice without there existing a danger of seeding ice formation in the body fluids. This 'goal' has been attained via development of organic antifreeze molecules (DeVries, 1971).

3.4.4.2 ORGANIC 'ANTIFREEZE' COMPOUNDS IN POLAR FISHES

The first hint that polar marine teleosts might contain organic antifreeze compounds was provided by the findings of Gordon *et al.* (1962) who reported that a significant fraction of the freezing point depression of the blood serum of certain Arctic fishes was due to an unidentified non-protein nitrogen fraction. In other marine teleosts, virtually all of the freezing point depression of the blood can be attributed to inorganic ions (*see* Dobbs and DeVries, 1975).

The first chemical characterisation of a fish 'antifreeze' molecule was achieved by DeVries and co-workers (DeVries, Komatsu and Feeney, 1970; Komatus, DeVries and Feeney, 1970; DeVries, 1971; Duman and DeVries, 1972; Lin, Duman and DeVries, 1972). In Antarctic nototheniid fishes of the genus *Trematomus* a family of glycoprotein antifreeze molecules is present which have molecular weights of from 2600 to 33 000 daltons. The repeating structure of the antifreeze molecules having molecular weights of 2600, 3500, and 8000 daltons is shown in *Figure 3.21*. These lower molecular weight antifreezes account for approximately 20% of the total antifreeze concentration on a weight basis.

All size classes of these glycoprotein antifreezes were found to have two curious effects on water/ice behaviour. First, the freezing point depressing abilities of the glycoproteins exceed those predicted on the basis of colligative relationships; a solution of the glycoprotein antifreezes lowers the freezing point of an aqueous solution some 200–500 times as much as an equal concentration of an ideal solute (DeVries, 1971). The glycoprotein antifreezes thus provide the fishes with a vastly increased resistance to freezing without the cost of greatly increased osmotic concentrations in the body fluids. The significance of the glycoprotein antifreezes we feel is that they eliminate a requirement that the fish come into osmotic conformity with seawater, a physiological adaptation which likely could wreak havoc with the cellular chemistry. For example, increasing ionic concentrations sufficiently to gain isotonicity with seawater would no doubt also require that many of the macromolecules of the fish change their properties so that, for example, their ion optima are brought into agreement with the new ion concentrations in the extra- and intracellular fluids.

A second interesting attribute of the glycoprotein 'antifreeze' compounds is their ability to lower the freezing point of a solution much more than they

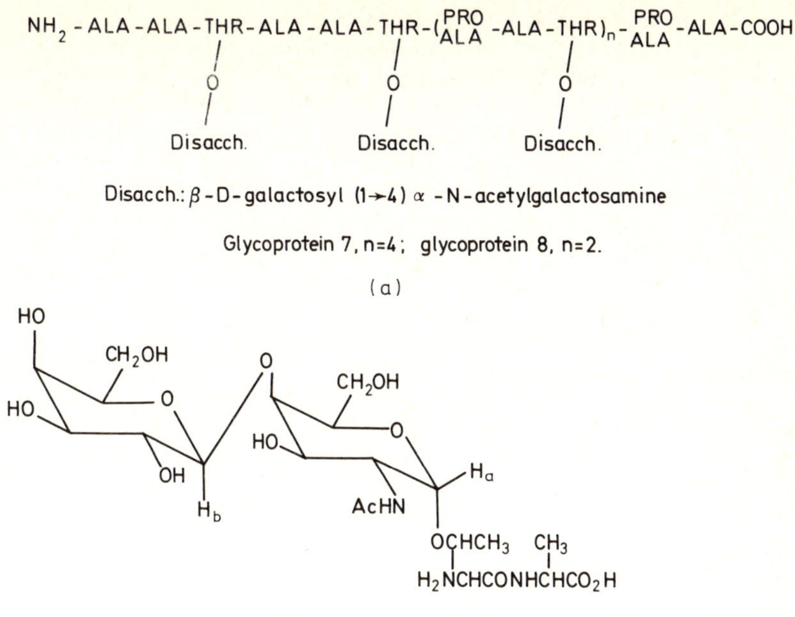

(b)

Figure 3.21(a) The structures of 'antifreeze' glycoproteins 7 and 8 (the most prevalent antifreezes) from the Antarctic fish, Trematomus borchgrevinki. *(b) Structure of glycodipeptide from subtilisin digestion of glycoproteins 7 and 8. (After Lin et al., 1972; courtesy Academic Press Inc.)*

reduce the melting point — a phenomenon termed 'thermal hysteresis' (Lin, Duman and DeVries, 1972). Again, the glycoproteins deviate sharply in their behaviour from so-called ideal solutes.

The structural bases of these effects on water behaviour are not fully understood, but it is clear that the hydroxyl groups on the glycoproteins are essential for antifreeze activity (Komatsu, DeVries and Feeney, 1970). When the hydroxyl groups are chemically blocked from interacting with water, the glycoproteins lose their special antifreeze properties.

A clue to the mode of action of the antifreezes has come from studies of the freezing-out behaviour of the antifreezes and other solutes (Duman and DeVries, 1972; Raymond and DeVries, 1972). When an aqueous solution of an ideal solute is frozen, the concentration of the solute in any portion of the solution which remains liquid is significantly increased, i.e. the solute is frozen-out of the ice lattice. Antifreeze molecules do not exhibit this behaviour unless they have been chemically modified in ways that lead to loss of their unusual abilities to alter freezing points. It therefore seems likely that the glycoprotein antifreezes exert their freezing-point-depressing effects by means of coating small ice crystals and preventing additional water molecules from joining the crystals.

A final aspect of the antifreeze story of some biological interest is the mechanism involved in regulating antifreeze synthesis in northern fishes which change their blood antifreeze concentrations on a seasonal basis. Duman and DeVries (1974a) have found that a long photoperiod is a necessary signal for triggering antifreeze removal from the blood in the northern flounder, *Pseudopleuronectes americanus*. Winter-acclimatised flounder did not lose antifreeze compounds when the photoperiod remained short but water temperatures were high. This finding suggests that control of antifreeze removal from the blood is via a fail-safe mechanism. Thus, unseasonably warm temperatures in the spring would not lead to loss of antifreeze until the day length was of sufficient length to tell the fish that further danger of freezing temperatures was past for the year. The synthesis of antifreeze during cold acclimatisation could be induced merely by lowering the holding temperature, however.

Current study of marine teleost antifreeze compounds is focusing on the functional and structural similarities and differences between the well characterised glycoprotein antifreezes of Antarctic fishes and the recently discovered functional analogues of these antifreezes which are present in Arctic fishes (Duman and DeVries, 1974a, 1974b, 1975). Initial observations (Duman, 1974; Raymond, Lin, and DeVries, 1975) indicate that the antifreeze molecules found in Arctic and Antarctic fishes are strikingly similar in some cases and extremely different in others. For example, antifreezes of the Antarctic fish *Trematomus* (*Pagothenia*) *borchgrevinki* and the northern tomcod (*Eleginus gracilis*) are both glycoproteins with highly similar amino acid compositions (Raymond *et al.,* 1975). In contrast, the antifreezes found in two other northern fishes, the sculpin, *Myosocephalus verrucosus,* and the winter flounder, *Pseudopleuronectes americanus,* appear to be almost entirely protein and to have a much wider variety of amino acids in their structure (Raymond, Lin and DeVries, 1975). Analysis of the three-dimensional structures of these different antifreezes will be extremely interesting, since in spite of their structural (compositional) differences, the glycoprotein and protein antifreezes appear to have very similar effects on ice formation.

3.5 CONCLUDING COMMENTS

In this chapter we have attempted to outline the major stresses imposed on marine organisms by changes in temperature, and the fundamental adaptive responses these organisms make to compensate for these stresses. While our emphasis has been primarily biochemical, the reader must not forget that biochemical adaptations frequently represent a 'last resort' response to environmental change. Thus it is often far easier for an organism to behaviourally or physiologically respond to a given stress than to restructure the basic chemistry of its cells and tissues.

When biochemical adaptations do occur, they often appear to be of three rather distinct types. First, the quantities of macromolecules or lower molecular weight substances responsible for effecting a process or forming a structure may be altered in adaptive manners. For example, enzyme concentrations may be increased during cold acclimation. Haemoglobin concentrations in poikilotherms may be reduced in cold-adapted aquatic species. Solute concentrations may be adjusted to alter freezing resistance.

A second adaptive strategy is qualitative in nature, as it involves new variants on molecular themes. Thus we find that enzyme homologues differ markedly and in apparently adaptive manners among species with different cell temperatures. Membrane phospholipids differ in fatty acid composition among differently thermally-acclimated specimens. Haemoglobin molecules have different oxygen binding affinities (Hochachka and Somero, 1973). In all of these qualitative restructurings, whether they occur over evolutionary or seasonal (lifespan) time courses, it appears that continued success in an environment demands more than simple adjustments in molecular concentrations; new molecular species, often requiring changes in genetic information, serve as a more satisfactory mechanism for coping with environmental change.

Lastly, an organism may adapt via modulating the activity of pre-existing macromolecules. This adaptive regulation of the activities of existing enzymes, for example, can involve chemical modulators (activators and inhibitors) and physical effects which achieve the same end. Thus the possibility that enzymes can exist in more than one conformational or aggregational state ('multistable' proteins) gives the organism a potential for spanning a wide environmental range with only a single type of enzyme, in terms of primary structure (amino acid sequence), which nonetheless can adopt a number of different functional characteristics. The extent to which multistable proteins contribute to environmental adaptation is not at present known. Certainly this is a fascinating phenomenon deserving of intensive study.

In examining all of these patterns of molecular adaptation, the comparative biochemist is in a unique position as a scientist. In an aesthetic sense, his study systems include organisms and phenomena whose beauty is perhaps the motivating factor behind his entry into science. In a creative sense, there can emerge from the study of adaptive mechanisms the clearest possible image of the course taken by molecular evolution. And, in times when those who choose to work with arcane marine species are often suspected of being too far from the main, accepted pathways of investigation, it is reassuring to remember that those who discover the subtle nature of variations on a biological theme are often in the best position to appreciate and communicate the fundamental nature of the theme or phenomenon *per se*.

REFERENCES

ATKINSON, D. E. (1969). 'Limitation of metabolite concentrations and the conservation of solvent capacity in the living cell', 29–43. In: *Current Topics in Cellular Regulation,* **I.** Ed. B. L. Horecker and E. B. Stadtman. Academic Press, New York

AYALA, F. J., HEDGECOCK, D., ZUMWALT, G. S. and VALENTINE, J. W. (1973). 'Genetic variation in *Tridacna maxima,* an ecological analog of some unsuccessful evolutionary lineages', *Evolution,* **27,** 177–191

BALDWIN, J. (1971). 'Adaptation of enzymes to temperature: acetylcholinesterases in the central nervous system of fishes', *Comp. Biochem. Physiol.,* **40,** 181–187

BALDWIN, J. and HOCHACHKA, P. W. (1970). 'Functional significance of isoenzymes in thermal acclimation: acetylcholinesterase from trout brain', *Biochem. J.*, **116**, 883–887

BARCROFT, J. (1934). *Features in the Architecture of Physiological Function.* Cambridge University Press, London, p. 40

BENESCH, R. E., BENESCH, R. and YU, C. I. (1969). 'The oxygenation of hemoglobin in the present of 2,3-diphosphoglycerate. Effect of temperature, pH, ionic strength, and hemoglobin concentration', *Biochem.*, **8**, 2567–2571

BEYER, R. F. (1972). 'Effects of low temperature on cold sensitive enzymes from mammalian tissues', 17–54. In: *Hibernation-Hypothermia: Perspectives and Challenges.* Eds. F. E. South, J. P. Hannon, J. R. Willis, E. T. Pengelley and N. R. Alpert. Elsevier, Amsterdam

BOWLER, K., DUNCAN, C. J., GLADWELL, R. T. and DAVISON, T. F. (1973). 'Cellular heat injury', *Comp. Biochem. Physiol.*, **45A**, 441–450

BRANDTS, J. F. (1967). 'Heat effects on proteins and enzymes', 25–72. In: *Thermobiology.* Ed. A. Rose. Academic Press, New York

BRETT, J. R. (1971). 'Temperature—animals-fishes', 513–560. In: *Marine Ecology,* **I.** Ed. O. Kinne. Wiley-Interscience, London

BROCK, T. D. (1967). 'Life at high temperatures', *Science,* **158,** 1012–1019

CALDWELL, R. S. and VERNBERG, J. F. (1970). 'The influence of acclimation temperature on the lipid composition of fish gill mitochondria', *Comp. Biochem. Physiol.,* **34,** 179–191

CAREY, F. G., TEAL, J. M., KANWISHER, K. W. and LAWSON, K. D. (1971). 'Warm-bodied fishes', *Am. Zool.,* **11,** 137–145

CLARK, M. G., BLOXHAM, D. P., HOLLAND, P. C. and LARDY, H. A. (1973). 'Estimation of the fructose diphosphatase-phosphofructokinase substrate cycle in the flight muscle of *Bombus affinis', Biochem. J.,* **134,** 589–597

DAS, A. B. (1967). 'Biochemical changes in tissues of goldfish acclimated to high and low temperature. II. Synthesis of protein and RNA of subcellular fractions and tissue composition', *Comp. Biochem. Physiol.,* **21,** 469–485

DEAN, J. M. (1969). 'The metabolism of tissues of thermally acclimated trout *(Salmo gairdneri)', Comp. Biochem. Physiol.,* **29,** 185–196

DEHNEL, P. A. (1955). 'Rates of growth of gastropods as a function of latitude', *Physiol. Zool.,* **28,** 115–144

DEVRIES, A. L. (1971). 'Glycoproteins as biological antifreeze agents in Antarctic fishes', *Science,* **172,** 1152–1155

DEVRIES, A. L., KOMATSU, S. K. and FEENEY, R. E. (1970). 'Chemical and physical properties of freezing point-depressing glycoproteins from Antarctic fishes', *J. Biol. Chem.,* **245,** 2901–2908

DOBBS, III, G. H. and DEVRIES, A. L. (1975). 'Renal function in Antarctic teleost fish', *Mar. Biol.,* (in the press)

DUMAN, J. G. (1974). 'The role of macromolecular antifreeze solutes in freezing resistance of cold water fishes'. Ph.D. dissertation, University of California, San Diego

DUMAN, J. G. and DEVRIES, A. L. (1972). 'Freezing behaviour of aqueous solutions of glycoproteins from the blood of an Antarctic fish', *Cryobiology,* **9,** 469–472

DUMAN, J. G. and DEVRIES, A. L. (1974a). 'The effects of temperature and photoperiod on antifreeze production in cold water fishes', *J. Exp. Zool.,* **190,** 89–97

DUMAN, J. G. and DEVRIES, A. L. (1974b). 'Freezing resistance in the winter flounder, *Pseudopleuronectes americanus', Nature,* **247,** 237–238

DUMAN, J. G. and DEVRIES, A. L. (1975). 'The role of macromolecular antifreeze in cold water fishes', *Comp. Biochem. Physiol.,* **52A,** 193–199

FOX, C. F. (1972). 'The structure of cell membranes', *Sci. Am.,* **226,** 30–38

FROEDE, H. C. and WILSON, I. B. (1972). 'Acetylcholinesterase', 89–114. In: *The Enzymes,* **5.** Ed. P. Boyer. Academic Press, New York

GOOCH, J. L. and SCHOPF, T. J. M. (1972). 'Genetic variability in the deep sea: relation to environmental variability', *Evolution,* **26,** 545–552

GORDON, M. S. (1968). 'Oxygen consumption of red and white muscles from tuna fishes', *Science,* **159,** 87–90

GORDON, M. S., AMDUR, B. H. and SCHOLANDER, P. F. (1962). 'Freezing resistance in some northern fishes', *Biol. Bull.,* **122,** 56–62

HASCHEMEYER, A. E. V. (1968). 'Compensation of liver protein synthesis in temperature acclimated toadfish, *Opsanus tau', Biol. Bull.,* **135,** 130–140

HASCHEMEYER, A. E. V. (1969a). 'Rates of polypeptide chain assembly in liver *in vivo:* relation to the mechanism of temperature acclimation in *Opsanus tau, Proc. Nat. Acad. Sci. (U.S.),* **62,** 128–135

HASCHEMEYER, A. E. V. (1969b). 'Studies on the control of protein synthesis in low temperature acclimation', *Comp. Biochem. Physiol.,* **28,** 535–548

HAZEL, J. (1972a). 'The effect of temperature acclimation upon succinic dehydrogenase activity from the epaxial muscle of the common goldfish (*Carassius auratus* L.). I. Properties of the enzyme and the effect of lipid extraction', *Comp. Biochem. Physiol.,* **43B,** 837–861

HAZEL, J. (1972b). 'The effect of temperature acclimation upon succinic dehydrogenase activity from the epaxial muscle of the common goldfish (*Carassius auratus* L.). II. Lipid reactivation of the soluble enzyme', *Comp. Biochem. Physiol.,* **43B,** 863–882

HAZEL, J. and PROSSER, C. L. (1970). 'Interpretation of inverse acclimation to temperature', *Z. Vergleich. Physiol.,* **67,** 217–228

HAZEL, J. and PROSSER, C. L. (1974). 'Molecular mechanisms of temperature compensation in poikilotherms', *Physiol. Rev.,* **54,** 620–677

HEBB, C., STEPHENS, T. C. and SMITH, M. W. (1972). 'Effect of environmental temperature on the kinetic properties of goldfish brain choline acetyltransferase', *Biochem. J.,* **129,** 1013–1021

HEINRICH, B. (1974). 'Thermoregulation in endothermic insects', *Science,* **185,** 747–756

HOCHACHKA, P. W. (1967). 'Organization of metabolism during temperature compensation', 177–213. In: *Molecular Mechanisms of Temperature Adaptation.* Ed. C. L. Prosser. *Am. Assoc. Adv. Sci.,* Washington D.C.

HOCHACHKA, P. W. (1968). 'Action of temperature on branch points in glucose and acetate metabolism,' *Comp. Biochem. Physiol.,* **25,** 107–118

HOCHACHKA, P. W. (1974a). 'Temperature and pressure adaptation of the binding site of acetylcholinesterase', *Biochem. J.,* **143,** 535–539

HOCHACHKA, P. W. (1974b). 'Temperature regulation at the cellular level', *Fed. Proc.,* **33,** 2162–2169

HOCHACHKA, P. W. and CLAYTON-HOCHACHKA, B. (1973). 'Glucose-6-phosphate dehydrogenase and thermal acclimation in the mullet fish', *Mar. Biol.,* **18,** 251–259

HOCHACHKA, P. W. and HAYES, F. R. (1962). 'The effect of temperature acclimation on pathways of glucose metabolism in the trout', *Can. J. Zool.,* **40,** 261–270

HOCHACHKA, P. W. and LEWIS, J. K. (1970). 'Enzyme variants in thermal acclimation trout liver citrate synthases', *J. Biol. Chem.,* **245,** 6567–6573

HOCHACHKA, P. W. and SOMERO, G. N. (1972). 'Biochemical adaptation to the environment', 100–156. In: *Fish Physiology* **VI.** Eds W. S. Hoar and D. J. Randall. Academic Press, New York

HOCHACHKA, P. W. and SOMERO, G. N. (1973). *Strategies of Biochemical Adaptation.* Saunders, Philadelphia

HOFER, R., LADURNER, H., GATTRINGER, A. and WIESER, W. (1975). 'Relationship between the temperature preferenda of fishes, amphibians and reptiles, and the substrate affinities of their trypsins', *J. comp. Physiol.,* **99,** 345–355

HOLETON, G. F. (1974). 'Metabolic cold adaptation of polar fish: fact or artefact', *Physiol. Zool.,* **47,** 137–152

INESI, G., MILLMAN, M. and ELETR, S. (1973). 'Temperature-induced transitions of function and structure in sarcoplasmic reticulum membranes', *J. mol. Biol.,* **81,** 483–504

ISMAIL-BEIGI, F. and EDELMAN, I. S. (1970). 'Mechanism of thyroid calorigenesis: role of active sodium transport', *Proc. Nat. Acad. Sci. (U.S.),* **67,** 1071–1078

JOHNSTON, P. V. and ROOTS, B. I. (1964). 'Brain lipid fatty acids and temperature acclimation', *Comp. Biochem. Physiol.,* **11,** 303–309

KARPATKIN, S. (1967). 'Soluble and particulate hexokinase of frog skeletal muscle', *J. Biol. Chem.,* **242,** 3525–3530

KOMATSU, S. K., DEVRIES, A. L. and FEENEY, R. E. (1970). 'Studies of the structure of freezing point-depressing glycoproteins from an Antarctic fish', *J. Biol. Chem.,* **245,** 2909–2913

KOSHLAND, D. E. Jr. and NEET, K. E. (1968). 'The catalytic and regulatory properties of enzymes', *Ann. Rev. Biochem.,* **37,** 359–410

LEVINS, R. (1968). *Evolution in Changing Environments.* Princeton University Press, Princeton, New Jersey

LEWIN, S. (1974). *Displacement of Water and Its Control of Biochemical Reactions.* Academic Press, New York

LIN, Y., DUMAN, J. G. and DEVRIES, A. L. (1972). 'Studies on the structure and activity of low molecular weight glycoproteins from an Antarctic fish', *Biochem. Biophys. Res. Comm.*, **46,** 87–92

LOW, P. S., BADA, J. L. and SOMERO, G. N. (1973). 'Temperature adaptation of enzymes: roles of the free energy, the enthalpy, and the entropy of activation', *Proc. Nat. Acad. Sci. (U.S.),* **70,** 430–432

LOW, P. S. and SOMERO, G. N. (1974). 'Temperature adaptation of enzymes: a proposed molecular basis for the different catalytic efficiencies of enzymes from ectotherms and endotherms', *Comp. Biochem. Physiol.,* **49B,** 307–312

LOW, P. S. and SOMERO, G. N. (1975a). 'Activation volumes in enzymic catalysis: their sources and modification by low-molecular-weight solutes', *Proc. Nat. Acad. Sci. (U.S.),* **72,** 3014–3018

LOW, P. S. and SOMERO, G. N. (1975b). 'Protein hydration changes during catalysis: A new mechanism of enzymic rate-enhancement and ion activation/inhibition of catalysis', *Proc. Nat. Acad. Sci. (U.S.),* **72,** 3305–3309

LOW, P. S. and SOMERO, G. N. (1976). 'Evolutionary trends in the catalytic activation, substrate binding, and structural properties of muscle pyruvate kinases', *J. Exp. Zool.* (In the press)

LYONS, J. M. and RAISON, J. K. (1970a). 'A temperature-induced transition in mitochondrial oxidation: contrasts between cold and warm-blooded animals', *Comp. Biochem. Physiol.,* **37,** 405–411

LYONS, J. M. and RAISON, J. K. (1970b). 'Oxidative activity of mitochondria isolated from plant tissues sensitive and resistant to chilling injury', *Plant Physiol.,* **45,** 386–389

MAETZ, J. and EVANS, D. H. (1972). 'Effects of temperature on branchial sodium-exchange and extrusion mechanisms in the seawater-adapted flounder *Platichthys flesus* L.', *J. Exp. Biol.,* **56,** 565–585

MASSARO, E. J. and BROOKE, H. E. (1971). 'Photoregulation of the expression of lactate dehydrogenase isozymes in *Fundulus heteroclitus* (L)', *Comp. Biochem. Physiol.,* **38B,** 327–332

MCMURCHIE, E. J., RAISON, J. K. and CAIRNCROSS, K. D. (1973). 'Temperature-induced phase changes in membranes of heart: a contrast between the thermal response of poikilotherms and homeotherms', *Comp. Biochem. Physiol.,* **44B,** 1017–1026

MESTER, R., IORDACHESCU, D. and NICULESCU, S. (1973). 'The influence of adaptation temperature on the behaviour of L-alanine: 2-oxoglutarate aminotransferase of the skeletal muscle of pond loach (*Misgurnus fossilis* L)', *Comp. Biochem. Physiol.,* **45B,** 923–931

MOON, T. W. (1975). 'Temperature adaptation: Isozymic function and the maintenance of heterogeneity', 202–220. In II. *Isozymes: Physiology and Function.* Ed. C. L. Markert. Academic Press

MOON, T. W. and HOCHACHKA, P. W. (1971). 'Temperature and enzyme activity in poikilotherms: isocitrate dehydrogenases in rainbow trout liver', *Biochem. J.,* **123,** 695–705

MOTAIS, R. and ISAIA, J. (1972). 'Temperature-dependence of permeability to water and to sodium of the gill epithelium of the eel *Anguilla unguilla'*, *J. Exp. Biol.,* **56,** 587–600

NEWELL, R. C. (1969). 'Effect of fluctuations in temperature on the metabolism of intertidal invertebrates', *Am. Zool.,* **9,** 293–311

NEWELL, R. C. and PYE, V. I. (1970a). 'Seasonal changes in the effect of temperature on the oxygen consumption of the winkle *Littorina littorea* and the mussel *Mytilus edulis* L.', *Comp. Biochem. Physiol.,* **34,** 367–383

NEWELL, R. C. and PYE, V. I. (1970b). 'The influence of thermal acclimation on the relation between oxygen consumption and temperature on *Littorina littorea* L.', *Comp. Biochem. Physiol.,* **33B,** 635–650

NEWELL, R. C. and PYE, V. I. (1971). 'Temperature-induced variations in the respiration of mitochondria from the winkle, *Littorina littorea* L.', *Comp. Biochem. Physiol.,* **40B,** 249–261

NEWSHOLME, E. A., CRABTREE, B., HIGGINS, S. J. THORNTON, S. D. and START, C. (1972). 'The activities of fructose diphosphatase in flight muscles from the bumble-bee and the role of this enzyme in heat generation', *Biochem. J.,* **128,** 89–97

NICKERSON, K. W. (1973). 'Biological functions of multistable proteins', *J. theor. Biol.* **40:** 507–515

NICKERSON, K. W. and DAY, R. A. (1969). 'Possible biological roles for metastable proteins', *Curr. Mod. Biol.,* **2,** 303–306

OHNO, S. (1970). *Evolution by Gene Duplication.* Springer-Verlag, Berlin

PATTON, J. (1975). 'The effect of pressure and temperature on phospholipid and triglyceride fatty acids of fish white muscle: a comparison of deepwater and surface marine species', *Comp. Biochem. Physiol,* **52B,** 105–110

PEISS, C. N. and FIELD, J. (1950). 'The respiratory metabolism of excised tissues of warm- and cold-adapted fishes', *Biol. Bull.,* **99,** 213–224

POTTS, D. C. and MORRIS, R. W. (1968). 'Some body fluid characteristics of the Antarctic fish, *Trematomus bernacchii*', *Mar. Biol.,* **1,** 269–276

PROSSER, C. L. (1973). *Comparative Animal Physiology.* W. B. Saunders, Philadelphia

PRUSINER, S. and POE, M. (1968). 'Thermodynamic considerations of mammalian thermogenesis', *Nature,* **220,** 235–237

RAY, P. H., WHITE, D. C. and BROCK, T. D. (1971). 'Effect of temperature on the fatty acid composition of *Thermus aquaticus*', *J. Bacter.,* **106,** 25–30

RAYMOND, J. A. and DEVRIES, A. L. (1972). 'Freezing behaviour of fish blood glycoproteins with antifreeze properties', *Cryobiology,* **9,** 541–547

RAYMOND, J. A., LIN, Y. and DEVRIES, A. L. (1975). 'Glycoprotein and protein antifreezes in two Alaskan fishes', *J. Exp. Zool.,* **193,** 125–130

ROOTS, B. I. (1968). 'Phospholipids of goldfish (*Carassius auratus* L) brain: the influence of environmental temperature', *Comp. Biochem. Physiol.,* **25,** 457–466

ROSSI-FANELLI, A. and ANTONINI, E. (1960). 'Oxygen equilibrium of hemoglobin from *Thunnus thynnus*', *Nature,* **186,** 895–896

SCHIMKE, R. T. (1969). 'On the roles of synthesis and degradation in regulation of enzyme levels in mammalian tissues', 77–124. In: *Current Topics in Cellular Regulation,* **1.** Ed. B. L. Horecker and E. R. Stadtman. Academic Press, New York

SCHOLANDER, P. F., FLAGG, W., WALTER, V. and IRVING, L. (1953). 'Climatic adaptation in Arctic and tropical poikilotherms', *Physiol. Zool.,* **26,** 67–92

SELANDER, R. K. and KAUFMAN, D. W. (1973). 'Genic variability and strategies of adaptation in animals', *Proc. Nat. Acad. Sci. (U.S.),* **70,** 1875–1877

SIDELL, B. D., WILSON, F. R., HAZEL, J. and PROSSER, C. L. (1973). 'Time course of thermal acclimation in goldfish', *J. Comp. Physiol.,* **84,** 119–127

SINENSKY, M. (1974). 'Homeoviscous adaptation. A homeostatic process that regulates the viscosity of membrane lipids in *Escherichia coli*', *Proc. Nat. Acad. Sci.,* **71,** 522–525

SINGER, S. J. and NICOLSON, G. (1972). 'The fluid mosaic model of the structure of cell membranes', *Science,* **175,** 720–732

SMITH, M. W., COLOMBO, V. E. and MUNN, E. A. (1968). 'Influence of temperature acclimatization on the ionic activation of goldfish intestinal adenosine triphosphatase', *Biochem, J.,* **107,** 691–703

SMITH, M. W. and KEMP, P. (1971). 'Parallel temperature-induced changes in membrane fatty acids and in the transport of amino acids by the intestine of goldfish (*Carassius auratus* L.)', *Comp. Biochem. Physiol.,* **39B,** 357–365

SOMERO, G. N. (1969a). 'Enzymic mechanisms of temperature compensation: immediate and evolutionary effects of temperature on enzymes of aquatic poikilotherms', *Am. Nat.,* **103,** 517–530

SOMERO, G. N. (1969b). 'Pyruvate kinase variants of the Alaskan king crab—evidence for a temperature-dependent interconversion between two forms having distinct and adaptive kinetic properties', *Biochem. J.,* **114,** 237–241

SOMERO, G. N. (1975a). 'Temperature as a selective factor in protein evolution: the adaptational strategy of "compromise" ', *J. Exp. Zool.,* **194,** 175–188

SOMERO, G. N. (1975b). 'The roles of isozymes in adaptation to varying temperatures', 221–234. In: *Isozymes Physiology and Function.* Ed. C. L. Markert. Academic Press, New York

SOMERO, G. N. (1975c). 'Enzymic mechanisms of eurythermality in desert and estuarine fishes', 168–187. In: *Environmental Physiology of Desert Organisms.* Ed. N. F. Hadley. Dowden, Hutchinson & Ross, Stroudsburg, Pa.

SOMERO, G. N. and DEVRIES, A. L. (1967). 'Temperature tolerance of some Antarctic fishes', *Science,* **156,** 257–258

SOMERO, G. N. and DOYLE, D. (1973). 'Temperature and rates of protein degradation in the fish *Gillichthys mirabilis*', *Comp. Biochem. Physiol.,* **46B,** 463–474

SOMERO, G. N., GIESE, A. C. and WOHLSCHLAG, D. E. (1968). 'Cold adaptation of the Antarctic fish *Trematomus bernacchii*', *Comp. Biochem. Physiol.,* **26,** 223–233

SOMERO, G. N. and HOCHACHKA, P. W. (1968). 'The effect of temperature on catalytic and regulatory functions of pyruvate kinases of the rainbow trout and the Antarctic fish *Trematomus bernacchii*', *Biochem. J.*, **110,** 395–400

SOMERO, G. N. and HOCHACHKA, P. W. (1971). 'Biochemical adaptation to the environment', *Am. Zool.*, **11,** 159–167

SOMERO, G. N. and LOW, P. S. (1976). 'Temperature: a "shaping force" in protein evolution'. In: *Biochemical Adaptation to Environmental Change,* Biochemical Society Symposium No. 41. Ed. R. M. S. Smellie. Academic Press, London (in the press)

SOMERO, G. N. and SOULÉ, M. E. (1974). 'Genetic variation in marine teleosts: a test of the niche-variation hypothesis', *Nature,* **249,** 670–672

SOULÉ, M. E. (1973). 'The epistasis cycle: a theory of marginal populations', *Ann. Rev. Ecology and Systematics,* **4,** 93–116

STEVENS, E. D. (1973). 'The evolution of endothermy', *J. theor. Biol.*, **38,** 597–611

STEVENS, E. D. and FRY, F. E. J. (1971). 'Brain and muscle temperatures in ocean caught and captive skipjack tuna', *Comp. Biochem. Physiol.*, **38A,** 203–211

TANSEY, M. R. and BROCK, T. D. (1972). 'The upper temperature limit for eukaryotic organisms', *Proc. Nat. Acad. Sci. (U.S.),* **69,** 2426–2428

THOMPSON, T. L., MILITZER, W. E. and GEORGI, C. E. (1958). 'Partial denaturation of a bacterial aldolase without loss of activity', *J. Bact.*, **76,** 337–341

USHAKOV, B. P. (1967). 'Coupled evolutionary changes in protein thermostability', 107–129. In: *Molecular Mechanism of Temperature Compensation.* Ed. C. L. Prosser. Am. Assoc. Adv. Sci. Washington, D.C.

VAN HANDEL, E. (1966). 'The thermal dependence of the rates of glycogen and triglyceride synthesis in the mosquito', *J. exp. Biol.*, **44,** 523–528

WILLS, C. (1973). 'In defense of naive panselectionism', *Am. Nat.*, **107,** 23–34

WILSON, F. R. (1973). 'Quantitating changes of enzymes of the Goldfish (*Carassius auratus* L.) in response to temperature acclimation: An immunological approach. Ph.D. Thesis, University of Illinois

WILSON, F. R., CHAMPION, M. J., WHITT, G. S. and PROSSER, C. L. (1975). 'Isozyme patterns in tissues of temperature-acclimated fish', 193–206. In: *Isozymes II: Physiology and Function,* Ed. C. L. Markert. Academic Press, New York

WILSON, F. R., SOMERO, G. and PROSSER, C. L. (1974). 'Temperature-metabolism relations of two species of *Sebastes* from different thermal environments', *Comp. Biochem. Physiol.*, **47B,** 485–491

WILSON, F. R., WHITT, G. S. and PROSSER, C. L. (1973). 'Lactate dehydrogenase and malate dehydrogenase isozyme patterns in tissues of temperature-acclimated goldfish (*Carassius auratus* L.)', *Comp. Biochem. Physiol.*, **46B,** 105–116

WOHLSCHLAG, D. E. (1964). 'Respiratory metabolism and ecological characteristics of some fishes in McMurdo Sound, Antarctica, 33–62. In: *Biology of the Antarctic Seas,* **1.** Ed. M. O. Lee. Am. Geophys. Union, Washington, D.C.

Four

Primitive respiratory adaptations

CHARLOTTE P. MANGUM
Department of Biology, College of William and Mary, Williamsburg, Virginia

4.1 INTRODUCTION

4.1.1 Preface

In the infancy of biochemistry forty years ago, the distribution of various compounds among animal phyla was catalogued for the purpose of corroborating orthodox phylogenies. Early infatuation with the results was quickly replaced by disillusionment which has persisted into the present. As recently as 1969, R. B. Clark (p. 62) warned of the 'apparent capriciousness' of biochemical and physiological features of annelids, and concluded that respiratory pigments, for example, have arisen many times.

Comparative biochemistry and physiology can contribute many insights into animal evolution if the results of each discipline are not considered in isolation. When the phylogenetic distribution of haemoglobins is viewed apart from the physiological advantages of enhancing the solubility of oxygen in body fluids and moving oxygen over large distances, then it is indeed puzzling. But if the retention of oxygen-carrying pigments in the circulatory system is selected positively only when they are quantitatively important in respiration, then one would expect to find them in animals (a) which live in habitats with low oxygen contents, (b) within which there is a large distance between sites of gas exchange with the external environment on the one hand and aerobic tissue on the other, and (c) in which rates of oxygen extraction from the environment are determined by the demands of aerobic metabolism. Undoubtedly there are additional physiological features of oxygen-carrying proteins that should be listed, but these three are sufficient to explain the occurrence of respiratory pigments in, for example, the infaunal classes echinoderms or phyla of lophophorates, but not in closely related epifaunal groups.

This chapter focuses upon the respiratory adaptations of the Annelida, with occasional reference to the related phyla Echiuroidea and Sipunculida. The same reasoning is helpful in understanding the presence or absence of oxygen carrying pigments in various species within these phyla (*see* p. 229).

But my goal is less to reach phylogenetic than adaptive conclusions. I have attempted to interpret respiratory pigment function against the background of other respiratory adaptations which determine *in vivo* operating conditions and thus to emphasise the pertinent aspects of oxygen binding.

The reader who is loyal to orthodox phylogenetic theory will recognise in this chapter many controversial assertions, only some of which are explicit. None of these positions is either original or unsupported; and none is truly essential to the argument. For example, the perennially uncertain phylogenetic position of the haemerythrin containing Priapuloidea and Brachiopoda favours neither the pigment's polyphyletic origins nor its homology. Annelids may or may not be the basal stock from which other respiratory pigment containing invertebrates arose, but they are not very far from it.

The peruser of bibliographies may also notice a bias in favour of recent works, often at the expense of older contributions that were classics in their time. The emphasis is made not out of disrespect for the awesome accomplishments of early workers, but rather in the belief that the technical advances of the past decade have resulted in a literature which is formidable to the non-specialist and for that reason, has not been assimilated into the body of knowledge presented in general texts.

In addition to this statement of intent, I should also clarify several points of terminology. While writers in North America and the United Kingdom usually assign all protohaemoproteins to the subsuming class 'haemoglobins', the term 'erythrocruorin' is widely used elsewhere to distinguish the large extracellular protohaemoproteins in annelids. Regardless of the interesting and often anachronistic history of the terminology, the distinction will be useful if the primary structure of these molecules proves to have little in common with that of intracellular haemoglobins. Although the evidence may be decisive by the time this volume reaches print, it is not so at this moment. I have made no distinction here, because the confusion might be unnecessarily aggravated by a premature change. A glossary of specialised terms used in various disciplines is given on p. 269.

I employ the taxonomic nomenclature given in Hartman's (1959, 1965) *Catalogue of the Polychaetous Annelids of the World* rather than prolong the use of outdated names. In this case, the evidence is decisive. If it is more familiar, however, an older name is given parenthetically.

Finally, I am grateful to my colleagues who generously made available to me their unpublished data and manuscripts. They include E. J. Boell, C. and J. Bonaventura, P. K. Chien, R. P. Dales, G. B. Kitto, L. J. Parkhurst, J. L. Scott, B. Seamonds, J. M. Shick, J. B. Sullivan, R. T. Terwilliger, S. N. Vinogradov, R. E. Weber and R. M. G. Wells. K. Johansen made many helpful suggestions.

4.1.2 The thesis

Discussions of the evolution of respiratory adaptations often explore the transition from the liquid to the gaseous medium—the water-air migration in arthropods or vertebrates. So many of the sophisticated mechanisms of respiratory and circulatory control evolved to accompany this important event. Presumably, evolutionary innovation was accelerated as animals exploited a new habitat that made different demands on the respiratory system than the old one.

An earlier period of respiratory adaptation has received little attention. It also accompanied the exploitation of a previously unoccupied niche and it was in many ways more profound. At least in the sense of their far-reaching consequences for the rest of animal history, the innovations were more bold than subtle, and the results more fundamental than refined. Specifically, these events occurred when vermiform animals began to penetrate more than a few millimetres into the soft bottom of the sea. The success of invasion of the new habitat is measured by the simple fact that their annelid progeny comprise over 75% of the macroscopic animals that inhabit the larger fraction of the earth's surface (Sanders, Hessler and Hampson, 1965).

Envisage the conditions of animal life immediately prior to exploitation of the infaunal habitat. Animals were metazoan; they had nerves, muscles, digestive and excretory organs; they engaged in bisexual reproduction and they probably controlled the timing of biological events with chemical messages. The larger individuals among them lived either in the water column, that homogeneous environment which offers little diversity to encourage speciation, or else they lived on the bottom where they still had to feed from the water column, which is a marginal economy. These epifaunal animals were sitting on top of a soft, particulate substratum containing so much organic matter that they could afford to be extraordinarily inefficient if they could only succeed in reaching it (George, 1964; Mangum, 1964; Hobson, 1967). After they dug into the bottom, no radical adaptations of the digestive system occurred until later phyla met different problems. Protection of these soft bodied animals was undoubtedly an additional advantage of penetrating the sand. Predatory attacks of one epifaunal species on another are known (Simon, 1965), but I know of no evidence indicating that annelids or lower metazoans have the sensory acuity to locate prey in the substratum. The escape may have been temporary, but it must have worked until predators became more skilled.

Physical advantages of the habitat also offered protection from environmental stress. Relative to air and water, sand has thermal insulating properties. In temperate zone intertidal habitats where the temperature overhead changes 3–5°C/day an animal living 30 cm in the soft bottom experiences a change of only 1.5°C/day (*Figure 4.1*). The locality where W. R. Rhodes and I recorded the temperature changes shown in *Figure 4.1* supports a large population of onuphid polychaetes (Mangum, Santos and Rhodes, 1968). In the several six months periods for which we succeeded in obtaining data, the temperature at the surface varied from −5.4°C in the early morning of a day in February 1972 to 32.8°C at the end of May 1973 But *Diopatra cuprea*, living half a metre in the bottom, experienced temperatures no lower than 0.7 and no higher than 29.7°C.

Moreover, when the osmotic concentration of the medium in estuarine habitats is catastrophically diluted, the worm underneath can become

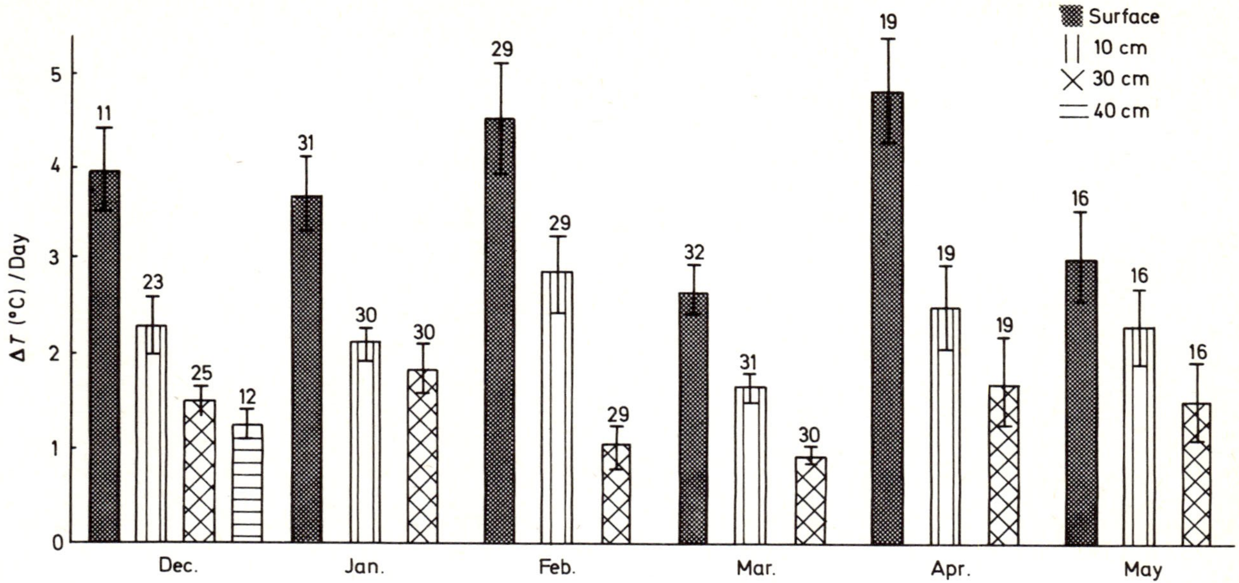

Figure 4.1 *Daily temperature changes (± S.E.) in the soft bottom of an intertidal habitat of the York River estuary in Virginia. Biota described previously by Mangnum* et al. *(1968). Data recorded continuously for a total of 152 days in the months of December to May of the years 1968, 1969, 1971, 1972 and 1973. Probes placed in the lower intertidal zone at the surface and at several depths below the surface of the substratum. Signal amplified by Atkins 10 channel temperature recording system. Discrepancies in N (given in parentheses for each depth) caused by occasional failure of the flip-flop switch to move the recording pen. Data collected by C. P. Mangum and W. R. Rhodes*

quiescent, and ignore the change for several days by ceasing to ventilate and thus retaining water of a higher osmotic concentration in its tube. Following the sudden decrease, in less than 24 hours, of salinity from 31 to 15‰ this response was observed in maldanid polychaetes (Mangum, 1964). Under these conditions the microhabitat inside the tube must become virtually anoxic, and the animal must switch over to anaerobic metabolism, which can sustain the lives of many species for several days, even at summer temperatures (Reish, 1955). Although the response may seem only to substitute death by asphyxiation for death by osmotic shock, periods of freshwater dilution longer than a few days occur rarely in estuaries and the anaerobic faculty is clearly adaptive.

The soft bottom has one great disadvantage for an organism that in the long run remains locked into the cellular machinery of aerobic metabolism. Very few marine sediments have any available oxygen below a few centimetres depth. *The greatest deprivation and the greatest instability that accrued from exploitation of the soft bottom was the loss of a microenvironment that remains constant in oxygen and virtually equilibrated to the atmosphere.*

The adaptations that enabled success in this low oxygen environment include:

1. Active ventilation of the microhabitat.
2. The gill, an organ that served originally to accomplish gas exchange with the external medium, although later it acquired additional functions.
3. The closed circulatory system, a set of tubular distribution channels which increased the efficiency of internal oxygen convection.
4. The heart, an organ evolved specifically to propel vascular fluid.
5. The red blood cell, containing oxygen-carrying pigments.
6. Three of the four known respiratory pigments. The fact of multiplicity is probably a strong argument for the independent origin of convected respiratory pigments within the polychaete annelids as they evolved various respiratory adaptations; with the exception of the gastropods, in which the multiplicity is found in freshwater species (usually considered poor candidates for phylogenetic ancestry); other classes of animals have only one.

When one considers this impressive list in comparison with later contributions to respiratory function, it is difficult to escape the conclusion that the advances are anything but capricious. Further innovations may be marvels of refinement but they were largely anticlimactic.

This chapter is a discussion of respiratory adaptations in a form that is zoologically close to the original, which has special qualities representing a compromise between the inherited material with which the annelids had to work and the unique demands of the new habitat.

4.2 VENTILATION

At least several species of burrowing oligochaetes ventilate the body wall by extending portions of the body into the overlying water column and undulating them in the ambient fluid. Not surprisingly, this rather dangerous behaviour pattern is less widespread than driving fluid through the burrow. Members of several polychaete families supplement ventilation of sites of gas exchange with ciliary currents, but the more common mechanism of driving fluid is muscular. An annelid worm is constructed as a double walled cylinder—a smaller tube contained within a larger tube and separated by a large coelomic space. The mass of the outer cylinder is more than half of total body weight in many sedentary worms, and it consists almost entirely of muscles which function in the locomotion of errant species. In species that maintain an essentially stationary position in a tube or burrow, however, peristaltic contractions of these muscles move fluid through the infaunal microhabitat. Relative to other activities, the energetic cost must be enormous. The activity can be usefully analysed in economic terms by expressing the profit margin (oxygen made available minus oxygen expended in the activity) at different levels of the factor limiting procurement (incurrent PO_2), because muscular ventilation in most annelids is punctuated by periods of rest. The analysis can be made from a continuous record of oxygen consumption ($\dot{V}O_2$) in which activity and rest are clearly demarcated. The increment in aerobic metabolism accompanying a burst of muscular contractions that traverse the length of the animal's body and thus push fluid through the burrow is somewhere between two- and fifteen-fold, depending on temperature and the particular habit of the species (Dales, 1969; Mangum and Sassaman, 1969; Hoffmann and Mangum, 1970; Coyer and Mangum, 1973; Mangum and Burnett, 1975). The virtual synonomy of ventilation with uninterrupted activity of sedentary annelids is perhaps not surprising; the worm's behavioural repertoire may very well be limited by the relentless demand for oxygen. However, the profit is very great. When the water column is nearly equilibrated with the atmosphere, which it usually is, a conventional muscular ventilator such as *Amphitrite ornata* maintains a comfortable margin of about 50% between the increment in oxygen combusted during ventilation activity and the volume extracted from the current (Mangum and Burnett, 1975).

The ventilation rhythm is quite pronounced. Typically it consists of bursts of muscular activity alternating with periods of rest, a feature that was cleverly documented by G. P. Wells (1950) in a series of experiments on various worms. The onset of a burst of pumping or its cessation, however, is not believed to be under simple reflex control. A precise feedback mechanism, triggered by a production variable such as O_2 or CO_2, is one of the refinements achieved only later in evolution. The annelid ventilatory rhythm appears to be governed by a pacemaker system associated with nerve nets located in the gut and ventral body walls (Wells, 1950). The effects of sensory input can be detected, however. When PO_2 or PCO_2 of the medium are progressively altered, less than extreme changes may induce a brief and transient modification of the amplitude of contractions, but not the frequency or duration parameters of the rhythm (Dales, Mangum and Tichy, 1970; Mangum *et al.,* 1975). When the progressive changes are carried to extremes, however, saturation of the medium with CO_2 or decreasing PO_2 to levels below 30 mm Hg abolishes the rhythm in some species (Dales, Mangum and Tichy, 1970; Mangum, 1970). The regions where these nerve nets are located can even be excised and studied *in vitro,* with much the same result. The parameters of the rhythm are not identical with those in the intact animal—the load on the muscle is quite different after such radical surgery—but the rhythm persists (Wells, 1950). Local autonomy and spontaneous rhythmic activity are, of course, physiological hallmarks of nerve nets wherever they occur (Passano, 1963).

The profit margin of oxygen from ventilation diminishes at lower levels of incurrent PO_2, but in *Amphitrite ornata* it does not disappear until the animal exhausts the supply. Water flow does not increase and yet oxygen extraction remains much the same, which suggests a compensatory adjustment of the circulatory system about which little is known (Mangum and Burnett, 1975). This relationship between profit and loss in muscular ventilation is not true of all annelids. Under normoxic conditions the onuphid polychaete *Diopatra cuprea* extracts less oxygen from the water current than many other species. The incurrent serves the additional function of carrying chemical stimuli which are essential to the animal's mode of feeding, and therefore the oxygen expenditure during ventilation seems almost profligate until one learns that the chemosensory function is abandoned at lower oxygen levels (Mangum, Santos and Rhodes, 1968; Mangum and Cox, 1971; Mangum and Burnett, 1975). The oxygen profit margin drops precipitously until it becomes insignificant at a water column PO_2 somewhat in excess of 25 mm Hg. At this point the worm shuts down ventilation and oxygen uptake entirely, and presumably relies on anaerobic pathways.

The ability to shut down aerobic respiration when it becomes uneconomical and to depend on anaerobiosis for prolonged periods (at least days) without suffering visible harm is not an annelid invention. It is widespread among aquatic invertebrates, and they do not always exhaust their oxygen supply first. The mechanism of metabolic control is not very well understood, and the phenomenon sometimes appears in an unpredictable fashion (Mangum and Van Winkle, 1973). J. M. Shick (personal communication) has found that aerobic shutdown in the echinoderm *Ctenodiscus* is effected by a combination of low oxygen and high H_2S—neither factor is sufficient by itself. How this synergism is manifested at the cellular level (*see* Chapter 5) is not known.

The character of the ventilation rhythm may be quite simple, as in the quill worm *Hyalinoecia tubicola* (*Figure 4.2*), or it may be complex, owing to the superimposition of different cycles. Although early studies demonstrated the often impressive magnitudes of water moved (*Table 4.1*), the exact respiratory implications of this vigorous activity have not been appreciated until recently. The earlier studies made predictions of oxygen conditions in the tube or burrow from separate measurements of oxygen uptake, at atmospheric PO_2, which is too high, and water flow (Mangum, 1963, 1964).

Table 4.1 VENTILATION RATES IN ANNELIDS, ECHIUROIDS, AND SIPUNCULIDS. TEMPERATURE IS VARIABLE FROM 11 TO 25°C, BUT APPROACHES THE ANNUAL MAXIMUM FOR THE PARTICULAR LATITUDE

Species	*Flow rate* ($ml\ H_2O/h$)	*Flow rate* ($ml\ H_2O/g\text{-}h$)	*Source*
Annelida			
Polychaeta			
Arenicolidae			
Arenicola cristata		11–27	Mangum (1976a)
A. marina	120–240	14–37	Van Dam (1938); Krüger (1964); Jacobsen (1967)
Chaetopteridae			
Chaetopterus variopedatus	480–600	111	Wells and Dales (1951); Dales (1969)
Glyceridae			
Glycera dibranchiata	32	11	Hoffmann and Mangum (1970)
Maldanidae			
Branchioasychis americana	<0.2	<0.23	Mangum (1964)
Clymenella torquata	3	60	Mangum (1964)
C. zonalis	2	80	Mangum (1964)
Petaloproctus socialis	<0.1	<1.5	Mangum (1964)
Nereidae			
Neanthes (=Nereis) virens	25		Lindroth (1938)
Onuphidae			
Diopatra cuprea	68	50	Mangum *et al.* (1968)
Hyalinoecia tubicola	0.5–9.0	5–23	Dales (1969); Dales *et al.* (1970)
Sabellidae			
Sabella pavonina			
ciliary	73	390	Dales (1957)
muscular	15	1.2	Wells (1953)
Serpulidae			
Hydroides norvegica			
ciliary	11	900	Dales (1957)
Myxicola infundibulum			
ciliary	286	100	Dales (1957)
muscular	0	0	Wells (1953)
Pomatoceros triqueter	27	1400	Dales (1957)
Salmacina dysteri	0.3	2090	Dales (1957)
Spirorbis borealis	0.2	950	Dales (1957)
Terebellidae			
Amphitrite ornata	106	35	Mangum *et al.* (1975)
Eupolymnia crescenti		20	Dales (1961b)
Neoamphitrite robusta		9	Dales (1961b)
Thelepus crispus		13	Dales (1961b)
Echiuroidea			
Urechis caupo	660–1740	49–129	Hall (1931); Redfield and Florkin (1931)
Sipunculida			
Phascolion strombi	1.2–7.8	11–55	Kristensen (1969)

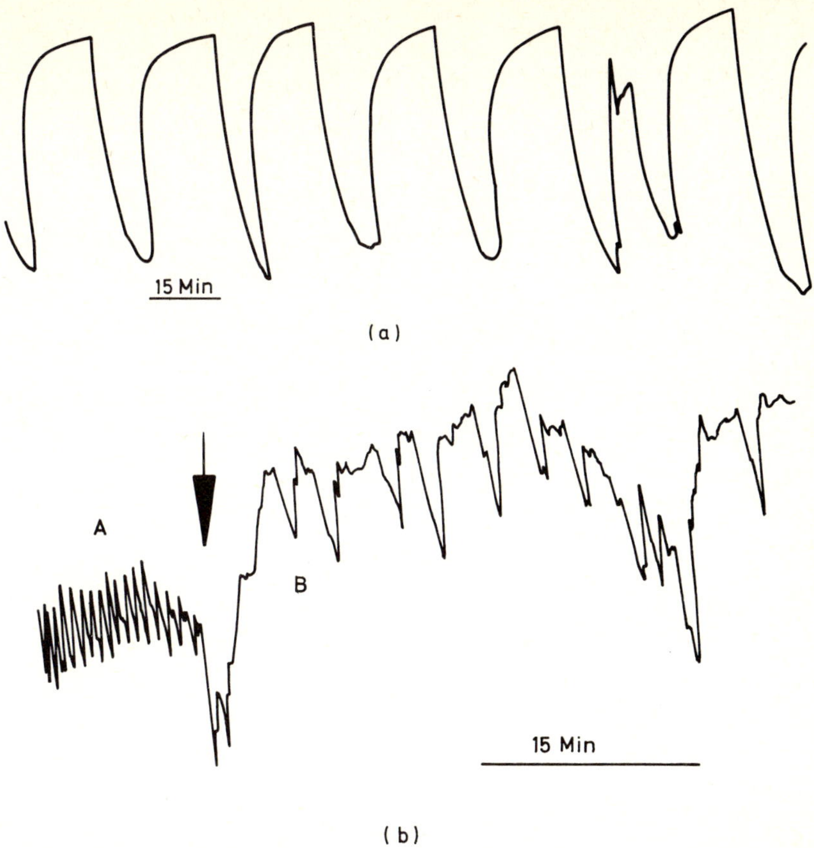

Figure 4.2 Kymographic recording of fluid movements generated by tubicolous annelids. (a) The onuphid polychaete Hyalinoecia tubicola *at 20–21°C. Deflection of the writing pen below baseline caused by movement of fluid into the tube; return of pen to baseline reflects cessation of fluid movement. Each burst of activity moves 1–2 ml H_2O through tube. Data from Dales* et al. *(1969). (b) The terebellid* Amphitrite ornata *at 22–24°C. A = Incurrent. Each deflection caused by movement of 1.0-1.5 ml H_2O through tube. B = Excurrent. At arrow, animal reversed its position in the tube*

Alternatively, microhabitat PO_2 was estimated from measurements of oxygen in point samples of tube water; the results were quite variable and rather low, probably because the samples reflected the rhythm but portrayed it poorly.

Continuous measurements of microhabitat PO_2 can now be made by inserting into the tube or burrow an oxygen electrode which is so small that it fits into a hypodermic needle. The continuous trace of PO_2 usually shows the same rhythmic fluctuations as the record of fluid movement (*Figure 4.3*). Its integral is a measure of the average oxygen level at a particular site in the microhabitat.

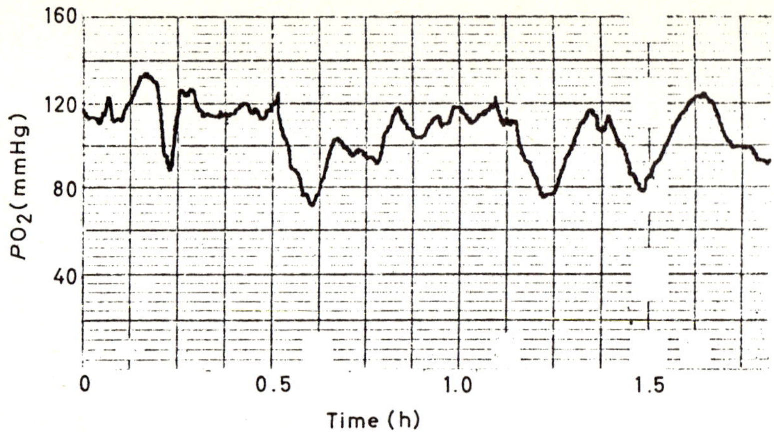

Figure 4.3 *PO_2 in the head shaft (excurrent) of a tube inhabited by* Amphitrite ornata *at 22–24°C. In this species, oxygen is extracted by the gills from the excurrent stream*

In respiratory physiology the analysis of fluid movements within and around animals often assumes that fluid movements are laminar, i.e. that fluid moves in coherent streamlines. However, the pattern of flow along the body wall of some annelids departs sufficiently from the model to be called turbulent, owing to the roughness of surfaces and the timing and complexity of forces generated in muscular contractions (Wells and Dales, 1951; Taylor, 1952). The distinction is important because the vortices formed during ventilation (Mangum and Cox, 1971) may either enhance the molecular diffusion of oxygen or it may result in the mixing of afferent and efferent fluids to a degree where PO_2 gradients are very small and net movements of oxygen are reduced. This kind of movement, called eddy diffusion, is intensively studied by hydrographers but it is often ignored by physiologists. Its importance in the respiratory function of ventilation in annelids has not been investigated.

Patterns of flow in tubes and burrows are extremely complicated, and they differ greatly in various species. Many annelids build tubes with separate inhalant and exhalant openings. In these species flow is always unidirectional, but the direction may change periodically. The pattern of incurrent flow appears to be laminar, but it changes considerably as the current moves past the contoured body surface (*Figure 4.2*). Disruption of the streamlines and hence mixing of fluid may be so great that it eliminates stable PO_2 gradients between the gill and postbranchial water in the excurrent. In some species flow is not partitioned; local eddies and vortices clearly result in mixing between incurrents and excurrents (Mangum and Cox, 1971). Consequently, concepts employed by vertebrate physiologists, such as P_iO_2 (PO_2 of inspired fluid) and P_eO_2 (PO_2 of expired fluid) may have a different meaning in the study of gas exchange by many invertebrates. The values for microhabitat PO_2 (*Table 4.2*) certainly approximate the oxygen levels at sites of gas exchange more closely than those for the water column above the

Table 4.2 OXYGEN LEVELS IN ANNELID AND SIPUNCULID TUBES AND BURROWS IN RELATION TO BODY FLUID PO_2 AND OXYGEN AFFINITY OF THE RESPIRATORY PIGMENT. DATA FROM MANGUM AND KONDON (1975), MANGUM *ET AL.* (1975), MANGUM (1976A, 1976b), WEBER AND MANGUM (IN PREPARATION)

Species	*Temperature* (°C)	*Water column PO_2* (mm Hg)	*Mean microhabitat PO_2* (mm Hg, ±S.E.)	*Mean body fluid PO_2* (mm Hg, ±S.E.)	P_{50} (mm Hg)
Polychaeta					
Arenicolidae					
Arenicola cristata	22	144–148	104	2–4	1.7–2.2
Glyceridae					
Glycera dibranchiata	18	155–159	120 (±11)	5 (±1)	7.4
Onuphidae					
Diopatra cuprea	19	122–128	73 (±9)		
Terebellidae					
Amphitrite ornata	23–24	140–145	75 (±4)	10 (±2)	10.0 (vascular) 2.6 (coelomic)
Sipunculida					
Phascolopsis gouldi	23	145–155	78 (±2)	7(±)	5.2
	10			15 (±1)	1.4

tube but the degree of approximation depends upon the particular functional combination of gill structure and fluid flow. For example, the PO_2 at the metamerically arranged gills of *Glycera dibranchiata* may be portrayed as a more or less monotonic decrease from the incurrent (= water column in *Table 4.2*) to the excurrent (= microhabitat in *Table 4.2*) values. In contrast, it is accurately expressed for *Amphitrite ornata* by the excurrent or microhabitat PO_2, because the gills are located anteriorly in the mixed fluid of the tube head shaft. Data for oxygen levels in the microenvironments of four species are summarised in *Table 4.2*. In general, microhabitat PO_2 is about half that in the water column. Most important, *at water column partial pressures obtaining in most natural habitats, microenvironmental oxygen levels do not remain low for very long and they do not reach anoxia as long as the tube or burrow is submerged.*

Because oxygen in the tube microenvironment is maintained at an intermediate level only with the considerable energetic expenditure of at least twice the resting rate of aerobic metabolism, adaptations reducing its dissipation to the surrounding anoxic sediments also appear in many forms. Burrowers representing the more primitive annelid families generally confine their transient tunnels to the upper regions of the substratum adjacent to the oxygen source overhead (or in some families, overtail). The animal fills a relatively large fraction of its burrow, and the convection distance between the overlying water column and the gill is short, thereby minimising loss of oxygen to the surrounding sand during transit. In contrast, highly adept tube builders such as *Diopatra cuprea* construct shafts composed of multiple layers of a compliant material, probably a form of onuphic acid (*see below*). The tube extends as much as a metre down into the soft substratum. The worm occupies a small fraction of its tube volume, and in an emergency the animal may retreat to the lower depths where it gains some immunity from physical state changes such as ice formation in the water column [that cold day in February 1973 (*see* p. 193) did not kill the annelid population]. The convection distance, however, is lengthened by severalfold when the animal resorts to this escape.

Most annelid tubes sustain an internal hydrostatic pressure, which permits the animal to work with the walls of the tube when its peristaltic or undulatory waves are driving fluid. Gas permeability may be very low but it is rarely zero; the exterior surface of the tube as well as several millimetres of contiguous sediment are usually oxidised. Zero oxygen permeability has been noted only for tubes of members of the family Chaetopteridae (Petersen and Johansen, 1967), a group of often large animals that penetrate to considerable depths in the substratum without the aid of a respiratory pigment (*see also* Section 4.7).

The physical and chemical properties of the mucous matrix of these remarkable tubes are poorly known. The very diversity of texture suggests that specific properties and their relation to the particular habits of the animal that synthesises the material will prove to be a fascinating inquiry.

The most carefully studied tube material is made by the quill worm *Hyalinoecia tubicola*. The principal component, aptly designated onuphic acid, is a macromolecule composed of large quantities of phosphorylated glucose residues together with small amounts of fucose. Dissociation of the molecule into subunits does not alter the relative proportions of constituents. This property, as well as the even distribution of labile linkages in partial hydrolysates, points to a more or less linearly arranged carbohydrate polymer with a repeating unit of about 6×10^3 daltons (Pautard and Zola, 1967).

The similarity of this substance, which also comprises about 70% of the material in chaetopterid tubes (Zola, 1967), to other carbohydrate polymers with well-known physical properties offers an irresistible analogy. *The solubility of oxygen in this class of compounds is high, but its diffusivity is very low**, resulting in oxidation of sediments within a few millimetres of space but with little loss of oxygen in zoological time.

4.3 THE GILL

Since the sedentary annelid lives in a chamber, little protection would be gained by enclosing the gill in a body recess and therefore it is always an evolution rather than an involution of the body wall (*Figure 4.5*). It may be perfused with fluid moved from and returned to an open coelomic space, or it may receive separate afferent and efferent branches of a vascular system (*see* Section 4.4). With only one known exception, annelid gills always end blindly, and therefore fluid must return to the source in the same set of tubes in which it entered. The gill may take the form of short fingerlike protrusions of the body wall from most of the animal's many segments (e.g. the bloodworm *Glycera dibranchiata, Figure 4.6*), or it may be a highly branched structure localised to a particular region of the body (e.g. the terebellid *Amphitrite ornata* in *Figure 4.5*). The diversity of gill form is perhaps one of the more notable examples of adaptive radiation among the various families; it is certainly one of their more pleasing visual qualities. Unlike the ventilatory stream, which is carefully maintained as a unidirectional current by most species, there is but one example in which afferent and efferent channels within the annelid gill are reinforced by anatomical partitions (Spies, 1973). And yet in many species separate currents exist. Although no partitions can be seen in cross sections of the *A. ornata* gill, the optical density of blood in living preparations (*Figure 4.5(a)*) suggests the presence of two flow cores. In species with intracellular haemoglobins that are oxygenated in the gill, simple visual observation of the red cells moving through these transparent structures reveals that flow, which is often caused by tracts of discrete ciliation, is consistently unidirectional. *Glycera dibranchiata* has simple unbranched gills metamerically repeated on each parapodium along the length of its body (*Figure 4.6(e)*). The afferent stream is dorsal and the efferent stream is ventral. Its close relative *G. americana* has substituted simply branched gills (*Figure 4.6(f)*), which increases the

*Isolated data describing the diffusion of molecular oxygen through plastic membranes of various thickness and composition abound in technical bulletins issued by manufacturers of physiological apparatus, but not in the scientific literature. Some detail can be found in Carritt and Kanwisher (1959), Carey and Teal (1965) and Slack (1971).

exchange surface from 21 to 28% of the total body surface area, or from 49 to 71 mm^2/gm wet weight. However, the simplicity of flow in a system of branched tubes, even one as rudimentary as this, must be less than it was in the unbranched gill.

When a unidirectional fluid moving through a system of tubes approaches a bifurcation, it is confronted with a region of increasing pressure at the branchpoint, i.e. the magnitude of the negative pressure gradient decreases. Flow in the main tube slows down, and that in the boundary layers on the branch tube walls is retarded; its direction may even be reversed. The magnitude of overall retardation varies directly with flow rate and branch angle, and inversely with tube size (Zamir and Roach, 1973). Consequently, the increase in gas exchange surface in a branched gill is achieved only at the expense of retardation of fluid flow and possibly the loss of directional homogeneity inside. In an undifferentiated tube with fluid moving simultaneously in two opposite directions, the mixing of afferent and efferent fluids must be enhanced, and the PO_2 difference between the two fluids reduced, by branching. This is probably the reason why the annelid gill became contractile.

In *G. americana* (but not *G. dibranchiata*) the gill is withdrawn every few seconds to a site within the parapodium by the negative pressure of ipsilateral muscle contractions in adjacent segments. The involution by internal suction results in periodic filling and emptying of the gill, thus enhancing the average PO_2 difference across the gill membrane. Additional complexity in gill branching, as in the onuphid *Diopatra cuprea* (*Figure 4.5(e)*), is accompanied by intrinsic contractility of the gill. The pattern of periodic filling and emptying may reach its ultimate development in the Terebellidae, a family characterised by several pairs of highly branched and sub-branched gills. In *Amphitrite ornata,* whose specific name is no coincidence (*Figure 4.5(a)*), the gills are so large that in aggregate they comprise 25–30% of the total body surface area but only 1.5–2.0% of total body weight. Expressed as area/body weight, these dimensions approximate those of the more highly evolved molluscan gill (Steen, 1971). Although the total volume of blood in this species is not known, we do know that gill contractions return to the internal vessels a volume of blood somewhere between 25 and 50% of the volume contained in the two largest vessels, which must be a large fraction of the total (Mangum *et al.,* 1975). Gill contractions, which are locally autonomous and therefore continue even when a filament is severed from the main branch, are probably effected by cells found on the walls of blood vessels throughout the vascular system (Parker, 1923). Consequently, the cost of this adaptation is an increase in the length of the diffusion path, or the thickness of the gill epithelium, from 6 μm in *G. americana* to 9–12 μm in *A. ornata.*

The direction of blood flow through the sabellid gill is believed to be reversible, an intriguing observation which appears to have escaped attention given to the reversible tunicate heart. Reversibility, which is regulated in tunicates by pressure changes (Kriebl, 1968), also reduces effects of blood mixing.

The trivial metabolic drag of the gill is graphically expressed by its small biomass. Its importance in overall oxygen uptake can be estimated by depriving the animal of its function. In *A. ornata* the gill supplies all of the oxygen to the animal's haemoglobin. Despite the total absence of impermeable skeletal elements, the path of oxygen entry into both vascular and coelomic fluid is largely confined to the thin-walled gills by the thickness and the absence of a circulatory supply to the body wall. Some 50–60% of the oxygen consumed by all tissues in animals acclimated to summer temperatures enters through these delicate structures (Mangum *et al.,* 1975). In contrast, the primitive fingerlike gills of *G. dibranchiata* supply only about 20% of its oxygen, a diminution that is probably identified with the character of body fluid movements as well as gill structure. Glycerids lack the well developed vascular system found in *A. ornata,* and the fluid moving through their gills is coelomic.

The conspicuous feathery gill of sabellids and serpulids (*Figure 4.5(f)*), which is protruded from the tube into the water column, and serpulids has been subjected to experiment on several occasions. The branchial crown, which generates ventilatory flow by ciliary instead of the muscular mechanisms more typical of the annelids, apparently serves the primary function of providing the animal's food rather than its oxygen, at least under the normoxic conditions at which the experiments have been conducted. This conclusion is supported by the very low rate of oxygen extraction (only 10%) from the ventilatory stream (Dales, 1961a). Although ciliary flow across the branchial crown is accompanied in most species by muscular ventilation of the body wall, which is enclosed within a tube, the two flow rates are quite disparate on a weight specific basis. The ciliary current (vol. fluid/wt) is six times greater than the muscular current, whereas oxygen uptake (vol. O_2/wt) by the branchial crown is only one-fourth of the total. In other words, oxygen uptake by the branchial crown compartment is 40% of the total, while VO_2 of the branchial crown is only 25% of the total (Dales, 1961a).

Functional comparisons of annelid gills with those of other kinds of animals cannot be made quantitatively on the basis of present information. The process of gas exchange in vertebrates is often expressed by numerical indices (Mangum, 1976c), permitting precise comparison and evaluation of the performance of the system. Some of these expressions require careful re-thinking and fundamental modification for the analysis of gas exchange in soft-bodied animals, because they tacitly assume that gas exchange is limited to the gill. Others require knowledge of the gas content of pre- and postbranchial body fluids, which is highly desirable but not yet available. Annelids with closed circulatory systems usually have separate afferent and efferent branchial vessels, but their small size has thus far prohibited anaerobic sampling. The very pertinence of these concepts to species with only coelomic and no vascular circulation is open to question.

Since their shape is not limited by rigid skeletal elements, the possibility exists that organs of gas exchange in annelids respond to environmental variables in a compensatory fashion. Tentacle extension in the sipunculid *Phascolopsis* (= *Golfingia*) *gouldi* and lung formation in the swampworm *Alma emini* are correlated with the cessation of environmental fluid movements rather than PO_2 or PCO_2 *per se* (Mangum and Kondon, 1975; Mangum, Lykkeboe and Johansen, 1975). More subtle responses of features such as surface area of the extensible gill, however, have not yet been investigated.

4.4 THE CIRCULATORY SYSTEMS

R. B. Clark (1964) has argued convincingly that the origin of large volumes of internal body fluid completely closed off from the external medium was a necessary *precedent* to penetration of the soft bottom; a high pressure fluid skeleton permits the development of an efficient digging organ. Therefore early annelids must have carried coelomic fluid with them into their tubes and burrows. The respiratory function of coelomic fluid, which is moved by combined ciliary and muscular actions, clearly increased after the exploitative event. The second circulatory system, a set of tubes often equipped with one to many fluid driving pumps, has little or no skeletal function and its volume is much smaller. Its fluid, blood, is believed to be circulated more efficiently and its oxygen transport function is consequently greater.

4.4.1 Structural design

In general the annelid vascular system consists of large dorsal and ventral vessels running the long axis of the body and lying well within the coelomic cavity rather than in tissue (*Table 4.3*). In the chlorocruorin containing serpulid *Mercierella enigmatica* (Skaer, 1974) the walls of the larger vessels are only one cell thick (less than 1 μm), indicating that the diffusion barrier between blood and coelomic fluid is slight. One to several hearts may be formed by evolutions or involutions of the dorsal vessel. Alternatively, the vessel may pulsate diffusely along its length owing to contractions of longitudinal muscle fibres in its ventral wall (Kermack, 1955). In either case peristaltic contractions of the vessel wall alter its volume in much the same way that contractions of the body wall alter the volume of coelomic fluid.

Annelid families with elaborate gills to enhance the extraction of oxygen from the ambient medium have also evolved a system of large vessels traversing the length of the body. However, deep tissues are virtually avascular*. Indeed, flow-through capillaries are restricted to a few families. The endings of small blood vessels in groups such as the Sabellidae and Terebellidae, which otherwise have highly developed vascular systems, penetrate only a few glandular structures; most of the vessels ramify on to surfaces of organs where their walls are contiguous with coelomic fluid as

*A recent work describes aspects of the vascular system of the serpulid *Mercierella enigmatica*, which is an interesting exception to this generalisation; it has the well-developed branchial crown which is typical of serpulids and sabellids, but its body wall is also vascularised (Skaer, 1974). It is possible that tissue vascularisation is an osmotic adaptation to the notably euryhaline distribution of the species (Skaer, 1974), or it may be a general feature of vascular morphology in the family, which is otherwise poorly known. In *Protula tubularia*, tissue vascularisation is confined largely to the thoracic membrane, which is located anteriorly and which may function as a supplementary gill (Fauvel, 1959).

Table 4.3 SIZE OF BLOOD VESSELS IN ANNELIDS. DATA FOR *MAGELONA* SP. FROM PHOTOGRAPHS OF SECTIONED MATERIAL SHOWN BY JONES (1968); ALL OTHER DATA FROM MATERIAL FIXED AND SECTIONED BY THE AUTHOR. REPRESENTATIVE RANGE GIVEN FOR LARGE VESSELS; MINIMUM DIAMETER GIVEN FOR CAPILLARIES

Species	*Vessel*	*Diameter* (μm)
Polychaeta		
Magelonidae		
Magelona sp.	dorsal	50–90
	ventral	200
	segmental loops	20
	loop shunts	9
Maldanidae		
Clymenella mucosa	dorsal	100
	ventral	70
	capillaries	13
C. torquata	dorsal	35–40
	capillaries	5
Petaloproctus socialis	dorsal	17–25
	ventral	17–25
	capillaries	7
Nereidae		
Nereis virens	dorsal	100–150
	capillaries	12
Onuphidae		
Diopatra cuprea	dorsal	100–125
	capillaries	12
Oligochaeta		
Lumbricidae		
Lumbricus terrestris	dorsal	150–300
	ventral	70–125
	capillaries	10
Achaeta		
Hirudidae		
Hirudo medicinalis	dorsal	150–175

well as respiring tissues (Fox, 1937; Thomas, 1940; Ewer, 1941; Mangum *et al.*, 1975). Conversely, annelids with the greatest development of tissue vascularisation belong to essentially gill-less groups like most families of oligochaetes (Stephenson, 1930; Mendes and Nonato, 1957) and the polychaete families Maldanidae (Pilgrim, 1966) and Nereidae (Nicoll, 1954). This correlation, together with the prevalence of these small vessel beds in superficial areas of the body wall and a density that is probably inadequate to supply oxygen uptake (Johansen and Martin, 1966), implies an origin of capillaries as instruments of oxygen procurement from the external environment rather than a means of distribution to tissue deep within the body. The extreme of this development may occur in glossoscolecid swampworms, which periodically form lungs by folding over the vascularised dorsal surface of the body wall (Beadle, 1957). The body wall of gill-less annelids often has a rich supply of small blood vessels, traditionally designated 'capillaries'. The quite accurate use of the term, which literally means small bore tubes, has probably obscured a functional peculiarity of the annelid vascular system. The terminals usually end as blind tubes or loops (Stephenson, 1930)—there is only one recorded example of flow-through capillaries in annelid vascular systems, and in this family (the Nereidae) they have apparently arisen within modern genera (Nicoll, 1954). In most species the movement of blood must be either tidal or simultaneously bidirectional in the interior vessels as well as in the blind ending gills (*see* Section 4.3). In either case there must be considerable mixing of afferent and efferent blood in many vessels. The same conclusion for coelomic fluid is unavoidable, although for different reasons.

4.4.2 Fluid flow

The flow of blood in vertebrate vessels is usually assumed to be laminar, although turbulence in the heart and aorta has long been known. Actually, the assumption of laminar flow is based on a few observations of the recovery of dyes in coherent streamlines after passage through the system, and the authors of modern medical texts discuss the presence of small degrees of turbulence (Folkow and Neil, 1971). Turbulent flow in the large vessels of rabbits is caused by branching (*see also* Section 4.3), and by the pulsatile flow pattern (McDonald, 1952). In the mammalian vascular system the periods of turbulence, which are predictable (Green, 1944), are too brief to achieve thorough mixing in normal animals, and hence the older observations on dye recovery. Pulsatile flow, changing cross-sectional area and rough surfaces, all of which expedite turbulence, are conspicuous features of the coelomic cavities of many groups of soft-bodied animals.

Fluid is moved in the coeloms of sedentary annelids partly by muscular contractions of the body wall and partly by longitudinal tracts of ciliation. The body wall is often transparent in small annelids and the paths of coelomic cells can be traced just as dyes are used in fluid mechanics. A single wave of muscle contraction passing across a particular group of segments in the mid-region of *Amphitrite ornata,* for example, appears to move the cells smoothly. However, the relaxation of these muscles and accompanying contraction of the circular muscles causes a local change in pressure of such magnitude that, for a fraction of a second, some of the cells are sucked back in the opposite direction. Coupled with the deformation of coelomic spaces and with the roughness of coelomic surfaces due to the presence of organs, this observation suggests that considerable mixing occurs (whether it is truly turbulent is an unanswered question). Red cell tracks can also be observed in young glycerids. They appear to be smooth in resting *G. americana.* When ventilation activity is initiated by the body wall muscles the gut also moves, but in a direction opposite to that of the body wall. The result is formation of small and transient vortices of red cells. If this eddy formation were characterised quantitatively, possibly by microcinematographic analysis, its real importance in respiration might become clearer.

The magnitude of fluid mixing in annelid circulatory systems cannot be estimated at present, and the absolute difference in PO_2 between sites of oxygen uptake and delivery remains unknown. However, the qualitative implication of the hypothesis, viz. that the PO_2 difference is small relative to that in more advanced circulatory systems, is almost mundane.

4.4.3 PO_2 and pH

Although little is known of the magnitude of fluid movements inside annelids, we do have some knowledge of rates of fluid movement relative to anatomical landmarks. For example, Johansen and Martin (1966) estimated from sequentially filmed angiograms that the volume of blood in the dorsal vessel spanning 12 segments of the giant earthworm *Glossoscolex giganteus* is renewed each second. The indirect estimate of blood flow according to the Fick principle yields the figures of 1–2 ml/kg-min in *Arenicola cristata* (Mangum, 1976a) and 3 ml/kg-min for *Glycera dibranchiata* (Mangum, 1976c). In addition, blood gas parameters can now be measured, at least in coelomic cavities and a few large vessels. When animals are exposed to various external partial pressures of oxygen, the curve describing changes in coelomic fluid PO_2 is a complex function. The pattern shown in *Figure 4.4* for *Glycera dibranchiata* is true of several other species of annelids and molluscs (Mangum and Kondon, 1975; Mangum *et al.*, 1975; Freadman and Mangum, 1976). Coelomic fluid PO_2 changes rapidly at higher external oxygen levels, and then much less rapidly at lower levels. Because coelomic fluid PO_2 determines the oxygenation state of the respiratory pigment, the

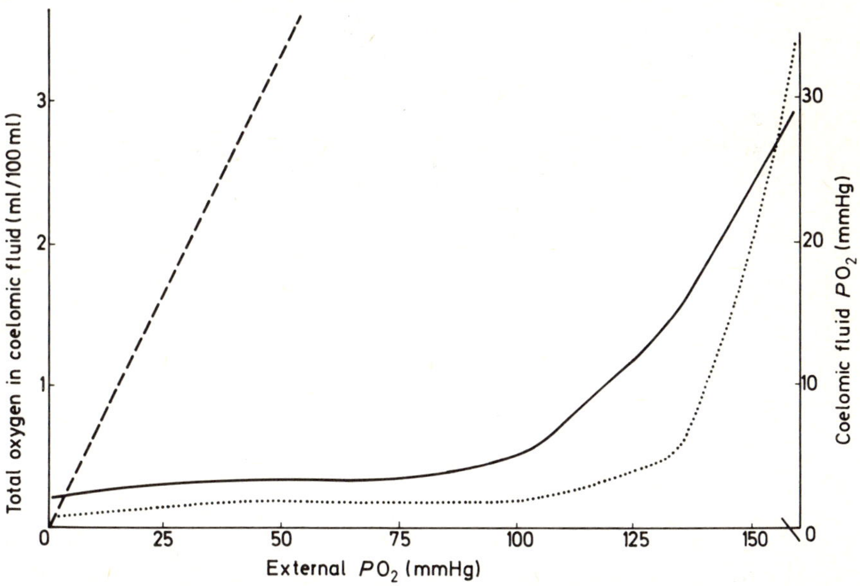

Figure 4.4 Changes in coelomic fluid PO_2 (dotted line) and total oxygen concentration of coelomic fluid (solid line) in the bloodworm Glycera dibranchiata *equilibrated to various external oxygen levels at 24–25°C. Dashed line represents oxygen isobar. PO_2 in submerged burrow (measured separately) is 120 mm Hg (Table 4.2). Data from Mangum and Carhart (1972) and Mangum (1976b)*

curve describing changes in total oxygen concentration of coelomic fluid has roughly the same shape (*Figure 4.4*), although the two are not identical because the relationship is nonlinear.

Since it is important that the small PO_2 differences between the two sites of gas exchange in coeloms induce changes in oxygenation of the respiratory pigment, the maximum slope of a nonlinear curve describing oxygenation *in vitro* should span the small *in vivo* PO_2 interval. The fit is approximately expressed by the relationship of P_{50} to coelomic fluid PO_2 when the animals are held at the oxygen levels found in their microhabitats (*Table 4.2*). Above P_{50} the oxygenation curve begins to asymptote, and below P_{50} the changes in dissolved oxygen are reduced. Therefore the agreement of these parameters for pigments which are well suited to transporting oxygen under operating conditions *in vivo* should be fairly close, as in the sipunculid *Phascolopsis* (= *Phascolosoma,* = *Golfingia*) *gouldi* at 23°C (at lower temperatures, however, haemerythrin may be of little use in oxygen transport; *see Table 4.2*). In contrast, if mean coelomic fluid PO_2 approximates P_{70} or P_{90} then the PO_2 difference at sites of oxygen uptake and delivery delimits a portion of the oxygen binding curve that changes at less than the maximum rate, and the oxygen transport function is accordingly diminished. This condition is apparently true of the terebellid polychaete *Amphitrite ornata,* where P_{50} of coelomic haemoglobin (*Table 4.7*) is much smaller than coelomic PO_2 (10 mm Hg). The very small quantities of haemoglobin in these unusual coelomic cells may function only to supply their own oxygen needs; oxygen transport seems to be accomplished primarily by vascular haemoglobin, which has an oxygen affinity that approximates coelomic fluid PO_2 (*Table 4.7*), and thus blood must transfer much of its oxygen to the coelom.

Table 4.1 summarises the available information on rates of fluid flow outside the organ of gas exchange in annelids and a single sipunculid. With the exceptions of a few large species in which afferent and efferent fluids can be separately sampled, quantitative information on fluid movement inside invertebrate animals is simply unavailable. The important quantity $\dot{V}_w/Q$, or the ventilation:perfusion ratio, is known for very few of the many different kinds of animals (Mangum, 1976c). To emphasise the importance of circulatory responses, however, we can compare the relationship between PO_2 in body fluids and in the ventilatory stream, and the change in this relationship at different external oxygen levels (*Table 4.4*). When $PO_{2bf}/PO_{2ext} = 1$, then body fluid PO_2 falls in exact linear proportion to external PO_2. When the quantity exceeds 1, body fluid PO_2 falls at a greater rate than external PO_2, and when it is less than 1, body fluid PO_2 falls more slowly than external PO_2.

The species listed in *Table 4.4* exhibit many of the possible forms of the response. In the two species of epifaunal sea urchins belonging to the genus *Stronglylocentrotus,* for example, body fluid PO_2 actually increases after an initial reduction of external PO_2. Since these animals do not actively move large volumes of water across the respiratory podia, and since the demand of aerobic metabolism changes very little over the same range of external PO_2 (Johansen and Vadas, 1967), then this relationship implies a compensatory response of body fluid flow. Conversely, coelomic fluid PO_2 in the

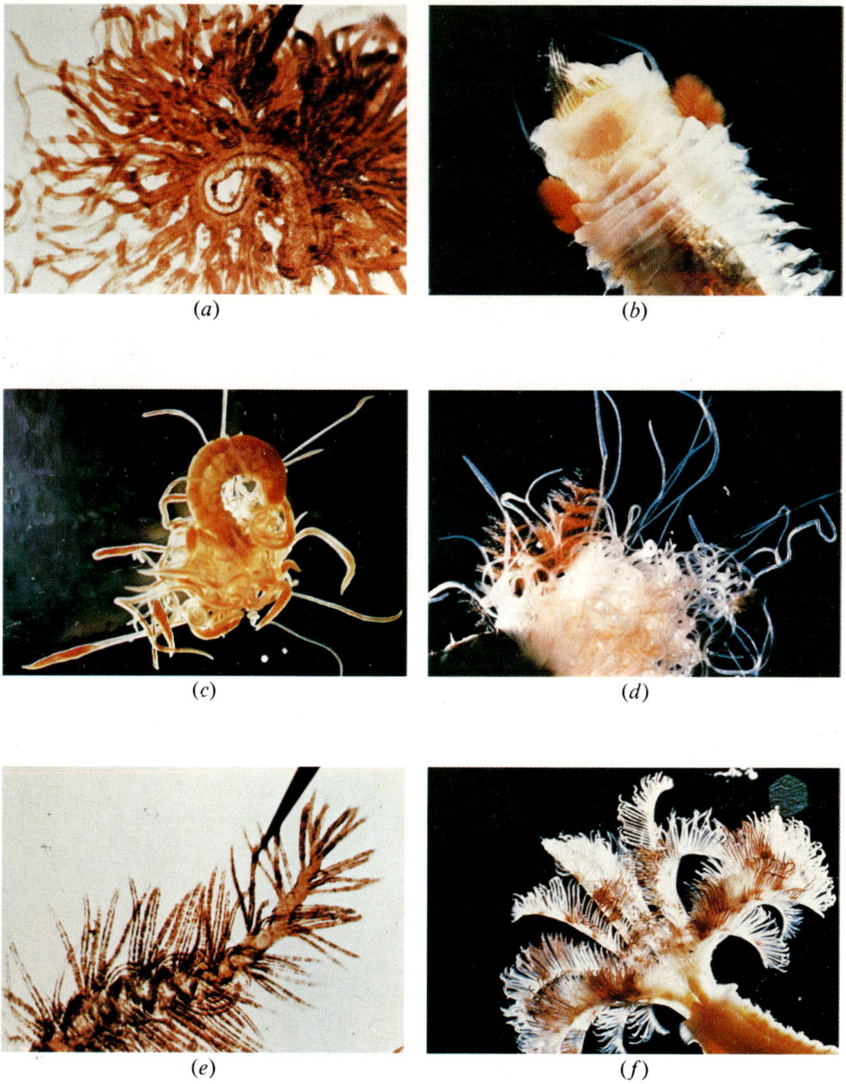

Figure 4.5 The annelid gill (*a*) Amphitrite ornata (*b*) Pectinaria gouldi (*c*) Enoplobranchus sanguineus (*d*) Pista maculata (*e*) Diopatra cuprea (*f*) Potamilla reniformis. *Figures 4.5* (*b*) *and* (*d*) *courtesy J. L. Simon; Figure 4.5* (*f*) *courtesy Gray Museum, Marine Biological Laboratory, Woods Hole*

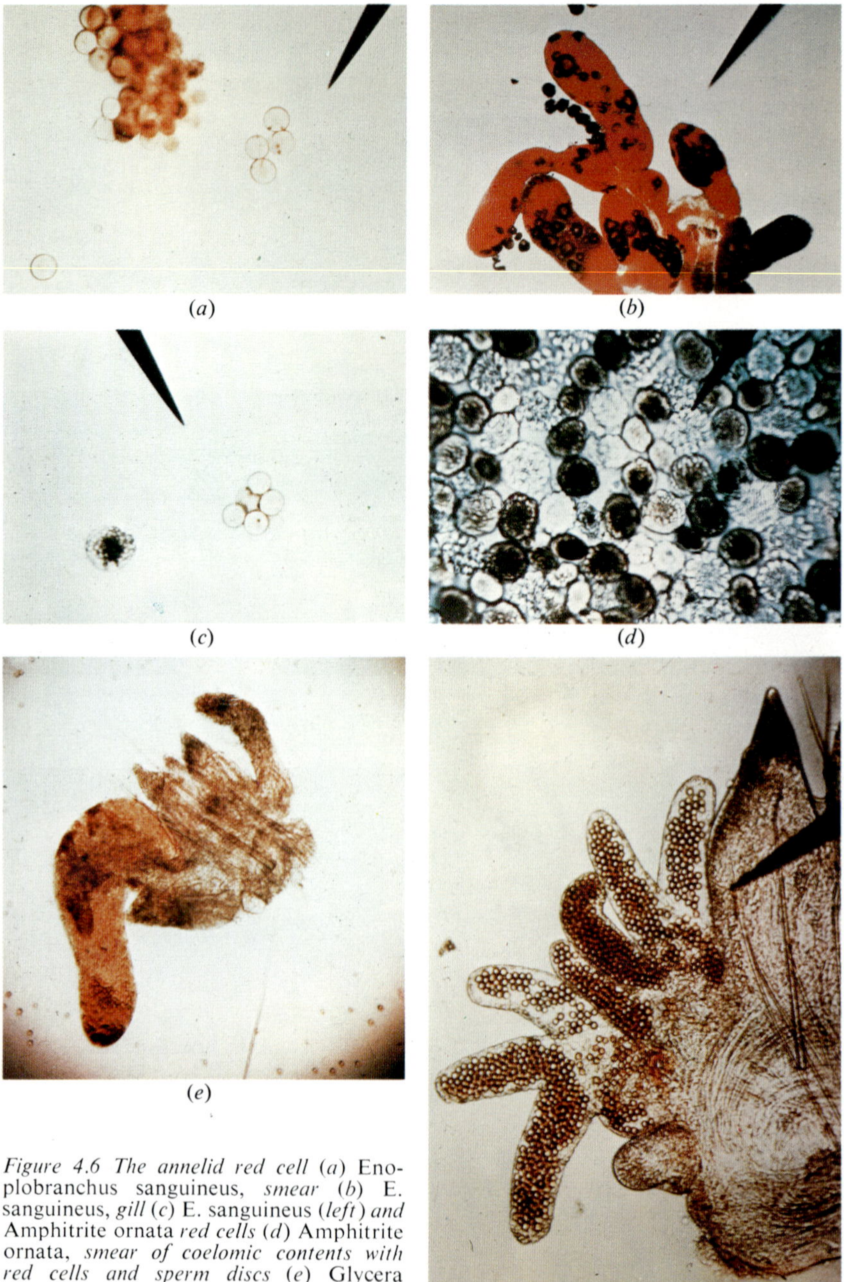

Figure 4.6 The annelid red cell (*a*) Enoplobranchus sanguineus, *smear* (*b*) E. sanguineus, *gill* (*c*) E. sanguineus (*left*) *and* Amphitrite ornata *red cells* (*d*) Amphitrite ornata, *smear of coelomic contents with red cells and sperm discs* (*e*) Glycera dibranchiata, *isolated parapodium with gills* (*f*) Glycera americana, *isolated parapodium with gill*

bloodworm *Glycera dibranchiata* declines precipitously at higher oxygen levels. Since the respiratory demand changes at the same rate as external PO_2 (Mangum and Van Winkle, 1973) and since the ventilation rate does not change, this result suggests a negative response by circulation. While the patterns for different species in *Table 4.4* are various, the changes are difficult to explain without invoking specific responses of fluid movements inside the animals. Our ignorance of quantitative aspects of circulation is probably the greatest gap in understanding invertebrate respiration.

In sabellids (Fox, 1937; Wells, 1953) and in the bloodworm *Glycera dibranchiata* (Mangum, 1970) circulation responds to low oxygen conditions not by an increase in fluid flow but by virtual cessation. Species such as bloodworms, with substantial oxygen reservoirs in the form of coelomic haemoglobin, may prolong at least partial aerobic metabolism for two hours or more. The oxygen combined with chlorocruorin, which never occurs in coelomic fluids, must have a far more limited life and therefore switchover to anaerobiosis must be complete in sabellids.

The acid-base balance of annelid body fluids is not controlled with the same precision as in vertebrates. Interspecific variation under the same environmental conditions is as great as 0.5 (Mangum, 1972, 1973; Wells, 1974). Intraspecific variation with temperature follows the rule of relative alkalinity in the sipunculid *Phascolopsis* (= *Golfingia*) *gouldi,* but not in the polychaetes *Arenicola marina, A. cristata* and *Glycera dibranchiata* (Mangum, 1973; Wells, 1974). In these species the effects of temperature on H^+ activity are either very small or entirely absent, which would seem to violate the laws of physical chemistry. The phenomenon in *G. dibranchiata* is explained by the proliferation of gametes in the coelom at low temperature, presumably adding acidic metabolites to coelomic fluid (Mangum, 1973). However, the blood of lugworms shows the reduction in the constant ΔpH/°C, both *in vitro* and *in vivo;* this highly adaptive feature (*see* Section 4.7.3) must be an intrinsic property of blood (Weber, 1972; Weber and Mangum, in preparation).

Intraspecific variation of body fluid pH with salinity has not been adequately studied in annelids. Preliminary measurements suggests that it does not occur in *G. dibranchiata* in the range 20–30‰, but that coelomic fluid pH in nereids varies inversely with acclimation salinities in the range 8–34‰.

In arthropods, salinity induced variation in blood pH may be:

1. Direct, as a result of the addition of CO_2 to the blood in dilute media (Fyhn, Petersen and Johansen, 1972).
2. Inverse, as a result of the input of ammonia to the blood when the cells adjust to a dilution by reducing the size of the free amino acid pool (Truchot, 1973; Weiland and Mangum, 1975).
3. Nonexistent, when aerobic metabolism does not change and intracellular osmolality is controlled by substances other than free amino acids (Mangum *et al.,* 1976).

A priori, each of these responses may be found in different species of annelids.

Table 4.4 THE CHANGE IN BODY FLUID PO_2 OF INVERTEBRATE ANIMALS EXPOSED TO VARIOUS EXTERNAL OXYGEN LEVELS

Species	*External PO_2 range* (mm Hg)	$\Delta PO_2\,bf/\Delta PO_2\,ext$	*Source*
Cnidaria	5–30	<0.01	Sassaman and
Ceriantheopsis americanus	30–75	0.6	Mangum (1974)
	75–159	<0.01	
Metridium senile	0–159	0.2[1]	Mangum and Van Winkle (1973)
Annelida			
Amphitrite ornata	5–30	0.2	Mangum *et al.* (1975)
	30–80	0.0	
	80–148	0.5	
Glycera dibranchiata	0–75	0.0	*Figure 4.4*
	75–130	0.7	
	130–159	1.6	
Sipunculida			
Phascolopsis gouldi			Mangum and Kondon (1975)
10°C	0–53	0.0	
	53–69	0.5	
	69–159	1.0	
23°C	0–59	0.0	
	59–108	0.3	
	108–159	1.0	

Mollusca			
Gastropoda			
Nassarius obsoletus[2]	0–159	0.4[1]	Kushins and Mangum (1971)
Lamellibranchа			
Noetia ponderosa	10–40	0.08	Freadman and Mangum (1976)
	80–110	0.5	
	110–159	*c.* 1	
Cephalopoda			
Octopus dofleini	91–143	*c.* 0.3–0.7	Johansen and Lenfant (1966)
Arthropoda			
Crustacea			
Cancer magister	120–159	*c.* 0.4–0.5	Johansen *et al.* (1970)
Echinodermata			
Asteroidea			
Pteraster tesselatus	100–145	*c.* 1	Johansen and Petersen (1971)
Echinoidea			
Strongylocentrotus droebachensis	0–80	1.0	Johansen and Vadas (1967)
	c. 80–135	0	
S. purpuratus	0–80	1.0	Johansen and Vadas (1967)
	100–140	0	
Holothuroidea			
Thyone briareus	0–70	0	Mangum and Van Winkle (1973)
	70–132	0.3	

[1]Slope of fitted regression line
[2]Data for PO_2 of gas bubble held in mantle cavity rather than body fluid PO_2

4.5 THE HEART

So little progress has been made in understanding the physiology of the annelid heart that anatomical descriptions still provide most of the clues to its function (Fauvel, 1959; Dales, 1963). The annelid heart takes many forms. If the term 'heart' is restricted to mean a discrete organ that supplies the fluid driving force, then hearts are absent from many families with otherwise well developed vascular systems; the vessels are often diffusely pulsatile. On the other hand, if the pacemaker activity of a specialised region of the circulatory system is the diagnostic feature, then hearts are common elements of the local segmental vascular systems in annelids (Nicoll, 1954). Presumably the fluid movements of greatest respiratory importance in gill-less species occur within a segment, and their direction is largely dorsoventral and lateral, between the epithelium and the organs within that segment. The more powerful fluid driving pumps generate forces in the anteroposterior direction, and the pattern of fluid flow depends on the position and the character of the gill. In *Arenicola marina* the paired hearts are expansions of lateral vessels that supply the digestive tract, and they appear to function largely in driving fluid from the gut sinus into the large ventral vessel, which is itself not contractile, and then into the gills (Kermack, 1955).

The persistence of structures such as the branchial hearts in modern eunicids suggests that vascular pumps in annelids had a metameric origin, like everything else. In any event, segmental circulation is clearly the primitive pattern. The position of hearts in virtually all of their many forms indicates that their major function is to move fluid through the organ of gas exchange with the external environment, whether it be a parapodial capillary bed or a blind-ending gill. The gill itself may be regarded a heart in some families; in terebellids the gill contracts with such force that its contents are virtually emptied.

Control of fluid pressure and the direction of fluid movement by a system of valves may have arisen within the serpulids as they became larger; serpulid valves are rings of sphincter muscle located externally to the vessels (Ewer, 1941). Valves assume their more customary form of endothelial flaps in the oligochaetes, where they are believed to play an important role in preventing mixing with the blood in the dorsal vessel (Stephenson, 1930). Both types are present throughout the well developed vascular system of magelonid polychaetes (Jones, 1968).

In the giant South American earthworm *Glossoscolex giganteus* the pressure in the dorsal vessel, which supplements the lateral hearts to drive fluid through the system, reaches values as high as 95 mm Hg. These values include the high hydrostatic pressures created in coelomic fluid by the powerful body wall muscles, which are superimposed upon those in the blood (Johansen and Martin, 1966). Pulse pressure is about 5–9 mm Hg.

Disagreement regarding the origin and control of the heartbeat in various annelids may reflect fundamental divergence although the experimental evidence is hardly conclusive. Investigators of species in which the system pulsates diffusely have often concluded that the beat is myogenic in origin

(Gaskell, 1914, 1919; Stephenson, 1930; Nicoll, 1954). In the achaetes this myogenic pulsation is modulated by both excitatory and inhibitory innervation (Gaskell, 1914), which is also found in most polychaetes examined. These conclusions are based on the persistence of the beat in isolated elements of the system as small as a single segment (Nicoll, 1954), as well as on pharmacological and anatomical evidence (Gaskell, 1914, 1919). On the other hand, the local expansion of the dorsal vessel known as a heart in *Arenicola cristata* yields an electrocardiogram characterised by rapid oscillations that resemble nerve action potentials rather than slow muscle potentials (Prosser, 1950). This finding implies a basic neurogenic pacemaker, as in arthropods. However, Johansen and Martin (1966) presented evidence that *in situ* stretch receptors govern the force of contraction by the hearts of *G. giganteus,* which are local; this evidence raises the possibility of myogenic modulation if not origin of the beat.

4.6 THE RED CELL

The perennial question of the adaptive significance of the red cell may be less puzzling if its origins are recalled. Haemerythrin, which appears in a small and homogeneous family of polychaetes, always occurs in cells. Chlorocruorin, found in four of the more highly evolved and specialised families, never does. Haemoglobin, however, occurs in many different families including the most primitive groups which lack closed circulatory systems and accomplish gas transport by moving coelomic cells between the sites of gas exchange. The origin of haemoglobin as a carrier in body fluids was very likely simultaneous with that of the red cell, and both events appear to have preceded the origin of the vascular system. Therefore an alternative and equally fruitful way of phrasing the question is: *Why was the red cell abandoned when the vascular system arose?*

Speculations on the adaptive significance of the red cell usually cite advantages pertaining to the physical properties of red cell suspensions: (a) abolition of the colloid osmotic pressure exerted by highly concentrated protein solutions, (b) reduction of fluid viscosity of a concentrated protein solution and (c) in annelids, protection of the oxygen carrying proteins in coelomic fluid from loss through the nephridia that open into the coelomic cavity. Several possibilities of relevance to metabolism and function of the respiratory pigment should be added to the list: (d) biosynthesis is more accurately regulated at the cell level than at a higher level requiring enteroreception and endocrine response, (e) ferrous haem proteins are more easily protected from oxidation and resultant loss of the ability to combine reversibly with molecular oxygen and (f) cofactors that modulate oxygen binding properties of respiratory pigments are localised in the red cell for ready mobilisation and sensitive metabolic control.

4.6.1 Colloid osmotic pressure

Until recently, knowledge of the colloid osmotic pressure of invertebrate body fluids was confined to estimates made from protein concentrations or oxygen carrying capacity (summarised by Mangum and Johansen, 1975). These estimates often led to vastly exaggerated values because they assumed a particular molecular weight of the colloids, or the same number of osmotically active colloidal particles, as in mammals. In fact the number may be either greater or smaller for a particular protein content, because molecular weight of invertebrate oxygen carrying pigments varies from 0.25 to 140 times that of Haemoglobin A. But the molecular weight of extracellular respiratory pigments is always more than that of Haemoglobin A, and therefore the number of particles is very much less than in mammalian erythrocytes (*Table 4.6*).

Since data on osmotic pressure of a solution of purified protein can be used to estimate molecular weight, a few measurements were made on annelid haemoglobins before the use of the ultracentrifuge became commonplace. If these substances are responsible for virtually the total colloid osmotic pressure of body fluids [an old supposition which is not entirely true (Mangum and Johansen, 1975)], and if measurements of colloid osmotic pressure were made at the *in vivo* concentration (the relationship between osmotic pressure and protein concentration is non-linear and difficult to predict), then reasonable conclusions can be inferred from the older data shown in *Table 4.5(A)*. Expressed as fractions of the total osmotic pressure of annelid body fluids, including the contribution of all osmotically active particles, the numbers are very small indeed (>0.15%). Extracellular haemoglobin in the blood of the lugworm *Arenicola marina* contributes less to total osmotic pressure than the plasma proteins of mammals (*c.* 0.5%).

Table 4.5 COLLOID OSMOTIC PRESSURE OF ANNELID HAEMOGLOBINS

Species	*Osmotic pressure* (mm Hg)	*Haemoglobin concentration* (g/100 ml)
A. Calculated, from data on purified compounds in known concentrations reported by Roche and Combette (1937), according to the Van't Hoff equation in the form $C = \frac{\pi}{RT}$, where π = osmotic pressure, R = gas constant, C = concentration and T = absolute temperature.		
Arenicolidae		
Arenicola marina	4.08	6.5 (WolveKamp and Vreede, 1950)
Capitellidae		
Dasybranchus caducus	35.60	3.6[1]
Glyceridae		
Glycera gigantea	13.40	3.6[1]
B. Measurements of unaltered body fluids by Mangum and Johansen (1975)		
Arenicolidae		
A. marina		
blood	1.55	
Nephtyidae		
Nephtys hombergi		
blood	0.78	
coelomic fluid	0.24	*c.* 0.2–0.4 (Clark, 1964)

[1]No measurements reported; value for *G. dibranchiata* substituted (Hoffmann and Mangum, 1970). This value is likely to be too high for *D. caducus*.

The real interest in colloid osmotic pressure is less the contribution of proteins to water balance with the external medium than to the balance between different fluid compartments within the animal. The Starling hypothesis, formulated in the context of the mammalian circulatory system, postulates that the movement of water across a biological membrane and into or out of a fluid compartment is governed by the balance between hydrostatic pressure (P) and colloid osmotic pressure (π) according to the expression:

$$P - \pi = (P_i \pm P_o) - (\pi_i \pm \pi_o)$$

where the subscripts denote the parameters inside (i) and outside (o) the compartment. The sign of the term on the left is determined by the magnitude of blood (or coelomic fluid) pressure (P) and the number of colloidal particles, which are too big to move freely through the membrane and which have an affinity for water*. Particles that move freely, such as ions and small molecules (whose upper size limit varies considerably for different membrane systems), do not exert an effective osmotic pressure. If the quantity $P - \pi$ is positive, small particles are squeezed out; if negative, small particles are sucked in. In a mammal with an equivalent haemoglobin solution instead of a red cell suspension, the tissues would be dried out.

The only available measurements of both parameters in the same annelid body fluid are for *A. marina* coelomic fluid, in which hydrostatic pressure is very high (10–70 mm Hg, depending on muscular activity) and colloid osmotic pressure is essentially zero (Mangum and Johansen, 1975). Coelomic fluid, which bathes the organs in the coelom and actually penetrates in between the fibres of body wall muscles, must be continuously hydrating the cells. *Glycera gigantea* and *Dasybranchus caducus* are both burrowing species without vascular systems and with red cells in coelomic fluid, in which hydrostatic pressures are likely to reach the same high levels as in *A. marina.* If the red cells were replaced by haemoglobin solutions at a concentration found in other glycerid species (which is probably an exaggeration for the capitellid *D. caducus*), colloid osmotic pressure (*Table 4.5*) would still be considerably lower than average hydrostatic pressure.

The problem of fluid balance in species with two fluid compartments is more complex. The volume of coelomic fluid is always much greater than that of blood (except perhaps in some of the primitive achaetes), and therefore the question may be more meaningfully phrased in terms of possible excesses in blood hydration rather than tissue desiccation. The only measurements of blood pressure in annelids were made on earthworms of the tropical species *Glossoscolex giganteus* (Johansen and Martin, 1966). The values for blood pressure cited in Section 4.5 include superimposed coelomic fluid pressures, but fluid balance is determined by the difference between pressures in the two compartments (*see above*). If diastolic pressure is at least the same as coelomic fluid pressure (which must be true because

*Hence the operational meaning of colloid osmotic 'pressure', which is simply the magnitude of hydrostatic pressure required to oppose this movement.

the vessels do not collapse), then an average of the minimum blood pressure is obtained by halving pulse pressure. These values are 9 mm Hg in the ventral vessel and 5 mm Hg in the dorsal vessel.

G. giganteus is so much bigger (body wet weight = 500 gm) than the species listed in *Table 4.5* that extrapolations to vascular systems in small worms may be unsafe. The body weight of *A. marina* whose blood was sampled for the data in *Table 4.5* was about 5 gm. However, the size of the annelid extracellular haemoglobins, and therefore the number of particles in equivalent solutions, is remarkably similar (*Table 4.6*). The colloid osmotic pressure of *G. giganteus* blood can be reasonably estimated from the data in *Table 4.5(B)* and its oxygen carrying capacity (Johansen and Martin, 1966). Oxygen carrying capacity, and therefore osmotic pressure, is 1–2 times the value in *Table 4.5(B)*, or 1.55–3.10 mm Hg. The small excess of P over π suggests that fluid moves from the blood into the coelom. There is no reason to suppose that the release of haemoglobin into extracellular fluid resulted in excessive blood hydration and tissue desiccation, and it may have been necessary to oppose drying out the blood. The margin is sufficiently small, however, to suggest a limitation of blood oxygen carrying capacity and positive selection for reducing the number of colloidal particles by polymerisation of haemoprotein subunits, which of course occurred.

4.6.2 Viscosity

The problem of fluid viscosity is so complicated that the inadequacies of present information preclude fruitful speculation in quantitative terms. A red cell suspension is a heterogeneous fluid whose flow properties are determined by the behaviour of the plasma, behaviour of the cells and interactions between both. The viscosity of mammalian blood is actually *greater* than that of an equivalent haemoglobin solution as long as it flows in tubes of about 80 μm diameter* or more (Cokelet and Mieselman, 1968; Schmidt-Nielsen and Taylor, 1968). In big tubes the flow properties of the red cells dominate, and their effect on fluid viscosity exceeds that of extracellular haemoglobin. However, in smaller tubes the viscosity of mammalian blood is lower than that of an equivalent haemoglobin solution (Snyder, 1973). The decrease, known as the Fåhraeus–Lindqvist phenomenon, is explained by the aggregation of the red cells in the core of the stream, allowing the plasma to flow freely along the tube walls. When only a few cells can fit abreast into a tube, the plasma flow dominates and consequently fluid viscosity is less. The viscosity of a red cell suspension, and presumably the critical tube size for the Fåhraeus–Lindqvist effect is influenced by mechanical properties of the cells such as their resistance to deformation (Murphy, 1967) and by hematocrit (Wells and Merrill, 1962). Although

*A recent summary of fluid flow studies in man, which admirably simplifies the subject for the non-specialist, gives the threshold as 150 μm diameter (Talbot and Berger, 1974).

small differences in red cell size do not influence the critical tube diameter for the Fåhraeus–Lindqvist effect (Snyder, 1973), differences as great as those found within the annelids and their relatives must do so.

The body fluids of annelids and most other animals either partly or wholly conform to changes in environmental variables such as temperature and salinity; therefore the effects of environmental change on fluid viscosity must be considered. The difference in the effects of thermal change on viscosity of haemoglobin solutions and red cell suspensions is very small. The viscosity of seawater, the composition of which is virtually the same as annelid plasma (except for haemoglobin), increases more than twofold when the temperature is reduced from 30 to 0°C. Over the same temperature interval, the change in viscosity of haemoglobin solutions at concentrations found in annelids is barely perceptible (Allison, 1965). The viscosity of seawater increases by less than 1% when the salt content is raised from 1 to 35‰, but a 50% dilution of human blood increases its viscosity by 30% (Murphy, 1967).

The influence of flow rate must also be considered. The flow of a heterogeneous fluid such as blood (but not that of a homogeneous protein solution) is non-Newtonian, i.e. viscosity is not independent of shear rate and hence flow velocity, but instead the two parameters vary inversely.

To summarise and simplify, the release of haemoglobin into an extracellular environment might reduce the circulatory workload in an animal (a) whose blood vessels are primarily large tubes, (b) whose blood contains a relatively small volume of cells, (c) in which the red cells are nucleated and therefore relatively resistant to deformation, (d) in which environmental variables such as temperature and salinity are not precisely regulated, if at all, and (e) in which fluid flow velocity is low. If the animal is better characterised by the opposites of each of these features, the circulatory work required to drive a red cell suspension might be less. The conditions which favour haemoglobin solutions seem to be more characteristic of annelids, but information on subjects such as flow rates, tube size (*Table 4.3*) etc. is neither sufficiently quantitative nor thorough enough to support a very convincing case. To decide whether the Fåhraeus–Lindqvist phenomenon is important in an animal, for example, one must know the proportion of tubes above and below the critical diameter and the energetic savings for each. This kind of accounting has been made for only one species, the domestic dog, in which the total driving force would be 40% greater if it had a haemoglobin solution rather than a red cell suspension (Snyder, 1973).

Two *de facto* arguments are perhaps more cogent: (a) In the single annelid family that has its oxygen carrying pigment in vascular cells, the Magelonidae, the cells are too small (1–2 μm) for the Fåhraeus–Lindqvist phenomenon to occur in any vessel except those forming loops in a few segments (*Table 4.3*). (b) Members of several families which have evolved vascular systems with extracellular haemoglobins have also retained red cells in the coelom, where the Fåhraeus–Lindqvist phenomenon cannot possibly occur. Fluid viscosity, then, cannot have been the crucial determinant in the retention of the red cell.

Table 4.6 MOLECULAR WEIGHT AND HAEM CONTENT OF HAEMOPROTEINS IN ANNELIDS AND ECHIUROIDS. APPROXIMATION MADE FROM SEDIMENTATION CONSTANTS GIVEN FOR SOME SPECIES

Species	*Molecular weight* Native molecule	*Molecular weight* Subunits	*Haem content* (% by weight)	*Source*
Polychaeta				
Arenicolidae				
Arenicola cristata	2.85×10^6	13×10^3	4.5–4.6	Waxman (1971); Vinogradov *et al.* (1974)
		50×10^3		
		$13–14 \times 10^3$ (2)		
A. marina	*c.* 3×10^6			Svedberg (1933)
Capitellidae				
Notomastus latericeus	34.5×10^3			Svedberg and Eriksson-Quensel (1934)
Cirratulidae				
Cirriformia sp.	3×10^6	18.5×10^3	3.08	Swaney and Klotz (1971)
		12×10^3		Vinogradov *et al.* (1974)
		50×10^3		
		$13–16 \times 10^3$ (3)		
Eunicidae				
Marphysa sanguinea	2.4×10^6	*c.* 200×10^3	2.24	Chew *et al.* (1965)
		2.5×10^5		
		c. $18–50 \times 10^3$		
Flabelligeridae				
Brada villosa	*c.* 3×10^6			Svedberg (1933)
Glyceridae				
Glycera americana	*c.* 18×10^3			Wilcovsky, Sullivan and Weber
	c. 60×10^3			(unpublished
G. dibranchiata	18.2×10^3			Padlan and Love (1968)
	$17–18 \times 10^3$			Mangum (1970)
	95×10^3			Mangum and Carhart (1972)
	$17–18 \times 10^3$			Vinogradov *et al.* (1970)
	c. 40×10^3			Vinogradov *et al.* (1970)
	17.7×10^3			Seamonds *et al.* (1971)
	125×10^3			Seamonds *et al.* (1971)

G. gigantea	18×10^3		Weber (1973)
	60×10^3		Weber (1973)
G. robusta	$48–50 \times 10^3$	17.6×10^3	Terwilliger *et al.* (1976)
G. rouxi (=goesi)	34×10^3		Svedberg (1933)
Lumbrinereidae			
Lumbrinereis fragilis	*c.* 3×10^6		Svedberg (1933)
Nereidae			
Nereis virens	*c.* 3×10^6		Svedberg (1933)
Pectinariidae			
Pectinaria belgica	*c.* 3×10^6		Svedberg (1933)
Sabellidae			
Eudistylia vancouveri	3.1×10^6		
	30×10^3		
	15×10^3		Terwilliger *et al.* (1975)
Sabella penicillus	*c.* 3×10^6		Svedberg (1933)
Spirographis spallanzani	2.8×10^6	$34–37 \times 10^3$ (2)	Antonini *et al.* (1962b); Guerritore and Zito (1971)
Scalibragmidae			
Polyphysia (=Eumenia) crassa	*c.* 3×10^6		Svedberg (1933)
Serpulidae			
Pomatoceros triqueter	$2–3 \times 10^6$		Svedberg and Eriksson-Quensel (1934)
Serpula vermicularis	*c.* 3×10^6		Svedberg (1933)
Terebellidae			
Amphitrite ornata			
coelomic	17×10^3		Weber *et al.* (1976)
Enoplobranchus sanguineus	17×10^3		Weber *et al.* (1976)
Pista pacifica			
coelomic	$17–18 \times 10^3$ (2)		Terwilliger and Koppenheffer (1973)
vascular	3.4×10^6	280×10^3	
		120×10^3	
		60×10^3	
		15.5×10^3	Terwilliger *et al.* (1975)
Thelepus crispus			
vascular	3.3×10^6		
	270×10^3		
	16×10^3		Garlick and Terwilliger (1974)

Table 4.6 *continued*

Species	*Molecular weight* *Native molecule*	*Subunits*	*Haeme content* (% by weight)	*Source*
Oligochaeta				
Eisenia foetida	*c.* 3×10^6			Svedberg (1933)
Limnodrilus gotoi	3.01×10^6			Yamagishi *et al.* (1966)
Lumbricus terrestris	3.45×10^6		3.08	Rossi-Fanelli *et al.* (1970)
	3.3×10^6	92×10^3		Chaincone *et al.* (1972)
	3.2×10^6	68×10^3		Weichelman and Parkhurst (1972)
		19×10^3		
		16×10^3		
	3.23×10^6	$24–28 \times 10^3$	2.78	Shlom and Vinogradov (1973)
		12×10^3		
		33×10^3		
		50×10^3		
		19×10^3		
		16×10^3		
		14×10^3		
Lumbricidae sp.	3.84×10^6	163×10^3		David and Daniel (1974)
		40.8×10^3		
		22×10^3		
Tubifex tubifex	3.01×10^6			Scheler and Schneiderat (1959)
Achaeta				
Haemopsis sanguisuga	*c.* 3×10^6			Svedberg (1933)
H. grandis		*c.* 35×10^3		Vinogradov *et al.* (1975)
		$12–16 \times 10^3$ (3)		
Hirudo medicinalis	*c.* 3×10^6			Svedberg (1933)
Placobdella sp.		13×10^3		Shlom *et al.* (1975)
		15×10^3		
		17×10		
		26×10^3		
Echiuroidea				
Urechis caupo	*c.* 65×10^3			Bonaventura and Kitto (1973)

4.6.3 Haemoglobin excretion

The postulated protection of the respiratory pigment from excretory loss is also an insufficient condition. Examination of the relation between the type of nephridium and the disposition of the haemoglobin molecule in more primitive families reveals too much diversity. Capitellid polychaetes have open metanephridia collecting from coelomic fluid and their haemoglobin is protected by its location within red cells, whereas haemoglobin dissolved in the coelomic fluid of nephtyds apparently does not filter through the closed protonephridia. Glycerid nephridia, however, do not open directly into coelomic fluid and yet their haemoglobin is cellular. Magelonid polychaetes, as well as members of two other animal phyla, the echinoderms and the phoronids, retain the red cell in fluids that are not filtered by excretory organs, which again suggests that the red cell has additional advantages.

4.6.4 Biosynthetic control

Little is known about the control of haemoprotein synthesis at the cell level, and no systematic studies of the process in species with intracellular haemoglobins have been undertaken. There is, however, a large body of evidence indicating that the synthesis of extracellular haemoproteins results in by-products that do not occur in healthy vertebrates (*see* Section 4.7). If anabolic control in annelids is similar to that in vertebrates, then the intracellular environment has the advantageous result of preventing production of porphyrins and haems that are not central to the pathway. This supposition is supported by the absence of these compounds in at least one species with only intracellular and no extracellular haemoglobins, *Glycera dibranchiata* (Mangum and Dales, unpublished).

4.6.5 Intracellular control factors

Characteristics of the vertebrate red cell such as the proximity and metabolic control of intracellular modulators refining the physiological functions of haemoglobin or of enzyme systems maintaining its valence state would seem to be a valuable feature of the intracellular environment. However, evidence is growing that annelid red cells do not contain specific modulators. The oxygen affinities of haemoglobins extracted from coelomic cells of the terebellids *Amphitrite ornata* and *Enoplobranchus sanguineus* are not altered by the addition of organic phosphates, nor are they different from oxygen affinities of the molecules when in the intracellular environment (Mangum *et al*., 1975). Interpretation of the data for glycerid bloodworms is more complex, the most probable inference from the comparison of oxygen affinities for intracellular and extracted haemoglobins of *G. dibranchiata* is that there is no difference (Mangum, 1976b). At present the comparison of oxygen binding properties of haemoglobins in red cells and in extracts has been made for only one invertebrate species other than annelids and sipunculids; the oxygen affinity of the haemoglobins in red cells of the arcid clam *Noetia ponderosa* does not differ from that of extracts (Freadman and Mangum, 1976). The origin of specific modulators, at least in haemoglobin-containing cells, may well have been a vertebrate improvement on the original theme.

The presence in annelid cells of enzymes catalysing the reduction of methaemoglobin or methaemerythrin has not been investigated. The absence of appreciable quantities of oxidised or denatured haeme compounds from the body fluids of freshly collected worms is notable, as is their presence in animals kept under poor conditions in the laboratory. Methaemoglobin or haemochromagen formation is an early sign of illness that follows quickly, for example, upon prolonged exposure to daylight in the laboratory (*see* Section 4.7). It is a classic symptom of chronic porphyria, which in sedentary worms is a normal state of health so long as they remain in the darkness of the soft bottom (Kennedy and Dales, 1958; Mangum and Dales, 1965). In nature ferric haemoproteins, whose origin is unknown, have been found only in the gut lumen (Phear, 1955). Aquatic annelids kept in water-saturated air in the laboratory often suffer haemoprotein oxidation.

A somewhat more subtle effect of the intracellular environment on respiratory pigment function has recently been revealed by measurements of the oxygen release properties of annelid and sipunculid red cells (Mangum and Kondon, 1975; Mangum *et al*., 1975). Despite the apparent absence of cooperative oxygen binding to these haemoglobins and to haemerythrins in extracts, the oxygenation properties of the substances in cells are not simple (*Figure 4.7*). There is a significant increase in the slope of an oxygen equilibrium curve about 50% oxygenation, and often a significant decrease below that level. The phenomenon is not an annelid peculiarity; it is a widespread if not universal feature of the red cell. Its adaptive significance to infaunal annelids is very clear, because it enhances each of the two major functions of coelomic cell pigments: (a) oxygen transport at higher oxygen levels, which prevail *in vivo* when the animal ventilates, and (b) oxygen storage at low PO_2's, which occur *in vivo* when ventilation ceases at low tide. The intracellular environment provides a refinement of simple haemoprotein function that results in more efficient gas exchange. *Figure 4.7* illustrates the quantitative importance of the change above 50% oxygenation. By transforming the ordinate units to absolute quantities of oxygen, it can be seen that the change in coelomic fluid PO_2 induces the release of 25 instead of 6 μl O_2.

The cells themselves are quite different from one another (*Figure 4.6*) and from those in mammals. Most annelid red cells are structurally simple and variable in size, even within an individual. Both haemerythrin- and haemoglobin-containing cells are rather small (1–40 μm diameter) discs. In side view they partly assume the familiar concave form, but the apparently incompressible nucleus causes a bulge at the centre. With the sole exception of haemerythrin-containing cells circulating in the closed vascular system of

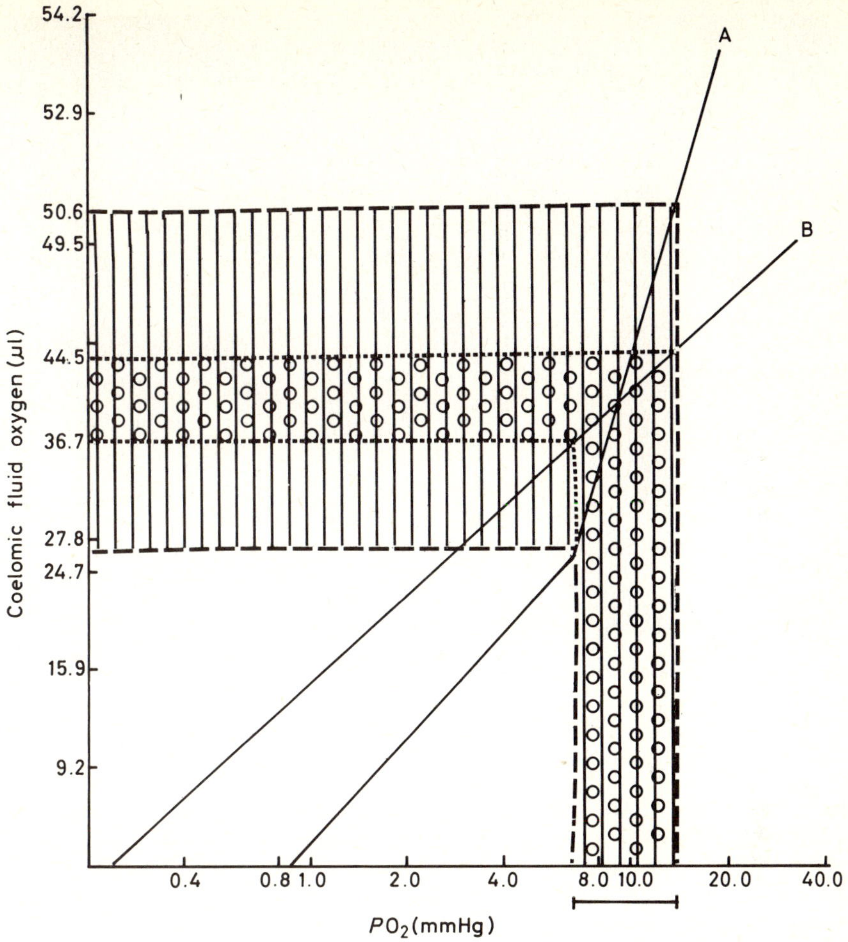

Figure 4.7 Oxygenation of purified extracts of coelomic haemerythrin from Phascolopsis gouldi *at 22°C in PO_4 buffer at pH 7.0–8.2 (dotted line). Oxygen release curve for coelomic cells at 23°C in borate buffered seawater at pH 7.58 (dashed line). Units of ordinate transformed from Hill expression to μl O_2 bound by the intracellular pigment at measured* in vivo *concentrations. Projection on ordinate from area marked with open circles gives volume of oxygen released by haemerythrin extracts; projection on ordinate from vertically hatched area gives volume delivered by haemerythrin in cells. Data from Mangum and Kondon (1975)*

the annelid family Magelonidae (which are exceptional in both their location and their contents) these cells are nucleated.

Typical cytoplasmic organelles can be identified (*Figure 4.8*). Rough endoplasmic reticulum is not found in *G. dibranchiata* red cells, but variable numbers of free ribosomes are scattered in the cytoplasm (Seamonds and Schumacher, 1972). While mitochondria are scarce, relative to other types of cells, the rate of oxygen consumption is considerably higher than those of vertebrate erythrocytes (Mangum and Carhart, 1972). The coelomic cells of

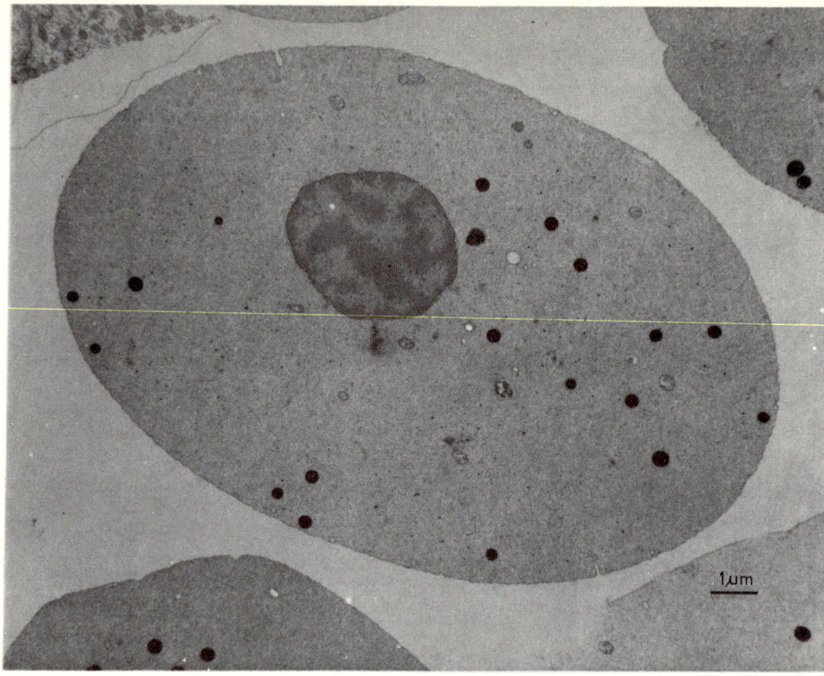

Figure 4.8 The red cell of the bloodworm Glycera dibranchiata. *Electron micrograph prepared by P. K. Chien*

Amphitrite ornata, whose major function is probably not respiratory despite the presence of small amounts of haemoglobin (Mangum *et al*., 1975), have an even higher rate of aerobic metabolism. The structure of the cells from a closely related species, which has been described in detail by Dales (1964), is very different from that of the haemoglobin- or haemerythrin-containing cells of any other group of animals (*Figure 4.6*).

Bloodworm cells actively incorporate labelled phenylalanine into protein, albeit at an unimpressive rate (Hoffmann and Mangum, 1970). In addition to haemoglobin, the cells synthesise low molecular weight RNA (Shafie *et al*., 1975). Near the Sôret band the integrated absorbance of intact cells of *Glycera americana* is fairly variable; one interpretation of this finding is that the haemoglobin content of a single cell is also variable (Cowden, 1966). Haemoglobin cannot be detected in the cell nucleus and nuclear contents do not communicate with the cytoplasm through large pores in the membrane, unlike in amphibians (Cowden, 1966; Dales and Pell, 1970).

'Pink' or dark red cells are found in members of the annelid family Magelonidae and the phylum Sipunculida. These cells, which contain haemerythrin, are poorly described in literature. In magelonid polychaetes they are very small (1–2 μm diameter) and anucleate — the only example outside of the vertebrates of a respiratory pigment in vascular blood cells and a rare example outside of the mammals of blood cells without nuclei. Pink cells in sipunculids are larger (6–32 μm in diameter) and usually mononucleate, although giant multinucleate cells are also present. They have a relatively low rate of aerobic metabolism, less than annelid red cells, and they contain an estimated 2 ng or 10^{10} molecules of haemerythrin (Mangum and Kondon, 1975).

4.7 RESPIRATORY PIGMENTS

4.7.1 Haemoproteins

Advocates of caprice in the course of haemoprotein evolution often point to the sporadic distribution of these molecules. Some annelid families have a respiratory pigment and others do not; some species within a family have one while others do not. Members of the remarkable genus *Serpula* test credulity by mixing haemoglobin and chlorocruorin in their blood (Fox and Vevers, 1960). Nonetheless, taxonomic whimsy does not mean that the invention of haemoglobin was superfluous. An annelid worm may be quite successful with no respiratory pigment in its body fluids, but it does not grow to be a very big worm and it does not penetrate very far into the soft bottom. The advantages of being a very big worm are not entirely obvious unless large size enabled some species to become predators when there were few competitors at that trophic level, but the advantages of filling the vacant soft bottom are clear (*see* pp. 193-195).

Among infaunal worms the most notable exception to the correlation of large body size with the presence of a respiratory pigment is *Chaetopterus variopedatus,* which has managed to become quite large (though not predatory) and to penetrate half a metre into the bottom without the aid of a respiratory pigment. It has done so by carrying heteronomous segmentation to an extreme, so that enormous fanlike expansions of the body wall drive copious volumes of water through the tube (*Table 4.1*). This activity, whose rate may be determined by nutritional rather than respiratory demands, is accompanied by a *15-fold increase* in aerobic metabolism at 15°C (Dales, 1969), more than three times the increment in *Amphitrite ornata* which has haemoglobin in its blood and coelomic fluid (Coyer and Mangum, 1973).

Another exception is tentative but interesting. While participating in the 1968 Bering Sea Expedition of R/V *Alpha Helix,* I found a large specimen of an unidentified species of *Glycera,* which had no haemoglobin in its numerous coelomic cells. The finding is not entirely unexpected, because members of several animal groups that inhabit cold, oxygen rich waters have atypically small amounts of respiratory pigment. Notable examples include the several species of ice fish, at least one of which has no haemoglobin at all (Rund, 1954), and the Alaska king crab *Paralithodes camtschaticus* which has less than one tenth the haemocyanin found in well fed temperate zone crabs (Mangum, unpublished).

Textbooks of animal physiology usually lump together the intracellular and extracellular haemoglobins into a single category, which contains molecules with the same haem group but with very different peptides. They also place chlorocruorin in a distinct category, based on the probably trivial modification of one of the eight side chains on the pyrroles in its haem (*Figure 4.9*). It is clear that this classification is highly artificial, from both biological and chemical points of view. *The extracellular haeme proteins, chlorocruorin and haemoglobin, have more in common with one another than either has with intracellular haemoglobin.* The statement is true of the structure, the physiological function and probably the evolutionary orgin of these pigments. In so far as present information permits, the more fundamental dichotomy between the extracellular and intracellular haem proteins is illustrated in the discussion that follows.

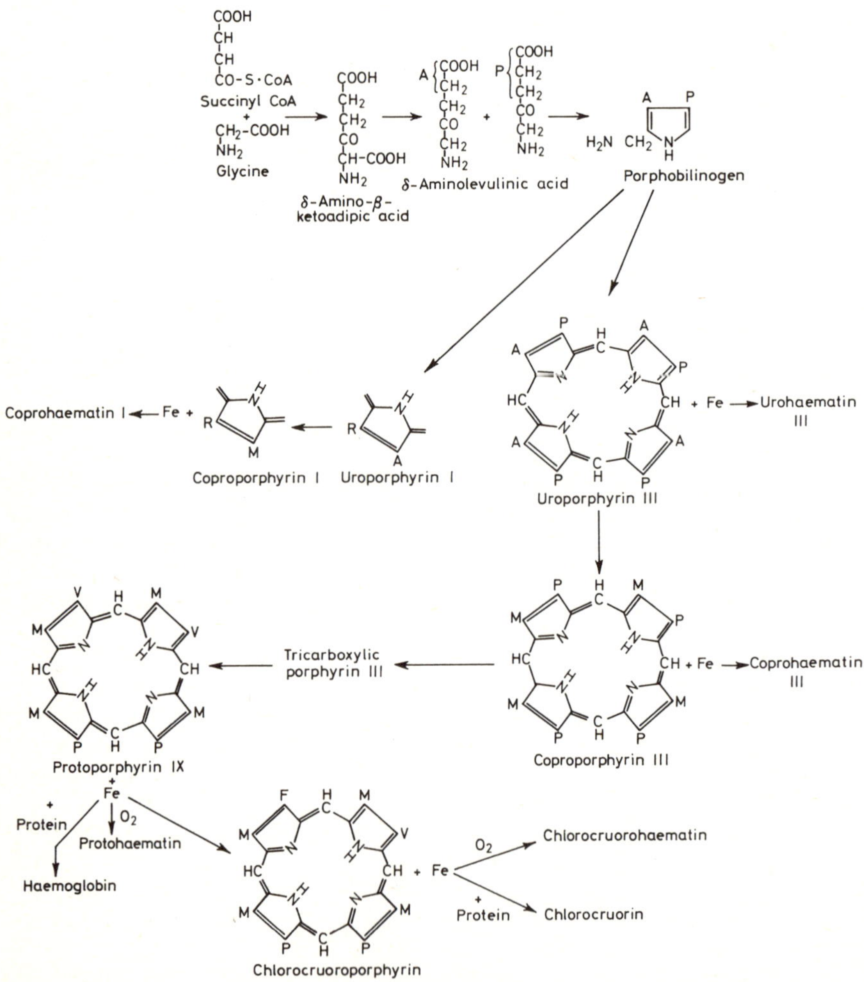

Figure 4.9. The biosynthetic pathway of haem in annelids. Modified from Mangum and Dales (1965)

4.7.1.1 BIOSYNTHESIS

The large extracellular haemoproteins are synthesised in tissue variously known as chloragogue, extravasal, intravasal or the heart body, depending on tradition and its anatomical location. Regardless of their anatomy, the tissues are believed to be homologous in the different classes of annelids and they apparently play the common role of manufacturing the respiratory pigment. Their importance in haemopoiesis was postulated in the last century on the evidence of a high iron content. More substantial evidence was presented by Kennedy and Dales (1958), who identified in them several by-products known from the vertebrate biosynthetic pathway.

In *Arenicola marina* the haemoglobin molecule is elaborated to its final form in Golgi channels which detach from the organelle as vesicles and migrate into the cytoplasm. The vesicles fuse to form large vacuoles full of haemoglobin, which are ultimately emptied into the bloodstream (Breton-Gorius, 1963). Although the anabolic process is believed to assume a cyclical pattern, its control is totally unknown.

The central steps in the elaboration of the complex heterocyclic structure protohaem from its aliphatic precusor δ-aminolevulinic acid have been demonstrated *in vitro* in preparations of oligochaetes (MacRae and Bogorad, 1958; Delkeskamp, 1964) and polychaetes (Kennedy and Dales, 1968). There is no reason to suppose that the pathway differs from that in vertebrates (*Figure 4.9*); indeed, many of the same iron storage compounds are found in the annelid tissues (Bessis and Breton-Gorius, 1960; Bessis, 1962). As the porphyrin ring is initially formed from the smaller pyrrole structure and then as the carboxyl side chains are successively modified, however, large excesses of various porphyrin compounds are produced (*Figure 4.9*). Only a fraction of the product remains in the mainstream of the pathway. Even more bizarre, the conversion of pyrrole to porphyrinogen results in production not only of the series III isomer, some of which is destined to become the prosthetic group of haemoglobin or chlorocruorin, but also the series I isomer, which has a different sequence of side chains and therefore cannot be used to make respiratory pigment (Kennedy and Dales, 1958; Mangum and Dales, 1965).

When these compounds are found in vertebrate animals they are regarded as errors of metabolism. Porphyrins with the centre of the complex ring free of a metal atom absorb so much light that their presence in appreciable quantity causes lesions in tissue. The pathological condition is known as porphyria and, although not a common malady, it is a serious handicap to an animal which is active in daylight.

The condition is tolerated as the norm in the infaunal annelids, probably because few of them ever see the light of day. The bodies of errant species, or worms that crawl about on the surface of the sand, and organs in sedentary species which are exposed to daylight, such as the branchial crowns in serpulids and sabellids, do not contain large amounts of free porphyrins. In sedentary species much of the porphyrin material is converted to corresponding metalloporphyrins, a process that considerably quenches the energy absorption and also forms dark brown screening pigment which accumulates in the body wall as the animal ages (*Figure 4.9*). This use of iron would be an intolerable extravagance in an animal that does not live and feed in an iron enriched environment, but it is not so wasteful in terrestrial soils and marine sediments (Mangum and Dales, 1965).

Although free porphyrins are far more common in subhominid mammals than often supposed (Kluver, 1944; Kennedy, 1970), the magnitude of porphyrin production must have diminished in evolution and the control of haemoglobin synthesis must have been tightened. In vertebrates the biosynthetic pathway is regulated by the feedback inhibition of protohaem on the production of ALA synthetase, the enzyme catalysing the formation of that first ring structure (*Figure 4.9*). Enzymes catalysing subsequent reactions are present in amounts that do not limit the product (Kappas and Granick, 1968). Dales and Pell (1970) noted that the removal of annelid haemoglobin from the cell releases inhibition and thus precludes the possibility of haemostatic control at this level. This insight underlines the point made in Section 4.6 that the question of why haemoglobin is often packaged inside red cells may not be as interesting as why it was ever released into the bloodstream. The evolution of the large extracellular haemoproteins may have been quite expensive in terms of anabolic economy.

And yet the very cyclical pattern of extravasal cell activity suggests that some form of control is exerted. Moreover, haemoglobin biosynthesis in at least one errant species, *Neanthes* (=*Nereis*) *arenaceodentata,* seems to be regulated under stress conditions, it responds to low oxygen levels with a compensatory increase (Raps and Reish, 1971). However, this response does not appear to occur in several other species (Fox, 1955; Brafield personal communication). In vertebrates a compensatory response to low PO_2 is induced by the release of feedback inhibition on the production of ALA synthetase (Simons and Boell, 1971). In annelids it is at least possible that control is exerted at the level of the finished product, the haemoprotein in the bloodstream, although this notion is entirely untested. This form of control, which would require enteroreception and endocrine response, would probably be less precise than a mechanism operating at the cell level.

Haemoglobin catabolism in annelids is unknown. My own interest in haeme metabolism arose from the puzzling distribution in several species of bile pigments, open chain tetrapyrroles produced by haem degradation in vertebrates (Mangum, 1962a). In the annelids, however, these compounds always occur in the meso- or saturated form, and they are derived from algal pigments present in the animal's food rather than its haemoglobin (Mangum, 1962b). While negative evidence is not very satisfying, I am prepared to venture the conclusion after a fifteen year search that protobilins do not occur in annelids and that haem is not degraded by the same route as in vertebrates. It may not be degraded at all; it may simply be carried by cells that move through the gut wall (Marsden, 1966) and released into the gut lumen as haemochromagen (Phear, 1955). It may be less expensive to lose iron in this way, than to catabolise the haeme molecule and conserve a metal that is in abundant supply.

The synthesis of intracellular haemoglobin and the concomitant question

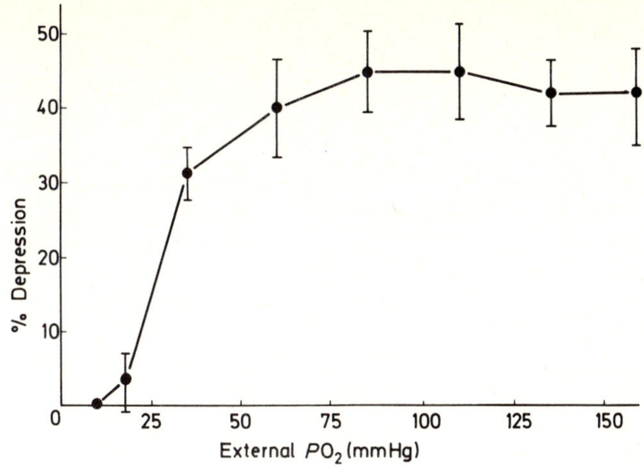

Figure 4.10 The depression of aerobic repiration at 22°C in Arenicola cristata *caused by blocking its haemoglobin with 0.2 ml CO/1. Experimental procedure described by Hoffmann and Mangum (1970); criteria for acceptance of data discussed by Mangum (1970)*

of red cell formation in annelids has received little attention. In families such as the glycerids with no vascular system, haemoglobin biosynthesis cannot occur in extravasal tissue or heart bodies. At the junction of the proboscis and the oesophagus bloodworms have tonguelike glandular structures that contain haem compounds, leading Raphaël (1933) to suppose that they might be organs of haemoglobin degradation. In a recent anatomical study, however, Michel (1970) concluded that the functions of these structures are neurosecretory and digestive. Loose masses grossly resembling extravasal tissue are invariably found in the same region of the coelomic cavity of *Glycera americana* and *G. dibranchiata.* When I sectioned them and sent the fixed preparations to R. P. Dales, however, he was unable to demonstrate the presence of haeme compounds. Aspects of the life history and metabolism of the annelid red cell would seem to be a fertile field of investigation.

4.7.1.2 ULTRASTRUCTURE OF EXTRACELLULAR HAEMOPROTEINS

The discovery that these enormous molecules can actually be observed and considerable detail of fine structure portrayed from electron micrographs (Roche, Bessis and Thiery, 1960) was most exciting. Indeed, the very elegant anatomical studies by Breton-Gorius (1963) quickly revealed details of the elaboration of haemoglobin in the extravasal cell. However, the electron dense image of the annelid haemoglobin molecule is not easily interpreted in terms of its chemical structure.

The extracellular haemoglobin molecules are a pair of superimposed hexagonal discs, 218–260 Å in diameter and 105–174 Å high (*Figure 4.11*).

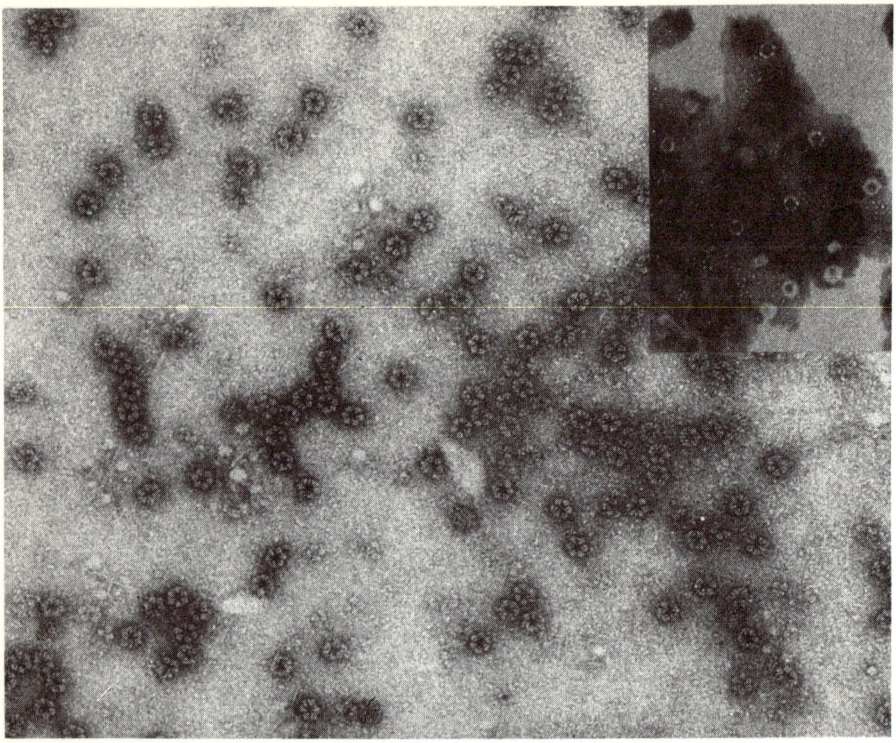

Figure 4.11 Fine structure of the vascular haemoglobin of Amphitrite ornata *negatively stained with 1% phosphotungstic acid at pH 6.7. Width of hexagons at parallel sides = 218 Å (N = 50); height of hexagon pair in side view = 105 Å (N = 18). Arrow directed at 12-layered stack. Insert shows spherical particles which appear after adjusting the pH with 1N NaOH to 8–9. Electron micrograph prepared by J. L Scott. Magnification × 59,500*

The six units of each disc surround a central depression 70–80 Å wide, each of the subunits is 70–80 Å in diameter and 100 Å long (Levine, 1963; Roche, 1965; Yamagishi *et al.*, 1966; Shlom and Vinogradov, 1973; *Figure 4.11*). Each of the six units of a hexagon is usually envisaged as a triad, although occasionally they appear to be quadrepartite (Yamagishi *et al.*, 1966; *Figure 4.11*).

The molecule appears as if it is composed of two principal subunits, 12 (= 2 + 6) secondary subunits and 36 (= 3 × 2 × 6) or 48 (= 4 × 2 × 6) smaller particles. In addition, the large central cavity of the hexagon may contain material, holding together the two members of the pair, which is distinct from the pair material itself (Levine, 1963). Most observers have described the central depression as a void, but Shlom and Vinogradov (1973) believe that material is present that does not comprise part of the hexagons, and they verge on suggesting that it may be one of the minor peptides they prepared from the earthworm molecule (*see* p. 245). Moreover, van Bruggen and Weber (1974) have observed a seventh subunit in the central depression of the molecule prepared from *Oenone fulgida*, a polychaete which belongs to the little known family Lysaretidae.

Although there are no qualitative differences between haemoglobins from members of the three major classes of annelids, the smaller extracellular haemoglobins found in gastropods and crustaceans do not exhibit this structure (Roche, 1965). The functional significance of quantitative differences between species of annelids is not yet clear. On the one hand haemoglobin from *Arenicola marina*, with a high degree of subunit interaction in oxygen binding, is a more compact molecule than that of *Lumbricus terrestris*, which is less cooperative in oxygen binding (Levine, 1963; *Table 4.7*). The vertical dimensions of the haemoglobin from *Amphitrite ornata* are much smaller than those of other molecules (*Figure 4.11*), however, and yet it shows little subunit interaction in oxygen binding (*Table 4.7*); its molecular weight is not precisely known.

When the hierarchy of fine structure is translated to the language of protein chemistry, the neat image of the molecule is destroyed. Fine structure can be used to generate predictions of the size of the peptide submultiples and the ultimate protomeric subunits of these giant haemoglobins, but the predictions have not yet been confirmed. While haemoglobins from the polychaetes *Arenicola cristata, Marphysa sanguinea*, and *Pista pacifica* dissociate to subunits with masses corresponding to one twelfth of the native molecule, possibly a single triad or tetrad, those from other members of the three major classes of annelids often do not (*Table 4.6*). Moreover, none of the chemical dissociation products have molecular weights equal to 1/2, 1/6, 1/36 or 1/48 × (3×10^6).

Nevertheless alterations of the native state of the molecule do result in the qualitative dimensional changes which are expected. The use of uranyl acetate instead of phosphotungstate for negative staining, or equilibration to a pH slightly below the isoelectric point, both of which precipitate the protein, cause an increase in hexagon diameter to 300 Å. Splitting the molecule by equilibration to high pH, by chemical agents such as urea or by an unknown spontaneous process that occurs when a solution is allowed to age, results in products composed of various numbers of twelfths (formerly the triads or tetrads), which then assume a somewhat swollen and globular form (Levine, 1963; Roche *et al*., 1963; Mangum and Scott, unpublished; *see Figure 4.11* insert). Finally, freezing and thawing, which often alters oxygenation properties, also induces shape irregularities of the hexagon. Reconstitution of the split products does not yield a structure that can be resolved by the electron microscope (Roche, 1965).

The blood haemoprotein of *Arenicola marina* dissociates only in part at high pH, but the molecules left intact no longer have the same oxygenation behaviour when they are separated from the split products by electrofocusing and returned to *in vivo* pH (Weber, 1970). More important to the present discussion, the cooperative behaviour of the molecules in a fraction consisting largely of single members of the hexagon pair are no different from those of the intact hexagon pair. Nor are those of another fraction consisting primarily of twelfths, although these particles tend to reaggregate into a larger molecule that may be either native or altered. These interesting

Table 4.7 OXYGENATION PROPERTIES OF ANNELID HAEMOPROTEINS

Species	P_{50} (mm Hg)	n	pH	$\frac{\Delta log\ P_{50}}{\Delta pH^1}$	Source
A. EXTRACTS					
A. Haemoglobins					
Polychaeta					
Arenicolidae					
Abarenicola claparedi	4.6	1) 2.3	7.4	−0.33	Weber (1971a)
		2) 3.5	7.4		
Arenicola cristata	1.62–2.63	5.0–6.7	7.6–7.9	−0.70	Allen and Wyman (1952)
	3.6–4.1	5.0–5.7	5.8–7.6	−0.032	Waxman (1971)
	1.7–2.8	1) 1–1.3		−0.34	Weber and Mangum (in prep.)
		2) 3.6–5.0			
A. marina	1.4–2.5	1) 2.12–2.62	7.00–7.55	−0.47–0.90	Weber (1970, 1971a, 1972)
		2) 3.35–4.70	7.00–7.55		
	3.0	1) *c.* 1	7.06		Economides and Wells (1975)
		2) 5.4	7.06		
Arenicolides branchialis	4.2	1) 2.5	7.0		Weber (1971a)
		1) 4.6	7.0		
Cirratulidae					
Cirriformia sp.	0.04–4.0	1.0–1.4	6.5–7.7	−1.5	Swaney and Klotz (1971)
Glyceridae					
Glycera dibranchiata					
light	5.2	1.0–1.2	7.4	−1.09[1]	Hoffmann and Mangum (1970); Mangum (1976b)
	4.95	1.08	6.05–8.40	0	Seamonds and Forster (1972)
	6.0–9.1	1.0	7.0–8.5	−0.45[1]	Mizukami and Vinogradov (1973)
heavy	10.2	1.2–1.5	7.4	0	Hoffmann and Mangum (1970); Mangum (1976b)
	5.00	0.94	6.05–8.40	0	Seamonds and Forster (1972)
	6.3–12.6	1.2–1.4	7.4–9.0	−0.19[1]	Mizukami and Vinogradov (1973)
mixture	7.00–7.37	1.04	7.4		Hoffmann and Mangum (1970); Mangum (1976b)
	7.25	1.02	6.05–8.40	0	Seamonds and Forster (1972)
G. gigantea					
mixture	13–16	1.8	6.25–9.25	0	Weber (1973)
Lysaretidae					
Oenone fulgida	11–15	1) 3.1	7.0–8.0	−0.16	Weber (1975)
		2) 1.8			

Lumbrinereidae					
Lumbrinereis tetraura	2.2–8.7	1) 1.6–5.0 2) 1.6–3.0	7.0–8.0	−0.6	Weber (1971a)
Nephtydae					
Nephthys hombergi					
coelomic	3.6–12.5	1.3–1.7			Weber (1971b)
vascular	10.2–16.8	1.2–1.8			
Nereidae					
Nereis sp.	11.5	0.9	7.0		Waxman (1975)
Nereis virens	1.5–10	1.1–1.2	6.68–7.33	0	Economides and Wells (1975)
Perinereis cultrifera	5.7	1) 1.5 2) 2.0			Weber (1971a)
Onuphidae					
Diopatra neapolitana	3.2–7.1	1) 2.0–3.0 2) 1.3–1.5	7.0–8.0	−0.35	Weber (1971a; 1975)
Opheliidae					
Travisia pupa					
coelomic	0.36	1	7.08–7.86	0	Manwell (1960a)
vascular	0.53–1.10	1−>1	7.03–7.48	−0.9	
Pectinariidae					
Lagis (=Pectinaria)					
koreni koreni	4.2	1) 1.9 2) 2.9			Weber (1971a)
Terebellidae					
Amphitrite ornata					
coelomic	2.7	1.0	6.25–9.05	0	Mangum *et al.* (1975); Weber *et al.* (1976)
vascular	10.0	1.3–1.6	5.81–7.90	0	
Enoplobranchus sanguineus	1.32	1.0	6.95–7.97	0	Mangum *et al.* (1975); Weber *et al.* (1976)
Eupolymnia crescenti	36	1.06	4.97–7.08	0	Manwell (1959)
Neoamphitrite robusta	30–50	1		0	Manwell (1963)
Pista pacifica					
coelomic	3.8	1.6	6–8	0	Terwilliger (1974)
vascular	25	1.5	6–8	0	
Terebella lapidaria					
vascular	3	1) 1.0 2) 2.7			Wells and Dales (1975)

Table 4.7 *continued*

Species	P_{50} (mm Hg)	*n*	*pH*	$\frac{\Delta log P_{50}}{\Delta pH^1}$	*Source*
Thelepus crispus					
coelomic	3.2	1.54	5.4–9.2	0	Garlick and Terwilliger (1974)
vascular	30–50	1–1.6	7.0–8.0	−0.49	Manwell (1963); Garlick and Terwilliger (1974)
Oligochaeta					
Allobophora terrestris	6				Haughton *et al.* (1958)
Alma emini	2.57–3.08	1) 0.97–1.23 2) 1.16–1.44	6.6–7.5	−0.1	Mangum *et al.* (1975)
Glossoscolex giganteus	7		7.5–7.8	small	Johansen and Martin (1966)
Lumbricus terrestris	3.5–4.8	1.81–1.84	7.21–7.72	−0.25	Manwell (1959)
	8				Cosgrove and Schwartz (1965)
	10–11	2.5	7.0		Shlom and Vinogradov (1973)
	3.9–6.5	4.6–5.4	7.1–7.9	−0.28	Waxman (1975)
Lumbricidae sp.	6.6	2.7	6.8		David and Daniel (1973)
Tubifex tubifex	0.67–2.29	1.9–2.5	6.02–8.56	0– −1	Scheler (1960)
Achaeta					
unidentified species	10.2–13.2	2.4–2.9	7.0		Waxman (1975)
B. Chlorocruorins					
Flabelligeridae					
Pherusa					
(=Stylarioides) inflata	24–80	1.70–1.89	6.97–7.48	−1.02	Manwell (1964)
P. plumosa	85–230	1.0	6.53–6.95	−1.03	Wells and Dales (1976)

Sabellidae					
Eudistylia vancouveri	39–140	1) 1.0 2) 4.7	7.00–7.93	−0.60	Manwell (1964)
Myxicola infundibulum	45–180	1) 4–5 2) <1	6.81–7.20	−1.54	Wells and Dales (1976)
Schizobranchia insignis	15–160	1) 1.0 2) 4.7	6.15–7.99	−0.56	Manwell (1964)
Spirographis spallanzani	15.8–78.1	1–5 (triphasic)	7.0–8.9	−0.45	Antonini *et al.* (1962a)
B. CELLS					
Glyceridae					
Glycera dibranchiata	6.20–9.45	0.80–0.83	6.8–7.4	0	Mangum and Carhart (1972)
G. gigantea	7.2–7.8	1.8			Weber (1973)
Terebellidae					
Amphitrite ornata	1.16	1.17	6.6		Mangum *et al.* (1975)
	2.60	1) 2.27 2) 0.85	7.3–7.9		
Enoplobranchus sanguineus	1.90	1.12	6.6		Mangum *et al.* (1975)
	1.33	1) 1.29 2) 0.66	6.8–7.8		
Terebella lapidaria	3–11	1.33–1.48	6.50–7.28	0	Wells and Dales (1975)

[1]This quantity is often given as $\varphi = \log P_{50}/7.4–7.0$. The values given here, however, were calculated for the whole pH range specified, because the interval 7.0–7.4 has little physiological significance in annelids, and because the data often do not permit the calculation of φ

results suggest that members of the hexagon pair do not interact in oxygen binding; nor do the six units of a single member of the pair. A similar conclusion for the haemoglobin of an unidentified lumbricid earthworm was reached by David and Daniel (1973), who showed that the split product with a sedimentation coefficient of 10 in the ultracentrifuge (= molecular weight of about 163×10^3 daltons) exhibits the same cooperativity in oxygen binding as the parent 60S molecules (*Table 4.7*). The oxygen affinity, however, was lowered (P_{50} = 8.9 mm Hg for 10S subunit and 6.6 mm Hg for 60S molecule). Terwilliger *et al*., (1975) found that the 280×10^3 particle of *Pista pacifica* is the smallest subunit that retains cooperativity.

David and Daniel (1974), with the collaboration of Ben-Shaul (1974), have recently postulated a very different quaternary structure for the haemoglobin of the Israeli lumbricid. Using optical measurements of the sedimentation pattern instead of the diffusion coefficient to compute molecular weight from sedimentation in the ultracentrifuge, they estimate that the native molecule (61.1S) weighs 3.84×10^3 instead of $2.7–3.0 \times 10^3$ (*Table 4.6*). Their electron micrographs show the familiar hexagons in flat view and they appear to show the hexagon pairs in side view. They agree with Yamagishi *et al.* (1966) and also *Figure 4.11* that the six units of the hexagons are tetrads rather than triads. They suggest that the native molecule is not a stack of two hexagons but rather four hexagons. The hypothesis is made to explain the molecular weight of peptide subunits computed from sedimentation behaviour. Specifically, if the molecule is composed of four principal subunits, 24 (= 4×6) secondary subunits and 96 (= $4 \times 4 \times 6$) tertiary subunits, then the 1/24th particle corresponds to the 10S peptide (= 163×10^3, or *c.* $\frac{3.84 \times 10^6}{24}$ daltons) obtained by alkaline dissociation of the native molecule. The 1/96th particle corresponds to a 3.5S (= 40.8×10^3, or *c.* $\frac{3.84 \times 10^6}{96}$ daltons) peptide.

These interesting findings await the test of further coordinated studies of sedimentation behaviour and the fine structure of split products. Although the point is not always clear in the original works, the estimates of $2.4–3.2 \times 10^6$ for the molecular weights of extracellular haemoproteins seem to have been calculated from the Svedberg equation, using D (diffusivity). As emphasised by David and Daniel (1974), high molecular weight compounds have very low diffusion coefficients, which are therefore difficult to determine accurately, and alternative methods are probably preferable. Optical measurements made on *Lumbricus terrestris* haemoglobin by Rossi-Fanelli *et al.* (1970) also yield an estimate appreciably higher than 3×10^6 (*Table 4.6*). Molecular weights of extracellular haemoproteins may be somewhat higher than previously supposed.

On the other hand, the evidence presented by David and Daniel (1974) for a four-layered quaternary structure does not agree with the conclusions of the several electron microscopists who have studied these molecules, and it is not supported with electron micrographs showing that arrangement. In the best micrographs (Breton-Gorius, 1963; Roche, 1965), side views very clearly show two layers separated by a small cleft. Plates often show stacking of the hexagon pairs into multiples of the two layers (*Figure 4.11*), but uneven numbers of discs are not observed and single discs occur only after treatments to induce dissociation (van Bruggen, in Weber, 1970). The diameter of the spherical particles observed on alkaline dissociation (*Figure 4.11,* insert) is similar to the height of a single hexagon (Levine, 1963; Roche *et al*., 1963), indicating that the two-layered structure usually regarded as the native molecule, cannot easily be resolved into four layers.

David and Daniel (1974) correctly predict the sedimentation coefficient of a 1/24th particle from an equation which requires computation of a term from the measured height of the molecule in electron micrographs. However, Ben-Shaul (1974) used uranyl acetate instead of phosphotungstate for negative staining, which results in precipitation of the protein and significantly greater dimensions of the hexagons (Levine, 1963). They report a hexagon diameter of 370 Å and a pair height of 237 Å. If the procedure did in fact alter protein structure, then the success of the prediction is not clear.

In any event, models of quaternary structure must have the supporting evidence of the size of peptides obtained as split products in the ultracentrifuge or on SDS gel, which must in turn be consistent with the subunits observed in electron micrographs of native molecules. They must also agree with electron micrographs of the molecule in both flat and side views.

Studies of chlorocruorin show few if any differences from extracellular haemoglobin. Electron micrographs of the native molecule are similar (Guerritore *et al*., 1965), and the sizes of split products are similar (Guerritore and Zito, 1971; Terwilliger and Terwilliger, 1975). Particles weighing about 30 $\times$ 10^3 daltons have been observed in electron micrographs after dissociation (Terwilliger and Terwilliger, 1975). At least two distinct peptides of this approximate size (34 $\times$ 10^3 daltons) have been detected (Guerritore and Zito, 1971); on further dissociation they break down into components of 14–15 $\times$ 10^3 daltons (Terwilliger *et al.,* 1975). The gross amino acid composition of chlorocruorin and extracellular haemoglobin appears to be more similar than that of extracellular and intracellular haemoglobin. Like extracellular haemoglobin and unlike its intracellular counterpart, chlorocruorin has one Fe atom per two units of peptide (Terwilliger *et al*., 1975).

4.7.1.3 CHEMICAL STRUCTURE

In the century since 1872 when E. R. Lankester presented spectroscopic evidence of the similarity of the chromophore of invertebrate and human haemoglobins, opinion on the structural affinity of the protein moiety has vacillated. As suggested above, the difficulty in resolving the point is due in part to the heterogeneity of the category 'haemoglobin'. Therefore the intracellular and extracellular haem compounds are discussed separately.

4.7.1.3.1 Intracellular haemoglobins

The molecular weight of haemoglobins extracted from annelid red cells ranges from 17–18 × 10³ in glycerids and terebellids to 125 × 10³ in *Glycera dibranchiata* (*Table 4.6*). The diversity in the two families reflects the adaptive exploration that students of annelids learn to expect. While coelomic cells in the terebellids contain haemoglobins of only one size and one or two electrophoretic mobilities (Terwilliger and Koppenheffer, 1973; Weber *et al*., 1976), the glycerids are less uniform. Their red cells may contain molecules of either one (*G. robusta*), two (*G. dibranchiata* and *G. gigantea*) or three (*G. americana*) different sizes, and one (*G. robusta*) to seven (*G. americana*) electrophoretic mobilities (Hoffman and Mangum, 1970; Weber, 1973; Terwilliger, Garlick and Terwilliger, 1976; Weber *et al*., 1976).

At least two other polychaete families, capitellids and opheliids, contain cellular haemoglobins whose structure and complexity are virtually unknown. Svedberg (1933) reported a haemoglobin of 34.5 × 10³ daltons in *Notomastus latericeus,* a member of the family Capitellidae. Unfortunately the function of haemoglobin in capitellids, which are known for their tolerance of low oxygen conditions (Reish, 1955), has not been investigated.

The conformation of the peptide chain of the major monomer from *G. dibranchiata* is similar to that of a subunit of mammalian haemoglobin (Padlan and Love, 1968). In addition, its primary structure has many similarities to various vertebrate haemoproteins (Imamura, Baldwin and Riggs, 1972). Only 23% of the amino acid residues are found in exactly the same place in the annelid monomer and in sperm whale myoglobin, and the departures include four of seven residues that are alike in all vertebrate haemoproteins. However, *almost half of the annelid residues are found in the same place as in some one of a variety of vertebrate haemoproteins.*

The polymer from *G. dibranchiata* has a different overall amino acid composition, suggesting that it is not a multiple of either the major or a minor monomer (Seamonds, Forster and George, 1971). Also, the sequence of the first 15 amino acids has only five residues in common with those of the major monomer (Imamura, Baldwin and Riggs, 1972). Finally, a minor polymeric component is still different, at least at the N-terminal segment.

Both the relative and the absolute quantities of these substances are highly variable. Coelomic cells of *G. dibranchiata* from southern New England in the summer contain nearly equal amounts of light and heavy haemoglobins, but those of animals collected in the early autumn from waters in northern New England contain less than one third as much polymer as monomer. Whether the difference is seasonal or geographic, genotypic or phenotypic, is unknown. A similar quantitative change in coelomic cell haemoglobin is found in *Amphitrite ornata* (Mangum *et al*., 1975). Favouring the genetic hypothesis is the fact of very different faunas at the twol locales, suggesting the interposition of barriers to gene flow between them. On the other hand, the concentration of coelomic cell haemoglobin in individuals of *Neoam-*

phitrite figulus taken from the same locality changes with season by a factor of two (Dales, 1964).

In contrast to the similarity of primary structure between glycerid and vertebrate haemoglobins, the monomeric haemoglobin in coelomic cells of the terebellid *Enoplobranchus sanguineus* shows little similarity to that of any vertebrate except the lamprey. Even more important, *the similarity between Enoplobranchus and lamprey haemoglobins is greater than that between Enoplobranchus and G. dibranchiata* (Weber *et al*., 1976). This result should introduce some caution into the renewed optimism over the use of simple biochemical evidence in constructing phylogenies.

Coelomic cells of the terebellid *Pista pacifica,* a member of a different subfamily from *Enoplobranchus,* contain two monomers separable by electrophoresis and by total amino acid composition (Terwilliger and Koppenheffer, 1973). The differences in amino acid composition between this species and bloodworms indicate that at least large portions of the peptide chains will prove to be dissimilar.

The multiplicity of haemoproteins in annelids is not easily understood, either in mechanistic or adaptive terms; it is not unparalleled in other aspects of annelid biology. Indeed, G. P. Wells once wrote (1961, pp. 230–231) of arenicolids that they '. . . are now merely radiating for the sake of diversity. Tired of selection, Nature has begun to doodle . . . But aimlessness is not necessarily unprogressive. Her game is a form of market research. Now and again she is bound to hit on something good enough to spread and put its rivals out of business'.

The superiority of the bloodworm sequence over that of the terebellid molecule may be inferred from its retention in evolution. However, it may be superior only in the context of later refinements rather than in the annelid red cell or in the soft bottom of the sea. The multiplicity may merely reflect the evolutionary experimentation that accompanied exploration of the new habitat.

4.7.1.3.2 Extracellular haemoproteins

The structure of the large extracellular haemoglobins and chlorocruorin is a far more difficult subject. After many years of obscurity, these interesting molecules are beginning to attract the attention of protein chemists. At high pH and also with the addition of urea, haemoglobin from *Lumbricus terrestris* dissociates into four polypeptide subunits, the largest of which breaks down further on SDS electrophoresis and mercaptoethanol into three smaller subunits. The hierarchy is represented by Shlom and Vinogradov (1973) as in *Figure 4.12.* Clearly, the protein is considerably more complex than previously supposed. Each of these peptide subunits is distinguished by its amino acid composition as well as its size. However, their relationship to the functional protomer, or the smallest subunit that displays all of the oxygen binding properties of the native molecule, is not yet known. Nor is the relationship of these subunits to the 128 haem chromophores of the intact protein known. As indicated in the discussion of quaternary structure (pp. 233–241), the relationship of peptide components to the dense bodies that appear in electron micrographs remains obscure.

Several studies of extracellular haemoglobins from other species suggest that some but not all of the native oxygen binding properties reside in a peptide that comprises one twelfth of the intact molecule, with a molecular weight of 200–300 × 10^3 (Weber, 1970; Weichelman and Parkhurst, 1972; Terwilliger *et al*., 1975). These particles can be dissociated further into two polypeptide chains with different amino acid compositions (*Table 4.6*). In *Arenicola cristata* they have masses of 13 × 10^3 and 14 × 10^3 daltons; either (a) the two subunits share a common haem group (Waxman, 1971), or (b) only one of the two possesses a haem group. In the Australian eunicid *Marphysa sanguinea,* one of the two dissociation products, about 200 × 10^3 daltons, is haem enriched and the other much smaller peptide, about 18–50 × 10^3, has none (Chew, *et al.,* 1965). However, the 22 × 10^3 peptide prepared by Daniel and David (1974) is believed to contain a haem group. While the size of individual peptides is not known, the iron content (0.22%) of haemoglobin prepared from the aquatic oligochaete *Tubifex tubifex* predicts a similar ratio of protein to ligand combining site. However, *the haem content explains only half of the iron atoms measured* (Scheler and Schneiderat, 1959), which implies that non-haem iron is present in considerable amounts. Whether this non-haem iron plays any role in oxygen combination, either adjunct or independent, is unknown. In contrast, Shlom and Vinogradov (1973) found similar ratios of protein to both iron and haem in earthworm haemoglobin. The confirmation of this feature of tubificid haemoglobin is extremely important to an understanding of the evolutionary origin of oxygen carrying pigments. If a peptide containing iron but no haem is in fact a subunit of some annelid haemoglobins and if it has any similarity to haemerythrins, then of course the phylogenetic distribution of these substances would be even less mysterious.

Vinogradov, Hall and Shlom (1974) have compared the subunits of dissociated haemoglobins from each of the three major classes of annelids. Extracellular molecules prepared from the oligochaete *L. terrestris,* the polychaetes *A. cristata* and *Cirriformia* sp.*, and the achaetes *Haemopsis grandis* and *Placobdella* sp. have in common only one small subunit of 12–13 × 10^3 daltons. A subunit of about 50 × 10^3 daltons occurs in both the polychaetes and in the earthworm. In the two polychaetes this peptide may be a heterodimer of chains weighing 13 and 16 × 10^3 daltons, but in the earthworm it consists of three separate peptide chains (*Table 4.6*). While the leeches apparently lack the 50 × 10^3 subunit, their haemoglobin dissociates in the presence of SDS and thiol into three or four smaller (12–6 × 10^3) subunits.

*Animals are apparently being furnished with the name *Cirraformia grandis* by a commercial supplier operating in the Gulf of Mexico. The annelid family Cirratulidae contains no genus with that spelling. It does include a genus *Cirriformia,* but the genus has no species *grandis.* There is a *Cirratulus grandis,* but it does not occur in the Gulf of Mexico. Meredith L. Jones of the US National Museum recently examined a large cirratulid collected by C. D. Long from the Gulf coast of northern Florida and concluded that either one of the two genera must be redefined to include this species, or else a new genus must be described. I shall refer to it as *Cirriformia* sp.

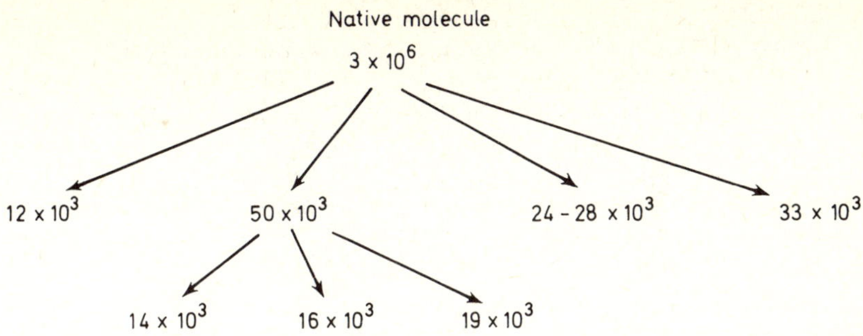

Figure 4.12 The relationship of the peptide subunits of haemoglobins from Lumbricus terrestris. *Data from Shlom and Vinogradov (1974)*

The structure of chlorocruorin, not as widely investigated, appears to be similar. Two distinct polypeptide chains, each with a haem group and a mass of 34–37 × 10^3 daltons, have been obtained by chemical dissociation. On further dissociation, peptides of 14–15 × 10^3 have also been detected. The largest dissociation product, one twelfth of the native molecule (= 220 × 10^3 daltons), is believed to be the functional protomer (Guerritore and Zito, 1971; Terwilliger *et al*., 1975; Terwilliger and Terwilliger, 1975).

4.7.1.4 OXYGEN BINDING AND RELEASE

The favourite data of comparative respiratory physiologists derive from the curve describing the oxygenation of an extract of a respiratory pigment. These curves are sources of important information to protein chemists, because they are intimately related to molecular structure. But the simplicity of oxygen binding data and the heavy reliance on them has probably retarded progress in understanding the role that respiratory pigments play in animals.

The essentials of oxygenation curves are reflected in the two constants (a) P_{50}, the partial pressure of oxygen at which the per cent saturation (Y) equals half, and (b) n, the slope of a curve after the data are transformed by a rather unusual mathematical procedure described by the empirically based Hill equation. The quantity log $\frac{Y}{1-Y}$ is plotted as a function of log PO_2, a procedure designed to linearise the data. In the literature one often encounters nebulous epithets applied to a pigment on the basis of its oxygen affinity, but the obscure relation of this property to an identifiable feature of the animal or its habitat has undoubtedly reinforced disillusionment with the zoological significance of comparative physiology and biochemistry. The variation in P_{50} shown in *Table 4.7*, for example, cannot be phrased in adaptive terms without thorough investigation of *in vivo* function.

Nevertheless, the oxygen affinity of a respiratory pigment is valuable knowledge if it is viewed in conjunction with answers to other questions.

They include:

1. What are the operating conditions of PO_2 in the microhabitat at the site of external gas exchange?
2. What is body fluid PO_2 under these conditions? (The volume of blood in all but the largest annelids is insufficient for reliable measurement with the smallest microelectrodes in general use, but the volume of coelomic fluid in many species is more than ample. Because the vascular system is often bathed by coelomic fluid this information may be pertinent to the role of blood pigments as well as those in coelomic fluid).
3. If the pigment is extracellular, are there substances in blood that modify its oxygen binding?
4. If the substance is intracellular, what are the effects of the intracellular environment on its respiratory function?
5. What is body fluid pH under normal operating conditions and at different times of year?
6. How does total oxygen content of body fluid change with PO_2, internal and external, *in vivo*?

Additionally, we would like to have information on pH and PO_2 at sites of oxygen uptake at the gill and delivery at the target, circulatory dynamics and red cell PO_2. Some of these measurements are feasible in a few very large annelids, but the species may be zoological oddities. The enumerated questions, however, can be answered by making routine laboratory measurements on representative species.

4.7.1.4.1 Intracellular haemoglobins

The oxygen binding properties of the small haem proteins extracted from cells are very much alike (*Table 4.7*), despite important differences in the experimental conditions. With the exception of the anomalous behaviour of the *Glycera dibranchiata* monomer at low pH (Hoffmann and Mangum, 1970; Mizukami and Vinogradov, 1973), values for P_{50} of monomers range only from 0.36 in the opheliid *Travisia pupa* (Manwell, 1960a) to 6.0 mm Hg found by Mizukami and Vinogradov (1973) for *G. dibranchiata*. The oxygen affinities of monomers extracted from the body wall muscles of *Arenicola marina* (Weber and Pauptit, 1972) and from the ventral nerve cord of *Aphrodita hastata* (Wittenberg, Briehl and Wittenberg, 1965) fall within this range also.

At the pH of coelomic fluid during ventilation, these substances generally show no evidence of subunit interaction ($n \simeq 1$), which is the obvious expectation of a monomer. At low pH however, Hoffmann and Mangum (1970) and Mizukami and Vinogradov (1973) found that oxygen affinity decreases, which is certainly an unexpected result (*Table 4.7*). This finding may only mean that monomers aggregate under the experimental conditions of low pH and low PO_2, although they do not do so at low PO_2 (Bonaventura and Kitto, 1973) or low pH alone (Mangum, unpublished). Biologically the point is unimportant because oxygen affinity remains unchanged at the same low pH when the substance is inside the cell (Mangum and Carhart, 1972). P_{50} of coelomic cell monomers from species other than glycerids is not affected by pH (*Table 4.7*) or by the presence of organic phosphates (Mangum *et al*., 1975). Coelomic cell haemoglobins larger than monomers and dimers appear to have distinctly lower oxygen affinities, which is the expected result (Hoffmann and Mangum, 1970; Mizukami and Vinogradov, 1973).

The earliest comparisons of oxygen equilibrium properties of annelid haemoglobins in cells and in extracts yielded no evidence that the function of these substances is modulated by specific factors inside the red cell. However, these studies were not made with both preparations under the same controlled physiological conditions, and different techniques were used for the optically heterogeneous cell suspensions and the optically homogeneous extracts (Hoffmann and Mangum, 1970; Mangum and Carhart, 1972; Weber, 1973).

More recent investigations of the intracellular haemoglobins of terebellids, made with both preparations in buffered seawater, indicate that these monomeric haemoglobins have the same oxygen affinities whether inside the cell or not, and that the addition of NaCl or organic phosphates to the medium does not alter the equilibrium with oxygen (Mangum *et al*., 1975; Weber *et al*., 1976). When the oxygenation of the red cells was measured with a physiological technique, the change in slope (n) described on p. 225 was detected; this phenomenon has been found in molluscan, avian and mammalian red cells with the same or with alternative techniques (references cited by Mangum *et al*., 1975). However when the oxygenation of these cells was measured optically, the change in slope was not detected (Weber *et al*., 1976). The phenomenon does not appear in measurements of haemoglobin extracts, regardless of technique, and so it is unlikely to be a result of the interaction of oxygen binding sites. Instead it must represent a change in the oxygen uptake or release by the haemoglobins in red cells, possibly related to the convection of substances in the cytoplasm or facilitated diffusion. It will be very interesting to learn whether it results from experimental conditions or whether it occurs *in vivo*.

The comparison of oxygenation properties of glycerid haemoglobins in cells and in extracts is seriously complicated by their heterogeneity. There is no evidence to decide whether monomers and polymers are in different cells or whether they are mixed in the same cells. Our operating hypothesis has always been that they are in the same cells and that they freely mix, but it is based only upon the principle established by William of Occam, and not on a single empirical fact.

The initial studies of *G. dibranchiata* haemoglobins yielded the expected results that the oxygen affinity of the monomeric haemoglobin is higher than that of the polymer, and that P_{50} of a mixture of the two is the same as that of a buffered red cell suspension (Hoffmann and Mangum, 1970; Mangum and Carhart, 1972; Mizukami and Vinogradov, 1973). However, they also yielded the anomaly that the oxygen affinity of the mixture was not intermediate between the values for the two components, but rather lower than either (Hoffmann and Mangum, 1970; Seamonds and Forster, 1972). The anomaly apparently arose from the lability of the polymer under the particular experimental conditions because it did not reappear when different procedures were used (Mangum, 1976b; Weber *et al.,* 1976). In all of the glycerids studied, the oxygen affinities of reconstituted mixtures behave as simple averages of the values for the separate components. More important, the use of preparations in buffered seawater and the same technique of measurement confirms the previous conclusion that oxygen affinity does not change when the components are extracted from the cells, purified and then remixed (Mangum, 1976b). In addition, Weber *et al.* (1976) found no appreciable effect of inorganic salts or organic phosphates on the oxygen affinity of extracts. The change in slope (n) of red cell oxygenation is very small and it does not occur in extracts; the phenomenon probably has little adaptive significance in this species (Mangum, 1976).

The importance of the red cell microenvironment in the physiological functioning of these early respiratory pigments, then, is not entirely clear. However, the available evidence argues strongly against the presence of specific modulators inside the red cells. Sensitive control of haemoglobin function in response to environmental or physiological variables does not seem to have been achieved by the annelids (or molluscs; Freadman and Mangum, 1976). On the other hand, most measurements suggest that the red cell environment may have a more subtle effect on haemoglobin oxygenation, possibly resulting from physical rather than chemical features; it is not understood, but it may be more important in animals that have their red cells in coelomic fluids (p. 225).

The intracellular haemoglobins (and haemerythrin) are believed to function in oxygen transport and also in oxygen storage, at least in infaunal species that must tolerate a severe depression of the oxygen level in their stagnant microhabitats when the tide goes out. Various calculations predict that the large amount of haemoglobin in coelomic fluid could support total $\dot{V}O_2$ for periods of 1–2 h (Hoffmann and Mangum, 1970; Mangum *et al.*, 1975). Measurements of the decline in coelomic oxygen when the worm is placed in a hypoxic medium indicate that the store is never really depleted, which is a highly adaptive response because it prevents haemolysis. The function of the oxygen store may be to maintain a small oxygen supply to key tissues, such as the nerve cord and the coelomic cells themselves, rather than to support overall aerobic metabolism (Mangum, 1976b).

4.7.1.4.2 Chlorocruorins

Oxygenation properties of the large vascular haemoproteins are not as uniform as those of cellular haemoglobins, which may reflect the functional possibilities of greater permutations when a molecule consists of numerous subunits of different kinds. From a biological viewpoint these properties are also more interesting in themselves, because they can be interpreted in the light of *in vivo* measurements without reference to various features of the intracellular environment.

The few chlorocruorins studied seem relatively similar to one another (*Table 4.7*). They have very low oxygen affinities — under some conditions the lowest of all respiratory pigments. If one is inclined towards extrapolations to *in vivo* function from *in vitro* measurements, this feature might imply a 'high tension pigment'. The results of Ewer and Fox (1940) indicate otherwise; participation of chlorocruorin in aerobic respiration changes very little from air saturation to quite low oxygen partial pressures. The futility of interpreting values for oxygen affinity in the light of gross aspects of the external environment is clearly illustrated by an anomaly reported by Wells and Dales (1975). The oxygen affinity of chlorocruorin from the flabelligerid *Pherusa plumosa* is so low that it is only 65% oxygenated at 159 mm Hg and what is believed to be *in vivo* pH (6.96 at 15°C). The measured blood pH is unlikely to be representative of the *in vivo* value at the gill; the blood was collected from the gut sinus, a prebranchial site, and the authors note the difficulty of procuring samples free of coelomic fluid. The uncertainty, however, emphasises the need for further studies of the function of chlorocruorin.

Very low oxygen affinities of sabellid and serpulid chlorocruorins are correlated with distinctive ventilation behaviour (*see* Section 4.2). These animals have a very highly developed gill (*Figure 4.5(f)*), which is used in filter feeding as well as gas exchange. Unlike most tubicolous annelids, the gill protrudes out of the tube and into the water column where the oxygen supply is rarely reduced much below atmospheric equilibration, except in estuarine habitats. Weight specific rates of ventilation in these families are higher than in other groups by an order of magnitude, probably because they are determined by nutritional rather than respiratory demands (*Table 4.1*). It seems likely that blood PO_2's are high in members of these families. This supposition must be tested by measurement, however, and it does not seem to be consistent with the finding of low blood pH (Wells and Dales, 1976).

No information on feeding and ventilation in the other families with chlorocruorin is available.

Oxygen equilibrium curves for sabellid and serpulid chlorocruorins exhibit a complexity true of most extracellular haemoglobins; the curves cannot be linearised by the Hill transformation. Instead, two and sometimes three distinct phases appear (*Table 4.7*). At lower partial pressures the Hill constant n equals 1, but at intermediate partial pressures the per cent oxygenation changes very rapidly, indicating extensive subunit interaction. At higher PO_2's the curve again assumes a smaller slope, although it does not descend to 1 (Antonini, Rossi-Fanelli and Caputo, 1962a).

The addition of urea, which dissociates the molecule to a product of about 200×10^3 daltons, possibly corresponding to the triads seen in electron micrographs, extends the lower phase (n_1) to intermediate partial pressures and thus lowers oxygen affinity. A high degree of subunit interaction persists at high partial pressures, although the overall oxygenation curve is quite different from that of the native molecule (Antonini, Rossi-Fanelli and Caputo, 1962b).

Flabelligerid chlorocruorin, whose structure is completely unknown, does not show analogous phase complexity and its subunits interact less during oxygenation (*Table 4.7*). Interestingly, it is the absence of these features that is responsible for the paradox of incomplete oxygenation at 159 mm Hg. The chlorocruorin of *Myxicola infundibulum,* for example, actually has a *lower* oxygen affinity than that of *Pherusa,* and the value of n differs very little when the substance is less than about 30% oxygenated. Above that level, the cooperativity of oxygen binding increases very greatly in *Myxicola* but not in *Pherusa* (Wells and Dales, 1976). Thus the biological significance of the phase changes may be much the same for the extracellular as for the intracellular haeme proteins: if the PO_2 range of the rapidly changing phase coincides with *in vivo* conditions, the oxygen transport function is enhanced.

Chlorocruorins are highly sensitive to the ionic composition of the solvent. Although pH does not affect either the slopes of oxygen equilibrium curves or their heterogeneity, the chlorocruorins of all three families studied are characterised by large Bohr shifts (*Table 4.7*). Since there are no data available for the difference in postbranchial and prebranchial pH, the significance of this property cannot be evaluated. One would expect that a spatial Bohr shift would be more important in these animals than in most other invertebrates, however, because they have a well developed system of large internal vessels and highly subdivided small vessels ramifying into a pinnate gill. The emphasis would be on oxygen uptake from the water column rather than its delivery to the tissues, since flow-through capillaries are not present (Ewer, 1941). A large increase in blood pH at the gill would explain the anomaly reported by Wells and Dales (1976), and also the selection of a pigment with a large Bohr shift in these families. If blood pH in chlorocruorin containing annelids does prove to be very low and if the pH difference between post- and pre-branchial blood is very great, the determinants of acid-base balance must be investigated anew. Species with extracellular haemoglobin have very small quantities of CO_2 and various carbonate compounds (Toulmond, 1970; Wells, 1973).

Like most respiratory pigments, the effect of salts on the oxygen affinity of chlorocruorin is opposite to that of H^+; the addition of inorganic salts increases the oxygen affinity of the pigment from *Spirographis spallanzani* (Antonini, Rossi-Fanelli and Caputo, 1962b). The possible physiological significance of this feature is discussed in Section 4.7.1.4.3.

Chlorocruorin from *S. spallanzani* resembles *Arenicola* haemoglobin in its reduced temperature sensitivity; $\Delta H = -4.5$ kcal/mole, as opposed to *c.* -12 kcal/mole for mammalian haemoglobins (Antonini, Rossi-Fanelli and Caputo, 1962b). This feature is almost certainly adaptive, but it cannot be interpreted in the light of other temperature dependent variables such as $\dot{V}O_2$, blood pH etc., which are not known.

4.7.1.4.3 Extracellular haemoglobins

The diversity of the oxygenation properties of the extracellular haemoglobins is almost overwhelming (*Table 4.7*). At the present state of knowledge they do not sort out into discrete classes that can be explained by molecular structure or understood in terms of physiological conditions. At first glance this multiplicity might be used to support the contention that experimentation is the major annelid contribution to respiratory function, and that at least some modern representatives inherited the least successful experiments.

Rather than summarise all of the various combinations of properties found in different species (*Table 4.7*), I shall confine the discussion to haemoglobins in two families that represent the extremes of the range.

These species include several members of the family Arenicolidae, studied recently by Toulmond (1970, 1973), Waxman (1971, 1975), Weber (1970, 1971, 1972), Wells (1973, 1974) and Mangum (1976a, 1976b); and several of the Terebellidae studied by Manwell (1959, 1963), Terwilliger (1974), Terwilliger and Koppenheffer (1973), Terwilliger *et al.* (1975), Mangum *et al.* (1975), Wells and Dales (1975) and Weber *et al.* (1976).

In vivo these haemoglobins have many features in common. High concentrations occur in large, well-developed blood vessels and they are oxygenated in branched gills, although the gills are found in the primitive segmental pattern in the arenicolids and in the more specialised anterior position in terebellids. At oxygen levels above 60 mm Hg and at 23°C they are responsible for 40–55% of oxygen uptake, slightly more in *Amphitrite ornata* than in *Arenicola cristata* (*Figure 4.10*) or *A. marina* (Krüger, 1959; Mangum, 1976a). At low temperature this fraction is reduced but the role of these haemoglobins is still easily discerned. The major difference between the two groups is that the role of haemoglobin oxygen uptake begins to diminish at a higher PO_2 in arenicolids than in terebellids, a trend opposite to that predicted by the *in vitro* oxygen affinity (*Table 4.7*). The volume of blood appears to be greater in arenicolids, even on a weight specific basis (Toulmond, 1971; Mangum *et al*., 1975).

In vitro, however, these haemoglobins behave quite differently. Arenicolid haemoglobins have a very high oxygen affinity, well within the range of values exhibited by the intracellular haemoglobins. Oxygen equilibrium curves are strongly polyphasic, showing low to moderate subunit interactions at low oxygenation and great interaction at high oxygenation. The magnitude of the Bohr effect is relatively large. For many years these properties have been noted in contrast with the lower oxygen affinity and lower cooperativity of mammalian haemoglobins. Their physiological significance lies less in the oxygen conditions of the microhabitat, which are not very low, than in the patterns of flow in the circulatory system. Oxygenated and deoxygenated blood is highly mixed in the major distribution channels of a lugworm, with the result that blood PO_2's are generally low and the PO_2 difference between post- and pre-branchial blood is very small. A pigment with a lower oxygen affinity or less cooperativity simply would not work very well in this primitive circulatory system (Mangum, 1976a, b).

Although the pH dependence of oxygen affinity is a widespread feature of oxygen carrying pigments, its adaptive significance to most animals has never been clear. The quantity $\Delta \log P_{50}/\Delta pH$ is a useful index in comparing *in vitro* properties, but it does not express the contribution of the phenomenon to oxygen transport. For purposes of physiological evaluation, the Bohr shift must be translated to terms that are relevant to aerobic respiration, such as the increment in $\dot{V}O_2$.

Traditionally the Bohr shift has been understood as an increase in deoxygenation of the pigment at the target organ, effected by the addition to the blood of CO_2. In arenicolids there is a consistent pH difference between post- and pre-branchial blood of about 0.1 (Mangum, 1976a), although the effective agent is not known. Toulmond (1970) and Wells (1973) found very little CO_2 in arenicolid blood. The Bohr shift, which is moderate in *A. cristata* ($\Delta\log P_{50}/\Delta pH = -0.3$ to -0.4), is responsible for about 13% of the oxygen transported by haemoglobin. This figure probably increases in *A. marina,* whose haemoglobin has a large Bohr shift ($\Delta\log P_{50}/\Delta pH = -0.9$), but it cannot be estimated because blood PO_2's are incompletely known (Mangum, 1976a).

There is another reason why a large Bohr shift might be important to an animal that lives in an unstable ionic environment. A reduction in the salt concentration of the medium from 35 to 18‰ (equivalent to the lower limit of salinity tolerance of many arenicolids) causes an equal change in the salt level of body fluids; these worms are osmotic conformers (Oglesby, 1973). The reduction of blood salt lowers oxygen affinity from about 4 to 8.5 mm Hg and increases cooperativity from about 3.2 to about 3.8 at pH 7 and 20°C (Everaarts and Weber, 1974). The shift in P_{50} might not seriously impair oxygenation at the gills, because of the concomitant change in n, but it might result in a loss of oxygen to the coelom as the blood moves through the branchial efferents, which are bathed by coelomic fluid. However, the reduction of salt in body fluids must also cause a reduction in the pool of intracellular free amino acids as intracellular fluids re-equilibrate with the dilute blood. While the response has not been investigated in arenicolids, approximately 40% of the salinity-induced changes in osmolality of nereid tissues are due to free amino acids (Freel, Medler and Clark, 1973; Mangum and Oglesby, in preparation). The free amino acid pool is believed to be kept low in some phyla by increased deamination at low salinity, thus resulting in an elevated ammonia level and concomitant increase in blood pH (Weiland and Mangum, 1975). *Because the changes in H^+ and salts occur simultaneously, and because their effects on P_{50} are opposite, the oxygen transport system remains largely in balance even though it functions in an unstable ionic environment.*

This balance has been termed enantiostatic rather than homeostatic, in that the standing condition results from opposing forces. We do not yet know whether it occurs in annelids; even though the excretion of ammonia increases at low salinity (Emerson, 1969), the level in the blood may remain unchanged. In crabs the excess ammonia appears to be eliminated by the gill rather than the excretory organ, and its output is linked to the salt pump that generates a hyperosmotic blood. As long as the salt pump is not activated, the level of ammonia in blood goes up and H^+ goes down, but ammonia output does not change; the rate of ammonia excretion increases only when the blood becomes hypersaline (Mangum *et al.,* 1976). The same pattern of ammonia output occurs in *Nereis succinea* (Oglesby and Mangum, in preparation). But in osmoconformers, in which NH_4^+ does not serve as a counter-ion in Na^+ uptake, the response of blood pH at low salinity would be difficult to predict. It would also be difficult to predict in species that do not utilise the free amino acid pool in low salinity adaptation to the degree found in many annelids and crustaceans.

In any event, the large salt effect on arenicolid haemoglobin may mean that its function changes in low salinities, or that the oxygen transport system may be stabilised by an enantiostatic balance of H^+ and salts.

The temperature sensitivity of arenicolid haemoglobins is more clearly adapted to its unstable habitat. The oxygen transport system of a thermal conformer is especially sensitive to environmental change, as illustrated by the following facts (*Figure 4.13*):

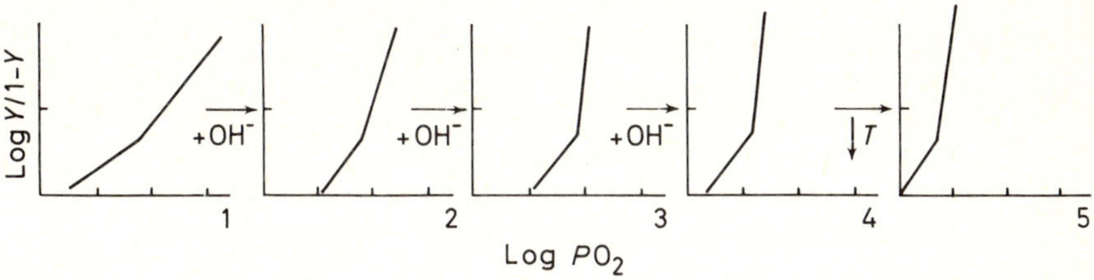

Figure 4.13 Effects of environmental variables on oxygen binding of annelid haemoglobins. Interaction of pH and temperature induced by temperature decrease. See text for explanation

1. The cooperativity of oxygen binding increases with pH (at least, within the physiological range).
2. The biphasic character of the oxygen equilibrium curve, or the ratio n_1:n_2, increases at high pH.
3. In many species blood pH increases at low temperature; H^+ activity is lowered.
4. Oxygen affinity of the respiratory pigment increases at low temperature; the heat of oxygenation (ΔH) is negative.

As a result of these four separate changes, other respiratory acclimations must occur to maintain the efficacy of the oxygen carrying pigment. Unless adaptation to low temperature involves compensations of circulation, ventilation or a qualitative change in the haemoglobin molecule itself (none of which are known), *a pigment which is well adjusted to its operating conditions at one season cannot remain so at other times of year.* If the carrier molecule is essential in maintaining the supply of oxygen to respiring tissue when metabolism is reduced in the cold, then any factor that minimises the temperature dependence of P_{50} and blood pH should be highly selected in the temperate zone.

The literature comparing the quantity ΔH for different species is difficult to evaluate because the thermally induced change in pH was almost certainly a tacit variable in the original experiments. If the solutions compared were studied in the same buffer, then at least the reported trends are correct though the magnitudes are not. If they were studied in a buffer that does not change very much with temperature, such as many widely used inorganic PO_4 systems, then the magnitudes are very nearly correct. However, studies of unbuffered blood or of haemoglobin extracts in most buffers include the concomitant effects of pH as well as temperature. *This criticism is pertinent to all of the studies of thermal effects cited in this chapter unless otherwise emphasised.* It is also pertinent to studies not mentioned here, unless the authors state explicitly that pH was measured *at* the experimental temperature (the pH of concentrated protein solutions cannot be accurately predicted or even measured by many types of electrodes) with an electrode designed for use with blood.

The data for arenicolids clearly indicate reductions of the temperature dependence of oxygen affinity (Weber, 1972; Weber and Mangum, in preparation) and blood pH (Mangum, 1973; Wells, 1974; Weber and Mangum, in preparation). ΔH for the haemoglobin of the subtidal Mediterranean species *Abarenicola claparedi,* whose habitat undergoes small changes in temperature, is slightly higher (−15.9 kcal/mole) than the values for many mammalian haemoglobins (*see above*). The values of ΔH for the eurythermal species *A. cristata* and *A. marina,* however, are only −6.6 and −5.3 kcal/mole respectively, even when the temperature dependence of pH is considered. Perhaps even more interesting (though inexplicable) is the reduced temperature sensitivity of blood pH. ΔpH/°C is 0.012 for *A. cristata* blood and 0.013 for *A. marina.* In glycerids, reduced temperature sensitivity of coelomic fluid pH is clearly not an inherent property of the fluid — it can be abolished by the appropriate experiment (Mangum, 1973). However, this property is intrinsic to arenicolid blood — it occurs *in vitro* as well as *in vivo,* and it seems to be effected by the haemoglobin molecule itself.

In contrast to arenicolids, the haemoglobins extracted from terebellid bloods have moderate to low oxygen affinities (*Table 4.7*). Phase heterogeneity of oxygen equilibrium curves is very small, as is cooperativity. *In vitro* oxygenation of the haemoglobin of *Amphitrite ornata* is unresponsive to pH changes from 5.81 to 7.97, to the addition of either organic phosphates or NaCl in physiological concentrations or to a small temperature change. Indeed, the only treatment that induces a significant change is a pH increase to unphysiological levels well in excess of the predicted *in vivo* condition at the coldest season, which has the effect of dissociating the molecule into its constituent subunits (*Figure 4.11*, insert). The absence of a significant change in P_{50} when the measurement temperature is lowered from 20 to 15°C may not mean thermal independence, but it does suggest that ΔH is small. In addition, measurements made in January, February and May on extracts of animals freshly collected at 8, 11 and 20°C are not different ($P > 0.05$), indicating that oxygen affinity does not acclimate to temperature change (Mangum *et al*., 1975).

In vivo the role of *A. ornata* haemoglobin is not diminished at 15°C, although its quantitative function does decline appreciably from more than 50 to about 20% of the oxygen consumed at 10°C. This pattern of diminished importance of the respiratory pigment at low temperature is fairly common in both annelids and sipunculids (Hoffmann and Mangum, 1970; Mangum and Kondon, 1975; Mangum *et al*., 1975). The opposite trend has been reported only for terrestrial annelids, where it is a somewhat surprising result because of a marked increase in oxygen affinity at low temperature; ΔH is −9.1 to −10.6 kcal/mole (Cosgrove and Schwartz, 1965). From an adaptive viewpoint this result is surprising, because one would not expect a *smaller* diffusion gradient between the air and the blood, or a higher blood PO_2 and consequent reduction in respiratory function, at low temperature. But again, our ignorance of circulation and *in vivo* operating conditions in earthworms limits the interpretation of these findings.

In *A. ornata* coelomic fluid PO_2 at low temperature is not known, but measurements of this parameter at 24°C reveal a very important relationship with P_{50}. Unlike *Arenicola cristata, mean coelomic fluid* PO_2 *in A. ornata exposed to oxygen levels that obtain in the microhabitat very nearly equals* P_{50} (*Table 4.2*). This finding means that blood flowing through the vessels, whose outer walls are only 1 cell thick and are bathed in coelomic fluid, delivers most of its oxygen to coelomic fluid; indeed this conclusion could almost be postulated on anatomical evidence of the paucity of capillaries in the vascular system.

Why the difference between the two families? Lugworms have a capacious coelomic cavity but for most of the year it carries few cells, none of which contain haemoglobin. In contrast, some 34% of the dry weight of an individual *Amphitrite ornata* consists of the cellular material circulating in its coelom. These cells include gametes as well as the intriguing red cells (*Figure 4.7*), which contain variable amounts of haemoglobin and undoubtedly have many other important functions (Dales, 1964). In other species of terebellids, the concentration of haemoglobin in coelomic cells is even higher. Unlike arenicolids, oxygen in the terebellids is transferred from the blood to coelomic haemoglobin, which has a much higher oxygen affinity than vascular haemoglobin (*Table 4.7*).

Physiologists and biochemists are fond of extrapolating from the molecule to the mudflat by categorising pertinent features of the habitat in terms of haemoglobin oxygen affinity. On this basis, arenicolid haemoglobin should be found in low oxygen habitats and terebellid haemoglobin in richer oxygen supplies. Actually, the reverse is close to the truth. Populations of lugworms reach their greatest densities in washed sediments with a larger particle size (Longbottom, 1970), and those of *Amphitrite ornata* in the finer sediments of more protected bottom. In this context, however, the truth is no more meaningful than the myth because both species ventilate their gills with fluid from the water column, which is well oxygenated.

More meaningful correlations of P_{50} can be made, first with microhabitat and then with body fluid PO_2, which are really reflections of the success of ventilation and gas exchange. At this level, the extrapolation begins to make sense. In a large container of sand kept under running seawater in the laboratory, *Amphitrite ornata maintains both a higher microhabitat and a higher coelomic fluid* PO_2 than *Arenicola cristata* (*Table 4.2*). The terebellids are vigorous ventilators of their tubes (*Table 4.1*); it would be interesting to know whether the particular design is worth the effort of a large increase in $\dot{V}O_2$ during the activity (Coyer and Mangum, 1973).

4.7.1.5 PARTICIPATION IN AEROBIC RESPIRATION

Alteration resulting in selective deprivation of function is a powerful experimental tool that has been little used in respiratory physiology, perhaps because of the acute awareness of physiologists that compensatory responses may mask primary effects.

The drug phenylhydrazine interferes with NADH reduction of

methaemoglobin in the vertebrate red cell, and its administration over a period of time induces haemolytic anaemia of such virulence that the red cells disappear from the blood (Cameron and Wohlschlag, 1969). Although it is not clear that the drug would interfere with the annelid red cell metabolism in the same way, the experiment might be useful in investigating the control of red cell proliferation and haemoglobin biosynthesis. In gauging the contribution of haemoglobin to respiratory function, however, it appears to be less useful than the classic carbon monoxide experiment. Like most drugs, the side effects of phenylhydrazine are only beginning to be known and the early reports do not elicit confidence in their simplicity. E. J. Boell (personal communication) finds that carbon monoxide blocking of a haemoglobin in the toad *Xenopus levis* causes no change in $\dot{V}O_2$ under normoxic conditions, whereas phenylhydrazine treatment elevates aerobic metabolism.

Careful controls can identify many pitfalls of the alternative experiment involving the use of carbon monoxide to block a functional haemoprotein. The possibility of overestimating pigment function due to CO poisoning of the cytochromes is a bit of a straw man (Mendes and Almeida, 1961), because the electron transport pigments have such a low affinity for the ligand (Seamonds *et al*., 1975). In our experience, CO poisoning of aerobic pathways has been detected only at partial pressures well below 10 mm Hg, which have rarely been included in experiments on intact animals.

The more likely artifact is underestimation of the haemoprotein contribution, due not only to compensatory responses. The use of an unnecessarily high CO concentration to induce COHb formation *in vivo,* which was common in the past, may result in an elevated rate of aerobic metabolism. Cytochromes have the ability to oxidise carbon monoxy compounds, a phenomenon that was discovered in insect tissues (Bodine and Boell, 1934) and is now known to occur in several annelid tissues (Johnson, 1942; Mangum and Carhart, 1972). The artifact can be avoided in most species by using an effective but appropriately low CO concentration. A soft bodied worm has no defence against the treatment other than circulatory shutdown, which apparently does not occur under the experimental conditions. Perhaps the most convincing tests of the experiment are the results from terebellid worms. Firstly, the effects of gill ligation cannot be statistically distinguished from those of CO blocking in *Amphitrite ornata,* indicating that oxygen transport by haemoglobin is effectively eliminated by both treatments and that the respiratory role of dissolved oxygen in the blood is small. Secondly, CO exposure causes a 25% reduction in VO_2 of *Enoplobranchus sanguineus,* which is graphically named, whereas it causes no change in the closely related species *Lysilla alba,* which has no haemoprotein (Mangum *et al*., 1975).

Since the experiment is usually performed on animals removed from their tubes so that the measured PO_2 is the same as that at the gill, a ventilatory compensation cannot occur. No control, however, can eliminate the possibility of an immediate compensation for the loss of a functional oxygen carrier by increased blood flow. This possibility has not been adequately investigated, although a delayed compensation of unknown nature was detected by Mangum *et al.* (1975). In teleost fish, an increase in cardiac output following phenylhydrazine induced anaemia is so great that it perfectly compensates for the loss of haemoglobin in oxygen transport (Cameron and Wohlschlag, 1969). While it seems intuitively unlikely that the primitive annelid system is capable of such responses, our knowledge of its adaptability is essentially non-existent.

An alternative experiment, designed to yield the same result, is commonly performed on large animals in which $\dot{V}O_2$ is virtually synonymous with the change in oxygen content of the blood after it returns from the tissues. Since almost all of the oxygen consumed in animals such as crabs and fish is taken up at the gill and transported to the mitochondria by blood, this figure provides an estimate of the role of the carrier molecule in aerobic respiration. In *Arenicola cristata,* which is big enough so that the measurement could be performed, haemoglobin carries more than 99% of the oxygen transported by blood (Mangum, 1967a). This figure grossly overestimates the importance of haemoglobin in aerobic respiration, however, because so much of the oxygen consumed enters directly into the cuticle and not into blood; the data in *Figure 4.10* are almost certain to be more nearly correct.

The absence of essential controls in the earliest CO experiments makes them difficult to evaluate, but results obtained more recently indicate that intracellular haemoglobin is responsible for some fraction between 20 (*Glycera dibranchiata*) and 42% (the terebellid *Enoplobranchus sanguineus*) of the oxygen consumed in water by aquatic polychaetes (Hoffmann and Mangum, 1970; Mangum *et al.*, 1975). Extracellular haemoglobin is responsible for 45 (*Arenicola cristata*) to 60% (*Nereis succinea*), and the presence of both forms for 50% of the oxygen consumed in water by *Amphitrite ornata* (Mangum *et al.*, 1975; Mangum, 1976a; C. Kendrick, unpublished data). In the bimodal oligochaete *Alma emini,* extracellular haemoglobin is responsible for about 38% of the oxygen consumed in air, and as much as 52% in water (Mangum, Lykkeboc and Johansen, 1975).

As Johnson (1942) very carefully showed, the high concentrations of CO used to block haemoglobin in the oligochaete *Lumbricus terrestris* cause elevation of $\dot{V}O_2$, and therefore the participation of haemoglobin is probably underestimated. Despite this reservation, depression of $\dot{V}O_2$ after exposure of various air breathing oligochaetes to high concentrations of CO ranges from 30 to 47% (Johnson, 1942; Mendes and Valente, 1953). The role of haemoglobin in the Achaeta is very poorly known; very high concentrations do not result in an overall change of aquatic oxygen consumption in two species but depress it by 18–25% in three others (Scheer, 1959). Unlike the results summarised above, this experiment was performed only on animals in air-saturated water. Using unspecified concentrations of CO, Wells and Dales (1975) found that the contribution of intracellular and extracellular haemoglobins in *Terebella lapidaria* to respiration in air is only 27%.

One must keep in mind the possibility that these figures may prove to be erroneously small, even when low (0.2–0.5 ml/l) concentrations of CO were used, owing to the occurrence of immediate circulatory adaptations. It is unlikely, however, that the magnitude of the error is very great. The geometry of an elongate vermiform animal means that it presents a large surface, which is either unvascularised or poorly vascularised, directly to the environment. Moreover, the magnitude of oxygen permeation from water into the cuticle must be considerably greater than that from blood into deep tissue, because the PO_2 gradient is so much larger. On *a priori* grounds alone, figures in the range 30–60% would be expected.

4.7.2 Haemerythrins

4.7.2.1 BIOSYNTHESIS

Nothing is known about the biosynthesis of haemerythrins. Sipunculids possess chloragogue tissue, which is believed to proliferate all types of coelomic cells including those with haemerythrin (Hyman, 1959). In magelonid polychaetes the blood cells are derived from the vessel walls (de Horne, 1949). Both situations are reminiscent of the role of annelid extravasal tissue in the biosynthesis of extracellular haemoproteins (*see* p. 231).

4.7.2.2. ULTRASTRUCTURE

Interpretation of the ultrastructure of sipunculid haemerythrins is more straightforward, probably because of its relative simplicity. Coelomic haemerythrins from *Phascolopsis* (= *Golfingia,* = *Phascolosoma*) *gouldi* have been studied by X-ray crystallography, and those of *Dendrostomum pyroides** by electron microscopy (North and Stubbs, 1974; J. Bonaventura *et al.,* in preparation). These molecules are conceived as a pair of tetragonal discs (50–70 Å diameter and 50 Å high), composed of spherical subunits (25–30 Å diameter). In the oxygenated state the four subunits of one member of the pair are superimposed upon the interstices of the other four, very much like the blastomeres of a spirally cleaving embryo. This arrangement permits maximal opportunity for subunit interaction, which can be detected in haemerythrin oxygenation although it is not very great. The effects of temperature on fine structure are not known, the electron micrographs were prepared with liquid nitrogen cooling.

4.7.2.3 PROTEIN STRUCTURE

Although few species have been examined, the primary structure of coelomic cell haemerythrin from sipunculids appears to be amazingly

*The specimens named *Dendrostomum pyroides* which are being supplied to investigators by a California company are mostly *D. zostericolum,* although some individuals may be *D. pyroides* (L. C. Oglesby, personal communication). Therefore differences in electrophoretic properties and amino acid compositions etc. may or may not reflect the interspecific divergence. Moreover, the haemerythrin studied by Manwell (1960b) is probably, but not certainly, the same as that studied by Klippenstein and co-workers and by Kitto and co-workers.

conservative. In most species, the native molecule, 108 + 10^3 daltons, is composed of eight identical subunits. Its amino acid composition is virtually identical in *Dendrostomum pyroides, Phascolopsis* (= *Golfingia* = *Phascolosoma*) *gouldi* and *Sipunculus nudus,* species which are as unlike as possible within this small and homogeneous phylum (Groskopf, *et al*., 1966; Klippenstein, Holleman and Klotz, 1968; Ferrell and Kitto, 1970). Moreover, the sequence of amino acids in *D. pyroides* and *P. gouldi* differs by only four of 113 residues (Klippenstein, Holleman and Klotz, 1968; Ferrell and Kitto, 1970). Interestingly, the primary structure of brachiopod haemerythrin does reflect the phyletic separation (Joshi and Sullivan, 1973). Coelomic haemerythrin from the Pacific sipunculid *Phascolosoma agassizi,* whose ultrastructure has not been described, is a trimeric molecule with a molecular weight of 40 + 10^3 and with three distinct subunits (Liberatore, Truby and Klippenstein, 1974). The properties of the forms separated by electrophoresis have not been correlated with those prepared by Manwell (1959), who reported two distinct oxygen affinities (*Table 4.8*).

In addition to the coelomic cell molecules, haemerythrin also occurs as a monomer in the proboscis retractor muscle and as a second, chemically distinct octamer in cells circulating in tubes running the length of the digestive tract and into anterior tentacles, which can be extruded into the water column. The tentacular system appears to be completely separate from the coelom, but older observations suggest that stained cells somehow find their way from one circulatory system into another (Hyman, 1959). If these observations are correct, the finding of distinct amino acid compositions is even more surprising. Ironically, the total amino acid composition indicates that coelomic, tentacular and myohaemerythrin within a species differ more from one another than does coelomic haemerythrin of separate species (Klippenstein, Van Riper and Oosterom, 1972).

4.7.2.4 OXYGEN BINDING AND RELEASE

The oxygen binding properties of haemerythrin extracts are fairly homogeneous within a phylum, but those of annelid haemerythrins are quite different from sipunculid haemerythrins, at least when they are in the cell (*Table 4.8*). Extracts of sipunculid coelomic cells at 20–25°C have a moderately high oxygen affinity and they usually show a very small degree of subunit interaction (*Table 4.8*). The exception is the North American Pacific coast species *Phascolosoma agassizi,* whose trimeric haemerythrin has a low oxygen affinity. Characteristically, these pigments are not affected by changes in pH, but P_{50} is very sensitive to temperature. *This generalisation is true even when the effects of temperature are considered separately from the thermally induced change in pH* (Mangum and Kondon, 1975). ΔH for haemerythrins is larger than that for haemoglobins and undoubtedly is of greater physiological importance. Consequently, this quantity and not $\Delta \log P_{50}/\Delta pH$ is given in *Table 4.8*. The effects of salts and various organic compounds have not been reported.

The thermal sensitivity of coelomic cell haemerythrin is so great that the

Table 4.8 OXYGENATION PROPERTIES OF HAEMERYTHRINS FROM ANNELIDS AND SIPUNCULIDS

Species	P_{50} (mm Hg)	*n*	*Temperature* (°C)	ΔH (kcal/mole)	*Source*
A. EXTRACTS					
Sipunculida					
Dendrostomum pyroides					
coelomic	4–5	0.99–1.10	25		Ferrell and Kitto (1970)
D. zostericolum					
coelomic	3.5	1.1	20		Manwell (1960b)
tentacular	15.0	1.2–1.3	20		
Phascolopsis gouldi					
coelomic	2.76	1.35	20		Kubo (1953)
	4	1.2	25	−17	Manwell (1959)
	5.0	1.4	25		De Phillips (1971)
	0.98	1.02	15		Mangum and Kondon (1975)
	3.07	0.92	22		
Phascolosoma agassazi					
coelomic	4		25		Manwell (1959)
	12		25		
Siphonosoma ingens					
coelomic	1.8	1	18.5		Manwell (1960a)
tentacular	1.0	1	18.5		
Sipunculus nudus					
coelomic	1.8		10		Bates *et al.* (1968)
	3.5	1.15	20	−13.5	
	8.0		29		

B. CELLS					
Annelida					
Magelona papillicornis	6.2	1.0	15		Wells and Dales (1974)
M. alleni	3.6		15		Wells and Dales (1974)
Sipunculida					
Dendrostomum zostericolum					
coelomic	4.5		20	−20	Manwell (1960a)
tentacular	40.0		20		
Golfingia elongata					
coelomic	4.0	1.2	15		Wells and Dales (1974)
Phascolopsis gouldi					
coelomic	1.36	(1) 3.35 (2) 1.26	10	−16.2	Mangum and Kondon (1975)
	1.88	1.17	15		
	5.17	(1) 3.20 (2) 1.38	23		

substance may very well function effectively in temperate zone animals for only a few warm months. In *Phasolopsis gouldi,* for example, the fit of microhabitat PO_2, coelomic fluid PO_2 and P_{50} is fairly good at 23°C (*Table 4.2*). The animal's ventilation activities, details of which are unknown, generate partial pressures averaging 77–81 mm Hg in the head shaft of the burrow. When the animal is exposed to these external PO_2's, coelomic fluid PO_2 is 6.5–7.5 mm Hg; P_{50} is 5.2 mm Hg. The effect of low temperature on ventilation could not be studied in the running seawater of our summer laboratory at Woods Hole. However, the change in temperature is unlikely to depress the activities of this cold temperate zone species so much that microhabitat partial pressures are *lower* at 10°C, which is the annual average for the latitude. Low temperature is far more likely to result in the same or somewhat *higher* oxygen levels in the burrow. This supposition is supported by the finding of little if any difference in the volume of fluid moved by *Phascolion strombi* when the temperature is varied between 15 and 22.5°C (Kristensen, 1969), although acclimated measurements may yield a different result. When *P. gouldi* is exposed to partial pressures higher than 68 mm Hg at 10°C, coelomic fluid PO_2 is 9 mm Hg and higher; P_{50} at 10°C is only 1.9 mm Hg and the haemerythrin is fully oxygenated at 15 mm Hg. Coelomic haemerythrin in sipunculids is probably a warm weather adaptation.

Unlike coelomic cell haemoglobins, the oxygen affinity of haemerythrin in intact cells is consistently lower than that of extracts, although the latter measurements were performed in the absence of salts (*Table 4.8*). Whether this result implicates the effect of specific cofactors in oxygen binding, or whether it reflects some other feature of the intracellular environment is not yet known. The concentration of ortho-phosphate in sipunculid coelomic cells is 0.2 μmoles/kg H_2O (Foster, 1974), much lower than the typical level in vertebrate erythrocytes.

The curve describing oxygen release by respiring coelomic cells is not linearised by the Hill transformation (*Figure 4.7*), just as those for haemoglobin-containing cells. The phase change may be even more complex here, although available procedures of data analysis separate only two phases at $P = 0.05$ (*Table 4.8*). In these animals the adaptive significance of the phenomenon is even clearer, although its explanation is equally obscure. As shown in *Figure 4.7,* a change in coelomic fluid PO_2 equal to that measured when animals are equilibrated to the mean burrow PO_2, induces the uptake or release of *four times* as much oxygen because haemerythrin occurs in cells. The change in total oxygen concentration of coelomic fluid *in vivo* with PO_2 is equally resistant to linearisation. Both in cells and in the intact animal the change in oxygenation is somehow enhanced at higher partial pressures, corresponding to those *in vivo* when ventilation is unimpaired at high tide (Mangum and Kondon, 1975).

Little is known about tentacular haemerythrin other than Manwell's (1960b) interesting insights into its oxygen transfer function. Indeed, the role of the tentacles in gas exchange is not clear in many sipunculids. They are small and their circulatory system is not very extensive. In *P. gouldi* the tentacles remain retracted within the animal at all except the lowest partial pressures, and we never saw them protruded from the burrow. However, the relationship of oxygen affinities of the two haemerythrins in *Dendrostomum zostericolum* (Manwell, 1960b) suggests that oxygen is transferred from the tentacles, which are extruded into the water column, to coelomic fluid.

The oxygen binding properties of annelid haemerythrins are known only from the recent work of Wells and Dales (1975) on the blood of the tiny magelonid polychaetes. In intact cells, their oxygen affinity is quite low even at 15°C, which approximates summer temperature in the habitat (*Table 4.8*). The finding of a low oxygen affinity pigment in a small animal is not surprising and it is consistent with the casual observations I once made on an undescribed species of *Magelona** collected from Hadley Harbor in Massachusetts. When several dozen worms were left in a bowl under a gentle stream of running seawater, the blood of these highly transparent animals appeared quite pink, characteristic of oxyhaemerythrin. Within 15–30 min of turning off the water, all traces of pink colouration had disappeared. The same experiment performed on the sipunculid *P. gouldi* requires 10–12 h for completion of the colour change, despite the animal's much larger size and thicker body wall. There is little doubt that annelid haemerythrin is readily oxygenated and deoxygenated *in vivo*.

4.7.2.5 PARTICIPATION IN AEROBIC RESPIRATION

The quantitative importance of haemerythrin, which does not combine with carbon monoxide, is not known. In the sipunculid worm *Phascolopsis gouldi* its *in vitro* properties are beautifully matched to *in vivo* operating conditions at 23°C, but they are so greatly modified by low temperature that the substance may be essentially a fair weather friend (*Table 4.2*). The volume of oxygen bound to haemerythrin in cells plus that dissolved in circulating coelomic fluid is 56 μl, which is a volume sufficient to supply the $\dot{V}O_2$ of a 5 g animal for approximately 30 min; this period is surely longer than the time required for the completion of circulation. Haemerythrin could supply 100% of the oxygen consumed by the animal, if its efficacy were not limited by convection. Almost certainly it plays a smaller role; most of the oxygen consumed must enter directly into respiring tissue without first crossing into coelomic fluid, since so much of the epithelial surface is contiguous with ambient rather than coelomic fluid (Mangum and Van Winkle, 1973). The actual contribution of haemerythrin is likely to remain a mystery in the immediate future.

The storage value of coelomic haemerythrin may be even greater than that of most coelomic haemoglobins. Predictions from first order kinetics suggest that the oxygen in coelomic fluid of *P. gouldi* can sustain measured $\dot{V}O_2$ for a period of about 2¼ h at 23°C and low PO_2 (Mangum and Kondon, 1975). When the prediction was recently tested by measuring the depletion of oxygen in coelomic fluid at a slightly lower temperature (20°C), the storage period observed was somewhat smaller but the agreement is fairly good (*Figure 4.14*).

*Which, according to Meredith L. Jones, will soon be transferred to the new genus *Maea*.

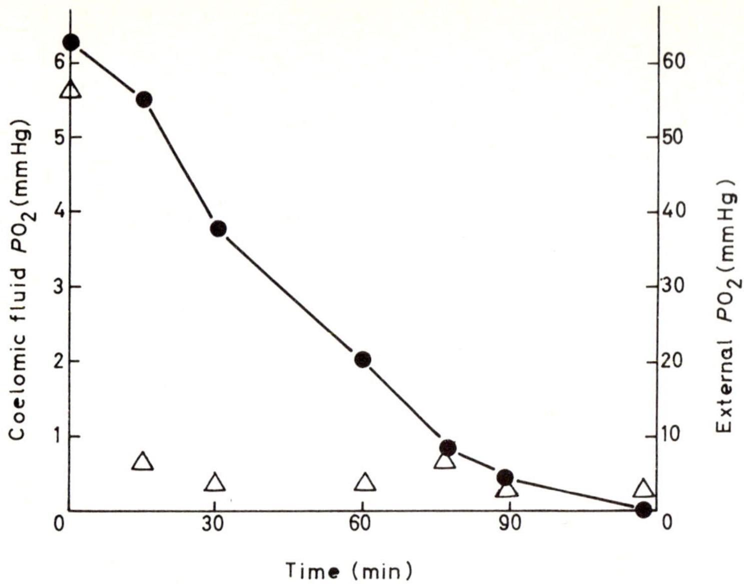

Figure 4.14 The decrease in coelomic fluid PO_2 (closed circles) when Phascolopsis gouldi *is transferred from water with a PO_2 approximating that in the burrow (68 mm Hg) to low oxygen (open triangles) water. Traces of oxyhaemerythrin disappeared only at time of final measurement (2 h). Temperature 21.5°C*

4.7.3 Velocity of ligand combination

Quite apart from oxygenation properties and their *in vivo* counterparts, there is a body of data which has been virtually ignored by comparative physiologists although it may prove to be useful in understanding haemoglobin function. These data derive from measurements of the kinetics of ligand combination, and the most interesting experiment in the present context is the time course of oxygen uptake or release by the respiratory pigments in the intact red cell. The measurement of oxygen uptake is made by placing a deoxygenated cell suspension in an atmosphere of oxygen, and that of oxygen release by placing an oxygenated suspension of red cells in an atmosphere of nitrogen.

The process of oxygen uptake involves the chemical reaction of haemoglobin and oxygen, and therefore it can be expressed by the constant of an equation describing a second order reaction:

$$\frac{d(HbO_2)}{dt} = k'_c \text{ (Hb) } (O_2)$$

where (HbO_2) is the molar concentration of oxyhaemoglobin, (Hb) is the molar concentration of deoxyhaemoglobin and (O_2) is the molar concentration of oxygen. Since K'_c is a time constant and since the reaction is very fast, it is usually assigned units of $M^{-1}s^{-1}$ ($\times 10^{-3}$). In the language of kineticists, the symbol (′) distinguishes the constant for 'oxygen on' from that for the 'oxygen off' reaction, designated k_c, and the subscript (c) distinguishes values for cell oxygen uptake or release from the analogous constants for haemoglobin extracts, designated k' and k. Because it is a less formidable experiment that yields information of pertinence to conformational changes of the molecule during the process of combination with ligands, the reaction with carbon monoxide is sometimes performed instead of that with oxygen. In those cases the constant is designated l, and it obviously has less physiological meaning *per se* although it may be quite useful for comparative purposes.

A summary of kinetic measurements made to date on annelid and sipunculid respiratory pigments is given in *Table 4.9*. Although the values are dependent upon both experimental temperature and pH, these conditions were omitted from *Table 4.9* because they are not essential to the present discussion. The information is available in the original sources, and the values of the constants are not as variable as they might appear from the ranges given in *Table 4.9*.

Velocity constants for the large extracellular proteins are quite variable,

Table 4.9 VELOCITY CONSTANTS FOR REACTIONS OF ANNELID HAEMOPROTEINS AND SIPUNCULID HAEMERYTHRINS WITH LIGANDS. TEMPERATURE AND PH GIVEN IN ORIGINAL SOURCE

A. COMBINATION OF HAEMOPROTEIN EXTRACTS WITH CARBON MONOXIDE

Species	l' ($M^{-1}s^{-1}$)	*Source*
Amphitrite ornata (cellular)	7.5×10^5	Weber *et al.* (1976)
Arenicola marina	0.29–0.46	Gibson (1955)
Cirriformia sp.[1]	0.21–1.30	Weichelman and Parkhurst (1973)
earthworm	0.22–0.41	Gibson (1955)
Enoplobranchus sanguineus	6×10^5	Weber *et al.* (1976)
Glycera dibranchiata		
monomers	1) $2.5–4.0 \times 10^7$ 2) $2.6–4.5 \times 10^7$	Seamonds *et al.* (1975)
Lumbricus terrestris	0.06–0.09	Weichelman and Parkhurst (1972)
Nephtys[2]	0.4	Gibson (1959)
Spirographis spallanzani	0.06–0.10	Brunori *et al.* (1965)

B. COMBINATION OF HAEMOPROTEIN EXTRACTS WITH OXYGEN

Species	k' ($M^{-1}s^{-1}$)	*Source*
Amphitrite ornata	3×10^7	Weber *et al.* (1976)
Arenicola marina	23×10^5	Gibson (1955)
Cirriformia sp.[1]	$220–570 \times 10^5$	Weichelman and Parkhurst (1973)
earthworm	23×10^5	Gibson (1955)
Enoplobranchus sanguineus	4.4×10^7	Weber *et al.* (1976)
Glycera dibranchiata		
monomers	1) 1800×10^5 2) 4100×10^5	Seamonds *et al.* (1975)

Table 4.9 *continued*

C. DISSOCIATION OF OXYHAEMOPROTEIN EXTRACTS

Species	*k* (s^{-1})	*Source*
Arenicola marina	19–30	Gibson (1955)
Amphitrite ornata (cellular)	150	Weber *et al.* (1976)
Cirriformia sp.	2.7–100	Weichelman and Parkhurst (1973)
earthworm	10–30	Gibson (1955)
Enoplobranchus sanguineus	110	Weber *et al.* (1976)
Glycera dibranchiata		
monomers	⩾13.8	Seamonds and Forster (1972)
polymers	⩾2.2	
Lumbricus terrestris	*c.* 1–13	Chiancone *et al.* (1972)
	32–42	Weichelman and Parkhurst (1972)
Spirographis spallanzani	6.5–20	Brunori *et al.* (1965)

D. COMBINATION OF HAEMOGLOBIN IN CELLS WITH OXYGEN AND CARBON MONOXIDE

Species	k'_c ($M^{-1}s^{-1}$)	l'_c ($M^{-1}s^{-1}$)	*Source*
Glycera dibranchiata	2.55×10^{-3}	2.20×10^{-3}	Seamonds and Forster (1972)

E. DISSOCIATION OF OXYHAEMERYTHRIN EXTRACTS

Species	*k* (s^{-1})	*Source*
Phascolopsis gouldi	2.27	Kung (1971)
Sipunculus nudus	67–74	Bates *et al.* (1968)

[1] *See* footnote on p. 244
[2] Probably *Nephtys hombergi*

and they seem to be correlated with oxygen affinity, although the correlation is not exact. Interpretation of the data is severely limited by our ignorance of circulatory dynamics; it will be interesting to learn whether the process of oxygen uptake by these molecules *in vivo* is affected by their reaction rates.

The most intriguing result presently available is the value of k'_c for red cells of the bloodworm *Glycera dibranchiata* (*Table 4.9D*). When kinetic constants are used to predict the requisite period for complete oxygenation of the haemoglobin in a mammalian red cell, the result is less than 1 s even when the partial pressure difference across the cell membrane is only 40 mm Hg and when the disc-like red cell is deformed to twice its average thickness (Moll, 1968). In order to generate comparable predictions for bloodworm red cells we must have one critical item of information that is lacking, viz. the intracellular haemoglobin content. Because bloodworm haematocrit is typically 59% and coelomic haemoglobin concentration 23.6% of that in human blood (Hoffmann and Mangum, 1970), the figure of 8 mM (=40% of that in the mammalian erythrocyte) is probably adequate for the present purpose. Whether we divide 8 mM by k'_c and thus predicate the oxygenation time on the experimental conditions of the stopped-flow apparatus, or whether we use the more abstruse calculus of finite differences (Moll, 1968), which entails a second uneducated guess of the average thickness of the bloodworm disc, is immaterial. The outcome of these predictions is that the *complete oxygenation of a bloodworm red cell is measured in a minimum of several seconds and possibly more than ten.*

The movement of red cells through the gas exchange organ of most annelids gives the general impression of a rather leisurely passage, certainly exceeding 10s in the terebellid *Enoplobranchus sanguineus* (Mangum *et al*., 1975). However, the movement of a cell through the simple gill of *Glycera dibranchiata* or the branched gill of *G. americana* requires 1–6 s, depending upon the location of the particular gill. In order to make the photograph in *Figure 4.6,* I was forced to wait several hours after isolating the parapodium; immediately afterwards I was unable to capture even the tracks of individual cells with an exposure of a few seconds. Moreover, when the body wall is opened and the paths of the red cells observed, they appear to course through only one gill and then to enter a local vortex in coelomic fluid, in which they travel laterally rather than anteriorly or posteriorly before returning to the gill — they do not follow the metameric pattern by moving repeatedly through the hundreds of sequential gills before delivering their oxygen on target. Therefore, *the rate of red cell oxygenation may be a factor that limits the animal's respiratory gas exchange.*

The smallest values of k in *Table 4.9c* predict that deoxygenation of the extracellular haemoproteins requires a maximum of about 1 s, as opposed to 0.02 s for human haemoglobin. This period is probably not limiting unless flow rates in the vascular system are a lot greater than believed to be. For example, the period between contractions of the major blood vessels of *Spirographis spallanzani* is 2–10 s (Ewer, 1941); the decay of the pulse pressure head is not known, but the observation suggests that one molecule remains in one place more than long enough to deliver its oxygen. The velocity constant may prove to be important in understanding why there are so few capillaries in deep tissue, however, where the flow would be expected to increase. It is at least conceivable that the deoxygenation process may be too slow.

4.8 SUMMARY

When annelid worms penetrated the soft bottom of the sea, metazoan animals encountered low oxygen conditions for the first time. The result of this exploitation of a new habitat was the introduction of most of the significant respiratory adaptations found in the animal kingdom. They include:

1. Ventilation, or the active movement of fluid across sites of gas exchange with the external environment. The ventilatory rhythm was generated by a pacemaker, with little sensory input from the outside controlling its timing. An on–off switch sensitive to environmental

variables was incorporated to prevent fruitless energy expenditure at low tide, but precise reflex control of the rhythm was a later refinement made by members of other phyla. The primary mechanisms of fluid convection were muscular, and their energetic cost was very great. As a result, substances with low gas permeability were evolved to line the burrow and to reduce the loss of oxygen to the surrounding sand.

2. The gill, an outward growth of the body wall which was not enclosed in a chamber because it was already protected by the burrow. The blood vessels inside were not separated into afferent and efferent channels. Consequently, gill branching entailed increased mixing of oxygenated and deoxygenated blood; its evolution was accompanied by the development of spontaneous contractility of the gill, which periodically emptied its contents into the internal vessels. The gill became the feeding organ in a few families, where it was ventilated extravagantly.
3. The closed circulatory system. Prior to the origin of the gill, it consisted in part of superficial capillaries which served as sites of gas exchange with the external rather than the internal milieu. After the gill was invented, they became far less important.
4. The heart, whose original function was to drive fluid through the blind ending gill.
5. The red cell, which is metabolically active and whose major functions were:
   (a) To control the production of respiratory pigment.
   (b) To permit refinements of respiratory pigment function. It was abandoned when the vascular system arose, possibly to reduce the circulatory workload of the primitive pump.
6. Three respiratory pigments. Chlorocruorin was a minor variation on extracellular haemoglobin, but it may have evolved to lower the oxygen affinity in response to the acquisition of a nutritive function by the gill, which was ventilated more profusely than the earlier haemoglobin containing gills. Haemerythrin, a more adventurous experiment, may have arisen to facilitate gas exchange in warm waters. Unlike chlorocruorin, however, it did not confer advantages which were beyond the capabilities of haemoglobin in one of its many forms; it was retained by only a few phyla. Both cellular and extracellular haemoglobins were able to function throughout the wide range of oxygen levels experienced in the soft bottom, but the quantitative participation of the extracellular substance in oxygen transport was much greater. The enhancement, however, was due more to convection efficacy in a vascular system than to an intrinsic feature of the molecule. Release of the molecule from the cell resulted in relaxation of biosynthetic control, and diminution of the oxygen storage function, which had been an important role of coelomic cell haemoglobin. The evolution of subunit heterogeneity, which accompanied release from the cell, permitted even greater refinements of the oxygen transport function than achieved within the red cell. In addition to the enhanced quantitative function accompanying increased convection, the extracellular haemoproteins acquired ion

sensitivity. As a result of H^+ dependence, the extraction of oxygen from the ventilatory stream may have increased in the highly developed gills of a few families.

4.9 GLOSSARY

branchial crown – a highly developed feeding and respiratory organ found on the anterior ends of members of the polychaete families Sabellidae and Serpulidae.

haemochromagen – ferrous iron metalloporphyrin with denatured or otherwise altered protein moiety.

infauna, epifauna – the animals living below and above, respectively, the water-substratum interface.

isoelectric focusing – the separation of proteins according to their isoelectric points in a combined density and pH gradient system.

mesohaem – iron metalloporphyrin with the following sequence of side chains on the four pyrrole rings: (1) methyl, (2) ethyl, (3) methyl, (4) ethyl, (5) methyl, (6) propionic, (7) propionic and (8) methyl (*see Figure 4.9*).

metanephridium – an excretory organ which opens to coelomic fluid by a funnel, although it is separated by a cell layer from the vascular system.

microhabitat, microenvironment – that portion of the habitat or environment of immediate physiological or ecological pertinence to the animal. The microhabitat of infaunal annelids is the tube or burrow.

protohaem – iron metalloporphyrin with the following sequence of side chains on the four pyrrole rings : (1) methyl, (2) vinyl, (3) methyl, (4) vinyl, (5) methyl, (6) propionic, (7) propionic and (8) methyl (*see Figure 4.9*).

protomer – the smallest peptide subunit of a respiratory pigment (in the present context) that exhibits the oxygen binding properties of the intact molecule.

protonephridium – an excretory organ consisting of one to several closed tubes whose lumen is separated by a cell layer from the body fluids.

SDS gel (sodium dodecyl sulphate polyacrylamide gel) – an esterified buffer support medium used in the separation of proteins and their subunits according to (in the present context) size.

$\dot{V}O_2$–the weight and time specific uptake of oxygen by an animal, a tissue, a cell or an organelle.

water column – a theoretical section of a natural body of water from the air –water interface to the water –substratum interface.

REFERENCES

ALLEN, D. W. and WYMAN, J. (1952). 'The oxygen equilibrium of hemerythrin of *Arenicola cristata*', *J. cell. comp. Physiol.*, **39**, 383–389

ALLISON, A. C. (1965). 'Properties of sickle cell hemoglobin, *Biochem. J.* **65**, 212–219

ANDREWS, J. D. (1973). 'Effects of tropical storm Agnes on epifaunal invertebrates in Virginia estuaries', *Ches. Sci.,* **14,** 223–234

ANTONINI, E., ROSSI-FANELLI, A. and CAPUTO, A. (1962a). 'Studies on chlorocruorin. I. The oxygen equilibrium of *Spirographis* chlorocruorin', *Arch. Biochem. Biophys.,* **97,** 336–342

ANTONINI, E., ROSSI-FANELLI, A. and CAPUTO, A. (1962b). 'Studies on chlorocruorin. II. Some physico-chemical properties of *Spirographis* chlorocruorin', *Arch. Biochem. Biophys.,* **97,** 343–350

BATES, G., BRUNORI, M., AMICONI, G., ANTONINI, G. and WYMAN, J. (1968). 'Studies on hemerythrin. I. Thermodynamic and kinetic aspects of oxygen binding', *Biochem.,* **7,** 3016–3020

BEADLE, L. C. (1957). 'Respiration in the African swampworm *Alma emini* Mich', *J. Exp. Biol.,* **34,** 1–10

BEN-SHAUL, Y. (1974). 'Electron microscopy of earthworm erythrocruorin', *J. mol. Biol.,* **87,** 101

BESSIS, M. (1962). 'L'hémosiderine et les mouvements du fer dans l'organisme', *Mouv. Rev. Francaise d'Hématol.,* **2,** 153–158

BESSIS, M. and BRETON-GORIUS, J. (1960). 'Aspects de la molécule de ferritine et d'apoferritine au microscope électronique', *C. r. Soc. Biol.,* **250,** 1360–1362

BODINE, J. H. and BOELL, E. J. (1934). 'Carbon monoxide and respiration. Action of carbon monoxide on respiration of normal and blocked embryonic cells. (Orthoptera)', *J. cell. comp. Physiol.,* **4,** 475–482

BONAVENTURA, J. and KITTO, G. B. (1973). 'Ligand-linked dissociation of some invertebrate hemoglobins', 493–507. In: *Comparative Physiology.* Eds. L. Bolis, K. Schmidt-Nielsen and S. H. P. Maddrell. North-Holland Publishing Company

BRETON-GORIUS, J. (1963). 'Étude au microscope électronique des cellules chloragogène d'*Arenicola marina* L. Leur role dans la synthèse de l'hémoglobine'. Doctoral dissertation, Universite de Paris, Masson et Cie. Paris

BRUGGEN, L. VAN and WEBER, R. E. (1974). 'Erythrocruorin with anomalous quaternary structure from the polychaete *Oenone fulgida', Biochim. Biophys. Acta,* **359,** 210–214

BRUNORI, M., GUERRITORE, D., ANTONINI, E., WYMAN, J. and ROSSI-FANELLI, A. (1965). 'Studia della clorocruorina. IV. Osservazioni sulla cinetica delle reazione della clorocruorina de *Spirographis spallanzanii* con i gas', *Publ. Staz. Napoli,* **34,** 521–527

CAMERON, J. N. and WOHLSCHLAG, D. E. (1969). 'Respiratory response to experimentally induced anaemia in the pinfish (*Lagodon rhomboides*)', *J. exp. Biol.,* **50,** 307–318

CHAPMAN, G. (1967). *The body fluids and their functions.* St. Martin's Press, New York, 70 pp

CAREY, F. G. and TEAL, J. M. (1965). 'Responses of oxygen electrodes to variables in construction, assembly and use', *J. appl. Physiol.,* **20,** 1074–1077

CARRITT, D. E. and KANWISHER, J. W. (1959). 'An electrode system for measuring dissolved oxygen', *Analyt. Chem.,* **31,** 5–9

CHAINCONE, E., VECCHINI, P., ROSARIA ROSSI-FANELLI, M. and ANTONINI, E. (1972). 'Studies on erythrocruorin. II. Dissociation of earthworm erythrocruorin', *J. mol. Biol.,* **70,** 73–84

CHEW, M. Y., SCOTT, P. B., OLIVER, I. T. and LUGG, J. W. H. (1965). 'Erythrocruorin of *Marphysa sanguinea*: isolation and some physical, physico-chemical and other properties', *Biochem. J.,* **94,** 378–383

CLARK, M. E. (1964). 'Biochemical studies on the coelomic fluid of *Nephtys hombergi* (Polychaeta: Nephtyidae), with observations on changes during different physiological states', *Biol. Bull.,* **127,** 63–84

CLARK, R. B. (1964). *Dynamics in Metazoan Evolution: the origin of the coelom and segments.* Clarendon Press, Oxford, 313 pp

CLARK, R. B. (1969). 'Systematics and physiology: Annelida, Echiura, Sipunculida', 1–68. In: *Chemical Zoology,* **5.** Eds. M. Florkin and B. T. Scheer. Academic Press, New York

COKELET, G. R. and MEISELMAN, H. J. (1968). 'Rheological comparisons of hemoglobin solutions and erythrocyte suspensions', *Science,* **162,** 275–276

COLMAN, C. H. and LONGMUIR, I. S. (1963). 'A new method for registration of oxyhemoglobin dissociation curves', *J. appl. Physiol.,* **18,** 420–423

COSGROVE, W. B. and SCHWARTZ, J. B. (1965). 'The properties and function of the blood pigment of the earthworm *Lumbricus terrestris', Physiol. Zool.,* **38,** 206–212

COWDEN, R. R. (1966). 'A cytochemical study of the nucleated, hemoglobin-containing erythrocytes of *Glycera americana', Trans. Am. micro. Soc.,* **85,** 45–53

COYER, P. E. and MANGUM, C. P. (1973). 'Effects of temperature on active and resting metabolism in polychaetes', 173–180. In: *Effects of Temperature on Ectothermic Organisms*. Ed. W. Wieser. Springer-Verlag, Heidelberg

DALES, R. P. (1957). 'Some quantitative aspects of feeding in serpulid fan worms', *J. mar. biol. Assoc. U.K.*, **36**, 309–316

DALES, R. P. (1961a). 'Observations on the respiration of the sabellid polychaete *Schizobranchia insignis*', *Biol. Bull.*, **121**, 82–91

DALES, R. P. (1961b). 'Oxygen uptake and irrigation of the burrow by three terebellid polychaetes', *Physiol. Zool.*, **34**, 306–311

DALES, R. P. (1963). *Annelids*. Hutchinson University Library, London. 200 pp

DALES, R. P. (1964). 'The coelomocytes of the terebellid polychaete *Amphitrite johnstoni*', *Q. J. micr. Sci.*, **105**, 263–279

DALES, R. P. (1969). 'Respiration and energy metabolism in annelids', 93–109. In: *Chemical Zoology* **4.** Eds. M. Florkin and B. T. Scheer. Academic Press, New York

DALES, R. P., MANGUM, C. P. and TICHY, J. C. (1970). 'Effects of changes in oxygen and carbon dioxide concentration on ventilation rhythms in onuphid polychaetes', *J. mar. biol. Assoc. U.K.*, **50**, 365–380

DALES, R. P. and PELL, J. S. (1970). 'Cytological aspects of haemoglobin and chlorocruorin synthesis in polychaete annelids', *Z. Zellforsch.* **109**, 20–32

DAM, L. VAN (1938). 'On the utilisation of oxygen and the regulation of breathing in some aquatic animals'. Doctoral dissertation, University of Groningen. 143 pp

DAVID, M. M. and DANIEL, E. (1973). 'Expression of cooperative oxygen binding at subunit level in earthworm erythrocruorin', *FEBS Lett.*, **32**, 293–295

DAVID, M. M. and DANIEL, E. (1974). 'Subunit structure of earthworm erythrocruorin', *J. mol. Biol.*, **87**, 89–101

DE HORNE, A. (1949). 'Le probleme des corpuscles du sang vasculaire de *Magelona papillicornis* F. Muller', *Arch. Zool. exp. gen.*, **86**, 41–49

DELKESKAMP, E. (1964). 'Über den porphyrinstoffwechsel bei *Lumbricus terrestris L.*' '*Zeitschr. vergl. Physiol.*, **48**, 400–412

DEPHILLIPS, H. A. (1971). 'Oxygen binding of haemerythrin', *Arch. Biochem. Biophys.*, **144**, 122–126

ECONOMIDES, A. P. and WELLS, R. M. G. (1975). 'The respiratory function of the blood of *Neanthes* (=*Nereis*) *virens* (sars) (Polychaeta: Nereidae)', *Comp. Biochem. Physiol.*, **51A**, 219–224

EMERSON, D. N. (1969). 'Influence of salinity on ammonia excretion rates and tissue constituents of euryhaline invertebrates', *Comp. Biochem. Physiol.*, **29**, 1115–1134

EVERAARTS, J. M. and WEBER, R. E. (1974). 'Effects of inorganic anions and cations on oxygen-binding of haemoglobin from *Arenicola marina* (Polychaeta)', *Comp. Biochem. Physiol.*, **48A**, 507–520

EWER, D. W. (1941). 'The blood systems of *Sabella* and *Spirographis*', *Q. J. micr. Sci.*, **82**, 587–620

EWER, R. F. and FOX, H. M. (1940). 'On the function of chlorocruorin', *Proc. roy. Soc. London B.*, **129**, 137–153

FAUVEL, P. (1959). 'Classe des annélides polychètes', 1–196. In: *Traité* de Zoologie, **5**, Ed. P. P. Grassé. Masson et Cie. Paris

FERRELL, R. E. and KITTO, G. B. (1970). 'Structural studies on *Dendrostomum pyroides* hemerythrin', *Biochem.*, **10**, 2923–2929

FOLKOW, B. and NEIL, E. (1971). *Circulation*. Oxford University Press, London. 593 pp

FOSTER, R. C. (1974). 'Comparative biochemical studies of osmoregulation in *Sipuncula*. I. Steady state characteristics of two sipunculids in full strength seawater', *Comp. Biochem. Physiol.*, **47A**, 855–866

FOX, H. M. (1937). 'On the blood circulation and metabolism of sabellids', *Proc. roy. Soc. Lond. B.*, **125**, 554–569

FOX, H. M. (1945). 'The oxygen affinities of certain invertebrate haemoglobins', *J. exp. Biol.*, **21**, 161–165

FOX, H. M. (1955). 'The effect of oxygen on the concentration of haem in invertebrates', *Proc. roy. Soc. Lond. B.*, **143**, 203–214

FOX, H. M. and VEVERS, G. (1960). *The Nature of Animal Colours*. Sidgwick & Jackson Ltd., London. 246 pp

FREADMAN, M. A. and MANGUM, C. P. (1976). 'Oxygenation of cellular haemoglobin in the arcid clam *Noetia ponderosa*', *Comp. Biochem. Physiol.* **53A,** 173–179

FREEL, R. W., MEDLER, S. G. and CLARK, M. E. (1973). 'Solute adjustments in the coelomic fluid and muscle fibers of a euryhaline, polychaete, *Neanthes succinea,* adapted to various salinities, *Biol. Bull.,* **144,** 289–303

FYHN, H., PETERSEN, J. A. and JOHANSEN, K. (1972). 'Eco-physiological studies of an intertidal crustacean, *Pollicipes polymerus* (Cirripedia, Lepadomorpha)', *J. exp. Biol.,* **57,** 83–102

GARLICK, R. L. and TERWILLIGER, R. C. (1974). 'Coelomic cell haemoglobin of the terebellid polychaete, *Thelepus crispus* Johnson. Structure and oxygen equilibrium', *Comp. Biochem. Physiol.,* **47A,** 543–554

GASKELL, J. F. (1914). 'The chromaffine system of annelids and the relation of this system to the contractile vascular system in the leech *Hirudo medicinalis*', *Phil. Trans. roy. Soc. B.,* **205,** 153–169

GASKELL, J. F. (1919). 'Adrenalin in annelids', *J. gen. Physiol.,* **2,** 73–85

GEORGE, J. D. (1964). 'Organic matter available to the polychaete *Cirriformia tentaculata* (Montagu) living in an intertidal mud flat', *Limnol. Oceanogr.,* **9,** 453–455

GIBSON, Q. H. (1955). 'Some observations on the reactions of two annelid haemoglobins with oxygen and with carbon monoxide', *Proc. roy. Soc. Lond. B.,* **143,** 334–342

GIBSON, Q. H. (1959). 'The kinetics of reactions between haemoglobin and gases, 2–51. In: *Progress in Biophysics and Biophysical Chemistry,* **9.** Eds. J. A. V. Butler and B. Katz. Pergamon Press, New York

GREEN, H. D. (1944). 'Circulation: physical principles'. In: *Medical Physics.* Ed. O. Glasser. Year Book Publ. Co., New York

GROSKOPF, W., HOLLEMAN, J. W., MARGOLIASH, E. and KLOTZ, I. M. (1966). 'Amino acid composition and terminal sequences of *Golfingia gouldi* hemerythrin', *Biochem.,* **5,** 3779–3782, 3783–3796

GUERRITORE, D., BONACCI, M. L., BRUNORI, M., ANTONINI, E., WYMAN, J. and ROSSI-FANELLI, A. (1965). 'Studies on chlorocruorin. III. Electron microscope observations on *Spirographis* chlorocruorin', *J. mol. Biol.,* **13,** 234–237

GUERRITORE, D. and ZITO, R. (1971). 'The terminal groups of chlorocruorin', *Biochim, Biophys. Acta,* **229,** 720–723

HALL, V. E. (1931). 'The muscular activity and oxygen consumption of *Urechis caupo*', *Biol. Bull.,* **61,** 400–415

HARTMAN, O. (1959). 'Catalogue of the polychaetous annelids of the world', *Allan Hancock Found. Occas. Pap.,* No. 23. 628 pp

HARTMAN, O. (1965). 'Supplement 1960–65 and index', *Allan Hancock Found. Occas. Pap.,* No. 23. 197 pp

HAUGHTON, T. M., KERKUT, G. A. and MUNDAY, K. A. (1958). 'The oxygen dissociation and alkaline denaturation of haemoglobin from two species of earthworm', *J. exp. Biol.,* **35,** 360–368

HOBSON, K. D. (1967). 'The feeding and ecology of two North Pacific *Abarenicola* species (Arenicolidae, Polychaeta)', *Biol. Bull.,* **133,** 343–354

HOCHACHKA, P. W. and SOMERO, G. N. (1973). *Strategies of Biochemical Adaptation.* W. B. Saunders Co., Philadelphia. 358 pp

HOFFMANN, R. J. and MANGUM, C. P. (1970). 'The function of coelomic cell hemoglobin in the polychaete *Glycera dibranchiata*', *Comp. Biochem. Physiol.,* **36,** 211–228

HYMAN, L. H. (1959). *The Invertebrata,* **5.** McGraw-Hill Book Co., New York. 783 pp

IMAMURA, T., BALDWIN, T. O. and RIGGS, A. (1972). 'The amino acid sequence of the monomeric hemoglobin component from the bloodworm *Glycera dibranchiata*', *J. Biol. Chem.,* **247,** 2785–2797

JACOBSEN, V. H. (1967). 'The feeding of the lugworm *Arenicola marina* (L.): Quantitative studies', *Ophelia,* **4,** 91–109

JEUNIAUX, C., DUCHATEAU, G. and FLORKIN, M. (1961). 'Variation de la composante amino-acide des tissus et euryhalinité chez *Perinereis cultrifera* Gr. et *Nereis diversicolor* (O. F. Müller)', *J. Biochem.* (*Tokyo*), **49,** 527–531

JOHANSEN, K. and LENFANT, C. (1976). 'Gas exchange in the Cephalopod, *Octopus dofleini*', *Am. J. Physiol.,* **210,** 910–918

JOHANSEN, K., LENFANT, C. and MECKLENBERG, T. A. (1970). 'Respiration in the crab *Cancer magister*', *Zeitschr. Vergl. Physiol.,* **70,** 1–19

JOHANSEN, K. and MARTIN, A. W. (1965). 'Circulation in the giant earthworm *Glossoscolex giganteus*. I. Contractile processes and pressure gradients in the large blood vessels', *J. exp. Biol.*, **43**, 333–347

JOHANSEN, K. and MARTIN, A. W. (1966). 'Circulation in the giant earthworm *Glossoscolex giganteus*. II. Respiratory properties of the blood and some patterns of gas exchange', *J. exp. Biol.*, **45**, 162–172

JOHANSEN, K. and PETERSEN, J. A. (1971). 'Gas exchange and active ventilation in a starfish, *Pteraster tesselatus*', *Zeitsch. vergl. Physiol.* **71**, 365–381

JOHANSEN, K. and VADAS, R. L. (1967). 'Oxygen uptake and responses to respiratory stress in sea-urchins', *Biol. Bull.*, **132**, 16–22

JOHNSON, M. L. (1942). 'The respiratory function of the haemoglobin of the earthworm', *J. exp. Biol.*, **18**, 266–277

JONES, J. D. (1963). 'The functions of the respiratory pigments in invertebrates', 11–89. In: *Problems in Biology*. Ed. G. Kerkut. Macmillan & Co., New York

JONES, M. L. (1968). 'On the morphology, feeding and behaviour of *Magelona* sp.', *Biol. Bull.*, **134**, 272–297

JOSHI, J. G. and SULLIVAN, B. (1973). 'Isolation and preliminary characterization of hemerythrin from *Lingula unguis*', *Comp. Biochem. Physiol.*, **44B**, 857–867

KAPPAS, A. and GRANICK, S. (1968). 'Steroid induction of porphyrin synthesis in liver cell culture. II. The effects of heme, uridine diphosphate, glucuronic acid and inhibitors of nucleic acid and protein synthesis in the induction process', *J. biol. Chem.*, **243**, 346–351

KENNEDY, G. Y. (1970). 'Harderoporphyrin: a new porphyrin from the Harderian glands of the rat', *Comp. Biochem. Physiol.*, **36**, 21–36

KENNEDY, G. Y. and DALES, R. P. (1958). 'The function of the heart body in polychaetes', *J. mar. biol. Assoc. U.K.*, **37**, 15–31

KENNEDY, G. Y. and DALES, R. P. (1968). 'Formation of uroporphyrin from porphobilinogen by the heart-body in polychaetes', *J. mar. biol. Assoc. U.K.*, **48**, 77–79

KERMACK, D. (1955). 'The anatomy and physiology of the gut of the polychaete *Arenicola marina* (L.)', *Proc. zool. Soc. Lond.*, **125**, 347–381

KLIPPENSTEIN, G. L., HOLLEMAN, J. W. and KLOTZ, I. M. (1968). 'The primary structure of *Golfingia gouldi* hemerythrin. Order of peptides in fragments produced by tryptic digestion of succinylated hemerythrin. Complete amino acid sequence', *Biochem.*, **7**, 3868–3878

KLIPPENSTEIN, G. L., VAN RIPER, D. A. and OOSTEROM, E. A. (1972). 'A comparative study of the oxygen transport proteins of *Dendrostomum pyroides*', *J. biol. Chem.*, **247**, 5959–5963

KLUVER, H. (1944). 'On naturally occurring porphyrins in the central nervous system', *Science*, **99**, 482–484

KRIEBL, M. E. (1968). 'Pacemaker properties of tunicate heart cells', *Biol. Bull.*, **135**, 166–173

KRISTENSEN, J. N. (1969). 'Irrigation in the sipunculid *Phascolion strombi* (Mont.)', *Ophelia*, **7**, 101–112

KRÜGER, F. (1959). 'Zur Wirkungsweise der Hämoglobins Versuche an *Arenicola*', *Verhandl. Deut. Zool. Ges. Münster.*, pp 348–351

KRÜGER, F. (1964). 'Messungen der Pumptatigkeit von *Arenicola marina* L. im Watt', *Helgol. Wiss. Meeresunters*, **1**, 70–91

KUBO, M. (1953). 'The oxygen equilibrium of hemerythrin and the Bohr effect', *Bull. Chem. Soc. Japan*, **26**, 189–192

KUNG, H. Y. (1971). 'Kinetic studies on haemerythrin', M.S. Thesis, University of Nebraska, Lincoln, Nebraska

KUSHINS, L. J. and MANGUM, C. P. (1971). 'Responses to low oxygen conditions in two species of the mud snail *Nassarius*', *Comp. Biochem. Physiol.*, **39A**, 421–435

LANKESTER, E. R. (1872). 'A contribution to the knowledge of haemoglobin', *Proc. roy. Soc.*, **21**, 70–81

LEVINE, O. (1963). 'Electron microscope observations on some 60S erythrocruorins and their split products', *J. mol. Biol.*, **6**, 95–101

LIBERATORE, F. A., TRUBY, M. F. and KLIPPENSTEIN, G. L. (1974). 'The quaternary structure of *Phascolosoma agassizii* coelomic hemerythrin', *Arch. Biochem. Biophys.*, **160**, 223–229

LINDROTH, A. (1938). 'Studien über die respiratorischen Mechanismen von *Nereis virens* Sars', *Zool. Bidr. Uppsala*, **17**, 396–497

LONGBOTTOM, M. R. (1970). 'The distribution of *Arenicola marina* (L) with particular reference to the effects of particle size and organic matter of the sediments', *J. exp. mar. Biol. Ecol.*, **5,** 138–157

MACRAE, E. K. and BOGORAD, L. (1958). 'Conversion of δ-aminolaevulinic acid to porphobilinogen by earthworms', *Anat. Rec.,* **131,** 577–578

MANGUM, C. P. (1962a). 'Source of dichromatism in two maldanid polychaetes', *Nature,* **195,** 198–199

MANGUM, C. P. (1962b). 'Environmental origin of mesobiliverdin in two maldanid polychaetes', *Am. Zool.,* **2,** 428

MANGUM, C. P. (1963). 'Studies on speciation in maldanid polychaetes of the North American Atlantic coast. III. Intraspecific and interspecific divergence in oxygen consumption', *Comp. Biochem. Physiol.,* **10,** 335–349

MANGUM, C. P. (1964). 'Activity patterns in metabolism and ecology of polychaetes', *Comp. Biochem. Physiol.,* **11,** 239–250

MANGUM, C. P. (1970). 'Respiratory physiology in annelids', *Am. Scient.,* **58,** 641–647

MANGUM, C. P. (1972). 'Temperature sensitivity of metabolism in offshore and intertidal onuphid polychaetes', *Mar. Biol.,* **17,** 108–114

MANGUM, C. P. (1973). 'Evaluation of the functional properties of invertebrate hemoglobins', *Neth. J. Sea Res.,* **7,** 303–315

MANGUM, C. P. (1967a). 'The oxygenation of hemoglobin in lugworms', *Physiol. Zool.,* **49** (In the press)

MANGUM, C. P. (1976b). 'Annelid hemoglobins: a dichotomy in structure and function'. Contribution to Olga Hartman Memorial Volume. Eds D. J. Reish and K. Fauchald, Allan Hancock Foundation Publ. Univ. So. Calif. Press., Los Angeles. (In the press)

MANGUM, C. P. (1976c). 'The analysis of oxygen uptake and transport in different kinds of animals (In preparation)

MANGUM, C. P., BOOTH, C. E., DEFUR, P. L., HECKEL, N., HENRY, R. P., OGLESBY, L. C. and POLITES, G. (1976b). 'The ionic environment of hemocyanin in *Limulus polyphemus,' Biol. Bull.* **150** (In the press)

MANGUM, C. P. and BURNETT, L. E. (1975). 'The extraction of oxygen by estuarine invertebrates', pp 147–163. In: *Ecophysiology of Estuarine Organisms.* Ed. F. J. Vernberg. Univ. South Carolina Press, Columbia, S.C.

MANGUM, C. P. and CARHART, J. A. (1972). 'Oxygen equilibrium of coelomic cell hemoglobin from the bloodworm *Glycera dibranchiata', Comp. Biochem. Physiol.,* **43A,** 949–958

MANGUM, C. P. and COX, C. D. (1971). 'Analysis of the feeding response to chemical stimulation in the onuphid polychaete *Diopatra cuprea* (Bosc)', *Biol. Bull.,* **140,** 215–229

MANGUM, C. P. and DALES, R. P. (1965). 'Products of haem synthesis in polychaetes', *Comp. Biochem. Physiol.,* **15,** 237–257

MANGUM, C. P. and JOHANSEN, K. (1975). 'The colloid osmotic pressure of body fluids of aquatic invertebrates', *J. exp. Biol.,* **63,** 661–671

MANGUM, C. P. and KONDON, M. (1975). 'The role of coelomic cell hemerythrin in the sipunculid worm *Phascolopsis gouldi', Comp. Biochem. Physiol.,* **50A,** 777–786

MANGUM, C. P., LYKKEBOE, G. and JOHANSEN, K. (1975). 'Oxygen uptake and the role of hemoglobin in the East African swampworm *Alma emini', Comp. Biochem. Physiol.,* **52A,** 477–482

MANGUM, C. P. and SASSAMAN, C. (1969). 'Temperature sensitivity of active and resting metabolism in a polychaetous annelid', *Comp. Biochem. Physiol.,* **30,** 111–116

MANGUM, C. P., SANTOS, S. L. and RHODES, W. R. (1968). 'Distribution and feeding in the onuphid polychaete *Diopatra cuprea* (Bosc.)', *Mar. Biol.,* **2,** 33–40

MANGUM, C. P., SILVERTHORN, S. U., HARRIS, J. L., TOWLE, D. W. and KRALL, A. R., (1976a). 'The relationship between blood pH, ammonia excretion and adaptation to low salinity in the blue crab, *Callinectes sapidus', J. Exp. Zool.,* **195,** 129–136

MANGUM, C. P. and WINKLE, W. VAN (1973). 'Responses of aquatic invertebrates to declining oxygen conditions', *Am. Zool.,* **13,** 529–541

MANGUM, C. P., WOODIN, B. R., BONAVENTURA, C., SULLIVAN, B. and BONAVENTURA, J. (1975). 'The role of coelomic and vascular hemoglobin in the annelid family Terebellidae', *Comp. Biochem. Physiol.,* **51A,** 281–294

MANWELL, C. (1959). 'Alkaline denaturation and oxygen equilibrium of annelid hemoglobins', *J. cell. comp. Physiol.,* **53,** 61–74

MANWELL, C. (1960a). 'Histological specificity of respiratory pigments. I. Comparisons of the coleom and muscle hemoglobins of the polychaete worm *Travisia pupa* and the echiuroid worm *Arhynchite pugettensis', Comp. Biochem. Physiol,* **1,** 267–276

MANWELL, C. (1960b). 'Histological specificity of respiratory pigments. II. Oxygen transfer systems involving hemerythrins in sipunculid worms of different ecologies', *Comp. Biochem. Physiol,* **1,** 277–285

MANWELL, C. (1963). 'The blood proteins of cyclostomes: a study in phylogenetic ontogenetic biochemistry', 372–455. In: *The Biology of Myxine.* Eds. A. Brodal and R. Fangë). Norwegian Government Press, Oslo

MANWELL, C. (1964). 'Chemistry, genetics and function of invertebrate respiratory pigments — configurational changes and allosteric effects', 49–119. In: *Oxygen in the Animal Organism.* Eds. F. Dickens and E. Neil. Pergamon Press, Oxford

MARSDEN, J. R. (1966). 'The coelomocytes of *Hermodice carunculate* (Polychaeta: Amphinomidae) in relation to digestion and excretion', *Can. J. Zool.,* **44,** 377–389

MCDONALD, D. A. (1952). 'The occurrence of turbulent flow in the rabbit aorta', *J. Physiol.,* **118,** 340–347

MENDES, E. G. and ALMEIDA, A. M. DE (1961). 'Carbon monoxide and oxygen uptake by the tissue: a study in the earthworm', *Bol. Fac. Cienc. Sao Paulo,* **25,** 489–499

MENDES, E. G. and NONATO, E. F. (1957). 'The respiratory metabolism of tropical earthworms. II. Studies on the cutaneous respiration', *Univ. Sao Paulo Fac. de Filos. Ciencas e Letras Bol.,* **223,** Zool. (21), 153–166

MENDES, E. G. and VALENTE, D. (1953). 'The respiratory metabolism of tropical earthworms', *Bol. Univ. Sao Paulo,* **18,** 91–102

MICHEL, C. (1970). 'Etude histophysiologique de la trompe d'annélides polychètes appartenant aux genres: *Eulalia, Phyllodoce, Glycera, Notomastus', Cah. Biol. Mar.,* **11,** 209–228

MIZUKAMI, H. and VINOGRADOV, S. N. (1973). 'Oxygen association equilibria of *Glycera* hemoglobins', *Biochem. Biophys. Acta,* **285,** 314–319

MOLL, W. (1968). 'The influence of hemoglobin diffusion on oxygen uptake and release by red cells', *Resp. Physiol.,* **6,** 1–15

MURPHY, J. R. (1967). 'The influence of pH and temperature on some physical properties of normal erythrocytes from patients with hereditary sherocytosis', *J. lab. clin. Med.,* **69,** 758–775

NICOLL, P. A. (1954). 'The anatomy and behavior of the vascular systems in *Nereis virens* and *Nereis limbata', Biol. Bull.,* **106,** 69–82

NORTH, A. C. T. and STUBBS, G. T. (1974). 'Crystallography of hemerythrin', *J. mol. Biol.,* **88,** 125–131

OGLESBY, L. C. (1969). 'Inorganic components and metabolism, ionic and osmotic regulation; Annelida, Sipunculida and Echiura', 211–310. In: *Chemical Zoology* **4.** Eds. M. Florkin and B. T. Scheer. Academic Press, New York.

OGLESBY, L. C. (1973). 'Salt and water balance in lugworms (Polychaeta: Arenicolidae) with particular reference to *Abarenicola pacifica* in Coos Bay, Oregon', *Biol. Bull.,* **145,** 180–199

PADLAN, E. A. and LOVE, W. E. (1968). 'Structure of the hemoglobin of the marine annelid worm *Glycera dibranchiata* at 5.5 Å resolution', *Nature,* **220,** 376–378

PARKER, G. H. (1923). 'Are there Rouget cells on the blood vessels of invertebrates?', *Anat. Rec.,* **26,** 303–305

PASSANO, L. M. (1963). 'Primitive nervous systems', *Proc. Nat. Acad. Sci.,* **50,** 306–313

PAUTARD, F. G. E. and ZOLA, H. (1967). 'Studies on onuphic acid. III. Principal structural features', *Carbohydr. Res.,* **4,** 78–81

PETERSEN, J. A. and JOHANSEN, K. (1967). 'Aspects of oxygen uptake in *Mesochaetopterus taylori,* a tube-dwelling polychaete', *Biol. Bull.,* **33,** 600–605

PHEAR, E. A. (1955). 'Gut haems in the invertebrates', *Proc. zool. Soc. Lond.,* **125,** 383–406

PILGRIM, M. (1966). 'The anatomy and histology of the blood system of the maldanid polychaetes *Clymenella torquata* and *Euclymene oerstedii', Proc. zool. Soc. Lond.,* **149,** 242-261

PROSSER, C. L. (1950). 'The electrocardiogram of *Arenicola', Biol. Bull.,* **48,** 254–257

PROSSER, C. L. and ZIMMERMAN, G. L. (1943). 'Effects of drugs on the hearts of *Arenicola* and *Lumbricus', Physiol. Zool.,* **16,** 77–83

RAPHAËL, C. (1933). 'Etude au trompe des glycères de le son organe excréteur d'hémoglobine', *Trav. Stat. Biol. Roscoff.,* **11,** 5–17

RAPS, M. E. and REISH, D. J. (1971). 'The effects of varying dissolved oxygen concentrations on the hemoglobin levels of the polychaetous annelid *Neanthes arenaceodentata', Mar. Biol.,* **11,** 363–368

REDFIELD, A. and FLORKIN, M. (1931). 'The respiratory function of the blood of *Urechis caupo*', *Biol. Bull.*, **61**, 185–210

REISH, D. J. (1955). 'The relationship of polychaetous annelids to harbor pollution', *Publ. Health Rept.*, **70** (12), 1168–1174

ROCHE, J. (1965). 'Electron microscope studies on high molecular weight erythrocruorins (invertebrate hemoglobins) and chlorocruorins of annelids', 62–80. In: *Studies in Comparative Biochemistry*. Ed. K. Munday. Pergamon Press, Oxford

ROCHE, J., BESSIS, M. and THIERY, J-P. (1960). 'Étude de l'hémoglobine plasmatique de quelques annélides au microscope électronique', *Biophys. Biochim Acta*, **41**, 182–184

ROCHE, J. and COMBETTE, R. (1937). 'Recherches sur l'erythrocruorines (hémoglobines d'invertébrés)', *Bull. Soc. Chem. Biol.*, **19**, 613–626

ROCHE, J., WURMSER, S., FINE, J. M. and AUTRAN, R. (1963). 'Nouvelles recherches sur l'hémoglobine (erythrocruorine) d'*Arenicola marina* L', *C. r. Soc. Biol.*, **157**, 1919–1921

ROSSI-FANELLI, M. R., CHIANCONE, E., VECCHINI, P. and ANTONINI, E. (1970). 'Studies on erythrocruorin. I. Physico-chemical properties of earthworm erythrocruorin', *Arch. Biochem. Biophys.*, **141**, 278–283

RUUD, J. T. (1954). 'Vertebrates, without erythrocytes and blood pigments', *Nature*, **173**, 848–853

SANDERS, H. L., HESSLER, R. R. and HAMPSON, G. R. (1965). 'An introduction to the study of deep-sea benthic faunal assemblages along the bay head Bermuda transect', *Deep-Sea Res.*, **12**, 845–867

SASSAMAN, C. and MANGUM, C. P. (1974). 'Gas exchange in a cerianthid', *J. exp. Zool.*, **188**, 299–306

SCHEER, M. (1959). 'Untersuchungen zur vergleichenden Stoffwechselphysiologie einheimischer Süsswasseregel (Hirudinea)', *Zeitschr. Vergl. Physiol.*, **42**, 20–42

SCHELER, W. (1960). 'Lichtabsorption and sauerstoffbindskurve des Häemoglobins von *Tubifex tubifex*', *Biochem. Zeitschr.*, **332**, 366–375

SCHELER, W. and SCHNEIDERAT, L. (1959). 'Über die Präparation und die Bestimmung des Molekular-gewichtes wie der Konzentration des Hämoglobins von *Tubifex tubifex*', *Acta Biol. Med. Germ.* **3**, 588–597

SCHMIDT-NIELSEN, K. and TAYLOR, C. R. (1968). 'Red blood cells: why or why not?', *Science*, **162**, 274–275

SEAMONDS, B. and FORSTER, R. E. (1972). 'Ligand equilibrium and kinetic characteristics of *Glycera dibranchiata* hemoglobins', *Am. J. Physiol.*, **223**, 734–738

SEAMONDS, B., FORSTER, R. E. and GEORGE, P. (1971). 'Physico-chemical properties of the hemoglobin from the common bloodworm *Glycera dibranchiata*', *J. biol. Chem.*, **246**, 5391–5397

SEAMONDS, B., FORSTER, R. E. and GOTTLIEB, A. J. (1971). 'Heterogeneity of the hemoglobin from the common bloodworm *Glycera dibranchiata*', *J. biol. Chem.*, **246**, 1700-1705

SEAMONDS, B., MCCRAY, J.A., PARKHURST, L. J. and SMITH, P. D. (1975). 'Oxygen and carbon monoxide kinetics of *Glycera dibranchiata* monomeric hemoglobin'. (In preparation)

SEAMONDS, B. and SCHUMACHER, H. R. (1972). 'Fine structure of erythrocytes of the common bloodworm *Glycera dibranchiata*', *Cytologia*, **37**, 359–363

SHAFIE, S. M., VINOGRADOV, S. N., LARSON, L. and MCCORMICK, J. J. (1976). 'RNA and protein synthesis in the nucleated erythrocytes of *Glycera dibranchiata*', *Comp. Biochem. Physiol.* **53B**, 85–88

SHLOM, J. M., AMESSE, L. and VINOGRADOV, S. N. (1975). 'Subunits of *Placobdella* hemoglobin', *Comp. Biochem. Physiol.*, **51B**, 389–392

SHLOM, J. and VINOGRADOV, S. N. (1973). 'A study of the subunit structure of the extracellular hemoglobin of *Lumbricus terrestris*', *J. biol. Chem.*, **248**, 7904–7912

SIMON, J. L. (1965). 'Feeding in the annelid *Eteone heteropoda*', *Q. J. Fla. Acad. Sci.*, **28**, 370–372

SIMONS, J. A. and BOELL, E. J. (1971). 'Normal and induced synthesis of δ-amino-levulinic acid synthetase in developing chick liver', *J. exp. Zool.*, **178**, 287–292

SKAER, H. LE B. (1974). 'The water balance of a serpulid polychaete *Mercierella enigmatica* (Fauvel). III. Accessibility of the extracellular compartment and related studies', *J. exp. Biol.*, **60**, 339–349

SLACK, K. V. (1971). 'Average dissolved oxygen measurement and water purity significance', *J. Water Poll. Control Fed.*, **43**, 433–446

SNYDER, G. K. (1973). 'Erythrocyte evolution: the significance of the Fahraeus-Lindqvist phenomenon', *Resp. Physiol.*, **19,** 271–278

SPIES, R. B. (1973). 'The blood system of the flabelligerid polychaete *Flabelliderma commensalis* (Moore)', *J. Morph.*, **139,** 465–490

STEEN, J. B. (1971). *Comparative Physiology of Respiratory Mechanisms.* Academic Press, London. 182 pp

STEPHENSON, J. (1930). *The Oligochaeta.* Clarendon Press; Oxford

SULLIVAN, B., BONAVENTURA, J. and BONAVENTURA, C. (1974). 'Functional differences in the multiple hemocyanins of the horseshoe crab *Limulus polyphemus* L.', *Proc. Nat. Acad. Sci.*, **71,** 2558–2562

SVEDBERG, T. (1933). 'Sedimentation constants, molecular weights and isoelectric points of the respiratory proteins', *J. biol. Chem.*, **103,** 311–325

SVEDBERG, T. and ERIKSSON-QUENSEL, I-B (1934a). 'The molecular weight of erythrocruorin. I.' *J. Am. Chem. Soc.*, **55,** 2834–2841

SVEDBERG, T. and ERIKSSON-QUENSEL, I-B (1934b). 'The molecular weight of erythrocruorin. II.', *J. Am. Chem. Soc.*, **56,** 1700–1706

SWANEY, J. B. and KLOTZ, I. M. (1971). 'Properties of erythrocruorin from *Cirraformia grandis*', *Arch. Biochem. Biophys.*, **147,** 475–486

TALBOT, L. and BERGER, S. A. (1974). 'Fluid-mechanical aspects of the human circulation', *Am. Scient.*, **62,** 671–682

TAYLOR, G. (1952). 'Analysis of the swimming of long and narrow annelids', *Proc. Roy. Soc. Lond.*, **A214,** 158–183

TERWILLIGER, R. C. (1974). 'Oxygen equilibria of the vascular and coelomic hemoglobins of the terebellid polychaete *Pista pacifica.* Evidence for an oxygen transfer system', *Comp. Biochem. Physiol.*, **48A,** 745–755

TERWILLIGER, R. C., GARLICK, R. L., TERWILLIGER, N. B. and BLAIR, D. P. (1975). 'Molecular weight of *Eudistylia vancouveri* chlorocruorin and its subunits', *Biochim Biophys. Acta,* **400,** 302–309

TERWILLIGER, R. C., GARLICK, R. L. and TERWILLIGER, N. B. (1976). 'Hemoglobins of *Glycera robusta:* structures of coelomic cell hemoglobin and body wall myoglobin', *Comp. Biochem. Physiol.* (In the press)

TERWILLIGER, R. C. and KOPPENHEFFER, T. L. (1973). 'Coelomic cell hemoglobins of the polychaete annelid, *Pista pacifica* Berkeley', *Comp. Biochem. Physiol.*, **45B,** 557–566

TERWILLIGER, R. C. and TERWILLIGER, N. B. (1975). 'Quaternary structures of annelid chlorocruorin and polymeric hemoglobins', *Am. Zool.*, **15,** 807

TERWILLIGER, R. C., TERWILLIGER, N. B. and ROXBY, R. (1975). 'Quaternary structure of *Pista pacifica* vascular hemoglobin', *Comp. Biochem. Physiol.*, **50B,** 225–232

THOMAS, J. G. (1940). *'Pomatoceros, Sabella* and *Amphitrite', LMBC Memoirs,* **33.** University of Liverpool Press, Liverpool. 88 pp

TOULMOND, A. (1970). 'Le fixation du dioxyde de carbone par le sang chez l'arénicole (*Arenicola marina* L., annélide, polychète)', *C. r. Acad. Sci. Paris* **270:** 1487–1490

TOULMOND, A. (1971). 'Détermination du volume des compartiments coelomique et circulatoire chez l'arénicole *Arenicola marina* (L.). Annélide polychaète', *C. r. Acad. Sci. Paris,* **272,** 257–260

TOULMOND, A. (1973). 'Time-related changes of blood respiratory variables in the lugworm *Arenicola marina* (L.)', *Resp. Physiol.*, **19,** 130–144

TRUCHOT, J-P (1973). 'Fixation et transport de l'oxygène par le sang de *Carcinus maenas:* variations en rapport avec diverse conditions de température et de la salinité', *Neth. J. Sea Res.*, **7,** 482–495

VINOGRADOV, S. N., HALL, B. C. and SHLOM, J. M. (1976). 'A primitive heme binding chain and subunit hemology in invertebrate hemoglobins', *Comp. Biochem. Physiol.* **53B,** 89–92

VINOGRADOV, S. N., MACHLIK, C. A. and CHAO, L. L. (1970). 'The intracellular hemoglobins of a polychaete', *J. biol. Chem.*, **245,** 6533–6538

WATERMAN, T. H. (1961). 'Comparative physiology', 521–593. In: *The Physiology of Crustacea* **2.** Ed. T. H. Waterman. Academic Press, New York

WAXMAN, L. (1971). 'The hemoglobin of *Arenicola cristata', J. biol. Chem.*, **246,** 7318–7327

WAXMAN, L. (1975). 'The structure of annelid and mollusc hemoglobins', *J. Biol. Chem.*, **250,** 3790–3795

WEBER, R. E. (1970). 'Relations between functional and molecular properties of annelid hemoglobins. Interaction between haems in the haemoglobin of *Arenicola marina* L.', *Comp. Biochem. Physiol.*, **35,** 179–189

WEBER, R. E. (1971a). 'Vergelijkende studier over haemoglobinen van Mediterrane polychaeten', *Koninkl. Nederl. Akad. van Wetens, Amsterdam,* **10,** 155–160

WEBER, R. E. (1971b). 'Oxygenational properties of vascular and coelomic hemoglobins from *Nephtys hombergii* (Polychaeta) and their functional significance', *Neth. J. Sea Res.,* **5,** 240–251

WEBER, R. E. (1972). 'On the variation in oxygen binding properties of haemoglobins of lugworms (Arenicolidae, Polychaeta)', *Proc. 5th Eur. Mar. Biol. Symp. Piccin. Publ., Padova,* 231–243

WEBER, R. E. (1973). 'Functional and molecular properties of corpuscular hemoglobin from the bloodworm *Glycera gigantea', Neth. J. Sea Res.,* **7,** 316–327

WEBER, R. E. (1975). 'Respiratory properties of haemoglobins from eunicid polychaetes', *J. Comp. Physiol.,* **99,** 157–160

WEBER, R. E., MANGUM, C., STEINMAN, H., BONAVENTURA, C., SULLIVAN, B. and BONAVENTURA, J. (1976). 'Hemoglobins of two terebellid polychaetes: *Enoplobranchus sanguineus* and *Amphitrite ornata'*. (Submitted)

WEBER, R. E. and PAUPTIT, E. (1972). 'Molecular and functional heterogeneity in myoglobin from the polychaete *Arenicola marina* L.', *Arch. Biochem. Biophys.,* **148,** 322–324

WEICHELMAN, K. J. and PARKHURST, L. J. (1972). 'Kinetics of ligand binding in the hemoglobin of *Lumbricus terrestris', Biochem.,* **11,** 4515–4520

WEICHELMAN, K. J. and PARKHURST, L. J. (1973). 'Kinetic origin of the pronounced Bohr effect in an annelid hemoglobin', *Biochem. Biophys. Res. Communic.,* **52,** 1199–1205

WEILAND, A. L. and MANGUM, C. P. (1975). 'The influence of environmental salinity on hemocyanin function in the blue crab, *Callinectes sapidus', J. exp. Zool.,* **193,** 265–274

WELLS, G. P. (1950). 'Spontaneous activity cycles in polychaete worms', *Symp. Soc. Exp. Biol.,* **4,** 127–142

WELLS, G. P. (1953). 'The respiratory significance of the crown in the polychaete worms *Sabella* and *Myxicola', Proc. roy. Soc. Lond. B.,* **40,** 70–82

WELLS, G. P. (1961). 'How lugworms move', 209–233. In: *The Cell and the Organism.* Eds. J. A. Ramsay and V. B. Wigglesworth. Cambridge University Press, Cambridge.

WELLS, G. P. and DALES, R. P. (1951). 'Spontaneous activity patterns in animal behaviour: the irrigation of the burrow in the polychaetes *Chaetopterus variopedatus* Renier and *Nereis diversicolor* O. F. Müller', *J. mar. biol. Assoc. U.K.,* **29,** 661–680

WELLS, R. E. and MERRILL, E. W. (1962). 'Influence of flow properties of blood upon viscosity-hematocrit relationships', *J. clin. Investi.,* **41,** 1591–1598

WELLS, R. M. G. (1973). 'Carbonic anhydrase activity in *Arenicola marina* (L.)', *Comp. Biochem. Physiol.,* **46A,** 325–332

WELLS, R. M. G. (1974). 'Hydrogen ion activity in polychaete body fluids', *Comp. Biochem. Physiol.,* **49A,** 567–574

WELLS, R. M. G. and DALES, R. P. (1974). 'Oxygenational properties of haemerythrin in the blood of *Magelona papillicornis* Muller. (Polychaeta: Magelonidae)', *Comp. Biochem. Physiol.,* **49A,** 57–64

WELLS, R. M. G. and DALES, R. P. (1975). 'Haemoglobin function in *Terebella lapidaria* (L.), an intertidal terebellid polychaete', *J. mar. biol. Assoc. U.K.,* **55,** 211–220

WELLS, R. M. G. and DALES, R. P. (1975). 'The respiratory significance of chlorocruorin', *Proc. 9th Ent. Mar. Biol. Symp.,* pp. 673–681. Ed. H. Barnes. Aberdeen University Press, Aberdeen

WITTENBERG, B. A., BRIEHL, R. W. and WITTENBERG, J. B. (1965). 'Haemoglobins of invertebrate tissue. Nerve haemoglobins of *Aphrodite, Aplysia* and *Halosydna', Biochem. J.,* **96,** 363–371

WOLVEKAMP, H. P. and VREEDE, M. C. (1940). 'On the gas binding properties of the blood of the lugworm (*Arenicola marina* L.)', *Arch. Neerl. Physiol.,* **25,** 265–276

YAMAGISHI, M., KAJITA, A., SHUKUYA, R. and KAZIRO, K. (1966). 'Quaternary structure of *Limnodrilus* hemoglobin', *J. mol. Biol.,* **21,** 467–472

ZAMIR, M. and ROACH, M. R. (1973). 'Blood flow downstream of a two-dimensional bifurcation', *J. theoret. Biol.,* **42,** 33–48

ZOLA, H. (1967). 'Sugar phosphate polymers in polychaete tubes and in mineralized animal tissues' *Comp. Biochem. Physiol.,* **21,** 179–183

Five

Enzyme and metabolic adaptations to low oxygen

P. W. HOCHACHKA
Department of Zoology, University of British Columbia, Vancouver

G. N. SOMERO
Scripps Institution of Oceanography, La Jolla, California

5.1 INTRODUCTION

Anyone familiar with the 'metabolic map' is aware that the initial channels of foodstuff degradation, e.g. the reactions of glycolysis, are fundamentally anaerobic schemes. The glycolytic reactions in which carbohydrates are oxidised are, of course, dehydrogenation reactions. Hydrogen is removed from triose phosphates, and NAD* is reduced to NADH, reactions which are totally independent of molecular oxygen. Similarly, the reactions of the pentose phosphate pathway, which provide pentose sugars and reducing power (NADPH) for biosynthetic processes include oxidation reactions which do not involve molecular oxygen. Only at the very final stages of electron transport is molecular oxygen actually required to support cellular oxidation of carbohydrates and other foodstuffs.

The use of molecular oxygen in energy metabolism is a late addition to the

*Abbreviations used:
AMP, ADP, ATP – adenosine mono-, di-, and triphosphate
NAD, NADH – nicotinamide adenine dinucleotide (oxidised and reduced forms)
NAD, NADPH – nicotinamide adenine dinucleotide phosphate (oxidised and reduced forms)
PEP – phosphoenolpyruvate
PK – pyruvate kinase
PEPCK – phosphoenolpyruvate carboxykinase
GAPDH – glyceraldehyde-3-phosphate dehydrogenase
LDH – lactate dehydrogenase
MDH – malate dehydrogenase
OXA – oxalacetate

'metabolic map' in two distinct senses. As discussed above, present day organisms reduce oxygen only during the final step of catabolism. In addition, when viewed from an evolutionary perspective, we find that the addition of an oxygen-utilising capacity to the anaerobic reactions of the cell is a relatively recent 'invention' (Wald, 1964). During a large part of biological evolution, metabolism was strictly anaerobic. The addition of oxygen-based oxidative metabolism could not occur until green plant photosynthesis had added sufficient amounts of oxygen to the earth's originally reducing atmosphere.

In exploring the differing abilities of marine organisms to survive under anoxic conditions, it seems useful to keep the outlines of the metabolic map and of metabolic evolution fresh in our minds. By so doing we are apt to appreciate better the central role played by the anaerobic core of metabolism, and we may avoid what seems to be an all too common prejudice among zoologists to regard anaerobiosis as a somewhat aberrant condition which at least multicellular organisms will choose to avoid at all costs. The approximately 18-fold increase in ATP production which has resulted from the addition of the Krebs citric acid cycle and electron transport schemes to the anaerobic core of metabolism does, of course, represent a major evolutionary breakthrough. However, in selecting a habitat or a 'life-style', an organism must always strike a compromise balance among a large array of environmental and physiological parameters. As in the case of temperature (*see* Chapter 3), an environment with unfavourable oxygen concentrations may yet be chosen by an organism if the other attributes of this habitat offer such favourable material for exploitation that a temporary or even a long-term reduction in metabolic efficiency is far outweighed by other gains. We will see, in fact, that a critically important role of adaptive processes involves schemes for allowing an organism to survive under highly unfavourable conditions relative to one environmental parameter so as to allow the organism to exploit effectively other environmental conditions.

The number of instances during evolution when organisms have 'chosen' to sacrifice metabolic efficiency to achieve other environmental ends is apt to astonish a biologist whose training in intermediary metabolism has been rat- or human-oriented. Among the invertebrates, impressive anaerobic capacities are found among the Cnidaria, Nemertina, Annelida, Mollusca, Arthropoda, Echinodermata and Urochordata (Mangum, 1973). Among the vertebrates one also finds extraordinary anaerobic performances. Turtles may dive for periods of several days (Jackson, 1968). Fish in ice-blocked bodies of water may live anaerobically for many months (Blazka, 1958). Weddell seals can remain submerged for more than an hour. Deep-diving whales exhibit even more impressive anaerobic abilities.

Before discussing the biochemical mechanisms utilised by multicellular marine organisms to cope with conditions of limited oxygen availability, we shall briefly focus attention on the environmental and physiological factors which lead to anoxia, i.e. to the unavailability of oxygen at the *cellular* level. With the exception of burrowing forms, some of whose respiratory adaptations have been discussed in the previous chapter, most of the marine organisms which are capable of high degrees of anaerobiosis live in environments where relatively large concentrations of oxygen are available. A set of one or more physiological constraints, rather than environmental oxygen levels, establishes the need for anaerobic metabolism. For example, a mussel may experience its highest environmental oxygen levels during anaerobiosis, during low tide the mussel is apt to be bathed with air. As pointed out in Chapter 1 the requirement for preventing water loss under these conditions is a more demanding necessity than the need to maintain an efficient oxidative metabolism. A diving mammal also swims in an environment relatively rich in oxygen. However, its mode of gas exchange precludes making use of environmental oxygen during dives. Thus the presence of an anaerobic habit does not denote the existence of an anoxic habitat in all cases. Anaerobic periods in the presence of relatively large amounts of oxygen are often characteristic of situations where (a) the respiratory apparatus is unable to extract oxygen, or (b) the level of activity demanded of an organism is so high that even abundant environmental oxygen is not sufficient to ensure adequate oxygen supply at the cellular level.

In describing molecular adaptations to anoxic cellular conditions, we will find that a major determinant of the adaptive mechanisms utilised by an organism is the length of the time period during which low oxygen stress is encountered. In addition, major distinctions will be seen between vertebrates and invertebrates. As a broad generalisation, we can state that both the (a) total anaerobic potential of a tissue and (b) the types of metabolic reactions which sustain energy metabolism under anoxic conditions strongly reflect the time course of anoxia. Organisms within both the invertebrate and vertebrate groups which are capable of sustained anoxic performance not only exhibit increased levels of enzymes associated with anaerobiosis, but in addition display a number of important 'metabolic inventions' which add additional enzymic pathways for energy extraction (ATP generation) to the so-called 'conventional' anaerobic scheme of glycolysis. Thus, in this chapter, we shall treat in order (a) the biochemical attributes of the initial sequence of anaerobic reactions, those involved in degrading glycogen to the level of lactic acid, which are at least largely a common denominator among all multicellular anaerobes, and then (b) the known additions which are superimposed on this basic catabolic scheme to facilitate longer-term anoxic excursions. We will find that, whatever pathway is being considered, certain common 'strategies' of adaptation will be important. Total concentrations of enzymes supporting anaerobiosis will, as one would predict, be high in efficient anaerobes. More interestingly, however, is the fact that the basic kinetic properties of enzymes supporting long-term anaerobiosis often appear especially tailored for supporting sustained energy production under anoxic conditions. We can therefore say that the enzymes of anaerobic pathways differ qualitatively as well as in concentration between organisms which are primarily aerobic and those which are able to sustain long periods of anoxia. Thus, as is often the case in studies of environmental adaptation, a close examination of the biochemical adaptations to anoxia can give us unparalleled insights into the 'strategies' of evolution at the molecular level.

5.2 GLYCOLYTICALLY-BASED STRATEGIES OF ANOXIA ADAPTATION

5.2.1 Biochemical requirements and solutions

In all cells that are able to sustain significant periods of anoxia, some provision is made (a) for a storage form of energy to be utilised during anoxia, (b) for the maintenance of redox balance, and (c) for the generation of high energy phosphate compounds (ATP equivalents). In many organisms, these three metabolic requirements are met by anaerobic glycolysis (*Figure 5.1*) where glycogen, the storage form of energy, is catabolised to the level of lactate during anaerobiosis. Redox balance is maintained by a functional 1:1 integration of GAPDH and LDH; the NAD utilised in the GAPDH oxidation is regained by LDH catalysed pyruvate reduction to lactate, and the scheme as regards NAD is cyclic and catalytic. Useful energy production in the form of ATP occurs at the PGK and PK reaction steps, per mole of glucose, a net of 2 moles of ATP being formed. Given this overall system, how do 'good' vertebrate anaerobes maximise it, or at least improve it, to support work under stressful conditions such as diving? Nature fortunately gives us some readily available clues to this problem for in all vertebrates the importance of anaerobic glycolysis varies greatly between tissues. From a careful comparison of tissues such as liver (which does not depend critically upon anaerobic glycolysis) with tissues such as white muscle (which during 'burst activity' derives essentially all its useful energy from anaerobic mechanisms), it becomes clear that nature 'tunes up' the glycolytic machinery in several important ways. Before these can be fully appreciated, however, it is important to review briefly our current understanding of the overall organisation and control of muscle glycolysis.

5.2.2 Multiple control sites in muscle glycogenolysis

Over the last decade or so, it has become apparent that control of glycolysis (indeed, control of other metabolic pathways as well) never resides at one key site, the so-called 'master reaction' of earlier literature. Rather, the pathway is broken up into various segments, in each of which there appears to be a key control reaction; during operation, control is transferred from site to site along the pathway, but we are not yet too certain of how this is organised in time. Is it sequential? Is it alternating, hopping forwards then backwards then forwards again? We do not know which alternative is correct. What we do know with a high degree of certainty, however, is that three key control sites appear over and over again in different species and in different tissues (Williamson, 1965; Scrutton and Utter, 1968; Sacktor, 1970; Hochachka *et al.*, 1970). The three sites are (a) glycogen phosphorylase, (b) phosphofructokinase (PFK), and (c) pyruvate kinase (PK), and in situations where glucose is an important alternative substrate for the pathway, hexokinase appears as an important regulatory site. These

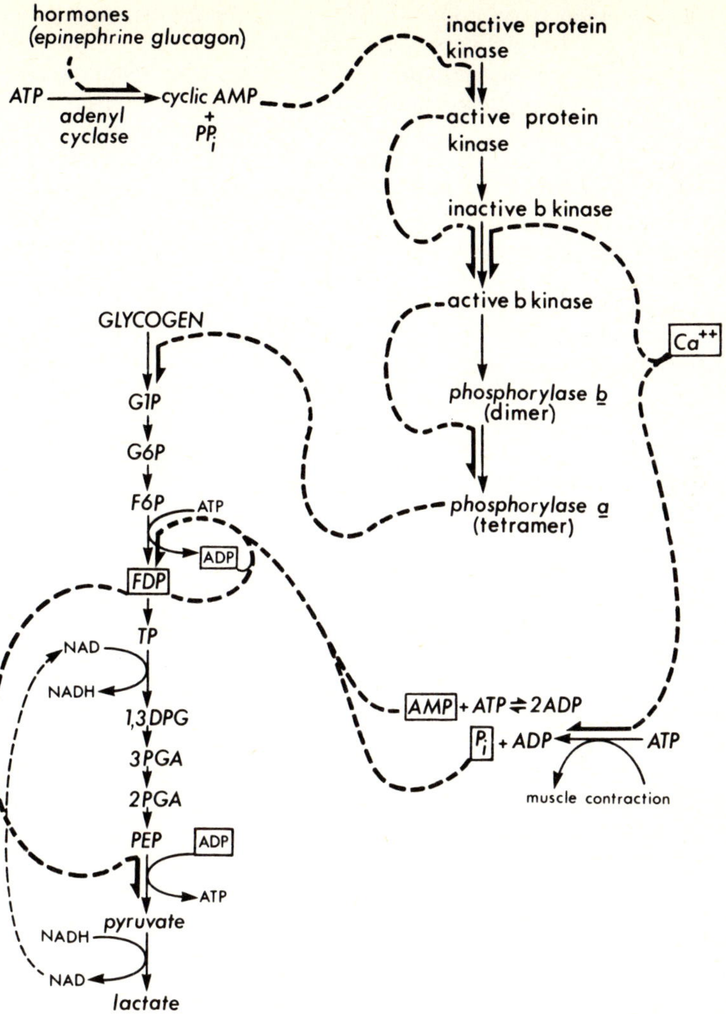

Figure 5.1 Metabolic map showing currently held concepts of glycolytic activation in skeletal muscle of vertebrate animals. Regulatory metabolites are connected by dashed lines with the enzyme steps which they activate; activation is indicated with a dark arrow. One aspect of this control diagram, FDP activation of pyruvate kinase, is thought to occur widely only among lower vertebrates; all other aspects are thought to be general, although certain characteristics are adjusted in diving vertebrates. (After Hochachka and Somero, 1973; courtesy W. B. Saunders & Co.)

enzymes share an important characteristic: under physiological conditions, they catalyse reactions that are in effect irreversible, for thermodynamic and/or kinetic reasons. Moreover, compared with other tissues, such as liver, they occur in much higher amounts in muscle and thus in part account for its greater glycolytic capacity (Scrutton and Utter, 1968). However, a higher amount of key enzymes does not account for the capacity of muscle glycolysis to swing from a low activity state almost instantaneously to a several hundred fold activated state (Danforth, 1965; Helmreich *et al.*, 1965). This characteristic, unique to skeletal muscle, depends not on the *amount* of any given glycolytic enzyme, but on the *kind* of enzyme present; that is, on its specific regulatory properties. Thus, most of the glycolytic enzymes in muscle occur not only in high concentrations, but also in more or less tissue specific form, and, if our reasoning is correct, understanding the way in which the three key enzymes of glycogenolysis are controlled and integrated should go a long way to explaining why muscle glycolysis is such a good 'anaerobic machine'.

5.2.3 Strategic positioning and control functions of glycogen phosphorylase

As is evident in *Figure 5.1,* glycogen phosphorylase is metabolically strategically positioned at the first step in the pathway and it initiates glycogen mobilisation. It is also physically placed strategically on to glycogen granules. From much *in vivo* and *in vitro* experimentation, it is now known to be under hormonal control (via a cascade control system) as well as under Ca^{2+} control. Time course of phosphorylase activation by hormones is in the order of minutes while Ca^{2+} activation, which depends upon muscle membrane depolarisation and can therefore be thought of as a neuronal-dependent activation mechanism, occurs in seconds or less (*see* Drummond, 1971, for a recent review). The Ca^{2+} activation appears to be of primary importance (particularly to diving vertebrates, where the blood flow and hence hormonal signals to muscle, are cut off during the dive) because it is thought to integrate metabolic events with mechanical (contractile) ones.

Upon membrane depolarisation, Ca^{2+} is thought to be released from binding sites on sarcoplasmic reticulum into the sarcoplasm at concentrations of about 2 μM. In addition to activating myosin ATPase and contraction, it directly activates phosphorylase *b* kinase (by greatly increasing its affinity for phosphorylase *b*) while simultaneously inhibiting phosphorylase phosphatase (*Figure 5.2*). The summed effect of Ca^{2+} release, then, is the 'flash activation' of glycolygen phosphorylase by (1) a direct activation of *b* kinase and thus conversion of (inactive) phosphorylase *b* to (active) phosphorylase *a*, and by (2) a specific inactivation of the phosphatase enzyme reconverting phosphorylase *a* to *b* (Heilmeyer *et al.*, 1970).

The conversion of phosphorylase *b* to *a* is now considered to be central to glycogen mobilisation in all vertebrate tissues, including muscle, but once in the active form, the level of enzyme activity still depends upon substrate and modulator concentrations. In muscle, the affinity of phosphorylase *a* for glycogen is unusually high, 50-fold higher, for example, than in the case of the brain enzyme (Lowry and Passonneau, 1966), and the muscle enzyme can therefore bind substrate with high efficiency. Moreover, the enzyme is further activated by AMP (5-fold activation with 0.1 mM AMP) which

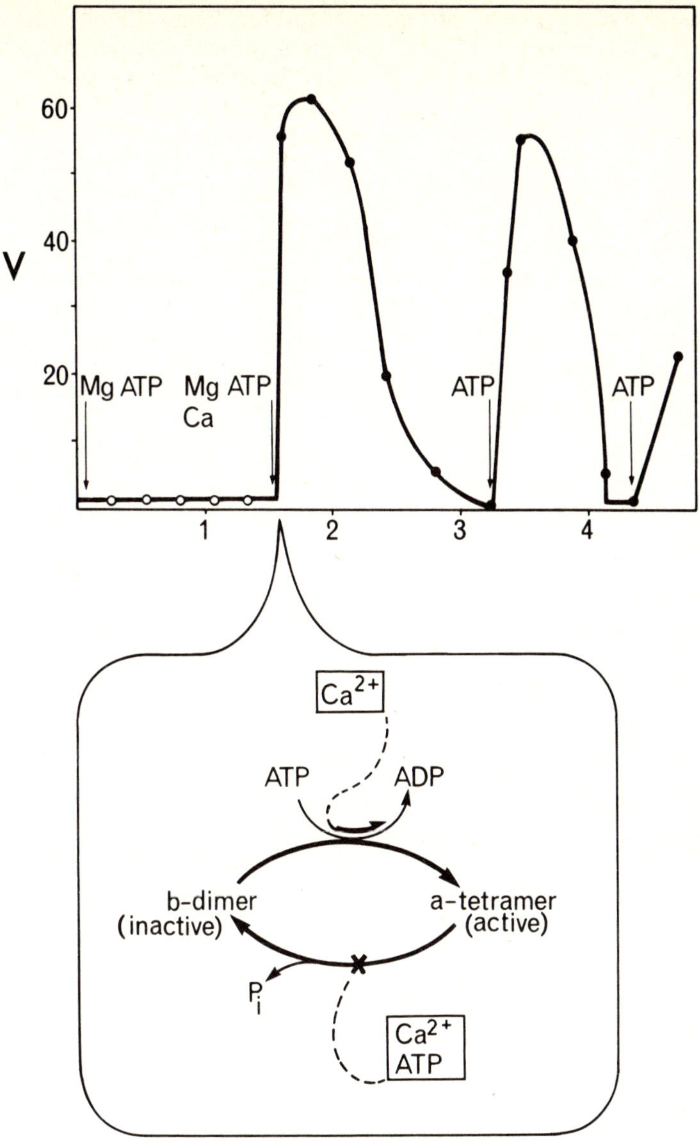

Figure 5.2 'Flash activation' of glycogen phosphorylase by Ca^{2+} and ATP as observed in glycogen particles isolated from rabbit muscle. Relative velocity is plotted against time in minutes, complete activation occurring well within the first seconds of addition of Ca^{2+} and ATP. ATP is required for phosphorylation of the b *dimer to the phosphorylase* a *tetramer, a reaction catalysed by phosphorylase* b *kinase. Ca^{2+} serves to increase by about 15-fold the affinity of this enzyme for its substrate, phosphorylase* b. *At the same time, Ca^{2+} and ATP are both required for inhibition of the reverse inactivating reaction, catalysed by a phosphatase and converting* a*-tetramer back to* b*-dimer phosphorylase. These mechanisms of flash activation are indicated below the graph. (Modified after Heilmeyer* et al., *1970)*

increases enzyme-substrate affinity still further. These kinetic properties strongly poise glycogen phosphorylase in the glycolytic direction despite the thermodynamically 'uphill' nature of the reaction and can set the stage for a glycolytic activation in muscle which surpasses by far that of any other tissue in the vertebrate body. To achieve this, the regulation of phosphorylase must be at least partially integrated with that of the next key control site in the pathway, phosphofructokinase.

5.2.4 Autocatalytic activation of muscle glycolysis probably depends on phosphofructokinase

Phosphofructokinase (PFK) catalyses the first committed step in glycolysis and as such has long been recognised as perhaps the most important single control site in glycolysis (*see* Mansour, 1972, for a recent review). A sufficient number of vertebrate tissues and species have now been examined to recognise a common control principle underlying all vertebrate PFK's. Thus for this enzyme *the two co-substrates, F6P and ATP, serve both as substrates* per se *as well as metabolite modulators*. One substrate, F6P, behaves as a typical positive modulator, while the co-substrate, ATP, behaves as an important negative modulator (*Figure 5.3*). All other regulatory metabolites exert their effects either by modifying enzyme-F6P affinity, or by modifying enzyme sensitivity to ATP, or more usually by modifying both F6P and ATP saturation kinetics (*Figure 5.3*).

Following activation of glycogen phosphorylase and myofibrillar ATPase, in normal skeletal muscle, rising levels of F6P, FDP, ADP, AMP, and P_i coupled with falling levels of creatine-P and ATP can lead to a very large PFK 'flare-up' when it is required. A central feature of this control system is that two of the positive modulators (FDP and ADP) are both products of the reaction; one of the positive modulators (F6P) is of course a substrate. Taken together, their regulatory effects lead to an autocatalytic, exponential rate of change from low activity states to high activity states, a characteristic that helps to explain the speed with which muscle glycolysis can be 'turned on'.

Parenthetically, one may add that these control properties of muscle PFK clearly reflect selective forces operating in muscle tissue. These control properties are not typically seen, or are less exaggerated, in other tissues of the vertebrate body such as liver, red blood cells, or digestive tract (*see,* e.g. Tejwani and Ramaiah, 1970). In most of these tissues, PFK catalytic activity is linear with time, whereas in muscle it of course follows an exponential product-activated pattern. In the case of most enzymes, including PFK from a protein-catabolising slime mould (Baumann and Wright, 1968), reaction products typically inhibit reaction velocity. Aside from this characteristic, other distinguishing features of muscle PFK compared with tissues such as the liver include an overall 'tighter' control by most organo-phosphate modulators and by citrate but a highly reduced sensitivity to ATP inhibition. Thus, for a given per cent change, muscle PFK requires about 1/10 as much ADP, AMP, or citrate as does the liver homologue; at

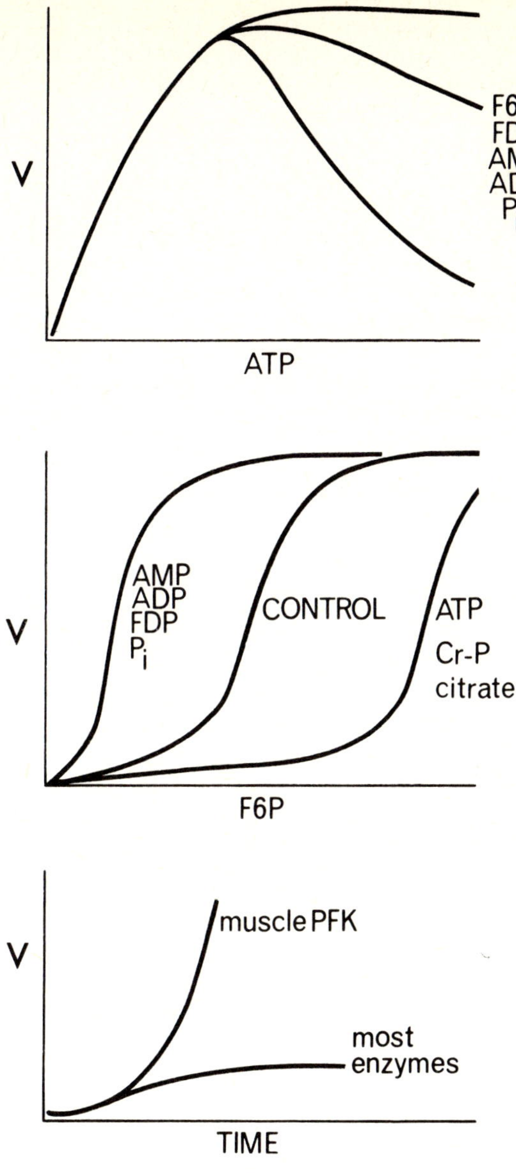

Figure 5.3 *Muscle PFK regulation is based on the fact that the substrates of the reaction both also behave as modulators. One of the substrates, ATP, becomes a potent inhibitor at high concentrations (upper graph); the other substrate, F6P, reverses this effect. F6P is also an activator in the sense that the binding of one molecule increases the enzyme affinity for the next, a property that leads to a sigmoidal saturation curve (middle graph). All other regulatory properties appear to be superimposed upon these two basic effects; thus all other regulatory metabolites (shown in the upper and middle graphs) either reverse ATP inhibition or increase enzyme-F6P affinity. A final point to note is that both products, FDP and ADP, are potent activators. This property, together with substrate (F6P) activation, leads to an autocatalytic activation of the enzyme with time (bottom graph)*

the same time, it requires 2–3 fold higher ATP concentrations to bring about the same percentage inhibition. As we shall argue below, some of the muscle PFK characteristics are further accentuated in 'good' vertebrate anaerobes such as divers.

Finally, the question arises as to how PFK catalytic rate is integrated with the activity of pyruvate kinase (PK), the next major regulatory enzyme in glycolysis. In most mammals studied, the major integration mechanism merely involves adenylate coupling; that is, ADP, the product of the PFK reaction, is a substrate of PK, and this in itself serves to automatically coordinate the activities of these two enzymes. In lower vertebrates (fishes, reptiles), PK is an allosteric enzyme under close metabolite regulation and FDP, the other product of the PFK reaction, serves as a potent feedforward activator of muscle PK, assuring nearly simultaneous activation of both enzymes (Somero and Hochachka, 1968; Storey and Hochachka, 1974a, c).

5.2.5 Maintenance of redox balance during anaerobic glycolysis in muscle

In general, redox balance during anaerobic glycolysis in muscle is maintained by a functionally 1:1 activity ratio between glyceraldehyde-3-P dehydrogenase (GAPDH) and lactate dehydrogenase (LDH), and this surely is the situation during early phases of glycolysis. Both enzymes occur in higher amounts in vertebrate muscle than in other tissues (Scrutton and Utter, 1968), and in rat muscle, for example, they occur in about a 1:1 ratio. Under extreme situations, the LDH reaction becomes limiting by mass action effects (White and Kaplan, 1972); at this time, if muscle glycolysis is to continue, the GAPDH oxidative step must have some other source of NAD. That source is usually considered to be the α-glycerophosphate dehydrogenase (α-GPDH) reaction, in which case α-glycerophosphate accumulates as an additional anaerobic end product (Williamson, 1965; Edington, Ward and Saville, 1973). Presumably, some controlling mechanism is available to 'turn on' α-GPDH at the correct time but at the time of writing we are aware of nothing definitive on this matter.

Not only is the amount of LDH present in skeletal muscle adjusted for a high glycolytic potential but so is the kind of LDH present (*see* Everse and Kaplan, 1974, for a recent review). Thus, it is now widely accepted that the muscle type of LDH tetramer shows at least two kinetic properties which suit it admirably for function in a tissue of high glycolytic potential: low enzyme-substrate affinity and low substrate inhibition. The latter effect prevents substrate inhibition of the reaction during rapid glycolysis, while the low enzyme-substrate affinity prevents pyruvate saturation of the enzyme and hence prevents pyruvate accumulation without limit during glycolytic activation. As a result, lactate concentration can rise to very high levels and muscle tissue sustains higher lactate accumulations than any other tissue in the vertebrate body.

It should also be noted that pyruvate inhibition of muscle LDH's is very temperature dependent. At temperatures above approximately 25°C, for example, the muscle LDH's of the estuarine fish *Gillicthys mirabilis* exhibit no pyruvate inhibition, whereas at lower temperatures pyruvate inhibition is substantial (Somero, 1973). These observations suggest that at low temperatures, when oxygen is plentiful and activity levels are apt to be low, the fish can rely almost solely on oxidative metabolism. Thus, an LDH which is substrate-inhibited and thereby directs pyruvate to the Krebs cycle appears adaptive. At higher temperatures, where oxygen levels are low and activity may be high, an LDH with the 'muscle type' kinetics discussed above appears advantageous.

5.2.6 Hallmarks that make muscle glycolysis a 'good anaerobic machine'

From the above considerations, we conclude that, among the vertebrates, muscle glycolysis is one of the most efficient 'anaerobic machines' invented by nature. In its evolutionary development, selection seems to have favoured two fundamental characteristics (*Table 5.1*):

Table 5.1 WHY MUSCLE GLYCOLYSIS IS A GOOD 'ANAEROBIC MACHINE'

Metabolic requirements	*Solutions*
1. High glycolytic potential	High glycogen levels High enzyme levels
2. Large % change from low to high activity states	Specific regulatory forms of glycolytic enzymes
3. Complete on–complete off catalytic behaviour	Multiple metabolite modulators Mechanisms for amplifying metabolite signals
4. Tolerance for high lactate accumulation	High buffering capacity pH insensitive enzymes Acid pH optima M_4 LDH

1. High enzyme concentrations and abundant quantities of storage substrate (i.e. glycogen).
2. Specific enzyme variants designed:
   (a) For large percentage swings from low to high activity states (up to several hundred fold activation).
   (b) For exponential rates of change from low to high activity.
   (c) For accumulation of large lactate quantities.

The first characteristic gives muscle a high glycolytic potential; the second characteristic brings that high potential under tight metabolic control.

5.2.7 Muscle glycolysis in marine mammals

The basic design of muscle glycolysis is so effective that when muscle of a diving mammal, such as the porpoise, is compared with an animal such as the common laboratory rat, or man, only a small number of modifications are observed, and these are all, in effect, elaborations on the theme already described. Thus, when one considers muscle enzyme concentrations within the glycolytic chain (*Figure 5.4*), the major differences between a marine mammal and the laboratory rat are (a) increased levels of phosphoglucomutase (PGM), aldolase, α-GPDH, and LDH, and (b) decreased levels of PK. A third notable change is unusually high levels of FDPase, a non-glycolytic step, which is nonetheless involved in glycolytic control (Storey and Hochachka, 1974a, and unpublished data).

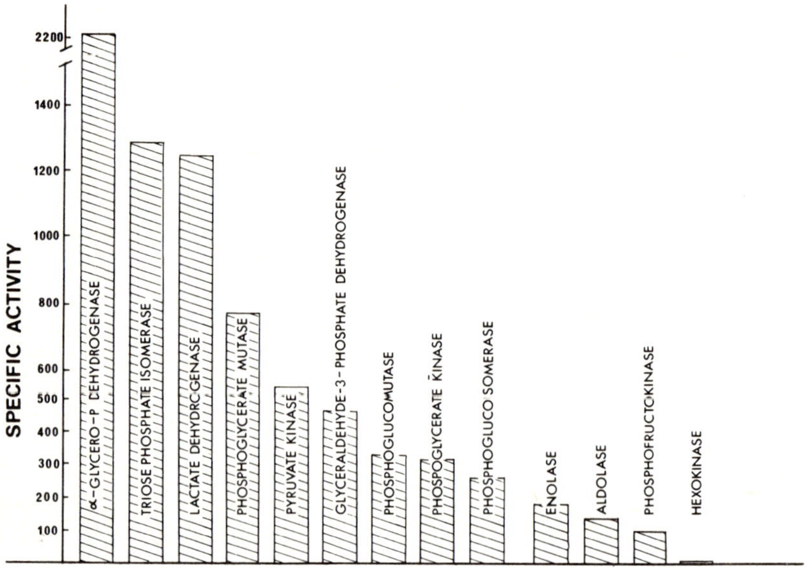

Figure 5.4 Enzyme profile of the glycolytic pathway in muscle of a marine mammal, the dolphin, Lagenorhynchus obliquidens. *Modified from Storey and Hochachka (1974c). The α-glycerophosphate dehydrogenase values are from Storey (unpublished data)*

On closer examination, the first set of observations can be readily explained. Thus, because muscle in marine mammals is cut off from blood circulation by peripheral vasoconstriction during diving, it must place a lesser reliance on blood glucose and a greater reliance upon muscle glycogen than would that of a terrestrial mammal; this requirement in turn is reflected in increased levels of PGM. Secondly, increased levels of aldolase contribute to the tight regulation of FDP levels, the latter of course is a key regulatory metabolite in the overall pathway. And thirdly, in marine divers, muscle cells must be prevented from becoming highly reduced, and this requirement is reflected in higher α-GPDH and LDH values. The high level of muscle FDPase and the low level of muscle PK, however, are not as easily explained.

5.2.8 Function of a high muscle FDPase activity in diving mammals

In the degree to which muscle glycolysis can oscillate between low activity and high activity states (between basal and maximally activated states), this multienzyme pathway is undoubtedly unique in the vertebrate body. In a relatively sluggish animal, such as the frog, it is possible to demonstrate that 200 to 300-fold glycolytic activation can occur in the sartorious muscle within seconds of electrical stimulation, and under extreme conditions a 600-fold activation can be obtained (Hochachka and Storey, 1975; Danforth, 1965). In fast swimming divers, such as the porpoise, one would anticipate at least a comparable capacity, both in terms of speed of response and in terms of the percentage activation. Achieving such large absolute activation calls for an essentially 'complete off – complete on' catalytic behaviour at key control sites such as at the F6P → FDP interconversion (Newsholme, 1972; Storey and Hochachka, 1974b). How this is achieved is not yet clear, because the concentration of no single regulatory metabolite changes by a large enough factor to account for the degree of activation observed. One possibility is that various metabolites act in a synergistic manner to bring about the required 'on–off' behaviour; to some extent, this certainly occurs, but the highest estimates of the degree of PFK activation that can be achieved by such means range between 200-fold (Storey and Hochachka, 1974b) and about 350-fold (Tejwani, Ramaiah and Ananthanarayanan, 1973). In obtaining these estimates, both studies have to assume a coordinated time course of change in the concentrations of various regulatory metabolites; any lag or 'slop' in the system (i.e. changes in positive and negative modulator levels being slightly out of balance), and these high values become greatly reduced. Even if they are accepted as physiologically relevant, they are still well below the potential requirements for PFK activation in fast swimming divers such as the porpoise, in 'burst' running of certain terrestrial animals, or in 'burst' flight patterns of birds such as the pheasant (Newsholme, 1972). Newsholme and his colleagues have argued that what clearly is required to account for the 'on–off' behaviour at sites such as the F6P → FDP interconversion is some sort of mechanism for amplifying metabolite 'signals'. Of a number of possibilities, muscle glycolysis seems to rely most upon an FDPase based amplification mechanism.

In physiological terms, FDPase catalyses a reaction which is the reverse of that catalysed by PFK. Although PFK is regulated by a large number of modulators, FDPase seems to be under the regulation of only one effector compound: AMP. AMP is a potent inhibitor of all FDPases thus far examined, except for bumble bee flight muscle where the enzyme is involved in a thermogenic function (Newsholme *et al*., 1972). When first discovered in muscle, the function of FDPase was unknown, and the enzyme's presence posed a perplexing problem since the simultaneous function of both enzymes in the same cell sets up a futile carbon cycle and a net ATP hydrolysis. That perhaps is precisely the point. Newsholme and his coworkers have argued that since both PFK and FDPase respond (in opposite manner) to at least one signal in common (AMP), the sensitivity of the overall F6P → FDP conversion will be far greater than if only PFK (or only FDPase) were AMP sensitive, or if only PFK were present in the cell. That is, a single signal aimed at any such two oppositely-directed reactions is greatly amplified if one enzyme is activated while the other is inhibited by that signal. The degree of amplification depends upon the rate of cycling/rate of glycolytic flux, and in muscle, the rate of cycling will of course be dramatically dependent upon the FDPase concentration. This situation seems important enough to illustrate with a set of simple calculations.

Consider two muscle types, one with low (0.1 arbitrary units of) FDPase activity, the other with high (5.0 units of) FDPase. Assume in both a basal resting F6P → FDP flux rate of 0.1 units. In the case of the low-FDPase muscle, a basal flux rate of 0.1 units depends upon 0.2 PFK units minus 0.1 FDPase units. Now a two-fold change in AMP concentration doubles PFK activity while simultaneously halving FDPase activity; the activated PFK rate is 0.4 units (i.e. 0.2×2) while the inhibited FDPase rate is 0.05 (i.e. 0.1/2). The net conversion rate (F6P → FDP) is now 0.35 units ($0.4 - 0.05$), representing a 350% increase. In the high-FDPase case, a basal flux rate of 0.1 units depends upon 5.1 PFK units minus 5.0 FDPase units. Assume that a two-fold change in AMP levels also leads to a doubling of PFK activity and a halving of FDPase activity; the activated PFK rate becomes 10.2 units, the inhibited FDPase rate becomes 2.5 units, and the overall activated (F6P → FDP) flux rate is 7.7 units. Compared to the basal rate of 0.1 units, this represents a 7700% change in net F6P → FDP conversion.

Clearly, for a given level of muscle PFK, the higher the FDPase, the greater the amplification of a given AMP signal. In this context, our observation that muscle FDPase/PFK ratios in porpoise are about 2–3 fold higher than in frog sartorius, or in a variety of other mammalian and bird muscles, can be fully appreciated. However, we have yet to explain the apparently paradoxical observation of relatively low pyruvate kinase levels in muscle of diving mammals.

5.2.9 The regulatory nature of muscle pyruvate kinase in diving mammals

An explanation for the comparatively low levels of PK within muscle of the porpoise had to await detailed kinetic studies of the enzyme. Others had observed that, when divers are treated as a single group, the levels of PK in muscle correlate with the length of diving each species is capable of achieving (Simon *et al*., 1974), and such a correlation between glycolytic capacity of the tissue and its PK titre in fact also holds for normal mammalian tissues (Simon and Robin, 1972). Unfortunately, Simon *et al*. (1974) fail to stress that within diving animals as a group PK concentrations are lower than in the common laboratory rat, and our studies of the porpoise confirm this observation (Storey and Hochachka, 1974a). What diving animals seem to have done at this locus is to accept an overall reduction in the activity of PK in favour of designing an enzyme which is much more sensitive to metabolite regulation. Thus, muscle PK in diving vertebrates, unlike muscle PK from terrestrial mammals, is under tight feedback inhibition by ATP, alanine, and probably citrate (Storey and Hochachka, 1974c), and under strong feedforward activation by FDP, which returns the PK maximum potential to the high range expected for a highly active glycolysis (Storey and Hochachka, 1974a). Moreover, as with other regulatory PK's, FDP not only directly activates the enzyme (by both K_m and V_{max} effects) but also strongly reverses inhibition by ATP, alanine, and citrate. These regulatory characteristics are in fact commonly observed in muscle PK's of lower vertebrates but appear to have been lost in most mammals. Diving animals have retained (or regained) this tight control over PK in part because of a high reliance upon glycolysis during diving, but mainly *because of important control requirements imposed upon muscle at the end of the dive, i.e. during anaerobic-aerobic transition, when muscle metabolism 'switches' from glycogen to other fuels.*

5.2.10 Metabolic fuels in muscle of marine mammals

Thus far in this discussion of metabolic adaptations for prolonged diving, we have oversimplified the situation by implying that glycogen is the sole carbon and energy source. During anaerobic portions of the dive that may be essentially true. However, when the animal is not diving, the preferred fuel is fat, and standard R.Q. values are in the range of 0.7 for most marine mammals thus far studied (Hochachka and Storey, 1975). To put it more accurately, then, an important consequence of the diving habit is a metabolic organisation that can oscillate efficiently between glycogen catabolism (during anaerobic portions of the dive) and fat catabolism (during steady state aerobic work, such as surface swimming, migrations, and so forth). In considering how this oscillatory behaviour is controlled it is convenient to look at the problem in terms of anaerobic-aerobic transition and vice versa.

5.2.11 How is lipid 'spared' during anaerobic glycogenolysis?

The problem of 'sparing' lipid during anaerobic metabolism is of course not unique to diving mammals. In better studied species, it is well established that fatty acid oxidation is 'turned off' during anaerobic glycolysis, but to date only one metabolite signal — lactate — has been found to play a role in integrating these events (*see* Drummond, 1971, for a recent review). Thus, when lactate levels increase, these serve to inhibit the mobilisation of triglyceride by inhibiting the first step in fat catabolism, that catalysed by lipase (*see Figure 5.5*). In addition, the mobilisation of adipose triglyceride is under hormonal control and this may contribute to the required integration between triglyceride and glycogen metabolism. Although neither mechanism has been studied in detail in any marine mammal, it is tempting to speculate that aerobic triglyceride catabolism in red and intermediate type fibres of the marine mammal (George and Ronald, 1973) is under hormonal control as shown in *Figure 5.5*, by direct effects on the high lipase content of these muscles (George and Ronald, 1973). During prolonged

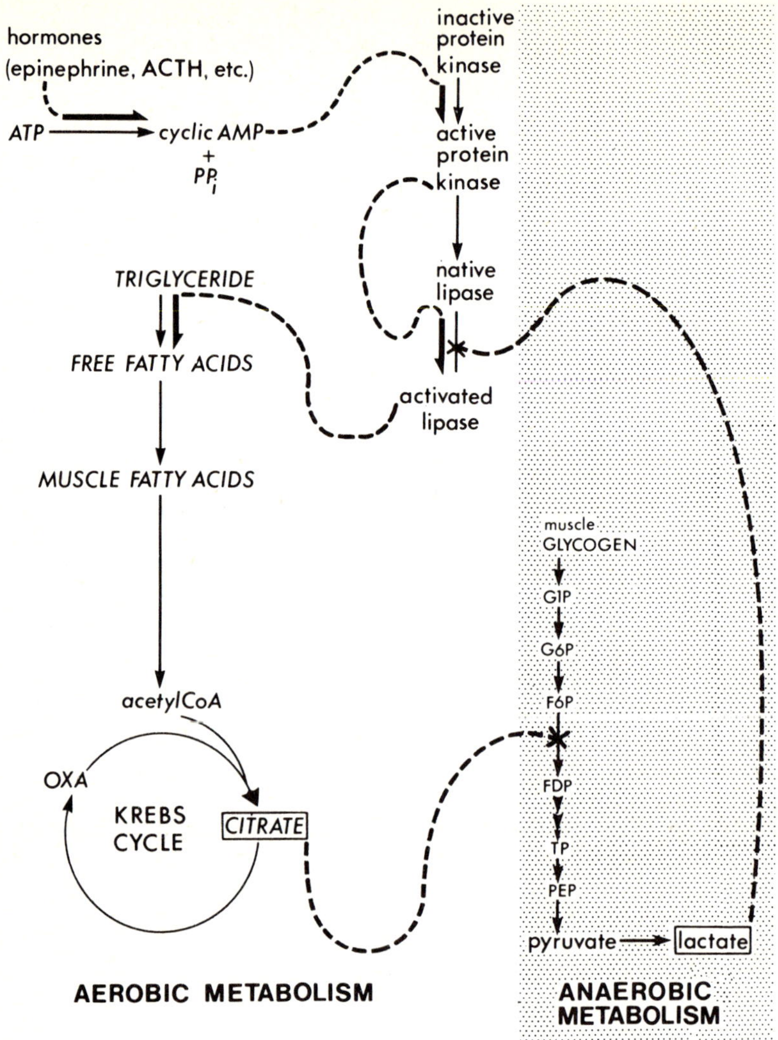

Figure 5.5 Control interactions between fat catabolism and glycogenolysis in muscle of common mammals such as the rat and man. Activation indicated by a dark arrow; inhibition, by a dark cross. (After Hochachka and Somero, 1973; courtesy W. B. Saunders & Co.)

diving, when blood flow to the muscle is shut off, such hormonal signals also would be automatically 'turned off' this leading to a drop in the ratio of active/inactive lipase. At the same time, rising lactate concentrations would serve to directly inhibit any lipase activity remaining, thus contributing to an effective 'sparing' of lipid at a time when glycogen fermentation is favoured. At the end of the dive, when O_2 is abundant, the diving mammal is faced with the opposite problem of turning off glycolysis at the same time as it is activating fat metabolism.

5.2.12 How is glycogen 'spared' during aerobic periods?

Fortunately, the answer to this question is better understood. In mammals in general, it is now clear that during anaerobic/aerobic transition, when fatty acid oxidation is initiated, a number of profound fluctuations in various Krebs cycle intermediates occur. Of these, the percentage increase in citrate concentrations is unusually high and this metabolite serves to feedback inhibit PFK, this effectively blocking glycolysis when that block is appropriate (*see,* e.g. Williamson, 1965). The same 'information channel' is used in various tissues of the vertebrate, but as we have pointed out, muscle PFK is unusually citrate sensitive (about 10 times more so than, for example, the liver homologue), and thus in muscle this control interaction is perhaps most effective. As far as we know, the same control mechanism at this locus in glycolysis also operates in tissues of diving vertebrates (Storey and Hochachka, 1974d), but whereas this seems to be a sufficient mechanism in muscle of typical terrestrial mammals, it is by no means the only way to 'turn off' glycolysis during aerobic periods in diving vertebrates. In vertebrate divers, pyruvate kinase is also an allosteric enzyme, and is highly sensitive to citrate; this would supply an additional means for blocking glycolysis during periods of fat catabolism (Storey and Hochachka, 1974c). A third and most important mechanism for blocking glycolysis at this time involves alanine inhibition of pyruvate kinase, but a full appreciation of the physiological significance of this effect requires a brief digression into the nature of Krebs cycle activation during fatty acid oxidation.

It is of course important to realise that the 'end product' of the β-oxidation spiral is acetylCoA, which is channelled into the Krebs cycle at the citrate synthase catalysed reaction. In the rat, during anaerobic/aerobic transition, activation of the β-oxidation spiral leads to a momentary piling up of acetylCoA as OXA reserves for citrate synthesis are inadequate (Safer and Williamson, 1973). In a diving animal such a limitation could be crippling. Thus, the diving habit leads in muscle to another important metabolic requirement: an efficient source of OXA that can be 'turned on' during fatty acid oxidation and Krebs cycle activation. The source of OXA is aspartate via the aspartate aminotransferase step. In marine mammals, such as the porpoise, the activity of this enzyme in muscle is up to 17 times higher than in terrestrial species (Owen and Hochachka, 1974), and its catalytic properties are such as to favour OXA production in the mitochondria during anaerobic/aerobic transition (*Figure 5.6*). Glutamate, produced in the reaction, in turn transaminates with pyruvate to regenerate α-KGA, a process leading to alanine accumulation. The *total amount of alanine accumulated under such conditions is equal to the summed increase in concentration of all Krebs cycle intermediates* (Safer and Williamson, 1973). That is a fundamental insight, for it emphasises that alanine is singly perhaps the 'best' metabolite signal of the degree to which the Krebs cycle is activated. It is therefore not surprising that alanine is such a good inhibitor of PK in diving vertebrates (Storey and Hochachka, 1974c), for the greater the degree of Krebs cycle activation, the greater the degree to which PK is alanine-blocked and carbohydrate reserves are 'spared' for anaerobic excursions (*Figure 5.5*).

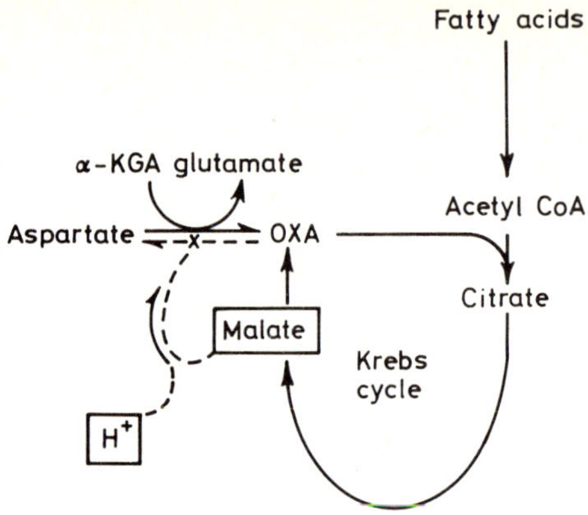

Figure 5.6 The favoured direction of aspartate aminotransferase function during the anaerobic/aerobic transition in diving vertebrates such as the porpoise. The aspartate affinity of the mitochondrial enzyme is about 5-fold higher than that of the cytoplasmic isozyme and it therefore competes effectively for intramitochondrial aspartate. Its K_m for OXA is about 10-fold higher than intramitochondrial OXA concentrations, a factor that also favours function in the direction of OXA production. Moreover, malate concentrations are increasing at this time, owing to Krebs cycle activation, and malate serves as a potent inhibitor of the backward reaction. A low pH occurring at the end of the dive further potentiates the malate control at this locus.

5.2.13 Summary: Key properties of muscle glycolysis in diving vertebrates

At this point, it is perhaps worth reiterating the basic theme running through the above discussion. First, muscle glycolysis even in the mundane laboratory rat, is already a most impressive 'anaerobic machine' and to improve further its capacity and efficiency in muscle of diving vertebrates seems to have involved only a modest number of modifications. Thus, the steady state concentrations of a few glycolytic enzymes are increased and this presumably reflects a higher overall glycolytic potential. To maintain control of this higher capacity, at least two additional modifications are now known: (a) muscle FDPase activity in divers is one of the highest thus far reported for any animal species (Storey and Hochachka, 1974a), the enzyme appearing to function in amplifying the AMP 'signal' for glycolytic activation, and (b) muscle pyruvate kinase, although occurring in lower specific activity, occurs as a regulatory enzyme, highly sensitive to feedforward activation by FDP and feedback inhibition by ATP, alanine, and citrate. The FDP feedforward activation presumably functions during aerobic/anaerobic transition occurring in the dive, while the feedback inhibition by ATP, citrate, and alanine (all acting in effect as 'end products' of aerobic, fatty acid catabolism) appears to function during anaerobic/aerobic transition at the end of diving. The latter characteristic emphasises another important consequence of the diving habit: a metabolic organisation that swings between an anaerobic, glycogen-based fermentation and an aerobic, fat-based oxidative metabolism. The control requirements imposed upon muscle by this metabolic organisation have led to the appearance of an unusually high level of aspartate aminotransferase. The mitochondrial form of this enzyme is designed to 'spark' the Krebs cycle by increasing OXA availability at the same time as acetylCoA is being produced by the β-oxidation spiral.

5.2.14 Anoxia tolerance of diving turtles

The kinds of molecular adaptations seen in diving mammals seem to reach their zenith in diving turtles, such as the green sea turtle (*Chelonia mydas*) and the red-eared turtle (*Pseudemys scripta*), which are capable of diving for many hours at a time, and, in some circumstances, for days at a time. These organisms come closer to becoming 'facultative anaerobes' than any other vertebrate group and it is therefore instructive to examine them in some detail.

Diving turtles as a group are several times more tolerant of anoxia than other reptiles, and are far more tolerant of anoxia than mammals. The green sea turtle, for example, can readily dive for at least two to several hours at a time (Hochachka *et al*., 1974) and is reputed to undergo 'resting' periods under water of at least several hours' duration. The red-eared turtle, *P. scripta,* survives dives as long as two weeks at 16–18°C despite a total lack of electron transport mediated O_2 consumption. During such anoxic dives of the red-eared turtle, blood glucose rises from 3 mM to about 60 mM, blood lactate rises to over 100 mM, and blood pH drops from 7.9 to 6.8 (*see* Storey and Hochachka, 1974c, d, for pertinent literature in this area). In the green sea turtle, following a two-hour anoxic dive, blood lactate concentrations rise to about 40 mM (Hochachka *et al*., 1974). Jackson (1968) has pointed out that after the first hour or so in a normal experimental 'dive' where the animal is fairly quiescent, all blood and tissue O_2 stores are fully depleted; yet the animal of course can continue its dive for many more hours on a glycogen-based fermentation whose measured capacity in caloric terms is about 15–20% of the animal's aerobic metabolism. Under such extreme diving conditions, *all the tissues of the body must be able to maintain their functions in anoxia.* Since the vertebrate heart and central nervous system typically display an absolute O_2 dependence, special attention has been focused on the heart of the diving turtle as an ideal vertebrate organ in which to sort out evolutionary mechanisms of anoxia adaptation. If our reasoning on this point is at all accurate, we would anticipate an overall metabolic organisation and control in the turtle heart rather comparable to that described above for skeletal muscle, possibly with even further exaggerations of a common theme. Is this expectation realised?

5.2.15 The anoxic turtle heart

Although the picture here is not yet entirely complete, there is a large enough body of information to indicate that we are on the right track. Thus, current information already confirms our observation that in compensating for temporary unavailability of O_2, a vertebrate activates anaerobic ATP yielding capacities by (a) increasing glycolytic potential, and (b) by modifying regulatory properties of key enzymes to keep that high potential under tight control. In diving turtles, the high glycolytic potential is seen both in glycogen and in enzyme levels. Thus, cardiac glycogen levels are 10 times higher in turtle than in terrestrial mammals and some two times higher than in diving mammals such as the seal (Daw, Wegner and Berne 1967; Kerem, Hammond and Elsner, 1973). This feature in itself creates a higher glycolytic potential and it is bolstered by high quantities of glycolytic enzymes. Key enzymes such as hexokinase, phosphorylase *a*, PFK, and LDH occur in substantially higher specific activities in turtle heart than in rat heart. Their integrated function is so efficient that transient changes in ATP/ADP ratios are not detectable during aerobic-anaerobic transitions (Hochachka and Storey, 1975). Whereas a drop in ATP concentration is an important means for de-inhibiting PFK and thus for 'turning on' glycolysis in the rat heart during aerobic-anaerobic transition, it is not a useful signal in the heart of a diving turtle; not surprisingly, turtle heart PFK is remarkably insensitive to ATP (Storey and Hochachka, 1974d). The usual regulatory role of ATP in this tissue is taken over by creatine phosphate, which is known to be rapidly depleted in anoxia (Clark and Miller, 1973), and which therefore supplies the tissue with a good measure of glycolytic requirements. Under aerobic conditions, creatine phosphate levels are high and serve to hold glycolytic rates low by potent PFK inhibition. In the absence of any other metabolic controls, a drop in creatine phosphate would serve to de-inhibit PFK and activate glycolysis. This de-inhibition, moreover, is greatly potentiated by FDP, one of the products of the PFK reaction. As FDP is known to momentarily accumulate during glycolytic activation, it leads to a further PFK activation and thus to an autocatalytic increase in the rate of its own production (*Figure 5.7*).

FDP control of glycolysis in the diving turtle is particularly pivotal, because, in addition to the above effects on PFK, it plays a key role in integrating PFK activity with that of PK, the next major control site in the glycolytic pathway (*Figure 5.7*). FDP control of PK is of two forms: firstly, it directly activates the enzyme by greatly increasing enzyme-substrate affinity, and secondly, it reverses and overrides inhibition of the enzyme by a variety of metabolites, ATP, alanine, and citrate probably being the most important. These control interactions are sufficient (a) to account for an exponential rate of change of PK activity during aerobic-anaerobic transition, and (b) to closely integrate the activities of PFK and PK, both major control sites in the glycolytic path (Hochachka and Storey, 1975).

In tissues such as the heart, which even in the diving turtle is supplied for as long as possible with oxygenated blood, important adjustments in lactate tolerance have occurred at least in part through evolutionary changes in heart-type LDH. Heart LDH is usually strongly substrate-inhibited so that whenever pyruvate concentrations rise, LDH is inhibited and pyruvate channelling into the Krebs cycle is in effect favoured; this characteristic is missing in turtle heart LDH, as in other diving species (Altman and Robin, 1969; Markert and Masui, 1970; Blix, 1971). Equally important, the LDH

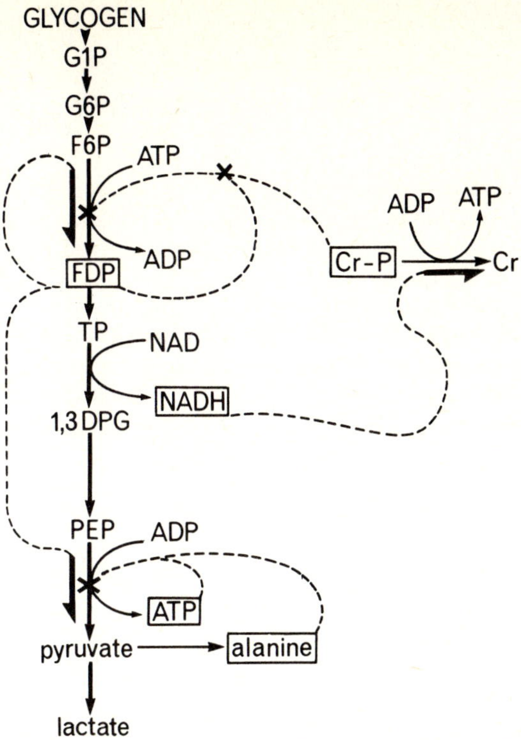

Figure 5.7 The diving turtle: control circuitry in glycolysis of the heart. Activation indicated by dark arrows; inhibition, by dark crosses. A major modification in this control set-up is the replacement of ATP inhibitory effects on PFK with creatine phosphate (Cr-P) inhibition. NADH activation of creatine kinase integrates creatine kinase activation with glycolytic activation. FDP takes on a particularly pivotal role in that it (1) reverses Cr-P inhibition, (2) product activates PFK, and (3) feedforward activates PK. Data from Storey and Hochachka (1974a, b) and from Storey (1975)

affinity for pyruvate decreases to the same range as in muscle. In other words, the kinetic properties of turtle heart LDH have been tailored to resemble the muscle isozyme, presumably because of the increased reliance of the heart upon anaerobic metabolism. In agreement with this conception, it can be readily demonstrated that the isolated turtle heart can sustain a (4 to 5-fold) greater contractile work load than can the rat heart under identical anoxic circumstances (Bing *et al*., 1972).

Through these impressive adjustments in the glycolytic machinery, the turtle can compensate for the temporary depletion of O_2 by a large increase in glycolytic production of ATP, and so can greatly extend the length of the dive as well as the amount of work that can be performed during the dive. However even in the diving turtle, where these mechanisms reach their zenith, the animal must re-surface sooner or later and repay his O_2 debt. Hence, his is a poor strategy for animals that invade anoxic environments on a sustained basis.

5.3 NON-GLYCOLYTIC MECHANISMS OF ANOXIA ADAPTATION

5.3.1 Storage substrates and anaerobic end products

In contrast to the vertebrates, many marine invertebrates have not become 'locked' into glycolysis as a sole device for anaerobic ATP formation. Rather, during anoxia they rely upon the *simultaneous* mobilisation of two energy sources — carbohydrates and amino acids. In consequence, they seldom produce lactate as a sole anaerobic end product; indeed lactate usually is not produced at all! Instead, a multiplicity of anaerobic end products are formed, the most important being (a) metabolic CO_2, (b) alanine, (c) succinate, and (d) propionate. Minor end products include other volatile fatty acids such as acetate, isovalerate, isobutyrate, and methylbutyrate (*see* Hochachka, Fields and Mustafa, 1973). How are these end products formed? What is their functional significance?

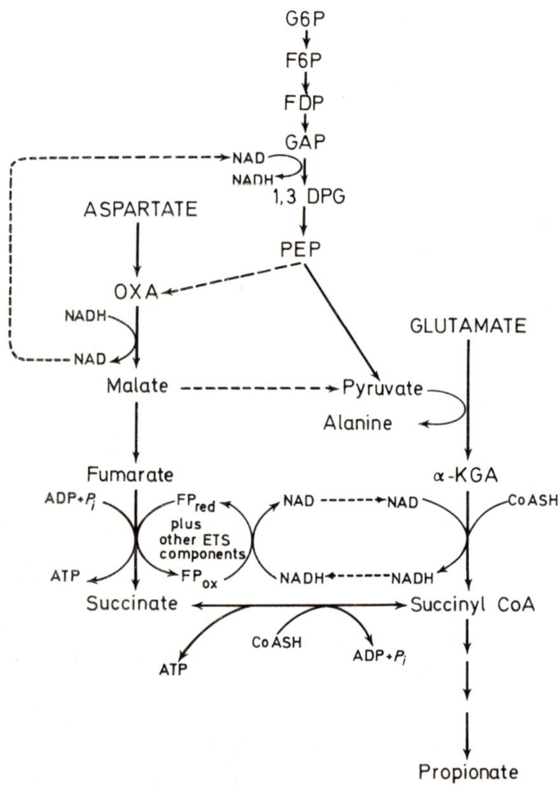

Figure 5.8 Mechanism of amino acid mobilisation both under aerobic and anaerobic conditions

5.3.2 Anaerobic metabolic organisation in bivalves

A detailed consideration of the available data from the oyster and other bivalves suggests a metabolic organisation (*Figure 5.8*) with at least four linear paths (Stokes and Awapara, 1968; de Zwann, 1976; Hochachka, 1976):

1. glucose→PEP→pyruvate→alanine→N-(1-carboxyethyl) alanine
2. glucose→PEP→OXA→malate→fumarate→succinate→→propionate
3. aspartate→OXA→malate→fumarate→succinate
4. glutamate→α-KGA→succinylCoA→succinate

In this organisation, the glycolytic pathway appears to be unchanged to the level of PEP, but at the PEP branchpoint the situation appears to depend upon the duration of anoxia (*Figure 5.9*). In isolated oyster hearts made anoxic for periods of up to an hour at 25°C, about 50% of glucose carbon flows to alanine, about 5% flows to succinate, while most of the rest appears in an unknown compound. Subsequently, Fields (1976) showed that the unknown compound is formed from pyruvate and alanine in an NADH-requiring enzyme reaction analogous to that catalysed by octopine dehydrogenase; N-(1-carboxyethyl)alanine is the presumed accumulating end product. Although a 1:1:1 depletion of pyruvate, alanine, and NADH has been clearly established, tests of the end-product structure are still in progress. This novel dehydrogenase occurs in highest titre in adductor muscle (about 70 μmole substrate consumed/min/g wet weight of muscle), at intermediate activities in heart, and lowest activities in mantle.

In addition, in the oyster heart, aspartate concentrations are high (about 15 mM), and these are depleted during anoxia (Collicutt, Fields and Hochachka, 1976). Most of the aspartate carbon flows to succinate; some accumulates as alanine. Currently, it appears that the OXA formed from either glucose or from aspartate behaves as a single metabolic pool, which is reduced to malate by cytoplasmic MDH. By comparison with other enzymes in oyster muscle, MDH occurs in high titre (about 100 units/g wet weight adductor muscle at 25°C) and, together with the above pyruvate-alanine dependent hydrogenase takes on the function of LDH in regenerating NAD for glycolysis. Not surprisingly, LDH is absent. Unlike the lactate formed in vertebrate tissues, the malate formed in oyster muscle does not accumulate, rather it is dehydrated to form fumarate which in turn is reduced to succinate in a reaction catalysed by 'fumarate reductase' and yielding a mole of ATP/mole of succinate formed. That is, fumarate in these tissues is thought to behave as a terminal electron acceptor (De Zoeten, Posthuma and Tipker, 1969).

To this point, it is important to emphasise, the system is in redox balance in the cytoplasm, but intramitochondrially, some oxidation reaction (or reactions) must be coupled with fumarate reduction. One candidate postulated for this job is the mobilisation of glutamate to α-ketoglutarate; the latter as substrate for α-ketoglutarate dehydrogenase is converted to succinylCoA and sets the stage for a substrate level phosphorylation in a reaction catalysed by succinic thiokinase:

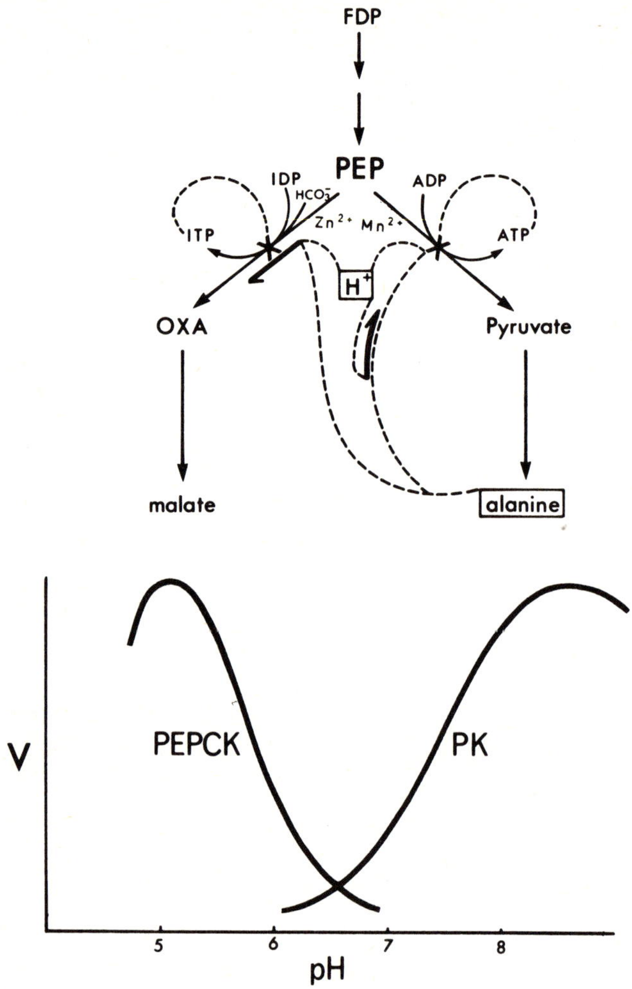

Figure 5.9 The PEP branchpoint in adductor muscle of the oyster. Under aerobic conditions, PEP is converted to pyruvate then catabolised to CO_2 and water by the Krebs cycle and electron transfer system. On transition to anoxia, alanine feedback inhibition, strongly potentiated by low pH, leads to PK inhibition with simultaneous feedback deinhibition of ITP-inhibited PEPCK. In the lower graph, relative velocity of the two competing reactions is plotted against pH; from the graph it is clear that dropping pH during anoxia also contributes to rechannelling PEP towards OXA at this branchpoint. (After Hochachka and Somero (1973), and Hochachka and Mustafa (1972)). In Mytilus, *a comparable control set up is believed to occur, but the transition appears to be of a more gradual nature (de Zwann, 1976). In adult* Ascaris, *PK is actually absent (Saz, 1971)*

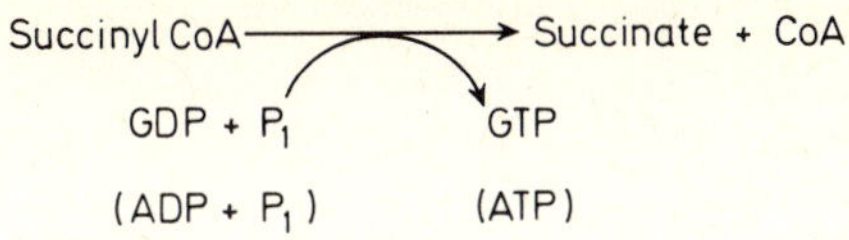

As in the Krebs cycle during aerobic metabolism, it is evident that in this scheme α-ketoglutarate dehydrogenase also must be functionally coupled in a 1:1 activity ratio with succinic thiokinase in order that CoASH be neither depleted nor accumulated (Hochachka, 1972; Hochachka, Fields and Mustafa, 1973). In oyster heart, recent studies (Collicutt, Fields, and Hochachka, 1976) have established that the glutamate → succinate path is substantially less active than the aspartate → succinate one; hence, for this tissue at least, the pathway certainly cannot represent a single, unique mechanism for supplying reducing equivalents to fumarate reductase. In other invertebrate facultative anaerobes, formally analogous pathways for the mobilisation of the branched chain amino acids (leucine, isoleucine, and valine) lead to the formation of a mole of ATP/mole of amino acid, with the release of volatile fatty acids (isovalerate, isobutyrate, methylbutyrate) as end products (*see* Hochachka, Fields and Mustafa, 1973). The ketocarboxylate dehydrogenase reactions in these pathways presumably would also form redox couples with fumarate reduction.

A close examination of *Figure 5.8* will indicate that as drawn this scheme (which ignores the pyruvate-alanine condensation reaction; its activity initially would presumably be limited by pyruvate and alanine) is in redox balance, if, and only if, for each 2 moles of PEP formed from glucose, 2 moles of aspartate and 2 moles of some α-ketocarboxylate (formed for example from glutamate, or one of the branched chain amino acids) are mobilised simultaneously. Indeed, such simultaneous mobilisation is insured by at least 2 mechanisms: (1) by the redox couples formed between MDH and triosephosphate dehydrogenase and between fumarate reduction and α-ketocarboxylate dehydrogenases and (2) by alanine aminotransferase. The latter, catalysing the reaction,

$$\text{pyruvate} + \text{glutamate} \rightarrow \alpha\text{-ketoglutarate} + \text{alanine}$$

also contributes to the coupling between carbohydrate and amino acid metabolism, since one substrate (pyruvate) derives at least in part from carbohydrate while the cosubstrate (glutamate) derives from the free amino acid pool. Furthermore, this coupling process explains one function for alanine as a major anaerobic end product in these organisms. Since the reaction is thermodynamically fully reversible, the kinetic properties of the enzyme in the oyster have been modified so as to favour unidirectional catalysis (Mustafa, 1975).

Mustafa has shown that in the forward direction, the oyster muscle enzyme displays an unusually high affinity for pyruvate but is largely unaffected by alanine (an apparent 'product activation' by alanine periodically observed was shown to be caused by contaminating amounts of the pyruvate-alanine dependent hydrogenase). In the reverse direction, the enzyme shows a low alanine affinity and is *product inhibited* by glutamate and probably by pyruvate (*Figure 5.10*). Thus, although thermodynamically

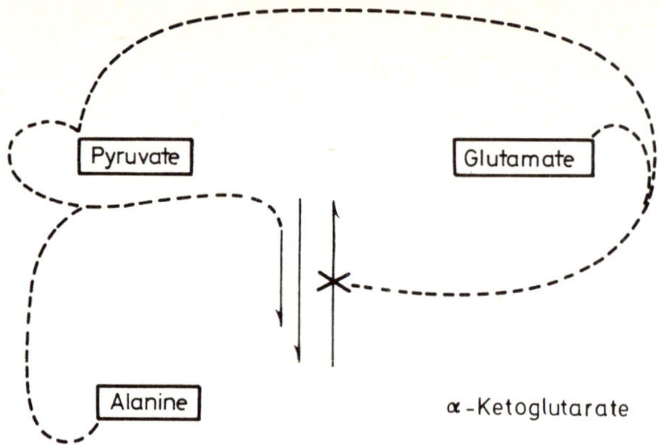

Figure 5.10 The control of alanine aminotransferase. Effective activation indicated by an arrow; inhibition by a cross. Two kinetic features, product inhibition by glutamate in the backward direction, and an extremely high affinity for pyruvate, can convert this enzyme reaction, which on thermodynamic grounds is fully reversible, into an essentially irreversible, one-way step. Data from Mustafa (unpublished data)

the reaction is freely reversible, the kinetic properties of the enzyme effectively promote unidirectional function for this kind of alanine aminotransferase. The pyruvate for the reaction arises either from pyruvate, if the pyruvate kinase step remains 'open', or from malate, a process catalysed by malic enzyme (Hochachka and Mustafa, 1972). Hence, it is evident that alanine formation may sometimes depend upon some exogenous source of malate. That source is aspartate, which is also fermented under these conditions; as aspartate concentrations fall alanine concentrations rise often in essentially a stoichiometric manner (DuPaul and Webb, 1971; Bayne, 1973). Aspartate mobilisation of course is initiated by a transamination:

$$\text{aspartate} + \alpha\text{-KGA} \rightarrow \text{glutamate} + \text{OXA}$$

The OXA is reduced to malate, as in the case of glucose fermentation. The reducing equivalents required for this reaction are regained by malic enzyme, and this reaction span thus is in redox balance. Finally, we come to the question of the origin of propionate which often accumulates as the major anaerobic end product in facultative anaerobic animals. Unfortunately, the data here are not too clear, although it seems that succinate is the ultimate source of propionate (De Zoeten, Posthuma and Tipker, 1969) and in *Mytilus* in prolonged (about 2–3 day) anoxia, propionate accumulates as a major end product (*see* de Zwann, 1976). Currently, we believe that malate and α-KGA enter the mitochondrion in exchange for succinate. Recent evidence on mitochondrial accumulation of anions in fact is consistent with this conception (Klingenberg, 1970); what is more, this transport coupling across the mitochondrial membrane stoichiometrically accounts for 2 moles of succinate formed per mole of malate and per mole of α-KGA entering the mitochondrion. The succinate released into the cytoplasm can be acetylated to succinylCoA, which can then be converted to propionylCoA and ultimately propionate. All the enzymes for this pathway occur in the cytoplasm and all are relatively reversible. Per mole of propionate formed by this route, 2 moles of ATP are netted. This is a substantial increase in ATP yield over schemes which end with succinate, and may explain why in many of these organisms propionate is often the major anaerobic end product formed (Saz, 1971; de Zwann, 1976).

5.3.3 Energy yield in anoxic oyster muscle

A comparison of the energy yield in oyster muscle relative to that of classical glycolysis is difficult because different substrates are used and different end products accumulate. Some of the substrates, such as aspartate, are not fermented by vertebrate muscle; propionate and other volatile fatty acids never are formed as anaerobic end products.

However, when the system is in redox balance (a presumed necessary condition for extended anoxic function), the overall yield of utilisable energy in the oyster muscle is 7 moles ATP/mole of G6P; simultaneously, 2 moles of aspartate and 2 moles of glutamate are converted to succinate. By comparison, the yield in mammalian muscle of course is 3 moles ATP/mole G6P. In considering the relative energetic efficiency in these organisms, it is useful to recall that in obligate anaerobes (such as the well studied *Ascaris lumbricoides*), PK is often not present (Saz, 1971). Deletion of this arm of the PEP branchpoint reduces glucose fermentation to a linear path, either G6P → succinate, or in some cases, G6P → propionate; in the first case, the energy yield is 5 moles ATP/mole G6P, while in the second case it probably is 7 moles ATP/mole G6P. That is, the trend in these organisms is for maximising energetic efficiency. Power output (yield of ATP/unit time) on the other hand, is probably fairly low. Isolated anoxic oyster hearts, for example, convert only about 1 μM glucose to alanine (aspartate to succinate)/g wet weight/s, equivalent to less than 1μM ATP/g/s. By comparison, trout muscle can convert 40 μM glucose to lactate/g/s during the first minute or two of burst work; this is equivalent to about 13 μM ATP/g/s, a value about an order of magnitude higher than observed in the oyster (*see* Hochachka, 1976, for further discussion of this area).

In summary, it appears that invertebrate facultative anaerobes utilise an exploitative strategy of anoxia adaptation allowing them to invade anoxic environments and sustain anoxic local conditions for time periods that as a fraction of their life time can be viewed as indefinite. The primary rule of design is an energy metabolism of relatively high efficiency (relatively high ATP yield/mole substrates) but low power output (low ATP yield/unit time), and these organisms are characteristically sessile or sluggish. Other features of this metabolism include:

1. High concentrations of multiple substrates (mainly carbohydrates and free amino acids) but relatively low levels of enzymes (allowing an efficient but low rate of fermentation).
2. Close regulation of the kind of enzyme present (e.g. PEPCK vs. PK, no LDH, a regulatory alanine aminotransferase, a 'fumarate reductase' etc.).

3. The use of mitochondrial metabolism for anaerobic purposes, a characteristic that singly, most strongly contrasts this metabolic organisation with highly O_2 dependent systems or classical glycolysis.

5.3.4 Conflicting metabolic demands imposed by simultaneous requirements for anaerobiosis and hyperosmotic regulation

In the introduction to this chapter we stressed that environmental adaptations to a particular physical, chemical or biological parameter must always be made within the context of the environmental situation as a whole, i.e. an organism cannot select its habitat strictly on the basis of a single parameter. The 'best' thermal regime, for example, may be highly unsatisfactory in terms of food availability or oxygen content. In this brief section of our chapter we wish to outline what appears to be a difficult metabolic problem for an invertebrate organism such as an estuarine mollusc which has an anaerobic metabolism like that of the oyster and which adapts to increasing osmotic concentration of its medium by adding increased concentrations of amino acids to its intracellular fluids.

The use of amino acids to adjust the intracellular osmolarity is a common 'strategy' among marine invertebrates (Hochachka and Somero, 1973; *see also* Chapter 6). Of critical importance in this process is the generation of high concentrations of glutamate, via the glutamate dehydrogenase (GDH) reaction:

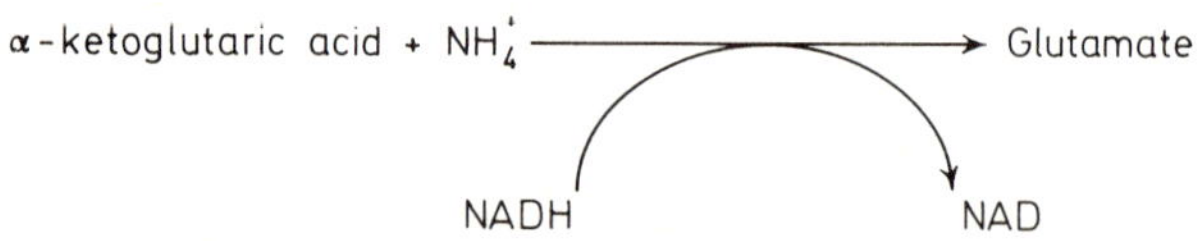

At this locus in metabolism we find a clear conflict between the demands imposed by anoxia and those imposed by increasing external (and blood) osmolarity. During anoxia, the mollusc requires a high turnover rate of α-KGA for energy metabolism. During hyperosmotic regulation, glutamate must be formed at the expense of α-KGA. The role of glutamate during hyperosmotic regulation is that of an amino group donor, for glutamate is the common intermediate through which amino groups are channelled to α-keto acids. Thus, during hyperosmotic regulation in many invertebrates, the amino group of glutamate is donated to pyruvate, forming alanine, or to other α-keto acids. Failure to maintain adequate glutamate concentrations during times of hyperosmotic stress would seem to preclude adequate osmotic regulation.

A second site of metabolic conflict between anaerobiosis and osmotic regulation is at the pyruvate kinase (PK) locus. In the anaerobic metabolism scheme of an organism like the oyster, decreased oxygen availability leads to the turning-off of PK (*Figure 5.4*), in order to direct PEP to OXA. During hyperosmotic stress, however, a high level of PK activity is required to generate pyruvate for alanine formation. Indeed, increases in intracellular potassium, which are likely to occur during hyperosmotic stress, will stimulate PK. During simultaneous stress from anoxia and increased osmotic content of the medium, the PK reaction would seem to be subject to a bewildering array of conflicting metabolic signals. Falling pH, owing to anoxia, would inhibit the enzyme; rising potassium content would activate the enzyme, and under these conditions it would seem very difficult to satisfy all metabolic and osmotic demands at once.

A further problem during simultaneous anoxic and osmotic stress would arise owing to the drawing-off of glycolytic intermediates for amino acid synthesis. 3-phosphoglyceric acid (which can be converted to serine and glycine) and pyruvate would be withdrawn from the catabolic channels just when a large glycolytic energy demand is occurring.

Lastly, redox balance might also be difficult to achieve under these conflicting demands for metabolic flow.

What 'solutions' to these problems might an estuarine mollusc or other invertebrate use? To our knowledge, this potential metabolic 'confrontation' has neither been appreciated nor studied. One approach to resolving this type of problem is suggested by the 'strategy' used in many other cases in which conflicting metabolic demands are handled by an organism, i.e. spatially separate the conflicting reactions. Thus, an organism having to degrade glucose and reform glucose from low molecular weight intermediates performs these tasks in different tissues. In other cases of metabolic conflict, different cellular compartments may be used. Perhaps in an invertebrate which might experience simultaneous anoxic and hyperosmotic conditions — and we should emphasise that such an experience seems likely to be uncommon — the reactions leading to anaerobic production of ATP and elevated amino acid levels are somehow separated in the cell or among different tissues, so the organism can satisfy both, potentially conflicting, demands on its metabolic reactions.

5.4 NON-GLYCOLYTIC MECHANISMS OF ANAEROBIOSIS IN VERTEBRATES

5.4.1 Introduction

To determine whether diving vertebrates such as turtles and seals are capable of channelling significant fractions of carbohydrate and amino acid along the pathways just described for certain invertebrates requires two types of investigation. First, a detailed look at the amounts and kinetic properties of the enzymes involved, for example, in directing PEP towards OXA is necessary. Second, measurement of the concentrations of anaerobic end product, such as succinate and alanine, can serve as an important clue as to whether the enzymes capable of sustaining the oyster-type of anaerobiosis are, in fact, operating in the anaerobic vertebrate.

Data of the second class are now appearing in the literature. Before discussing these data, one point should be stressed. Succinic acid, one of the major end products of the elaborate anaerobic scheme of organisms like the oyster and therefore one of the key indices of the type of anaerobic activity occurring in the organism, is an important component of the Krebs cycle reaction and is not, like lactate, a dead-end product. The lactate formed during anaerobiosis is largly channelled through the gluconeogenic reactions to reform glucose (in the vertebrates, this reaction sequence occurs largely in the liver). Lactate removal from the blood is a relatively slow process which is highly dependent on the rates of activity of the gluconeogenic reactions which, in turn, are dependent on high energy phosphate compounds regenerated following return of oxygen.

For succinate, a very different fate occurs when oxygen supplies return. Being a mainline rather than a dead-end product, succinate is not flushed out of the cells during anaerobiosis except in relatively small quantities. When oxygen returns, succinate can be rapidly utilised by all cell types in the Krebs cycle sequence. To detect succinate accumulations, two experimental approaches are possible. First, one could measure intracellular succinate concentrations immediately after anaerobiosis. Second, one could measure blood succinate immediately after anaerobiosis in an organism which greatly reduces blood supply to a particular tissue during anaerobiosis. Return of oxygen and return of blood flow to the tissue will lead to a rapid and transient flushing-out of at least a small portion of the succinate formed during anaerobiosis.

In this context, we examined blood concentrations of various metabolites prior to and following diving in the green sea turtle, the common harbour seal, the sea lion, and the porpoise (Hochachka *et al*., 1974). We found that when O_2 availability to working muscle in these diving animals is limited by peripheral vasoconstriction, the muscle ferments carbohydrate and amino acids simultaneously, in effect coupling two additional energy-yielding reactions to those of glycolysis. Multiple anaerobic end products accumulate as a result. Succinate is the chief end product of anaerobic amino acid catabolism, alanine is a minor end product, while pyruvate and lactate are produced by glycolysis. During recovery following diving, increased blood concentrations of all four metabolites can be readily measured (*Figure 5.11*).

5.4.2 Quantitative significance

What, then, is the quantitative significance of amino acid fermentation in the diving vertebrate? It will be noted (*Figure 5.11*) that blood succinate concentrations following diving are about 1/100 the concentrations of lactate. If we assume that the lactate : succinate concentration ratio in the blood accurately reflects the tissue ratio, then amino acid fermentation produces about 1/100 as much ATP as does glycolysis. However, any estimate of its contribution to anaerobic energy metabolism that is based on blood succinate concentrations must approach an absolute minimum, and it is therefore clear that any further assessment of the contribution of amino acid fermentation to the diving energy budget of these animals must await muscle biopsy studies.

In this connection it is worth emphasising that such studies have been

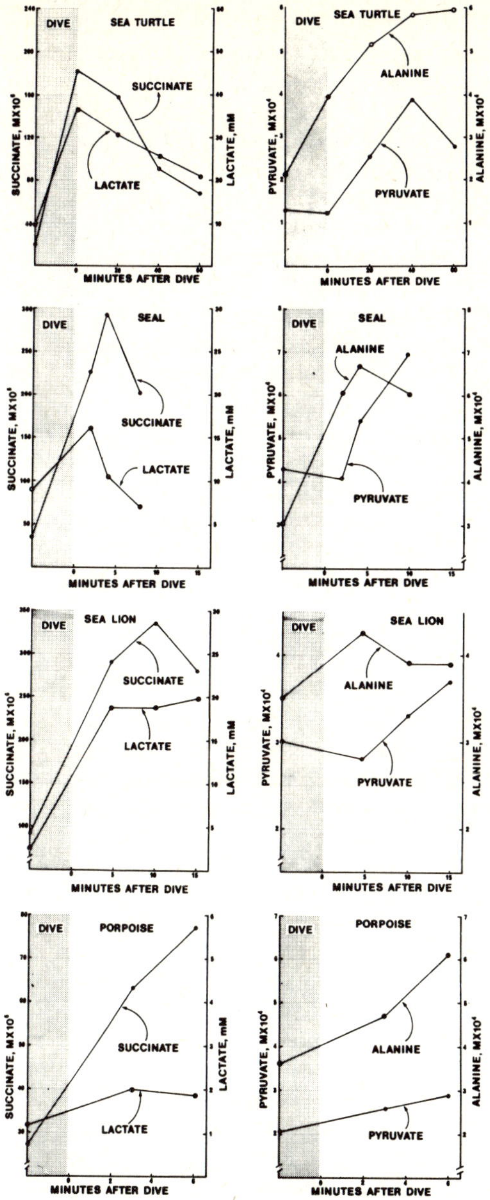

Figure 5.11 The effect of diving on the venous blood concentrations of succinate and lactate (left graphs) and of pyruvate and alanine (right graphs) in the sea turtle, the harbour seal, the sea lion, and the porpoise. Diving time periods and conditions given in Hochachka et al. *(1974)*

done on other mammals, such as the rat (Penney and Cascarano, 1970; Kandrashova and Chahoverts, 1971), the guinea pig (de Silva and Cazorla, 1973), and the diving turtle (Penney, 1974), as well as in another reptile, *Testudo hermanni* (Arillo and De Giuli, 1970). In many instances of anoxic or hypoxic stress, succinate has been shown to accumulate, but peak concentrations again are 1–2 orders of magnitude lower than are those for lactate. K. B. Storey has argued that this is a 'biologically sensible' strategy for an animal that repays an oxygen debt following anoxic excusions. His argument (Storey, personal communication) emphasises that the conversion of PEP to succinate by the oyster pathway yields 2 moles of ATP/mole of succinate formed, while the conversion of PEP to succinate by the aerobic (Krebs cycle) route yields 11 moles of ATP/mole of succinate formed. That is, if the animal can afford to 'wait out' the anoxia by storing pyruvate (as lactate) and then catabolising that pyruvate to succinate by aerobic routes, it gains over 5 times the amount of useful energy than it would if it converted pyruvate to succinate during actual anoxia. For this reason, Storey argues, we may find that amino acid fermentation is only of peripheral importance to energy metabolism in most vertebrate species. Although this conclusion is consistent with small free amino acid pools in vertebrate muscles and may therefore be valid with regard to ATP production, it may overlook an important potential role of amino acids in redox regulation during the dive.

5.4.3 Role of alanine and aspartate amino transferases in muscle redox balance

Whereas the above pathways may not significantly contribute to overall energy metabolism, they appear to play a highly significant role in maintenance of redox balance in glycolysis towards the end of diving. At such times, lactate concentrations are already high, so high that through mass action effects further pyruvate → lactate conversion rates become retarded and pyruvate either is transaminated to alanine or accumulates; following diving, pyruvate is washed out into the blood and increased levels can be readily measured in several diving species (*Figure 5.11*). This situation leaves glycolysis out of redox balance (per μmole of pyruvate accumulating, a μmole of NADH must be oxidised by some reaction other than that catalysed by LDH) and could not be tolerated by a diving animal if its dive is to continue. Owen and Hochachka (1974) have proposed that in porpoise muscle this situation is at least partially resolved during extreme anoxia by a functionally 1:1 coupling between alanine and aspartate aminotransferases. For this purpose, alanine aminotransferase occurs in porpoise muscle at concentrations up to 15-fold higher than in terrestrial mammals (Owen and Hochachka, 1974), and it effectively competes for pyruvate; as a result, alanine accumulates as an additional anaerobic end product in the porpoise (Hochachka *et al.,* 1974). Owen and Hochachka (1974) suggested that it is coupled to aspartate aminotransferase, which also occurs in unusually high titre, in order to account for the correlation between alanine accumulation and aspartate depletion (Hochachka, Fields and

Mustafa, 1973; Owen and Hochachka, 1974; Hochachka *et al*., 1974). In this scheme, glutamate and α-KGA would be depleted only to the extent to which the two pathways go to completion; i.e. to the extent to which succinate accumulates. If the pathways do not go to completion, glutamate and α-KGA would appear to be 'tumbled' between alanine and aspartate aminotransferases. Furthermore, this arrangement sets the stage for MDH catalysed reduction of OXA (the alternate product of the aspartate aminotransferase step) to malate. It assures a stoichiometric relationship between pyruvate accumulation and malate accumulation. That is, it assures a mechanism that in effect 'turns on' MDH to the degree necessary for balancing redox in the glycolytic path, because *the signal (pyruvate accumulation) for turning on this transaminase couple is also the measure of the degree to which the system is out of redox balance.* For this reason, we would anticipate that the absolute concentration changes in pyruvate, alanine, aspartate, plus the summed concentrations of malate, fumarate, succinate should all be in the same range, but that these need show no relationship with lactate accumulations. A close examination of the data in *Figure 5.11* will indicate that such in fact is the case. Thus, in muscle of the diving mammal, Nature seems to have designed an elegant transaminase-based mechanism for assuring that glycolytic function can be extended well beyond the inherent limitations of the last step in the pathway — that catalysed by LDH and leading to the production of lactic acid.

5.5 CONCLUDING COMMENTS AND GENERALISATION

As 'standard equipment', all organisms are supplied with a core of metabolic reactions which do not depend on the availability of molecular oxygen. The 'option' of aerobic metabolism has enabled organisms to attain levels of metabolic efficiency and physiological activity far in excess of those levels characteristic of organisms which lack the capacity to degrade nutrients to CO_2 and H_2O. Nonetheless, a diverse array of animals are able to sustain their energy needs for long time periods in the absence of oxygen at the cellular level. Their 'strategies' for accomplishing these feats are largely the additions of metabolic 'extras' to the pre-existing anaerobic reactions common to all organisms.

In overview terms, we can regard anaerobic adaptations at the enzymic level to entail but a small number of changes. First, the concentrations of enzymes and substrates for anaerobic reactions such as those of glycolysis may be raised to relatively high levels. Second, the kinetic properties of the enzymes of anaerobic pathways may be altered to promote (a) high rates of catalysis and (b) high regulatory efficiencies, such that rapid and quantitative shifts from low to high activity are possible. Lastly, organisms may increase their anaerobic 'options' by adding additional reactions to further the efficiency of energy (ATP) extraction and reduce the toxicity of the end products of anaerobiosis.

Although we are now able to appreciate the basic 'strategies' of anaerobiosis, we are still relatively ignorant about the detailed applications to which these basic mechanisms of adaptation have been put, especially in the case of vertebrates. Often our ignorance in cases like these stems largely from the narrow, non-comparative approach normally used in teaching biochemistry. The 'metabolic map' normally presented to the beginning biochemistry student is an abstraction, that either deletes or fails to consider the many routes and by-ways of metabolism used by 'lesser' organisms, and gives a distortedly simple view of the metabolic landscape. By examining the manners in which different marine organisms thrive under anoxic conditions, we can perhaps achieve an unique appreciation of both the complexity and the aesthetics of this landscape.

REFERENCES

ALTMAN, M. and ROBIN, E. D. (1969). 'Survival during prolonged anaerobiosis as a function of an unusual adaptation involving LDH subunits', *Comp. Biochem. Physiol.,* **30,** 1179–1187

ARILLO, A. and DE GIULI, A. M. (1970). 'Variazioni del ciclo di Krebs in anaerobiosi. I. Studi su *Testudo hermanni', Bollettino dei Musei e Degli Ist. Biol. Dell'Univ. de Genova,* **38,** 43–63

BAUMANN, P. and WRIGHT, B. E. (1968). 'Phosphofructokinase in a slime mold', *Biochem.,* **7,** 3653–3659

BAYNE, B. L. (1973). 'Aspects of the metabolism of *Mytilus edulis* during starvation', *Proc. 7th European Marine Biol. Symp.*

BING, O. H. L., BROOKS, W. W., INAMDAR, A. N. and MESSER, J. V. (1972). 'Tolerance of isolated heart muscle to hypoxia: turtle vs. rat', *Am. J. Physiol.,* **223,** 1481–1485

BLAZKA, P. (1958). 'The anaerobic metabolism of fish', *Physiol. Zool.,* **31,** 117–128

BLIX, A. (1971). 'Lactate dehydrogenases in diving mammals', *Comp. Biochem. Physiol.,* **40A,** 805–809

CLARK, V. M. and MILLER, A. Jr. (1973). 'Creatine phosphate levels in the anoxic turtle heart', *Comp. Biochem. Physiol.,* **44A,** 55–61

COLLICUTT, G. (1975). M.Sc. Thesis, University of British Columbia, Vancouver

COLLICUTT, J., FIELDS, J. H. A. and HOCHACHKA, P. W. (1976). 'Anaerobic metabolism of oyster heart', *Comp. Biochem. Physiol.* (In the press)

DANFORTH, W. H. (1965). 'Activation of glycolytic pathway in muscle', 287–297. In: *Control of Energy Metabolism.* Ed. B. Chance, R. Estabrook and J. R. Williamson. Academic Press, New York

DAW, J. C., WEGNER, D. P. and BERNE, R. M. (1967). 'Relationship between cardiac glycogen and tolerance to anoxia in the western painted turtle, *Chrysemys picta* (Bellii)', *Comp. Biochem. Physiol.,* **33,** 69–74

DESILVA, E. M. and CAZORLA, A. (1973). 'Lactate, α-GP, and Krebs cycle in sea-level and high altitude native guinea pigs', *Am. J. Physiol.,* **224,** 669–672

DE ZOETEN, L. W., POSTHUMA, D. and TIPKER, J. (1969). 'Intermediary metabolism of the liver fluke, *Fasciola hepatica', Hoppe-Seyler's Z. Physiol. Chem.,* **350,** 683–690.

DE ZWANN, A. (1976). 'The metabolism of invertebrate facultative anaerobes', *Br. Biochem. Soc. Symp.,* **41.** (In the press)

DRUMMOND, G. I. (1971). 'Microenvironment and enzyme function: control of energy metabolism during muscle work', *Am. Zool.,* **11,** 83–97

DUPAUL., W. D. and WEBB, K. L. (1971). 'Free amino acid accumulation in isolated gill tissue of *Mya arenaria', Arch. Int. Physiol. Biochim.,* **79,** 327–336

EDINGTON, D. W., WARD, G. R. and SAVILLE, W. A. (1973). 'Energy metabolism of working muscle: concentration profiles of selected metabolites', *Am. J. Physiol.,* **224,** 1375–1380

EVERSE, J. and KAPLAN, N. O. (1974). 'Lactate dehydrogenases: structure and function', *Adv. Enzymology.* Ed. A. Meister. **37,** 61–133

FIELDS, J. H. A. (1976). Ph.D. Thesis, University of British Columbia, Vancouver

GEORGE, J. C. and RONALD, K. (1973). 'The harp seal, *Pagophilus groenlandicus.* XXV. Ultrastructure and metabolic adaptation of skeletal muscle', *Can. J. Zool.,* **51,** 833–858

HEILMEYER, L. M., MEYER, F., HASCHKE, R. and FISCHER, E. H. (1970). 'Control of phosphorylase activity in a muscle glycogen particle', *J. biol. Chem.*, **245,** 6649–6656

HELMREICH, E., DANFORTH, W. H., KARPATKIN, S. and CORI, C. F. (1965). 'The response of the glycolytic system of anaerobic frog sartorius muscle to electrical stimulation', 299–312. In: *Control of Energy Metabolism.* Ed. B. Chance, R. Estabrook and J. R. Williamson. Academic Press, New York

HOCHACHKA, P. W. (1972). 'Enzymatic adaptations to deep sea life', *Oregon State Univ. Biol. Colloquium,* Oregon State University Press. (In the press)

HOCHACHKA, P. W. (1976). 'Design of enzymatic and metabolic machinery to fit life style and environment', *Br. Biochem. Soc. Symp.,* **41,** 3-31

HOCHACHKA, P. W., FREED, J. M., SOMERO, G. N. and PROSSER, C. L. (1970). 'Control sites in glycolysis of crustacean muscle', *Int. J. Biochem.,* **2,** 125–130

HOCHACHKA, P. W., FIELDS, J. and MUSTAFA, T. (1973). 'Animal life without oxygen: basic biochemical mechanisms', *Am. Zool.,* **13,** 543–555

HOCHACHKA, P. W. and MUSTAFA, T. (1972). 'Invertebrate facultative anaerobiosis', *Science,* **178,** 1056–1060

HOCHACHKA, P. W., OWEN, T. G., ALLEN, J. F. and WHITTOW, G. C. (1974). 'Multiple end products of anaerobiosis in diving vertebrates', *Comp. Biochem. Physiol.,* **50B,** 17-22

HOCHACHKA, P. W. and SOMERO, G. (1973). *Strategies of Biochemical Adaptation,* 18–76. W. B. Saunders Press, Philadelphia, PA.

HOCHACHKA, P. W. and STOREY, K. B. (1975). 'Metabolic consequences of diving in animals and man', *Science,* **187,** 613-621

JACKSON, D. (1968). 'Metabolic depression on O_2 depletion in the diving turtle', *J. Appl. Physiol,* **24,** 503–509

KANDRASHOVA, M. N. and CHAHOVERTS, N. R. (1971). 'Succinic acid in skeletal muscle during intense activity and rest', *Doklady Acad. Nauk SSR,* **198,** 243–246

KEREM, D., HAMMOND, D. and ELSNER, R. (1973). 'Tissue glycogen levels in the Weddell seal', *Comp. Biochem. Physiol.,* **45A,** 731–736

KLINGENBERG, M. (1970). 'Transport of cations across the mitochondrial membrane', *Essays Biochem.,* **6,** 125–159

LOWRY, O. and PASSONNEAU, J. (1966). 'Brain phosphofructokinase', *J. biol. Chem.,* **241,** 2268–2276

MANGUM, C. P. (1973). 'Responses of aquatic invertebrates to declining O_2 conditions', *Am. Zool.,* **13,** 529–542

MANSOUR, T. (1972). 'Phosphofructokinase', *Current Topics Cell. Regulation,* **5,** 1–47

MARKERT, C. L. and MASUI, Y. (1970). 'Lactate dehydrogenase in the penguin', *J. exp. Zool.,* **172,** 121146

MUSTAFA, T. (1975). 'The catalytic and regulatory properties of adductor muscle alanine aminotransferase from the oyster', *Comp. Biochem. Physiol.* (In the press)

NEWSHOLME, E. A. (1972). 'Control of phosphofructokinase in muscle', *Cardiol.,* **56,** 22–30

NEWSHOLME, E. A., CRABTREE, B., HIGGINS, S. J., THORNTON, S. D. and START, C. (1972). 'The activities of FDPase in flight muscles of the bumblebee and the role of this enzyme in heat generation', *Biochem. J.,* **128,** 89–97

OWEN, T. G. and HOCHACHKA, P. W. (1974). 'Purification and properties of alanine and aspartate transaminases from dolphin muscle', *Biochem. J.,* **143,** 541-553

PENNEY, D. G. (1974). 'Effects of prolonged diving during anoxia in the turtle *Pseudemys scripta elegans*', *Comp. Biochem. Physiol.,* **47A,** 933–941

PENNEY, D. G. and CASCARANO, J. (1970). 'Anaerobic rat heart', *Biochem. J.,* **118,** 221–227

SACKTOR, B. (1970). 'Control mechanisms in intermediary metabolism of insect flight muscle', *Adv. Insect. Physiol.,* **7,** 267–347

SAFER, B. and WILLIAMSON, J. R. (1973). 'Mitochondrial-cytosolic interactions in perfused rat heart', *J. biol. Chem.,* **248,** 2570–2579

SANADI, D. R. and FLUHARTY, A. L. (1963). 'The energy-yielding oxidation of NADH by fumarate', *Biochem.,* **2,** 523–528

SAZ, H. (1971). 'Facultative anaerobiosis in the invertebrates: Pathways and control systems', *Am. Zool.,* **11,** 125–135

SCRUTTON, M. C. and UTTER, M. F. (1968). 'Regulation of glycolysis and gluconeogenesis in animal tissues', *Ann. Rev. Biochem.,* **37,** 249–302

SIMON, L. M. and ROBIN, E. D. (1972). 'Relationship between pyruvate kinase activity and glycolytic capacity', *Int. J. Biochem.*, **3,** 329–335

SIMON, L. M., ROBIN, E. D., ELSNER, R., VAN KESSEL, A. L. G. J. and THEODORE, J. (1974). 'A biochemical basis for differences in maximal diving times in aquatic mammals', *Comp. Biochem. Physiol,* **47B,** 209–215

SOMERO, G. N. (1973). 'Thermal modulation of pyruvate metabolism in the fish *Gillichthys mirabilis:* the role of lactate dehydrogenase', *Comp. Biochem. Physiol.,* **44B,** 205–209

SOMERO, G. N. and HOCHACHKA, P. W. (1968). 'The effect of temperature on the catalytic and regulatory properties of pyruvate kinases of the rainbow trout and the Antarctic fish, *Trematomus', Biochem. J.,* **110,** 395–400

STOKES, T. and AWAPARA, J. (1968). 'Alanine and succinate as end products of glucose degradation in some invertebrates', *Comp. Biochem. Physiol.,* **25,** 883–892

STOREY, K. B. and HOCHACHKA, P. W. (1974a). 'Glycolytic enzymes in muscle of the pacific dolphin: role of pyruvate kinase in aerobic-anaerobic transition during diving', *Comp. Biochem. Physiol.,* **49B,** 119–128

STOREY, K. B. and HOCHACHKA, P. W. (1974b). 'Activation of muscle glycolysis: a role for creatine phosphate in phosphofructokinase regulation', *FEBS Lett.,* **46,** 337–339

STOREY, K. B. and HOCHACHKA, P. W. (1974c). 'Enzymes of energy metabolism in a vertebrate facultative anaerobe. Turtle heart pyruvate kinase', *J. biol. Chem.,* **249,** 1423–1427

STOREY, K. B. and HOCHACHKA, P. W. (1974d). 'Enzymes of energy metabolism in a vertebrate facultative anaerobe. Turtle heart phosphofructokinase', *J. biol. Chem.,* **249,** 1417–1422

TEJWANI, G. A. and RAMAIAH, A. (1970). 'Properties of phosphofructokinase from the jejunum', *Biochem. J.,* **125,** 507–512

TEJWANI, G. A., RAMAIAH, A. and ANANTHANARAYANAN, M. (1973). 'Regulation of glycolysis in muscle. The role of ammonium and synergism among the positive effectors of phosphofructokinase', *Arch. Biochem. Biophys.,* **158,** 195–199

WALD, G. (1964). 'The origins of life', *Proc. Natl. Acad. Sci. (USA),* **52,** 595–611

WARREN, L. G. and POOLE, W. J. (1970). 'Biochemistry of the dog hookworm. Nature and origin of the excreted fatty acids', *Exp. Parasitol.,* **27,** 408–416

WHITE, H. B. III and KAPLAN, N. O. (1972). 'Separate physiological roles for two isozymes of NAD-linked glycerol-3-phosphate dehydrogenase in chicken', *J. molec. Evol.,* **1,** 158–172

WILLIAMSON, J. R. (1965). 'Metabolic control in the perfused rat heart', 333–346. In: *Control of Energy Metabolism.* Ed. B. Chance, R. Estabrook and J. R. Williamson. Academic Press, New York

Six

Physiological adaptation to life in estuaries

A. P. M. LOCKWOOD
Department of Oceanography, University of Southampton

6.1 INTRODUCTION

The marine environment encompasses a wide range of conditions in respect of temperature, oxygen levels and salinity. It is rare, however, for the properties to change locally with any speed and, when this does happen, as a result of exceptional meteorological conditions, considerable mortality often occurs in affected areas (Brongersma-Sanders, 1957). For example, the warm current passing southwards from the Gulf of Panama occasionally extends its range down the South American coast beyond 12°S and into the area normally occupied by the cold Peruvian current. Massive kills of marine life follow such visitations of 'El Nino'. Conversely, unusually cold water conditions, such as occurred round British coasts in the winter of 1962/3 can also result in mortality of some species. Abrupt dilution of the water, as produced on the Great Barrier Reef at Bowen following heavy rain in 1918 proved fatal to many oceanic organisms and the reef had still not fully recovered by 1958.

In contrast with the relative stability of the sea, the waters of estuaries, and in particular the brackish ponds and ditches of salt marshes, are characterised by sudden and often extensive changes of salinity and temperature, *Figure 6.1(a)* (*see also* Chapter 1). In addition, a measure of oxygen depletion can occur in some brackish waters following temperature changes, or in the presence of a heavy organic load.

Local geographic, meteorological and hydrological conditions determine the magnitude and rate of change of salinity in estuaries and the latter may range in type from the virtually stable salinity gradient state, found in an inland sea such as the Baltic (*Figure 6.1(b)*), to the marked changes occurring during each tidal cycle in a salt-marsh gully or at Spring Tides in salt marsh pools. Organisms inhabiting such physiologically demanding

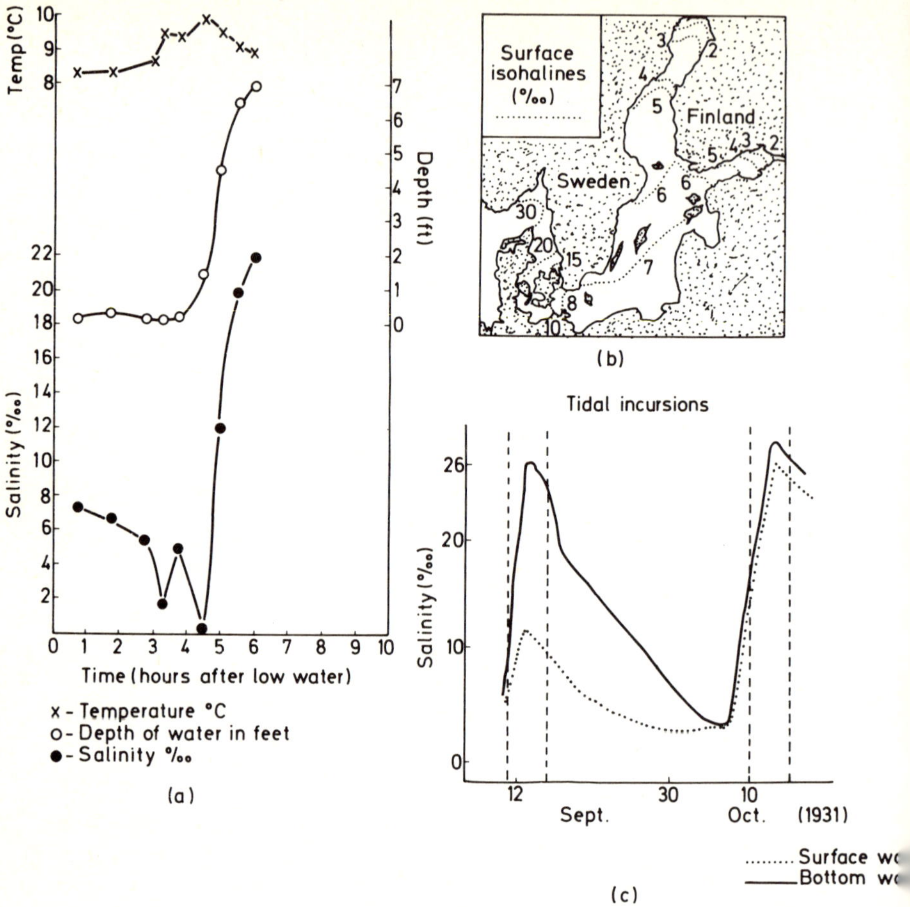

Figure 6.1 Temporal and spatial changes in salinity in various brackish water habitats. (a) Salt marsh gully in the estuary of the River Test, UK illustrating extreme changes of concentration during a single tidal cycle (after Ralph, 1965). (b) Surface isohalines in the Baltic Sea illustrating graded salinity change spatially. (c) Salinity change in a salt marsh pool over a semi-lunar period. (After Nicol, 1935; courtesy Cambridge University Press)

environments must be adapted to maintaining the body fluid concentration, volume and ion content at a level compatible with metabolic function of the cells.

Numerous review articles have considered the steady state relationship between the body fluids of euryhaline* and relatively stenohaline† forms after acclimation to a range of salinities and have discussed the physiological mechanisms involved in regulation and the influence of external factors on these mechanisms (e.g. Krogh 1939; Potts and Parry, 1964b; Beadle, 1957; Kinne, 1967; Lockwood 1962, 1968). In most estuarine conditions,

*Euryhaline = with wide ranging salinity tolerance.
†Stenohaline = with restricted salinity tolerance.

however, it is probably unusual for non-planktonic organisms to remain sufficiently long in a single body of water to reach the steady state appropriate to a particular salinity. Their physiological mechanisms must in fact be adapted to cope with continuous or irregular fluctuations of varying degrees of magnitude and rate. Survival in such circumstances is dependent on versatility of response within an overall non-steady state. In this chapter therefore special attention will be given to responses following change in conditions rather than to the steady state conditions alone and, where appropriate, attention will be drawn to the way in which physiological processes present in stenohaline marine animals may have been adapted, hypertrophied or modified by euryhaline forms.

6.2 TOLERANCE AND MECHANISMS OF REGULATION IN BRACKISH WATERS

The great majority of triploblastic marine invertebrates have blood which is isotonic or almost isotonic with the seawater they inhabit and their intra-cellular fluid is isosmotic with the blood. The ionic concentration of the extra-cellular fluid is generally relatively similar to that of the medium, though with some dynamically maintained differences (*Table 6.1*).

About half to one third of the osmotic concentration of the cells is accounted for by inorganic ions (*Table 6.2*), the remainder being due to the presence of small organic molecules, particularly free amino acids.

Dilution of the medium creates an osmotic gradient across the body

Table 6.1 RATIO OF CONCENTRATION OF IONS IN EXTRA-CELLULAR FLUID TO THE CONCENTRATION IN THE MEDIUM

	Na	K	Ca	Mg	Cl	SO_4	
Mollusca							
Eledone	0.89	1.23	1.08	1.03	0.854	1.50	(Hayes and Pelluet, 1947)
Venus	1.104	0.925	2.105	0.923	1.17	1.16	(Cole, 1940)
Annelida							
Amphitrite	0.98	1.43	1.007	1.09	0.99	1.01	(Cole, 1940)
Arenicola	—	1.39	1.17	1.0	1.0	0.92	(Bialaszewicz, 1933)
Arthropoda							
Carcinus	1.11	1.21	1.27	0.358	0.998	0.572	(Webb, 1940)
Callinectes	1.02	1.26	1.28	0.184	0.914	0.356	(Cole, 1940)
Cancer	1.004	1.20	1.186	0.648	0.974	0.740	(Cole, 1940)

Table 6.2 mM/kg MUSCLE FIBRE WATER. *NEPHROPS* DATA FROM ROBERTSON, (1961), *CARCINUS* FROM SHAW (1958B)

	K	Na	Cl	Mg	Ca	*ATP*	*AP*	m.osm/kg
Nephrops								
abdominal flexor	188	24.5	53.1	20.3	3.72	13.2	117.8	1037
Carcinus								
carpopodite muscle	146	35	5.3	17	5	9	82	983

Table 6.3 DECLINE IN THE NUMBER OF SPECIES OF SOME MOLLUSC GROUPS WITH DECREASED SALINITY IN THE BALTIC (FROM JAECKEL, 1952)

Approx. salinity	*Region*	*Scaphopoda*	*Bivalvia*	*Prosobranchs*	*Cephalopoda*	*Opisthobranchs*
35‰	North Sea	11	189	210	32	141
25‰	Kattegat	1	92	101	14	61
20‰	Danish Belts	1	42	40	5	28
8‰	Outer Baltic	–	11	13	–	6
4‰	Gulf of Bothnia	–	4	1	–	3

Table 6.4 CONCENTRATION OF INTERSTITIAL WATER IN SAND IN THE BED OF A STREAM CROSSING THE SEA-SHORE (AFTER REID, 1930; 1932)

	Stream water	*2" in sand*	*4" in sand*	*6" in sand*
High tide mark	0.35‰	2.25‰	1.55‰	12.42‰
150 yds below high water	1.8‰	16.4‰	17.45‰	24.9‰
Low water (250 yds below high water)	8.08‰	32.57‰	34.34‰	35‰

surface of normally isotonic marine forms and consequently results in net water entry, swelling and dilution of the body fluids.

Oceanic and neritic species tend to be rather sensitive to such dilution of the medium even when salinity gradients are relatively stable; a point which is well illustrated by the diminution in the number of mollusc species present as passage is made from the North Sea to the Central Baltic (*Table 6.3*).

Such tolerance of dilution of the medium as is possessed by offshore marine forms may be based largely on passive acceptance of short term cellular swelling rather than on specific adaptations. Passive tolerance alone is insufficient however to permit true penetration of estuaries and the colonisers of such demanding environments, though mostly derived from marine ancestors, are all in their way physiological entrepreneurs capable not only of surviving wide variations in the chemical and physical parameters of their environment, but also of being able to respond rapidly to any change in a particular parameter.

The attributes of species normally occurring in estuarine waters generally include one or more of the following:

1. Detection and avoidance of changes in salinity and oxygen.
2. Tolerance of extreme conditions on a short term basis.
3. Physiological and morphological adaptation to salinity, temperature and oxygen change.

Maintenance of any species in estuaries is dependent in addition on mechanisms designed to prevent loss of the larval stages to the sea in the net seaward movement of water. These may include:

4. Reduction in length of larval life or suppression of the larval phase.
5. Responses of the larvae to salinity, state of the tide and pressure which, coupled with variation in activity, tend to maintain them in water which is not moving seaward.

6.2.1 Detection and avoidance of unfavourable conditions

Physiological adaptations to a fluctuating environment take a finite period to complete and are often supplemented by behavioural responses which enable animals to delay, avoid or moderate exposure to extreme conditions. Estuarine bivalves such as *Mytilus edulis* close the shell valves when in seawater which is diluted suddenly and thus delay internal concentration changes, though following acclimatisation the species can tolerate salinities below 5‰. Similarly *Littorina littorea* withdraws into its shell on exposure to 25% seawater (Todd, 1964). Mud-dwelling forms may take advantage of the fact that the interstitial water in the substratum tends towards the average of the overlying water (*Table 6.4*) and retreat into their burrows or pull in siphons to avoid extreme conditions (*see also* Chapter 4).

Species which do not burrow tend to display selectivity when given a choice of media indicating that they can sense the concentration.

Two forms of selection occur: (a) preference for a medium within the overall range of salinities tolerated and (b) preference for a medium of a salinity close to that to which the individual has previously been adapted.

The first type of response lacks sophistication since, though it will tend to keep the organisms within a viable salinity range, it will not necessarily result in the ideal choice of medium to meet the immediate physiological requirements of the animal. For example, even after previous desiccation the shore crab *Pachygrapsus crassipes* tends to select 100% seawater when given a choice of 150%, 100% and 50% seawater, though 50% seawater would tend to restore the blood concentration towards the normal level more rapidly (Gross, 1957).

Another shore crab *Porcellana platycheles* (mid- to sub-littoral) shows preference in its choice of media only when placed in salinities outside its normal tolerance range. It will move into the more concentrated of two media when in low salinities (<40‰) and the less concentrated medium when in high salinities (>160‰) (Davenport, 1972a). *Corophium volutator* is somewhat more selective, preferring concentrations in the range 10–30‰ even though it can survive indefinitely in concentrations from 2‰ to 50‰. However, the narrower choice range is adaptive in so far as it represents a selection for concentrations within which growth and moulting frequency are maximal (McLusky, 1970a).

The type (b) response is shown by animals, such as the amphipod *Gammarus zaddachi,* which inhabit niches where salinity changes may be rapid and extensive. The estuarine bivalve *Scrobicularia plana* behaves in a similar manner tending to open their shells more readily when placed in a medium of similar concentration to that to which they have previously been acclimatised rather than to one which is more concentrated or more dilute (Freeman and Rigler, 1957). Preference for a medium similar to that to which an animal is already acclimatised (Lagerspetz and Mattila, 1961) must minimise the need for short term physiological adaptation.

Organisms living in the interstitial water of beaches in regions where they may be influenced both by water from the terrestrial water table and by saline incursions also show from their behaviour that they can detect salinity gradients (*see also* Chapter 1). The behaviour of the harpacticoid *Parastenocaris* from Baltic beaches indicates strong salinity preferences within a narrow range. When given a choice of sand saturated with water of various salinities it is repelled by 10‰ and 5‰ and selects media in the range 2.5–0.1‰ (Jansson, 1967).

Porcellana does not differentiate between sucrose isomotic with seawater and seawater itself though it does choose the former in preference to deionised water. It seems likely therefore that the assessment of the medium, at least by this crab, is based on the osmotic concentration rather than on any ionic parameter (Davenport, 1972a).

Removal of the antennal flagella has little effect on salinity preference. Ablation of the antennular flagella impairs the ability of *Porcellana platycheles* to choose between two concentrations though they still favour 100% seawater if this is one of the choices offered. Similarly droplets of diluted seawater placed on the flagellum of the antennule of the crabs *Portunus* and *Podophthalmus* elicit a nervous response which varies according to the salinity used (Van Weel and Christofferson, 1966). Additional support for the implication of the antennules in salinity detection comes from the observation that *Ligia occidentalis* tests pools with these organs (Abbott, 1939) and that removal of antennules and antennae abolishes the ability of *Asellus* and *Gammarus oceanicus* to respond to salinity gradients (Lagerspetz and Mattila, 1961). However, it is not improbable that chemo-sensory regions responding to salinity reside in other appendages also since T. E. Shaw (unpublished data) observes that *Ligia* may test the medium with its anal circi and Davenport and Wankowski (1973) have noted that *Porcellana platycheles,* when out of water, tests the medium with the legs, particularly legs 2 and 3, before re-immersing itself. Selection of 80% or 100% seawater is significantly greater than for more dilute media after immersion of the legs only.

Localised regions of the body sensitive to external concentration also occur in molluscs. Isolated osphradium-visceral ganglion preparations from the sea slug *Aplysia* display sensitivity to osmotic changes in the bathing medium. Response is mediated by a specific nerve axon after a change of only a few per cent in the medium concentration implying that sense organs capable of monitoring concentration are present in the osphradium (Stinnakre and Tauc, 1969). In another mollusc, *Nodlittorina granularis* the foot adjacent to the operculum appears to be cation sensitive, particularly with respect to Mg^{2+} and Na^{+} ions. (Ohsawa and Tsukuda, 1955).

6.2.2 Tolerance of extreme conditions on a short term basis

A number of organisms can tolerate short term exposure to extreme conditions which they would be unable to survive on a continuous basis. The classical example of such a case is the flatworm *Procerodes (Gunda) ulvae,* an animal colonising small streams crossing tidal shores in regions where there is exposure twice a day successively to fresh water and near 100% seawater. Extended survival in fresh water is dependent on the presence of calcium ions and in their absence *Procerodes* eventually disintegrates. However, survival is possible where the exposure to soft fresh water is only temporary pending the return of the tide (Pantin, 1931). Doubtless there are many other species which may survive in media too dilute for long term exposure during the inter-tidal period, increasing the body ion levels when the salinity rises and showing a net loss during the period of low tide when exposed to fresher water.

An extreme and entertaining example of the use of fluctuating salinities in the invasion of dilute media is furnished by the crab *Callinectes sapidus* colonising the St. John River in Florida. During the summer months the crab penetrates some 100 miles up the river whose salinity, at only some 150 ppm chloride, is too low to permit continuous regulation by the animal. However, in the river there are periodic pools supplied by saline ground water and here the crabs apparently 'tank up' with salt before proceeding further upstream. *Callinectes* does not penetrate up the neighbouring Suwannee and Santa Fe rivers which lack such saline springs (Odum, 1953).

6.2.3 Physiological and morphological adaptation to salinity change

Euryhaline organisms either maintain the body fluids at a concentration different from that of the media over part of their tolerance range (*Osmoregulators*) or allow the body fluids to become iso-osmotic with the media (*Osmoconformers*) (*Figure 6.2(a)*).

Osmoregulators fall in to two categories: those which are hypertonic to the medium when adapted to low salinities and more or less isotonic at high concentrations (*'Hypertonic regulators', Figure 6.2(b)*) and a more limited category of forms including the euryhaline teleosts, some isopods, mysids, prawns, and the annelid *Marphysa gravelyi,* which maintain themselves hypotonic to high salinities and hypertonic to low salinities (*Hyper-hypotonic regulators, Figure 6.2 (c)*).

A wide measure of variability occurs in the degree of hypertonicity or hypotonicity maintained and consequently in extreme cases there is only a marginal distinction between osmoconformers and osmoregulators.

The principal physiological mechanisms adapting euryhaline species to wide ranging concentrations include some or all of the following:

1. Volume regulation and flexibility in the rate of urine production.
2. Regulation of intracellular free amino acid and inorganic ion levels so as to maintain cell volume within narrow limits.
3. Maintenance of the body fluids hypertonic to dilute media by:
   (a) Active transport of inorganic ions into the animal to replace ions lost by diffusion across the body surface and in the urine.
   (b) Production of urine hypotonic to the body fluids.
   (c) Reduction in surface permeability to water and salt.

The emphasis placed on individual regulatory mechanisms varies from species to species but it is clear from the multiplicity of forms which have succeeded in colonising brackish and fresh waters that the physiological and biochemical techniques necessary for survival in dilute media have evolved many times in separate groups.

The clear implication of such repeated development of comparable systems is that the basic apparatus for such processes as the regulation of amino acids, active transport of ions at the body surface etc., are already present in marine forms subserving other functions and that natural selection has merely acted to modify and hypertrophy such existing systems.

6.2.3.1 VOLUME REGULATION IN ESTUARINE WATERS

Following dilution of the medium the degree of physical expansion resulting from osmotic water intake is generally greater in soft bodied forms than in those such as the crustacea and arachnids, with exoskeletons and also tends to be larger in stenohaline than in comparable euryhaline species. Among annelids even relatively euryhaline species such as the Indian polychaetes *Diopatra variabilis* and *Marphysa gravelyi,* which tolerate 5‰→28‰, may increase in weight by as much as 40–50% when transferred suddenly to 6‰

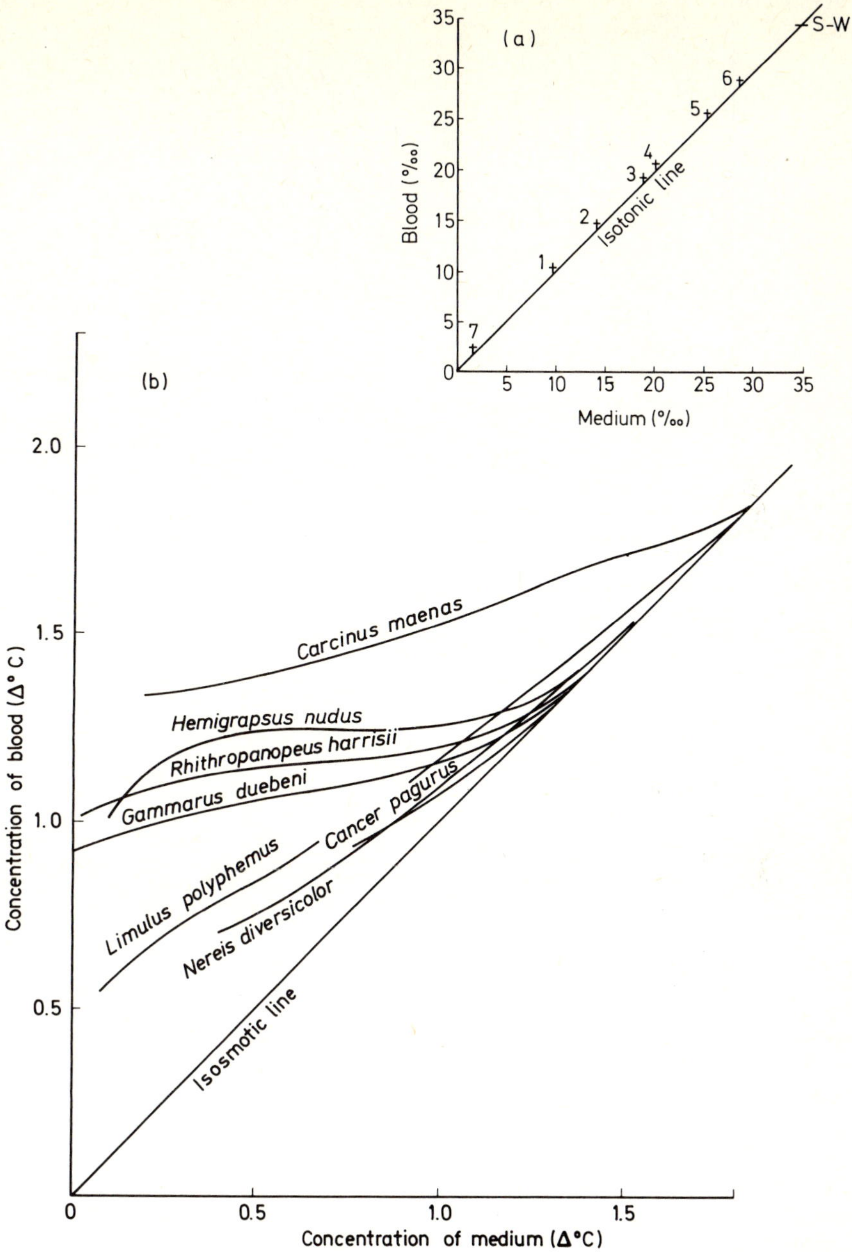

Figure 6.2 The relationship between blood concentration and medium concentration in various euryhaline species. (a) Approximate limits of survival for various osmoconformers: (1) Callianassa californiensis *(Thompson and Pritchard, 1969); (2)* Buccinum undatum *(Staarland, 1970); (3)* Eupagurus bernhardus *(Davenport, 1972); (4)* Porcellana platycheles; *and (5)* P. longicornis *(Davenport, 1972a); (6)* Maia squinado *(Duval, 1925); (7)* Mercierella enigmatica *(Skaer, 1974). (b) Forms regulating hypertonically in dilute media but isotonic at high salinities.*

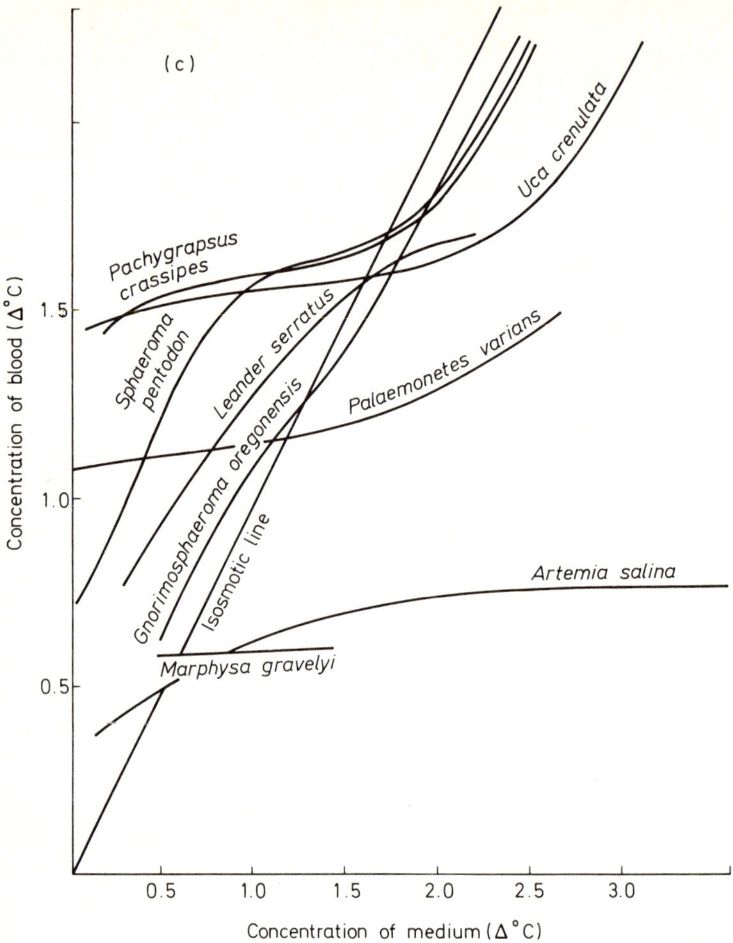

Figure 6.2 (c) Forms regulating hypertonically in dilute media and hypotonically at high salinities

(Krishnamoorthi and Krishnaswami, 1966; and Krishnamoorthi, 1963) (*Figure 6.3*). Crustacea are unable to expand to such an extend, relatively stenohaline forms such as *Galathea squamifera* and *Porcellana longicornis* generally dying after a weight increase of some 12% (Davenport, 1972b) though they are physically incapacitated by the swelling before this point is reached.

Size, with its effect on the surface to volume ratio, as well as permeability, is of importance in determining the rate of swelling and hence the likely fate of stenohaline forms in response to short term decrease in external salinity. Thus the large Spider crab, *Maia,* swells at a rate of some 4%/hour when transferred to 20% seawater whilst the smaller *Galathea, Porcellana longicornis* and *Eupagurus bernhardus* all increase in weight by about

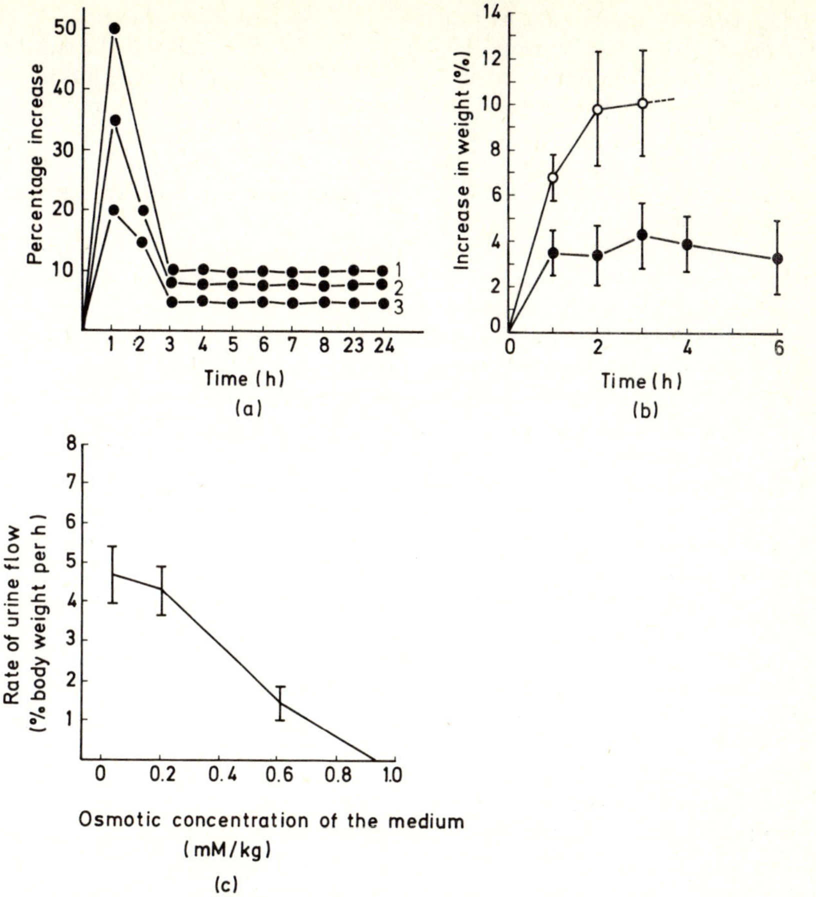

Figure 6.3 Changes in volume after exposure to dilute media (a) The annelid Diopatra variabilis *after sudden transfer from seawater to (1) 8.62‰, (2) 13.7‰ and (3) 20.72‰. (After Krishnamoorthi, 1963; courtesy Indian Academy of Sciences). (b) Weight changes of the crab* Porcellana platycheles *with (open circles) and without (closed circles) the nephropore openings blocked after transference to 60% seawater. Means and 95% confidence limits for 10 crabs. The dotted line represents a period after death. (After Davenport, 1972b; courtesy Cambridge University Press). (c) Urine flow rate of the amphipod* Gammarus oceanicus *in different salinities. Vertical lines are 2 × the standard errors. (After Werntz, 1963; courtesy The Biological Bulletin)*

12%/hour on transfer to 60% seawater. The copepod *Acartia tonsa* may even physically burst when exposed suddenly to 20% seawater though it will tolerate such a dilution if acclimatised more slowly (Lance, 1965).

Loss of salt across the body surface and in the urine plus the diluting effect of the water taken up by osmosis tend to decrease the osmotic gradient and slow the water entry. In addition the ability to vary the urine flow rate markedly is an important adaptive feature in estuarine species.

Marine Crustacea in seawater produce a urine volume equivalent to about 3–15% of their body weight/day; *Carcinus maenas* 3.6% (Shaw, 1961a),

4.7% (Webb, 1940), *Pachygrapsus* 3.9% (Gross and Marshall, 1960), *Cancer* 3–10% (Robertson, 1939) but such rates can be dramatically increased in the euryhaline forms on exposure to dilute media. Thus in 50% seawater *Pachygrapsus* is estimated to produce a urine volume equivalent to 58% of the body weight daily (Gross and Marshall, 1960) some fifteen times the rate in seawater whilst a comparable increase occurs in urine output when the euryhaline *Gammarus oceanicus* is exposed to dilute media (Werntz, 1963; *Figure 6.3(c)*).

Examination of the rate of loss of the inert marker ^{51}Cr EDTA from the body when *Gammarus duebeni* is in seawater and after transfer to a dilute medium indicates that adjustment to the rate of flow of urine can occur with considerable rapidity. In most animals the flow rate has reached the new maximum level within five minutes of the dilution of the medium, though occasionally individuals take longer to effect the change.

By similar means, provided that the osmotic gradient is not too large, the net uptake of water may be contained, excess water excreted and the body volume returned to near the normal value in soft bodied forms (*Figure 6.3(a)*) as well as in crustaceans. Although perhaps obvious, the importance of such increased urine production is indicated by the fact that the crab *Porcellana platycheles* which normally tolerates transfer from 100 to 60% seawater dies within four hours in the lower concentration if the urinary pores are blocked (*Figure 6.3(b)*; Davenport, 1972). The hermit crab *Eupagurus bernhardus* will, like *Porcellana platycheles,* survive in 60% seawater. However, it differs from the latter in tolerating a much greater degree of swelling. Water taken in is accommodated largely by the expansion of the soft abdomen and even when the excretory pores are blocked the animal only dies after the weight increase has reached some 30% (Davenport, 1972).

Rapid water entry with expansion of the body represents an acute risk only to highly permeable marine forms since, if they survive the period of initial expansion, the osmotic gradient between blood and media will decline as salt is lost across the body surface and in the urine. On gradual exposure to reduced salinities most stenohaline forms therefore remain more or less isosmotic with the medium until the problems which dilution entails at the cellular level ultimately prove fatal. Some euryhaline forms (*Figure 6.2(a)*) remain isosmotic over a considerable salinity range.

6.2.3.1.1 Volume regulation in forms isosmotic with the medium

Once conformers have come to osmotic equilibrium with their medium they may appear to have no overt osmoregulatory problems, but it is important not to overlook the fact that they do regulate the body water content within narrow limits and that they must in most cases take into the body sufficient water for the purpose of urine production.

Urine production in the lobster *Homarus* is reported (Burger, 1957) to be in part dependent on the colloid osmotic pressure of the blood and anuric or oligouric lobsters can be stimulated to increase urine flow after injection of colloid into the haemolymph. However, such control over water entry by means of regulation of colloid osmotic pressure would not be expected to lend itself readily to the sensitivity of response necessary to ensure both continuing volume regulation and reaction to acute situations such as large volume losses through haemorrhage. Evidence for an alternative system of bringing water into isosmotic forms is discussed on p.358. It suffices here to state that not only is urine flow rate in the amphipod *Gammarus duebeni* higher, when the animal is in seawater, than would be anticipated from the size of the osmotic gradient, but also that flow declines when ion uptake is inhibited. It seems probable, therefore, that part of the volume of fluid ultimately excreted enters in association with ion transport. The changes in ion transport which follow reduction in blood volume in both Crustacea (Lockwood, 1970) and gastropods (Greenaway, 1970) support this conclusion.

A considerable measure of accuracy in volume-controlling mechanisms is implied by the fact that the degree of expansion which occurs in both the euryhaline crab *Callinectes sapidus* (Haefner and Schuster, 1964), and in *Gammarus duebeni* (Lockwood and Inman, 1973c) at moult is virtually independent of the salinity of the medium (and hence osmotic gradient) in which ecdysis occurs.

Control of volume regulation in *Buccinum* is disturbed by treatment with eserine. The drug causes relaxion of the body wall musculature, decrease in urine production and increased concentration of osmotically active substances in the blood which, together, result in a swelling of the body (Akerlund and Fänge, 1972). Whether the eserine causes failure of peripheral volume receptors or of central interpretation remains to be established.

Possibly the origin of the use of ion movements in regulating internal water levels lies in systems such as that found in *Hydra* where unidirectional ion passage appears to control the cell water level. The cells of *Hydra* are some 40 m.osmoles hypertonic to fresh water and consequently some means of preventing osmotic water inflow is necessary. Contractile vacuoles are absent but it is found that (a) the organism takes up tracer sodium from the medium (Lilly, 1955) (b) the concentration of the enteron fluid is similar to that of the cells (c) *Hydra* contracts at frequent intervals expelling fluid from the enteron and (d) if a thread is tied round the column preventing such expulsion of fluid the animal swells (Marshall, 1968). Alternatively if the column is cut and allowed to regenerate, the cylinder will initially have no opening; though, after initial swelling, it will contract causing a rupture and release of fluid (Macklin, Roma and Drake, 1973). Marshall (1968) and Macklin, Roma and Drake (1973) conclude that volume regulation is based on a transport of ions into the enteron to maintain the latter at a concentration equivalent to or greater than that in the cells. Thus, excess water passes from the cells into the enteron and is subsequently expelled (*Figure 6.4*).

6.2.3.2 CELL VOLUME REGULATION AND FREE AMINO ACID METABOLISM

It is generally understood that the body cells of organisms approximate in osmotic concentration to the extra-cellular fluid and that they are relatively

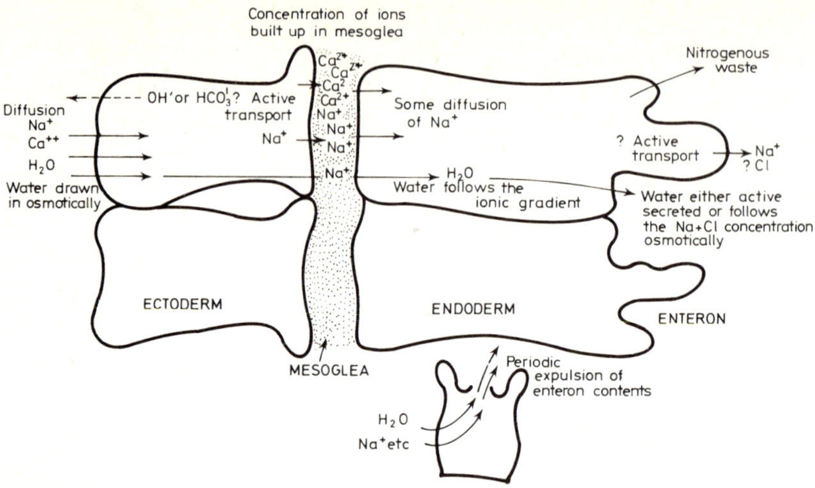

Figure 6.4 Postulated movement of water and ions across the body wall of Hydra. *(After Marshall, 1968; courtesy School Science Review)*

permeable to water. Consequently dilution of the blood is liable to result in water uptake into cells by osmosis if measures are not taken to adjust the intracellular concentration.

The theoretical consequences of failing to make such an adjustment are drastic. Consider a hypothetical marine form whose cells act as perfect osmometers and whose overall volume remains constant. P. C. Croghan (unpublished data) has shown that on transference to a dilute media the cells of such a form would expand to fill the entire internal space when

$$\frac{C_b}{C_{b_0}} = \frac{V_{a_0} - V_{b_0}}{V_{a_0}}$$

where C_b is the final blood concentration, C_{b_0} is the initial blood concentration, V_{a_0} is the overall body volume and V_{b_0} is the initial blood volume. Thus, if no means of regulating cell volume were to be present, quite small dilutions of the blood would result in a reduction of the extracellular fluid volume and circulatory collapse would follow any large drop. For example, an animal with an initial blood volume of 30% of the total volume would be expected to have a zero blood volume when the blood concentration had fallen to only 70% of its initial value.

Mere tolerance of cellular swelling is therefore inadequate to permit extended penetration of animals into estuarine waters though there are some species which survive a limited degree of dilution without exercising accurate regulation of cell volume. Thus the gastropod *Buccinum undatum,* which generally lives in salinities of 20‰–30‰, has some 60% of the total body water in the cells when acclimatised to 33‰ but about 80% in the cells after a week in 11‰ (Staarland, 1970; *Figure 6.5).*

Among normally euryhaline species any appreciable increase of cell volume following dilution of the medium is probably confined to soft-bodied

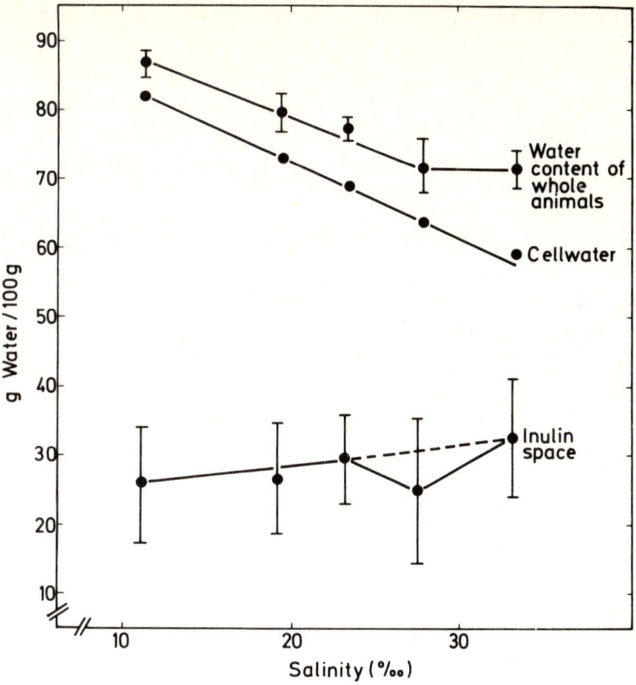

Figure 6.5 Inulin space, total body water and cell water of the common whelk at different salinities, indicating that, though the cell water content and total water content of Buccinum *increase when the medium is diluted, the blood volume declines. (After Staarland, 1970; courtesy Pergamon Press Ltd)*

forms and even then is usually marked only towards the lower limit of the tolerance range. Crustacea show more limited water uptake by the cells; there is only a 3% change in the water content of the muscles of *Carcinus* on transfer from 100% to 40% seawater (Shaw, 1958b; Austin, 1973) and a corresponding change of about 5% occurs when the crab *Pachygrapsus crassipes,* previously acclimatised to 150% seawater, is transferred to 50% seawater (Gross, 1957b). Small changes such as those shown by *Carcinus* and *Pachygrapsus* are, however, compatible with practically complete volume regulation. If water is caused to move into a cell to occupy the space vacated by intercellular osmotically active substances which are actively or passively removed when the blood is diluted there should, theoretically, be an increase in the water content of a cell on a weight basis even though the overall cell volume (the important factor from the point of view of mechanical function and packing) remains constant (Lange and Mostad, 1967). Indeed measurement of volume, as opposed to the water content alone, of the muscle cells of *Eriocheir sinensis* indicates that there is close similarity between the values in fresh water and seawater (Bricteaux-Gregoire *et al.,* 1962).

Volume regulation in response to changes in extracellular concentration is effected by adjusting the internal osmotic concentration of cells. However, the extent of capabilities in this respect vary. Comparison of the behaviour of muscle fibres from a range of stenohaline and euryhaline lamellibranchs (Lange, 1970) indicates that, although individuals of both groups display some measure of ability to vary the amount of osmotically active substances in the muscle cells when the salinity of the media is changed, only the more euryhaline species such as *Cardium edule* and *Mya arenaria* regulate the osmotic activity of the cells so that the overall change is negligible after adaptation to 40% seawater. In more stenohaline forms such as *Pecten septemradiatus, Venerupis rhomboides* and *Dosinia exoleta* water entry into the muscles, after any major dilution of the blood, more than compensates for occupation of space vacated by osmotically active components. Consequently on dilution of the media these forms, like *Buccinum,* suffer actual cellular swelling, with all the disadvantages which this entails. As might perhaps be anticipated accurate regulation of cell volume in the euryhaline forms is not restricted to muscle cells. It has, for example, also been observed in the gill cells of *Mytilus edulis* (Lange, 1968b).

A variety of substances contribute to the osmotic activity of cells but quantitatively the most important are inorganic ions and free amino acids (*Table 6.5*).

Table 6.5 OSMOTICALLY ACTIVE CONSTITUENTS OF *ERIOCHEIR* MUSCLE (AFTER BRICTEUX-GREGOIRE *ET AL.*, 1962)

	Eriocheir muscle (mM/kg)		
	Animals from F-W[1]	*Animals from S-W*[2]	*Difference*
Inorganic ions Cl, Na, K, Mg, Ca	203.5	483.4	279.9
Total Amino acids	157.9	340.7	182.8
Taurine	17.3	20.7	3.4
TMO	47.6	74.8	27.2
Betaine	17.8	13.9	−3.9

[1]F-W=fresh water
[2]S-W=seawater

If cells are to maintain their volume when the concentration of the blood changes then the concentration of some or all of these osmotically active substances must be appropriately varied to prevent osmotic shifts of water between the cell and extra-cellular fluid. Naturally, osmoconformers must effect larger changes for any given dilution of the medium than osmoregulators.

The need to maintain the electrical potential gradient across the surface of nerves and muscles places limitations on the degree to which shifts in the intracellular inorganic ion concentration can contribute to this process. In a euryhaline form such as *Carcinus* the membrane potential of the muscles remains practically constant whilst the osmotic concentration of the blood is varied in the range 580 to 200mM/l NaCl (which is approximately the normal viable limits of the crab) and the ratio of blood potassium concentration to cell potassium is kept substantially unaltered (Shaw, 1958a).

The chloride ion concentration of cells is generally regulated by the membrane potential:

$$E = RT\,1\text{n}\,\frac{(Cl_o)}{(Cl_i)}$$

where E is the transmembrane potential in volts, R is the gas constant (8.2 joules/mol.) T is the absolute temperature and Cl_i and Cl_o are the concentration of chloride inside and outside the cell.

If the electrical integrity of the cells is maintained over a wide range of external media then it would be expected that the ratio $(Cl_o)/(Cl_i)$ would also remain approximately constant. Comparison of related amphipods from different environments suggests, as might be expected, that regulation of this ratio is good in the euryhaline species, *Gammarus duebeni* and *Gammarus locusta,* but is less adequate in the marine and fresh water stenohaline species *Grammarus pulex* and *G. obtusatus (Figure 6.6).*

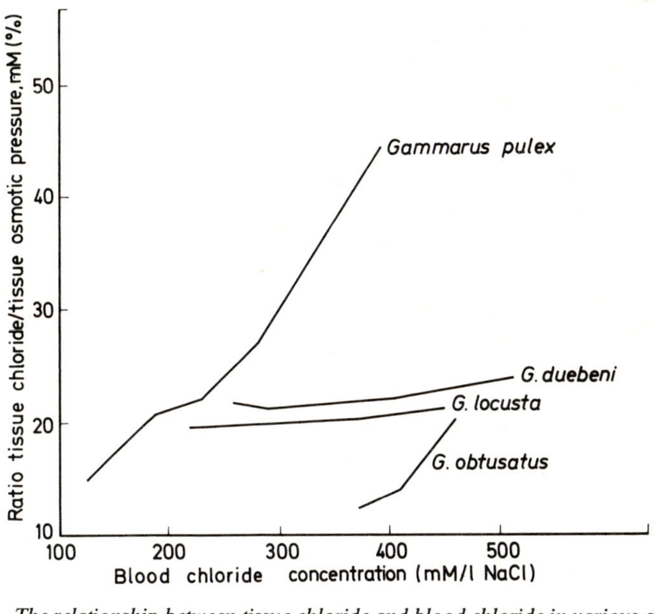

Figure 6.6 The relationship between tissue chloride and blood chloride in various amphipods illustrating that the ratio Cl_i/Cl_o is maintained more constant over a range of media in the euryhaline species Gammarus duebeni *and* G. locusta *than in the stenohaline* G. obtusatus *and* G. pulex. *(After Beadle and Cragg, 1940; courtesy R. J. Skaer)*

As a consequence of the restrictions placed on the adjustment of ion levels much of the additional regulation of cell osmotic concentration usually devolves upon amino acids, though other organic substances such as taurine, betaines and trimethylamine oxide also contribute to a lesser extent. However, the arachnid *Limulus,* which displays wide powers of tolerance in the range 20–200% seawater, differs from the general pattern since a major part of the cellular osmotic adjustment is due to non-protein nitrogen exclusive of amino acids, urea and trimethylamine oxide (*see also* Chapter 2). The components involved are as yet unknown (Robertson, 1970).

On exposure of most euryhaline forms to dilute media the cell free amino acid concentration declines (*Figure 6.7*). The effect is fully reversible and the animals regain the initial amino acid level on re-acclimatisation to full strength seawater (*Table 6.6*).

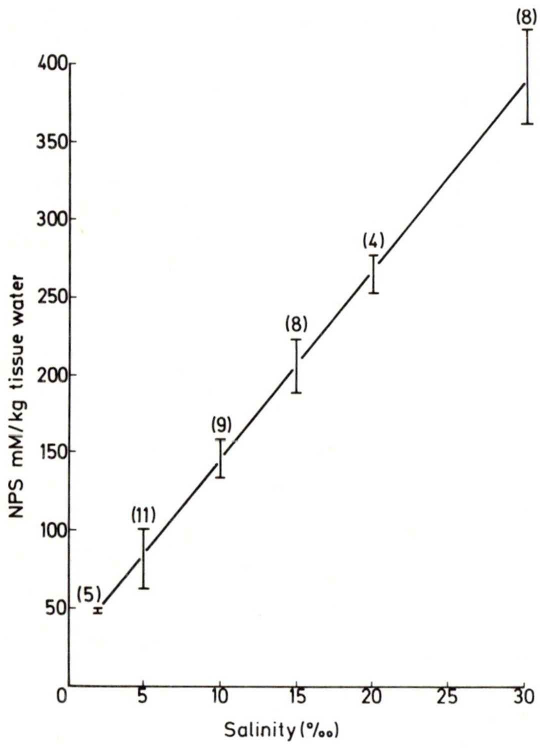

Figure 6.7 Variation in the muscle content of ninhydrin positive substance (mainly amino acids) with salinity of the medium in the clam Mya arenaria. *(After Virkar and Webb, 1970; courtesy Pergamon Press Ltd)*

Such corrective adjustment of the cell free amino acid level on exposure of the animal to a dilute medium is of widespread occurrence in both relatively stenohaline neritic forms and euryhaline species, though it is only pronounced in the latter. Regulation to at least some degree has been observed in vertebrates Gordon (1965), Baxter and Ortiz (1966) and Lange and Fugelli (1965) and in most of the invertebrate phyla *inter alia,* Mollusca, *Cardium, Mya,* (Lange, 1970), *Macoma inconspicuata* (Emerson, 1968); sipunculids *Golfingia gouldii* (Virkar, 1966) and polychaete annelids *Perinereis cultrifera* and *Nereis diversicolor* (Jeuniaux *et al*., 1961); *Neanthes*

Table 6.6 FREE AMINO ACIDS IN WHOLE CRAB (μM/20g FRESH WEIGHT *CARCINUS*) AT DIFFERENT TIMES AFTER TRANSFER OF THE ANIMALS FROM 11 TO 38‰ SEAWATER (AFTER SIEBERS *ET AL.*, 1972)

Substance	*Salinity 11‰*	*0.5 days in 38‰*	*1 day in 38‰*	*3 days in 38‰*	*10 days in 38‰*
Phospho-serine + Phospho threonine	1.96	1.47	2.17	1.94	2.13
Taurine	244.08	250.25	292.82	282.75	319.26
Aspartic acid	11.25	13.78	13.02	13.49	15.47
Threonine	18.33	24.56	19.10	21.30	20.68
Serine + asparagine	63.08	81.12	89.61	88.15	154.92
Glutamic acid	24.90	37.74	34.27	33.82	35.57
Proline	40.94	89.18	49.45	121.89	269.38
α-amino adipic acid	4.81	6.24	9.09	9.10	6.42
Glycine	88.09	107.58	110.53	205.52	241.60
Alanine	104.02	154.25	174.35	281.61	335.00
α-amino butyric acid	1.66	2.29	1.63	1.94	3.20
Methionine	14.79	16.39	8.93	5.26	8.78
Isoleucine	29.88	32.41	14.97	27.17	17.54
Leucine	44.56	60.41	27.27	43.73	26.94
Tyrosine	60.59	64.82	43.98	51.35	30.41
Phenylalanine	28.37	35.57	20.56	25.82	13.31
Lysine	46.66	68.40	42.78	48.13	21.80
Histidine	5.02	10.47	12.88	8.35	5.64
Ammonia	24.08	25.59	27.23	18.72	16.80
Arginine	142.89	192.00	221.08	191.76	117.4
7 undetermined	29.26	34.64	41.00	31.47	28.48
TOTAL	1031	1343	1276	1550	1717

arenaceodentata (Abarti and Reish, 1972); *Arenicola marina* (Duchateau-Bosson, Jeuniaux and Florkin (1961), *Nephthys caeca* (Emerson, 1968); Echinoderms *Asterias rubens* (Jeuniaux, Bricteux-Gregoire and Florkin, 1962); Crustacea, *Carcinus* (Shaw, 1958b); *Sphaeroma rugicauda* (Harris, 1969); *Eriocheir sinensis, Leander serratus,* (Florkin, 1962), *Leander squilla* (Stoner and Dunham, 1970).

Nevertheless the ability to vary overall cell amino acid concentration is not universal, particularly amongst normally marine species. Thus, the prosobranch mollusc *Thais emarginata* shows little change in the concentration of free amino acids/dry unit weight muscle on reacclimatisation from 100 to 75% seawater and similarly a population of *Acmaea scutum,* which are likely to experience salinity changes from 15‰ to 30‰ on an annual basis scarcely varies the ninhydrin positive substance/unit dry weight muscle when transferred from 100 to 50% seawater (Emerson, 1968).

6.2.3.2.1 The mechanism of amino acid variation

The free amino acid composition of muscles varies rather widely both between species and also at the level of the individual (*Tables 6.7* and *6.8*) and it is also not uncommon for some degree of variation to occur between the levels of the individual amino acids in the muscles of different individuals kept under similar conditions in seawater (*Table 6.9*).

Table 6.7 COMPARISON OF FREE AMINO ACIDS IN TISSUES OF VARIOUS ORGANISMS ADAPTED TO SEAWATER

	mM/100g of fresh tissue							
	Arenicola[1]		*Perinereis*[2]		*Asterias*[3]		*Leander*[4]	
	S-W[5]	*50% S-W*	*S-W*	*50% S-W*	*S-W*	*60% S-W*	*S-W*	*30% S-W*
Alanine	7.45	2.20	3.43	1.17	0.17	—	1.69	0.26
Arginine	0.02	0.07	0.02	0.01	0.13	0.10	2.58	2.07
Aspartic acid	1.38	1.46	0.72	0.66	0.11	0.05	0.18	0.05
Glutamic acid	1.04	0.64	1.48	0.79	0.14	0.17	0.32	0.11
Glycine	22.46	9.96	17.71	9.69	16.3	9.5	11.2	9.5
Histidine	0.12	0.37	0.16	0.06	0	0	0	0
Isoleucine	0.05	0.02	0.09	0.04	Tr	Tr	0.21	Tr
Leucine	0.07	0.03	0.12	0.05	Tr	Tr	0.34	Tr
Methionine	0.03	0.01	0.21	0.07	—	—	—	—
Phenylalanine	0.04	0.03	0.04	0.03	Tr	Tr	Tr	0
Proline	—	—	2.53	1.76	0	0	2.17	0.64
Threonine	0.19	0.09	0.79	0.36	Tr	Tr	0.21	Tr
Valine	0.06	0.02	0.20	0.11	Tr	Tr	0.37	Tr
Asparagine	—	—	—	—	0.08	0.11	0.14	Tr
Taurine	—	—	—	—	3.9	2.2	2.56	2.32
Serine	—	—	—	—	Tr	Tr	0.55	0.12
Glutamine	—	—	—	—	0.23	0.11	0.56	0.16
Lysine	0.18	0.15	0.08	0.04	Tr	Tr	0.16	0.05
Tyrosine	0.03	0.01	0.06	0.04	Tr	Tr	Tr	0

[1] Duchâteau-Bosson *et al.* (1961)
[2] Jeuniaux *et al.* (1961)
[3] Jeuniaux *et al.* (1962)
[4] Florkin (1962)
[5] S-W=seawater

Table 6.8 COMPARISON OF FREE AMINO ACID LEVELS IN THE TISSUES OF VARIOUS ORGANISMS ADAPTED TO SEAWATER TO SHOW THE DEGREE OF VARIATION

	mg amino acids/100gm fresh tissue in seawater					
	Perinereis[1]	*Asterias*[2]	*Leander*[3]	*Eriocheir*[4]	*Carcinus*[5]	*Arenicola*[6]
Alanine	305.7	15	150	734.3	182.7	663.6
Arginine	2.8	23	450	464.4	630.9	3.2
Aspartic acid	96.4	15	24	110.9	51.8	183.7
Glutamic acid	217.3	20	47	457.9	529.9	153.6
Glycine	1329.6	1300	840	1045.4	755.2	1685.7
Histidine	24.6	0	0	22.4	1.6	17.9
Isoleucine	11.8	Tr	27	36.3	22.1	6.4
Leucine	15.4	Tr	44	47.9	34.4	9.6
Lysine	11.1	Tr	23	65.6	28.3	25.6
Methionine	30.8	—	—	36.7	49.0	4.7
Phenylalanine	6.8	Tr	Tr	11.7	7.5	6.4
Proline	290.7	0	250	1561.6	563.1	0
Threonine	94.3	Tr	25	76.0	39.6	23.0
Tyrosine	10.5	Tr	Tr	9.3	5.9	4.1
Valine	24.4	Tr	43	50.1	38.2	7.5
Asparagine		10	18	—	—	—
Taurine	—	490	320	—	—	—
Serine	—	Tr	58	—	—	—
Glutamine	—	33	83	—	—	—

[1] Jeuniaux *et al.* (1961)
[2] Jeuniaux, Bricteux-Gregoire and Florkin (1962)
[3] Jeuniaux, Bricteux-Gregoire and Florkin (1961)
[4] Duchâteau-Bosson and Florkin, (1962)
[5] Duchâteau-Bosson, Florkin and Jeuniaux (1959)
[6] Duchâteau-Bosson, Jeuniaux and Florkin, M. (1961)

Table 6.9 VARIATION BETWEEN THE AMINO ACID COMPOSITION OF THE MUSCLES OF THREE INDIVIDUAL FEMALE *ERIOCHEIR SINENSIS* (CHINESE WOOL HANDED CRABS) FROM SEAWATER (AFTER DUCHÂTEAU AND FLORKIN, 1962). VALUES IN mg/100 μg FRESH MUSCLE

	1	*2*	*3*
Alanine	959.2	914.9	505.0
Arginine	717.0	848.0	415.5
Aspartic acid	61.4	64.4	105.7
Glutamic acid	484.2	411.9	329.9
Glycine	628.3	717.3	1089.5
Histidine	47.0	19.4	36.6
Isoleucine	24.0	14.6	32.3
Leucine	31.6	24.3	39.7
Lysine	7.7	2.4	54.8
Methionine	47.0	51.0	39.7
Phenylalanine	26.8	17.4	29.0
Proline	364.5	304.0	1613.8
Threonine	43.7	21.9	62.0
Tyrosine	24.9	12.2	7.9
Valine	37.9	25.5	56.7
K^+mg/100g tissue	428.9	448.4	321.0

To some extent such individual differences may be attributed to other internal or external factors; both stages in the moult cycle in Crustacea (Duchâteau-Bosson, Florkin and Jeuniaux, 1959) or low oxygen tension in the medium (Abarti and Reisch, 1972) can affect the relative abundance of individual muscle amino acids. However, study of a race of the worm *Neanthes arenoceodentata* inbred for 30 generations indicates that individual variation is still present even when animals of the same age are maintained on a uniform diet at constant conditions in respect of temperature, light, and salinity (Abarti and Reisch, 1972). It seems, therefore, that very precise regulation of the individual amino acids does not occur. Perhaps, however, some variation is to be expected as different proteins are fabricated or broken down and, as far as cell volume regulation is concerned, it is presumably immaterial which precise components contribute to the overall osmotic activity.

Most of the commonly occurring amino acids are present in the free amino acid (FAA) pool. However, in general, it is the non-essential amino acids which provide both the bulk of the pool and the major part of any osmotic adjustment in response to salinity change. Glycine, glutamic acid, alanine, proline and aspartic acid are commonly amongst the dominant substances present. Arginine is also well represented in Crustacea but plays no role in osmotic adjustment — presumably because much of it is present as the phosphagen arginine phosphate, an immediate energy store.

Quantitatively the major contribution to osmotic adjustment in *Carcinus* comes from alanine, proline and glycine (*Table 6.7*) and the same three amino acids also dominate the regulation of the amino acid pool in response to salinity variation in the shrimp *Crangon crangon* (Weber and Van Marrewijk, 1972). However, although one or more of these three amino acids usually plays the principal role in adjustment they are not necessarily all three important simultaneously. Thus in *Arenicola,* alanine and glycine dominate but proline is of little significance (Duchâteau-Bosson, Jeuniaux and Florkin, 1961) whilst in *Asterias* such amino acid change as can occur is almost entirely accounted for by glycine with a minor contribution from taurine (Jeuniaux, Bricteux-Gregoire and Florkin, 1962). In general, taurine has been less frequently measured, but when examined has been found to be a major contributor in some Crustacea (*Sphaeroma;* Harris, 1969), some molluscs (*Buccinum;* Staarland, 1970) and (*Mytilus;* Lange, 1968a). In *Mytilus,* taurine accounts for about one quarter of the total ninhydrin positive material when the animals are in 100% seawater. In 5‰ however it is virtually absent from the cells (Lange and Mostad, 1967). Taurine is the end-product of the metabolism of sulphur-containing amino acids and as such may perhaps be considered as being comparable to an excretory product. Its use as an osmotic regulator in molluscs etc. may therefore perhaps spare more valuable amino acid (Lange, 1968b).

Decrease in the free amino acid levels of cells is commonly accompanied by a temporary increase in the rate of loss of nitrogenous compounds from the body and conversely when the free amino acid pool is being increased the nitrogen loss is decreased (Florkin *et al.*, 1964). Most of these changes can be accounted for by variations in the rate of release of ammonia, e.g. the crab *Eriocheir* (Florkin *et al.*, 1964) and *Carcinus* (Austin, 1973; *Figure 6.8*) the annelid *Nephthys caeca,* the bivalve *Macoma inconspicua,* and the echinoderms *Strongylocentrotus dröbachiensis* and *Eupentacra quinquesemita* (Emerson, 1968). Such changes in the loss of NH_3 imply that regulation of intra-cellular concentration principally involves degradation of amino acids rather than polymerisation within the cell into peptides or proteins. This conclusion is further supported by the fact that when

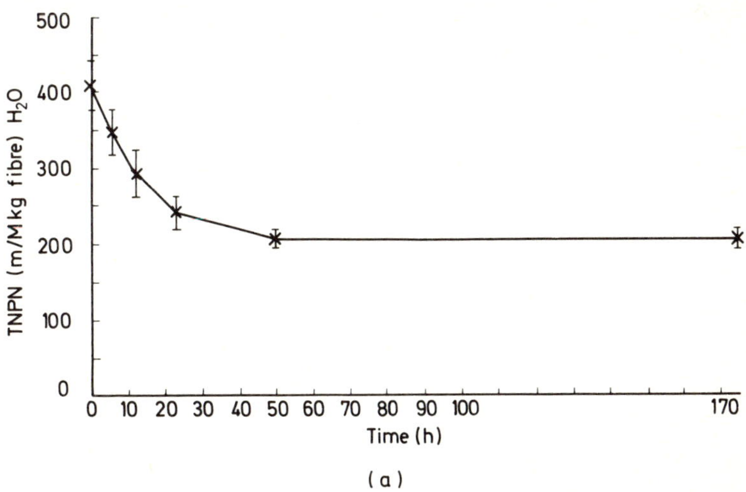

Figure 6.8 (a) Time course of decline in muscle amino acid levels after transference of Carcinus *from 100 to 50% seawater (TNPN = Total non protein nitrogen). (After Austin, 1973)*

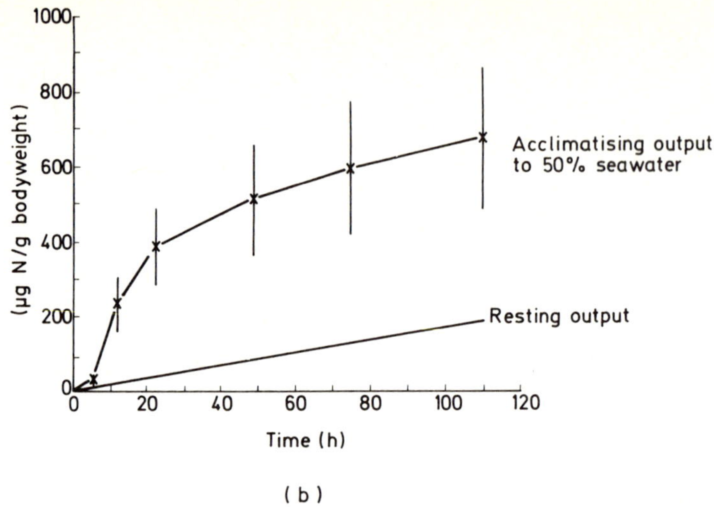

Figure 6.8 (b) Cumulative non-protein nitrogen release to the medium from Carcinus *after transference of the animals from 100 to 50% seawater. (After Austin, 1973)*

Eriocheir is transferred from fresh water to seawater the total (protein + free amino acid) amounts of alanine and proline in the muscles increases. Net synthesis of at least these two substances must therefore have occurred during re-acclimatisation to seawater (Florkin *et al*., 1964).

Peptide formation may, however, be of functional significance in the salinity-moderated amino acid adjustments in the foot cells of the snail *Melanopsis trifasciatus* (Bedford, 1971). Apart from the possibility of peptide formation within cells, three suggestions have been advanced to explain the changes in cell amino acid following dilution of the blood: (a) deamination of the amino acids within the cell (b) loss of amino acids from the cell to the blood followed by transport in the blood to a tissue where deamination occurs, and (c) loss of amino acid from cells and subsequent polymerisation to increase haemolymph protein. In (a) and (b) the ammonia resulting from deamination is thought to be carried in the blood to the respiratory surfaces where it diffuses out. The theories postulate similar biochemical processes for the formation or breakdown of the free amino acids; they differ primarily as to the principal site where this is presumed to occur.

The free amino acids are considered to be formed by the amination of appropriate organic acids. The four pathways of principal importance are probably (*Figure 6.9*):

α-ketoglutarate → glutamic acid
pyruvate → alanine
oxalo-acetate → aspartic acid
3 phosphoglycerate → glycine

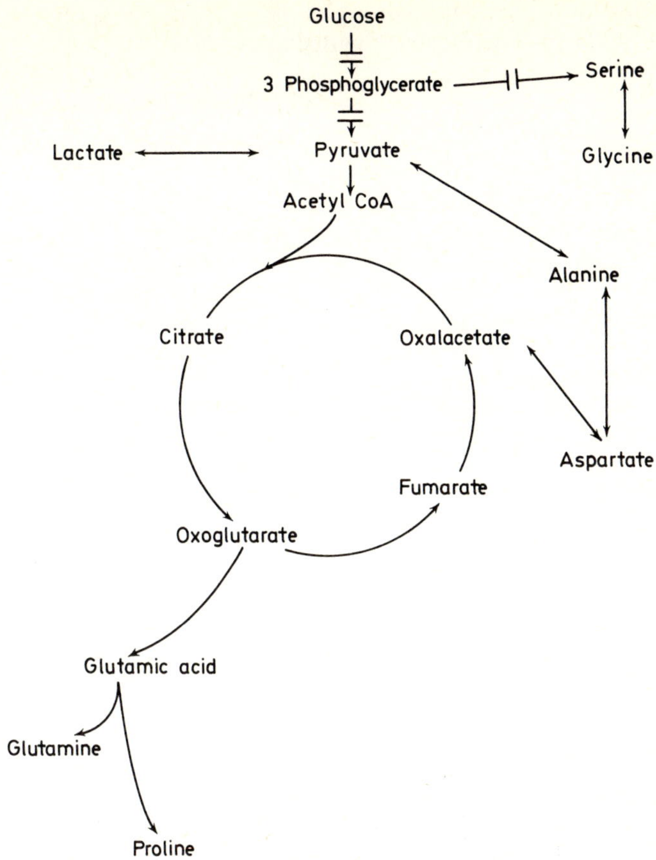

Figure 6.9 Some metabolic pathways involved in amino-acid synthesis

Regulation of the non-essential amino acid concentration in cells is thought by Florkin and Schoffeniels (1969) to be due to two main processes:

1. Modification of the activity of the pathways responsible for synthesis and degradation of amino acids.
2. Modification of the enzyme systems involved in the control of the fate of reducing equivalents in the cell.

A fascinating feature of amino acid control in euryhaline forms is the way in which inorganic ions directly influence the enzyme systems responsible for catabolism and anabolism and so establish positive feedback regulation (*see also* Chapter 2).

6.2.3.2.2 Intracellular metabolism of amino acids

The enzyme L-glutamate: NAD oxidoreductase (=glutamate dehydrogenase) is responsible for the amination of α-ketogluterate to form glutamine in the presence of reducing equivalent provided by NADH.

$$\mathrm{NADH} + \alpha\text{-ketoglutarate} + \mathrm{NH_4} \rightleftharpoons \mathrm{GDHNAD^+} + \text{L-glutamate} + \mathrm{H_2O}$$

NADP can substitute for NADH in this reaction but the initial velocity of the reaction is however greater with the latter.

It seems probable that the enzyme activity of glutamic dehydrogenase is normally directed towards the formation of the amino acid rather than its breakdown since ammonia is not produced if excess glutamate is provided as the substrate. However, the enzyme is influenced by the concentration of inorganic ions in the incubation medium. Study of the rate of disappearance of reduced diphosphopyridine nucleotide (NADH) in the presence of the enzyme (Schoffeniels, 1968) indicates that increased cation concentration tends to result in increased enzyme activity. The optimal concentration of sodium is at about 50mM/l for a fresh water form *Astacus* and 500 mM for the marine species (*Eriocheir*).

Another enzyme affected by rising ion levels is lactic dehydrogenase which catalyses the reaction:

$$\text{pyruvate} + \mathrm{NADH} + \mathrm{H^+} \xrightarrow{\mathrm{LDH}} \text{lactate} + \mathrm{NAD}$$

and tends to favour the formation of lactate. Rising NaCl inhibits this enzyme, thus tending to increase the availability of NADH for amino acid formation.

In an environmental context it is of interest that whereas the lactate dehydrogenase of the euryhaline *Eriocheir* is influenced in this way by NaCl, irrespective of the level of pyruvate present, this is not true of the equivalent enzyme from the stenohaline *Homarus* (Schoffeniels, 1968).

3-glycerophosphate dehydrogenase, which is involved in the transfer of reducing equivalents to the cytochrome chain, is also influenced by ion levels. It seems likely, therefore, that the changing NaCl levels in cells which follow changes in blood concentration may directly influence amino acid formation through selective control of the availability of NADH or NADPH to production of amino acids or to the respiratory system as appropriate (Florkin and Schoffeniels, 1969).

$$\mathrm{NADH} \begin{cases} \rightarrow \text{glutamate} + \mathrm{NAD} \\ \rightarrow \text{cytochrome system} \\ \rightarrow \text{lactate} + \mathrm{NAD} \end{cases}$$

Examination of the effects of inorganic ions on other enzyme systems involved directly or indirectly in amino acid formation or breakdown indicates that although variation in the ion levels influence the activity of various lyase and dehydrogenase enzymes, there is no consistent difference between the effect on enzymes of the lobster *Homarus* or of the relatively more euryhaline species *Astacus* (Gilles, 1969). In both animals increasing NaCl tends to decrease the activity of isocitrate and malate dehydrogenase:

$$\text{pyruvate} + \mathrm{CO_2} + \mathrm{NADPH} \rightleftharpoons \text{malate} + \mathrm{NADP}$$

thus tending to decrease utilisation of NADPH whilst it increases the activity of another malate dehydrogenase controlling the reaction:

$$\text{malate} + \text{NAD} \rightleftharpoons \text{oxaloacetic} + \text{NADH}$$

which might be expected to favour subsequent glutamic acid production by providing the oxaloacetic precursor. Inorganic ion levels appear to have little effect on the activity of aspartate amino transferase in either lobster or crayfish (Gilles, 1969) and the same is also true of alanine amino-transferase (Huggins and Munday, quoted by Gilles, 1969). Thus, since rising NaCl levels tend to inhibit malate and serine hydrolyases, amino acid breakdown is decreased. Coupled with the increase in glutamic acid production the overall effect of rising intracellular NaCl would be expected to produce a raised internal amino acid level (*Figure 6.10*).

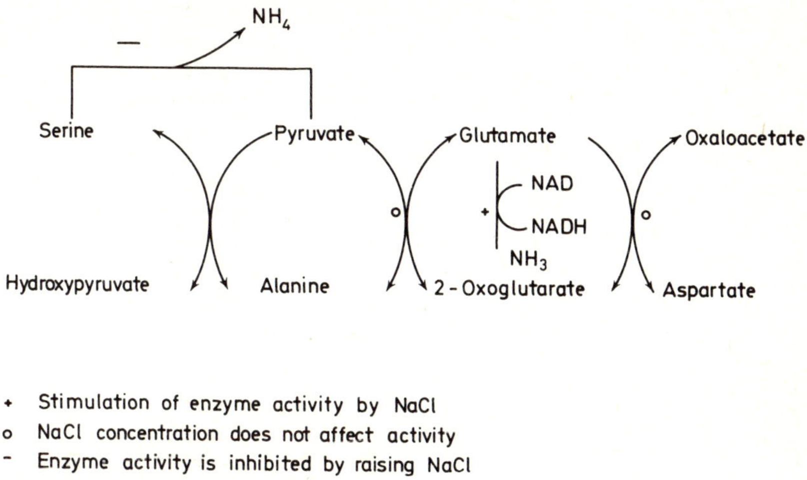

Figure 6.10 The role of NaCl in directing various enzyme systems towards the production and maintenance of amino acids in cells. (After Gilles, 1969; courtesy Arch. int. Physiol. Biochim.)

The levels of taurine, proline, alanine, aspartic and α-glutamic acid all increase when nerves from *Eriocheir* adapted to fresh water are isolated and placed into 100% seawater (Gilles and Schoffeniels, 1969), which implies, since the cell protein levels remain constant, both that amino acid formation occurs at the level of individual cells and that hormones are not necessary to initiate or maintain the process (Schoffeniels, 1960). However, examination of the loss and uptake of amino acids from cells indicates that intracellular synthesis and degradation are not the only factors contributing to the FAA level in cells.

6.2.3.2.3 Loss and uptake of amino acids by cells

In seawater some loss of proline and aspartic acid occurs from isolated nerves. When the incubating medium is diluted the loss of proline is greatly increased and so too is the loss of essential amino acids. Permeability changes probably account for this increased loss of the essential amino acids from the tissue. Glutamate, alanine, taurine, aspartic acid, serine and glycine all tend to decrease in the nerves but since they do not increase in the medium it is apparent that they must either have been deaminated or transaminated with subsequent degradation. This would correlate with the two observations that NH_4 loss from the cells is increased on dilution and that the amount of proline decrease in the nerves is *less* than the amount which appears in the medium (Gilles and Schoffeniels, 1969). Isolated ventricular cells of *Modiolus* also release amino acids to the medium on dilution (Pierce and Greenberg, 1972); taurine, glycine and alanine being particularly prominent in this case.

Tracer studies indicate that similar release of free amino acids from cells on dilution also occurs *in vivo*. ^{14}C-glycine, injected into *Carcinus,* is taken into the cells but if the animal is then transferred from 100 to 50% seawater the activity in the blood subsequently rises sharply for a time before declining once more. No such increase in blood ^{14}C levels occurs if crabs initially in 35 or 50% seawater are placed in 100% seawater (Austin, 1973).

Labelled glycine in the blood is also taken up into the hepatopancreas of *Carcinus* but conversely to the situation in other cells, the rate of uptake *increases* as the blood is diluted, (Austin, 1973). Presumably the hepatopancreas is involved in deamination of free amino acids released from other cells.

During the period of adaptation which follows transfer of organisms from seawater to a more dilute medium there is a substantial increase in the rate of release of ammonia both from the cells, (Gilles and Schoffeniels, 1969) and from the body (Emerson, 1968; Florkin *et al*., 1964; Austin, 1973; Jeuniaux and Florkin, 1961) whilst conversely ammonia release from the body declines during the period of re-acclimatisation to higher salinities. In *Carcinus* ammonia release remains relatively normal for a few hours after transfer from 100 to 50% seawater, then rises steeply between 5 and about 20 hours, when it returns to near the normal resting level (*Table 6.10*).

Table 6.10 TOTAL NON-PROTEIN NITROGEN (TNPN) OUTPUT RATE (μg/g BODY WEIGHT/h) AFTER TRANSFER OF *CARCINUS* FROM 100 TO 50% SEAWATER. OVER 90% OF TNPN IS AMMONIA (AFTER AUSTIN, 1973)

Hours since transfer	5.5	12	22	49	75	110
TNPN	6.6	23.6	19.3	4.4	3.5	2.2

Transfer of *Carcinus* from 11 to 38‰ salinity results in a sharp decrease in the levels of free amino acids in the blood despite the fact that the concentration in the body fluid as a whole is rising (Siebers *et al*., 1972). It appears likely, therefore, that uptake of free amino acids from the haemolymph into cells supplements the ability of cells to aminate organic acids to form amino acids *de novo.* The simultaneous drop in blood NH_4^+ levels is presumably a reflection of the amination process. The same authors also suggest that breakdown of blood protein may supply some amino acids for cell uptake.

The fact that isolated muscles from the euryhaline crab *Callinectes* regulate their volume well in hypotonic incubation media but only lose volume on exposure to hypertonic saline (Lang and Gainer, 1969) also seems to indicate that uptake of amino acids from the blood forms an important part of muscle free amino acid regulation (Weber and Van Marrewijk, 1972).

During the process of acclimatisation from 11 to 39‰ the trehalose in *Carcinus* rises some six-fold and this largely accounts for an approximate doubling of the total sugar concentration in the whole body fluid during osmotic adjustment (Siebers *et al*., 1972). Such a change contributes only marginally to overall cell balance and its precise metabolic function remains uncertain.

It seems clear, therefore, that intracellular changes in free amino acids are brought about both by anabolic and catabolic processes within the cell and by uptake and loss of amino acids across the cell surface. Presumably the relative importance of the two mechanisms will be found to vary from cell to cell. The overall effect of cell amino acid regulation is to permit rather accurate regulation of cell and blood volume regulation over a wide range of salinities in the more euryhaline forms; no change in extracellular space (^{131}I-diatrizoate space) can be detected in the amphipod *Gammarus duebeni* in the range 100 to 2% seawater (Lockwood and Inman, 1973b), in *Carcinus maenas* (inulin space) in the range 11.5–39.5‰ salinity (Siebers and Lucu, 1973) or in *Neanthes succinea* between 100 and 20% seawater (inulin space) (Freel, Medler and Clark, 1973).

In general it appears that development of the means of regulating the cell volume as the medium is diluted from seawater is also commonly associated with the ability to tolerate salinities in excess of that of seawater. For instance, Mars (1950) finds that molluscs capable of surviving in low salinities also tolerate high salinities (*Table 6.11*).

Table 6.11 SALINITY TOLERANCE RANGES OF SOME MOLLUSCS FROM ETANGS IN THE SOUTH OF FRANCE (AFTER MARS, 1950)

Species	*Mean concentration in salinity range* (‰)	*Range* ‰ ± *from mean*
Muricopsis blainoillei	37	2
Rissoa ventricosa	34	4
Ocenebra erinaceus	30	9
Gibbula adamsoni	27	12
Mytilus galloprovincialis	25	13
Loripes laetus	28	15
Bradydontis marioni	24	18
Cardium edule	32	28

6.2.3.3 REGULATION OF THE BODY FLUIDS CONCENTRATION HYPERTONIC TO THE MEDIUM

Regulation at the cellular level alone is inadequate to permit triploblastic forms to penetrate dilute brackish water or fresh water since normal cellular function necessitates a suitable external ion level (though the conformer *par excellence, Mercierella enigmatica* (serpulid polychaete), is practically isosmotic down to 50 mosmoles (Skaer, 1974)). In consequence all forms inhabiting dilute media maintain the body fluids more concentrated than the surroundings. The degree of hypertonicity displayed both in fresh water and in brackish water varies widely (*Figure 6.2(b)*) though, in the Crustacea, there is a tendency for the species of larger body size to have a higher osmotic gradient between blood and media than do smaller, related forms occupying the same general salinity range. Also, as might be anticipated, groups such as the molluscs and worms which have a relatively high surface permeability to water and inorganic ions tend to maintain smaller gradients than do the relatively less permeable Crustacea. Nevertheless even some of the euryhaline worms have a relatively high blood concentration in dilute media; *Nereis limnicola* (=*Neanthes lightii*) from Lake Mercred in California (2.6 mE/1 C1) have a blood concentration of 143 mE/1 C1 (Smith, 1957). A number of forms, including euryhaline teleost fish, some crabs, branchiopods, mysids, prawns, isopods and worms are hypertonic to media of low salinity and hypotonic to the medium at high salinity (*Figure 6.2(c)*).

Three factors must be considered in relation to the ability of animals to regulate themselves hypertonic to their medium: (a) permeability to water, (b) permeability to inorganic ions and (c) active uptake of ions. In addition, some forms can reduce renal ion loss by the production of urine hypotonic to the blood. Regulators maintaining themselves hypotonic to saline media do so by drinking the water and secreting excess ions across the body surface.

6.2.3.3.1 Surface permeability

Irrespective of whether they are regulators or conformers brackish and fresh water species tend in general to be less permeable to water and inorganic ions than related species, of similar body size, which are restricted to the sea.

6.2.3.3.2 Permeability to water

Comparison of non-marine with marine decapod Crustacea clearly illustrates the tendency for the former to reduce surface permeability. Thus Rudy (1967) has found that the permeability constants for water exchange in the marine crab *Macropipus depurator,* the estuarine and shore crab *Carcinus maenas* and the fresh water crayfish are, respectively, in the relationship 2.39, 0.79 and 0.20. Similarly, the brackish water isopod *Sphaeroma rugicauda* in 2% seawater exchanges water almost ten times more slowly than does the marine *Idotea linearis* (Lockwood and Inman, unpublished results) whilst the fresh water race of *Mesidotea entomon* from Lake Vättern is less permeable than either (Lockwood and Croghan, in the press).

Reduction in permeability has the advantage to a regulating form that it decreases the amount of water taken into the body by osmosis and hence the rate of ion loss during subsequent removal of excess water in the urine.

Decrease in permeability might at first sight appear unnecessary for an osmoconformer since, when the animal is in osmotic equilibrium, there will be little tendency for net transfer of either water or ions across the body surface other than under the influence of colloid osmotic pressure or indirectly through the effects of electrical gradients on electro-endosmosis. Presumably, however, the selective advantage of the degree of permeability reduction that does occur in such forms lies in the slowing of the rate of internal concentration change following *variation* in external salinity so that additional time is gained in which cellular osmotic adjustments may be effected.

In addition to the general differences in permeability between species inhabiting marine and non-marine environments some euryhaline species can vary their permeability to water according to the medium they are in. *Carcinus maenas* and another shore crab, *Hemigrapsus nudus,* which have comparable salinity tolerances, both show some decline in apparent

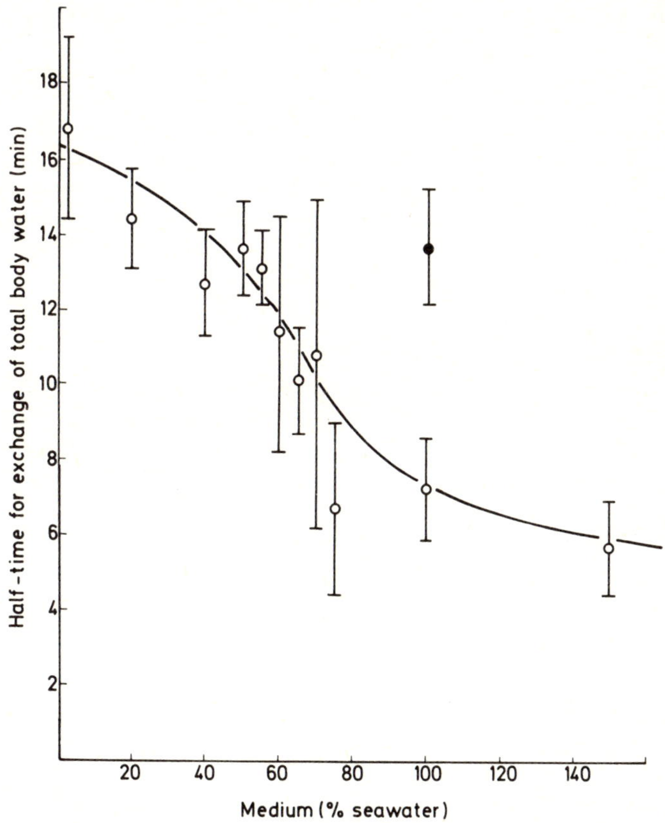

Figure 6.11 Reduction of apparent permeability to tritiated water in relation to dilution of the medium in Gammarus duebeni. *Vertical bars are 2 × the standard deviation. The solid dot is for animals exposed to a mannitol solution isotonic with seawater. (After Lockwood and Inman, 1973a; courtesy R. J. Skaer)*

permeability to water when the salinity of the medium is decreased from 100 to *c.*40% seawater (Smith, 1970d; Smith and Rudy, 1972). The still more euryhaline crab *Rhithropanopaeus harrisi* displays a somewhat larger variation in apparent permeability over the salinity range 95% seawater to 1% seawater (Smith, 1967) though not so great as in the amphipod *Gammarus duebeni* whose apparent permeability in fresh water is some 2.5 times less than in seawater, (Lockwood, Inman and Courtenay, 1973; *Figure 6.11*). The euryhaline worm *Nereis diversicolor* also displays a decrease in apparent permeability to water in dilute media (Smith, 1970).

Measurements of permeability using D_2O or T_2O are notoriously unreliable because of interference by such factors as isotopic differences (Smith and Rudy, 1972) unstirred layers (Dainty and House, 1966) or passage of water through narrow pores (Koeford-Johnsen and Ussing, 1953) but comparison of the urine flow with the net entry of water predicted from T_2O studies do indicate that in *Gammarus* at least the tracer fluxes give an approximation to the actual diffusional flow (Lockwood and Inman, 1973a).

Changes also occur in the apparent permeability to water in teleost fish in relation to salinity though the change is in the opposite sense to that of the invertebrates since the fish show a *decrease* in permeability on passing from fresh water to seawater (Potts *et al.*, 1967; Evans, 1969; Motais *et al.*, 1969). The necessity for fish to limit water loss by osmosis when in seawater possibly explains this difference, but hypotonic regulation in high salinities does not seem to result in an obligatory decline in permeability since the prawn *Palaemonetes varians* has a relatively constant apparent permeability in 120% seawater, 70% seawater and 10% seawater, media in which it is respectively hypotonic, isotonic and hypertonic (Rudy, 1967). Likewise the intertidal blenny *Pholis gunnellus* (teleost) does not vary water permeability in relation to salinity (Evans, 1969).

Artemia salina, the hypotonic regulator *par excellence,* doubtless owes part of its ability to survive in high salinities to an unusually low permeability to water, $T_{1/2}$ = 240 min (Smith, 1969; Ussing quoted by Krogh, 1939). It is also interesting to note in the same context that the water permeability of the euryhaline amphipod *Gammarus duebeni* is lower than that of the fresh water species *Gammarus pulex* again perhaps a reflection of the special adaptations required by a brackish water form to counter sudden changes in salinity rather than to meet the needs of the ultimate steady state. A further example of such specialised adaptation, also from the same animal, is that on transference from a low salinity to seawater the permeability initially declines still further and only gradually changes to the more permeable state generally found in fully adapted animals in seawater.

Some degree of facultative control may be exerted over permeability to water since removal of the eyestalks of the Mexican fresh water crab *Pseudotelphusa jouyi* (Thompson, 1967) is reported to increase the apparent permeability to tritiated water whilst ligaturing the base of the eyestalks increases the rate of water uptake by the crayfish *Procambarus clarkii* (Kamemoto and Ono, 1967) and by the crab *Metopograpsus messor* when it is hypertonic to the medium (Kato and Kamemoto, 1969). In the land crab *Gecarcinus* the apparent permeability of the foregut and passage of water and ions towards the blood is increased by extracts of the thoracic ganglion mass (Mantel, 1968). Nevertheless, it would perhaps be premature to believe that hormonal effects can be solely responsible for *all* the observed change in water permeability in relation to salinity since in *Gammarus* permeability constants appropriate to the dilute medium are established within (at most) five minutes following transfer to a low salinity; a time so short as to cast some doubts on the primacy of a hormonal regulating system Lockwood and Inman, 1973a). Observations by Saleé and Vidrequin-Deliege (1967) that stimulation of the brachial plexus of toads results in changes in the potential difference across the skin and in the ionic permeability of the skin, suggests that there might be some merit in examining the relationship between potential difference and apparent water permeability in euryhaline forms.

Other factors tending to affect water fluxes include temperature (Smith

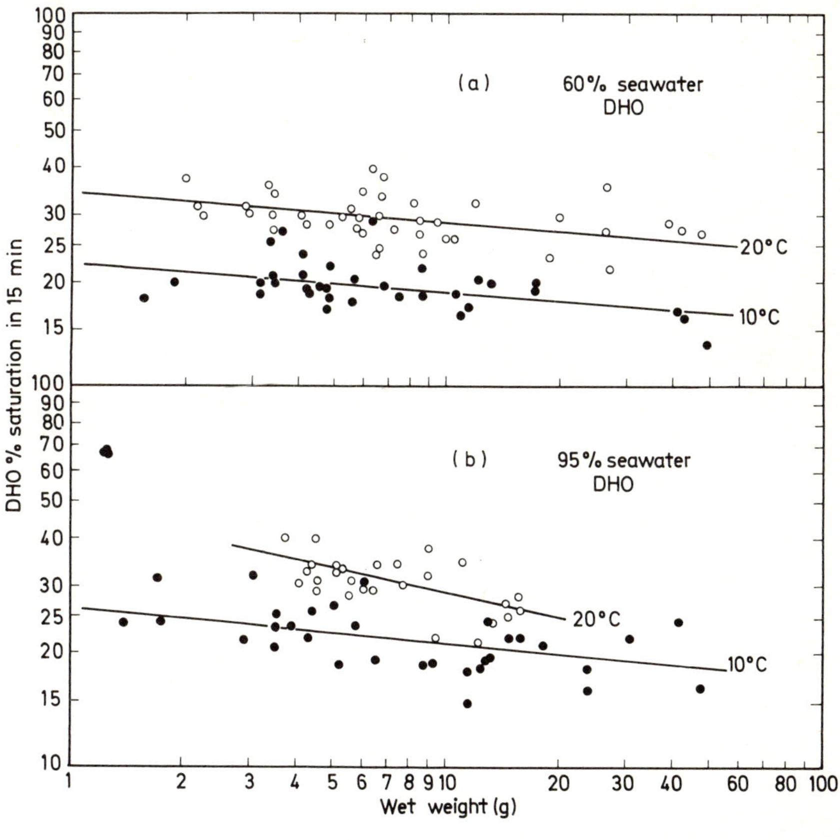

Figure 6.12 Uptake of deuterium oxide (D_2O) by Hemigrapsus nudus *in a 15 min period, showing the effect of temperature, salinity and body size on the overall exchange. (After Smith and Rudy, 1972; courtesy The Biological Bulletin)*

and Rudy, 1972; Evans, 1969), moult (in crustaceans) (Lockwood and Inman, 1973) and calcium concentration of the medium (in fish) (Potts *et al*., 1967).

The Q_{10} for influx of D_2O or T_2O in the crab *Hemigrapsus nudus* is about 1.62 (*Figure 6.12*) in the temperature range 10–20°C and Evans (1969) has similarly found a Q_{10} of approximately 2 for euryhaline teleosts.

The apparent permeability to water increases by a factor of about two when the euryhaline amphiphod *Gammarus duebeni* moults. This increase is about the same as that shown by the neritic marine isopod, *Idotea linearis,* which implies that the evolution of adaptational mechanisms for life in dilute media has not extended to decreasing changes in permeability at moult though more species must be examined before any definitive conclusion can be reached on this point (Lockwood and Inman, 1973c).

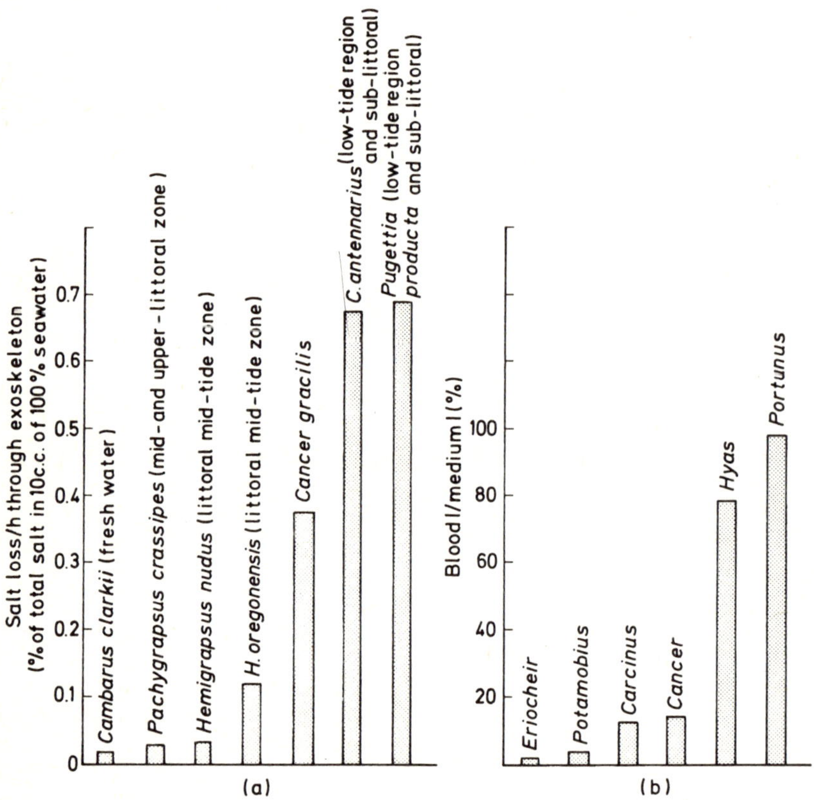

Figure 6.13 The ionic permeability of the exoskeleton of Crustacea from different environments showing the restricted permeability of brackish water and shore forms (after Lockwood, 1962 from Gross, 1957 and Nagel, 1934). (a) Relative permeability of the exoskeleton; the values are the means of three determinations with a gradient of 50% seawater across a portion of cuticle (permeability data from Gross, 1957b; shore distribution from Ricketts and Calvin, 1948). (b) Ratio of iodine in the blood to that in the medium 2½ h after placing various species in seawater containing sodium iodide. (After Nagel, 1934). Courtesy Cambridge University Press

6.2.3.3.3. Permeability to inorganic ions

The surface permeability to inorganic ions is reduced in euryhaline forms by comparison with related brackish water species. Nagel (1934) demonstrated that the rate of penetration of iodide into euryhaline and fresh water Crustacea was slower than that into sub-littoral marine forms whilst Gross (1957b) found a comparable relationship in the permeability of the cuticle and epidermis to salt of species from a range of habitats (*Figure 6.13*). Similarly in the annelids the permeability of the brackish water *Nereis diversicolor* to chloride is less than that of the marine *N. virens* (Jørgensen and Dales, 1957) and *N. diversicolor* is also less permeable to sodium than the more marine *Perinereis cultrifera* (Fretter, 1955). Conversely, on exposure to distilled water *N. limnicola* (which can survive and reproduce in fresh water for extended periods) loses salt more slowly than *N. diversicolor* itself (Smith, 1957).

Salt loss encompasses both loss in the urine and across the body surface but, at least in the larger crustaceans, it is the latter which tends to account for the major part of the total. Thus, in the Chinese wool-handed crab *Eriocheir sinensis,* the surface loss accounts for some 86% of the total (Krogh, 1938), in the crayfish *Austropotamobius* it is 90–92% (Shaw, 1959b; Bryan, 1960) and in the African fresh water crab *Potamon niloticus* blocking the excretory pores for 3 hours makes little difference to the overall rate of salt loss (Shaw, 1959a). Similarly in the worm *Nereis diversicolor* integumental loss is at least twice as great as the urine loss (Smith, 1970a).

Decrease in surface permeability results in a diminution of the specific loss rate in euryhaline Crustacea (*Table 6.12*) which thus in turn decreases the amount of work which has to be expended in replacing ions which have been lost by diffusion and in the urine.

Examination of the rate of sodium loss in terms of mM/l Cl per hour indicates the same feature (*Table 6.13*).

The isopod *Mesidotea entomon* and amphipod *Gammarus duebeni* are of interest since both have races well established in fresh water in addition to the main brackish water stocks. In both species the individuals colonising fresh water show a markedly slower rate of salt loss than do their brackish water relatives *Figure 6.14*.

To hypotonic regulators ion penetration down the concentration gradient presents a potential problem and appropriately *Palaemon serratus* is reported to effect a marked reduction in ion permeability when regulating the body fluids hypotonic to supra-normal salinities, i.e. 42‰ (Spaargaren, 1972).

Responses of the Crustacea to Ca^{2+} levels in the media are variable. *Carcinus* shows a marked decline in sodium efflux at a salinity of 15.9‰ when the Ca^{2+} level is increased by 5.10 mM/l (Lucu, 1973) but in *Gammarus pulex* (freshwater) and *G. duebeni* (brackish water) sodium loss rates do not appear to be influenced by the level of calcium in the medium. Ammocoete larvae of the lamprey in dilute media lose Na^{+} more rapidly in the absence of Ca^{2+} (Morris and Bull, 1968) and sodium efflux is also increased in the euryhaline teleost *Fundulus kansae* when the Ca^{2+} content of the media is lowered (Potts and Fleming, 1971). In teleosts also it appears

Table 6.12 RELATIONSHIP BETWEEN SPECIFIC LOSS RATE AND HABITAT IN VARIOUS DECAPOD CRUSTACEANS (VALUES FROM SHAW, 1961b)

		Habitat	*Blood (sodium)* (mM/l)	*Specific loss rate* (μM/h)
Crabs	*Carcinus maenas*	Marine and brackish water	300[1]	891
	Eriocheir sinensis	Estuarine and fresh water	280	153
	Potamon niloticus	Fresh water	259	27
Crayfish	*Autropotamobius fluviatilis*	Fresh water	186	4.7

[1] In 40% seawater

$$\text{Specific loss rate} = \frac{\text{Observed loss } (\mu\text{M/50g/h})}{\left(\frac{\text{Weight}}{50}\right)^{2/3}}$$

Table 6.13 (ADAPTED FROM SUTCLIFFE, 1968)

	Habitat	*Av. Wt.* (g)	*Na loss rate* (mM/l blood/h)	*Blood (Na)* (mM/1)	*Medium* (mM/l Na)	*T* (°C)
[1] *Carcinus maenas*	S-W[14]–B-W[15]	50	51	300	180	15–20
[2] *Pachygrapsus crassipes*	S-W –B-W	24	43	280	190	15
[3] *Eriocheir sinensis*	B-W –F-W	153	6.0	280	10	15
[4] *Potamon niloticus*	F-W[16]	15	2.3	259	0.5	24
[5] *Palaemonetes varians*	B-W	0.15	51.5	204	10	15
[6] *Palaemonetes antennarius*	F-W	0.15	13.7	177	0.5	15
[7] *Asellus aquaticus*	F-W	0.06	2.2	137	0.4	15–22
[8] *Sphaeroma rugicauda*	B-W		53.1			
[8] *Sphaeroma serratum*	S-W		96.9			
[13] *Mesidotea entomon* (F-W race)	F-W	0.25	8.8	260	0.17	10
[9] *Daphnia magna*	F-W	0.002	4.7	65	0.3	20
[10] *Triops longicaudatus*	F-W	0.5	3.2	74	0.25	25
[9] *Marinogammarus finmarchicus*	S-W	0.055	57.0	*c.*300	60–120	
[9] *M. obtusatus*	S-W	0.036	80.0	—	60–120	
[9] *G. tigrinus*	B-W	0.030	20.0	220	10	
[11] *G. duebeni*	B-W	0.071	10.9	273	10	
[9] *G. zaddachi*	B-W	0.048	13.7	252	10	
[11] *G. pulex*	F-W	0.047	4.9	135	0.3–0.5	
[12] *G. lacustris*	F-W	0.048	4.0	135	0.3–0.5	
[9] *Crangonyx pseudogracilis*	F-W	0.005	7.1	*c.*130	0.3	10

[1] Shaw (1961a)
[2] Rudy (1966)
[3] Shaw (1961b)
[4] Shaw (1959a)
[5] Potts and Parry (1964a)
[6] Parry and Potts (1965)
[7] Lockwood (1959)
[8] Harris (1970)
[9] Sutcliffe (1968)
[10] Horne (1966)
[11] Sutcliffe (1967)
[12] Sutcliffe and Shaw (1967a)
[13] Croghan, P. C. and Lockwood, A.P.M. (unpublished data)
[14] S-W=seawater
[15] B-W=brackish water
[16] F-W=fresh water

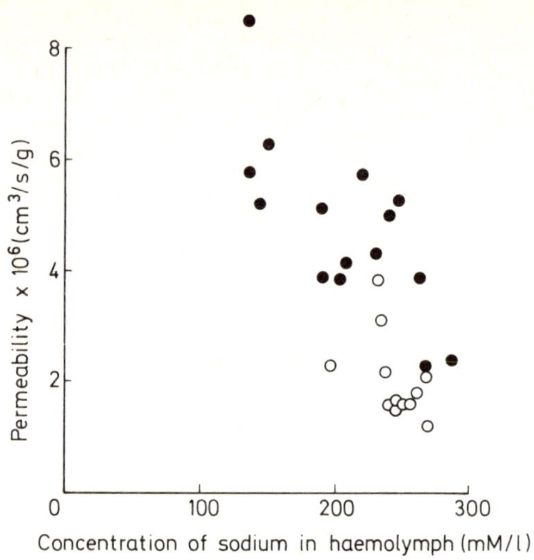

Figure 6.14 Comparison of the permeability to sodium in the Baltic (Asko) race (closed circles) and fresh water race (open circles) (Lake Malaren) of the isopod Mesidotea entomon. *(After Croghan and Lockwood, 1968; courtesy R. J. Skaer)*

that the hormone prolactin from the pituitary plays a major role in limiting the permeability to inorganic ions, and hence the loss of NaCl, when the fish are in fresh water (Potts and Fleming, 1971).

6.2.3.3.4 Hypotonic urine

Calculations based on steady state thermodynamic considerations suggest that it is less wasteful of energy to produce urine hypotonic to the blood than to lose ions during isotonic urine production and subsequently re-adsorb them from the medium (Croghan, 1962). For hypertonic animals living in low and fluctuating salinities the development of the ability to conserve ions by the formation of dilute urine may also represent an evolutionary expression of the old adage 'a bird in the hand . . . etc.'.

Marine invertebrates produce urine which is isotonic with the blood. In some cases, as in the gastropods *Acmaea scutum* (Webber and Dehnel, 1968) and *Nerita fulgurens* (Little, 1972) there are only minor differences in the ionic constitution of the blood and urine. Where marked disparities occur between the ionic composition of the blood and medium it is, however, usual for the excretory organ to participate in maintaining such differences by conserving ions which are concentrated in the blood and expediting the excretion of those which are reduced in the blood (*Table 6.14*).

In the case of *Carcinus* supposedly non-secreted markers such as inulin, diatrizoate and ethylene-diamine tetra-acetic acid are concentrated in the urine; thus implying that water and all other ions have been re-adsorbed (Riegel *et al.*, 1974) even though the urine remains isotonic with the blood. Re-absorption of water declines proportionally both if the urine flow rate is increased (as when the medium is diluted) or if the animal is treated with the inhibitor ethacrynic acid.

Table 6.14 THE ROLE OF THE EXCRETORY ORGAN IN CONTRIBUTING TO THE MAINTENANCE OF DIFFERENCES BETWEEN THE IONIC COMPOSITION OF THE BLOOD FROM THE MEDIUM (AFTER RAMSAY, 1961)

		Na	K	Ca	Mg	Cl	SO_4
Eledone (octopus)	(B)/(M)%	97	152	107	103	102	77
	(U)/(B)%	102	90	87	89	97	136
Carcinus (crab)	(B)/(M)%	110	117	108	34	104	61
	(U)/(B)%	95	78	94	390	98	224

(M), (U), (B) = concentration in medium, urine and blood respectively

Some modification of the relative rates of ion and water movement would confer on such a system the ability to produce hypotonic urine. A trend in this direction is seen in the euryhaline crab *Pachygrapsus crassipes* which is reported (Prosser, Green and Chow, 1955) to display a small measure of urinary hypotonicity at times.

The ability to produce urine more markedly hypotonic to the body fluids, and thus to conserve ions whilst eliminating water, has clearly evolved many times since it is present in many unrelated freshwater animals: *Limnaea pereger* (Picken, 1937); *Theodoxus fluviatilis* (Little, 1972); *Viviparus viviparus* (Little, 1965); *Anodonta cygnaea* (Florkin and Duchâteau, 1949); *Lumbricus terrestis* (Ramsay, 1961); *Gammarus pulex* (Lockwood, 1961); the Atyid shrimp *Syncaris pacifica* (Born, 1968); *Austropotomobius* (Bryan, 1960) etc. The faculty has been less studied in euryhaline species but production of urine more dilute than the blood has been measured *inter alia* in brackish water amphipods *G. duebeni* (Lockwood, 1961), *G. fasciatus* (Werntz, 1963), *Corophium volutator* (McLusky, 1968), the worm *Nereis diversicolor* (Smith, 1970c; *Table 6.15*) and in the euryhaline prosobranch *Potamopyrgus jenkinsi* (Todd, 1964).

Table 6.15 OSMOTIC CONCENTRATION OF MEDIUM, COELOMIC FLUID AND URINE OF *NEREIS DIVERSICOLOR* (AFTER SMITH, 1970c)

Medium	*Coelomic fluid* (mM/l NaCl)	*Urine* (mM/l NaCl)	*Medium* (mM/l NaCl)
Baltic S-W[1] (*c*.95 mE(l Cl)	178	150	101.2
Diluted Baltic water (*c*. 30mE/l Cl)	150.9	90.3	36.8
Diluted Baltic water (*c*. 10 mE/l Cl)	130.2	78.3	18.0
Diluted Baltic water (*c*. 5 mE/l Cl)	119.6	59.5	5.8

[1] S-W=seawater

The capacity to produce hypotonic urine appears in at least some forms to be related to the length of the excretory duct. Thus in the gammarids, forms with long ducts produce more dilute urine than those with short ducts, *Table 6.16*. Similarly the worm *Lycastis indica*, which inhabits dilute brackish water and can live for months in fresh water, has a relatively larger nephridium than worms such as *Perinereis nuntia* and *Nereis chilkaensis*, which live in marine and strongly saline waters (Krishnan, 1952).

Table 6.16

	Natural habitat[1]	*Length of tubule*[2] (mm)	*Acclim. medium*	*Blood* (mM/l)	*Urine* (mM/l NaCl)
Gammarus locusta	25–35‰	1.6	50% S-W[3]	440	440
Gammarus duebeni	0.1–40‰	3.0	F-W[4]	260	40–50
Gammarus pulex	F-W	4.0	F-W	150	5–10

[1] Based on Bassindale (1942)
[2] Values for 12 mm individuals (Hynes, 1954)
[3] S-W=seawater
[4] F-W=fresh water

Hypotonic urine formation in brackish water forms would be expected to be primarily a useful adaptation to hypertonic species with high water permeability at the body surface and to small animals, i.e. those having a large surface to volume ratio. In both cases a large proportion of the total body ion content would be lost in a short period if the urine remained isotonic with the body fluids when the medium was suddenly diluted. Provided that the loss of inorganic ions across the body surface is not large, the production of hypotonic urine will delay drop in blood concentration following dilution of the media and so permit time for regulatory adjustments at the cellular level. The role of the excretory organ in this respect is clearly shown in the case of *Gammarus duebeni.* This amphipod inhabits small pools on salt marshes, rockpools above high tide level and similar sites where it may be exposed both to hypersaline waters and to the risk of sudden dilution of the medium by rain water. When fully acclimatised to media in the range 2% seawater to 160% seawater the animal produces urine hypotonic to the haemolymph only when the water is more dilute than about 40% seawater (*Figure 6.15(a)*). However, the physiological response in non-steady state conditions is very different. On sudden transference from 160% seawater to fresh water the animals start producing urine hypotonic to the blood within about two hours at a time when the blood concentration *is still in excess of 100% seawater* (*Figure 6.15(b)*). Such an 'anticipatory' response on the part of the control systems regulating urine concentration does much to lessen the rate of decline of blood concentration in these circumstances (Lockwood, 1964). A comparable 'anticipatory' response in respect of the active uptake of sodium from the media is shown both by *G. duebeni* and the estuarine isopod *Sphaeroma rugicauda* (cf. p. 356).

6.2.3.3.5 *Active transport of inorganic ions*

Active transport of inorganic ions against the electro-chemical gradient to replace ions lost by diffusion and in the urine is a general feature of euryhaline organisms. The rate of transport is influenced by (1) physiological factors within the animal, including:

(a) the balance between different ion species in the blood,
(b) the overall blood concentration,
(c) effects engendered by sudden dilution of the medium,

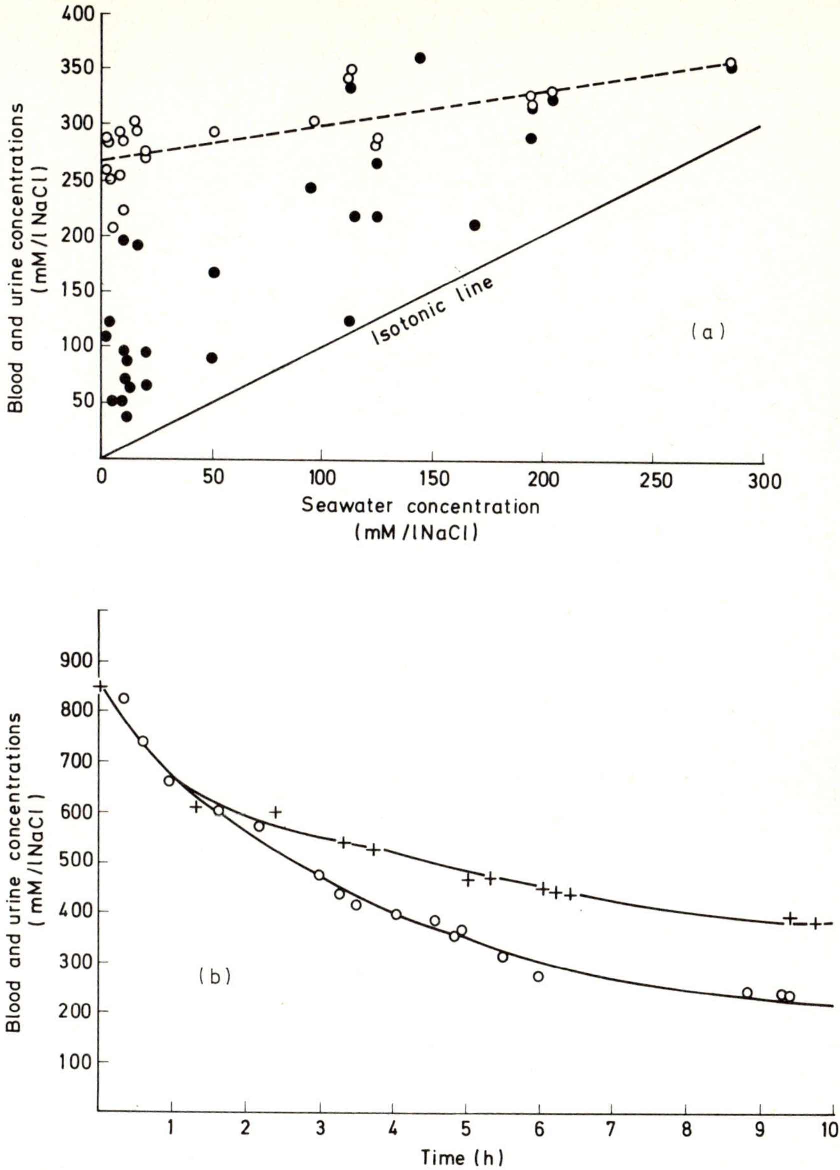

Figure 6.15 Hypotonic urine formation by Gammarus duebeni. *(a) In animals fully acclimatised to the medium hypotonic urine is produced at salinities lower than c.40% seawater. Open circles = blood; closed circles = urine. (b) Dilute urine is produced at high blood concentrations when animals have been transferred from a high salinity to fresh water. Open circles = urine; crosses = blood. (After Lockwood, 1961; courtesy R. J. Skaer)*

(d) blood volume,
(e) processes occurring in association with ecdysis (Crustacea),

and by (2) physical and chemical features of the environment whose effects are mediated via the transporting mechanism. This latter category includes:

(f) cations (other than those being transported) and pH,
(g) temperature,
(h) concentration of the ion being transported in relation to the affinity of the transport mechanism for the ion.

(a) Ion balance The rate of loss of different ion species varies. In the crayfish for instance, the loss of chloride may be only 72% of the sodium loss rate (Shaw, 1960) and consequently it is necessary that the systems regulating different ions should have independence of activity. Such independence has been demonstrated on *Eriocheir* which can take up chloride from *inter alia* NaCl, KCl, NH_4Cl and Ca Cl_2 and sodium from NaCl, Na_2SO_4 and Na HCO_3 (Krogh, 1939; Shaw, 1960).

Effect of inbalance in ion ratios: Disturbance of the internal ion balance results in changes in rate of transport of one ion relative to another, e.g. when *Eriocheir* is maintained for a time in $NaHCO_3$ the chloride level in the blood falls. On subsequent return to sodium chloride the crab takes up chloride faster than sodium, the reverse of the normal situation, until the haemolymph ion ratios have been restored to normal (Shaw, 1960).

(b) Effect of blood concentration on rate of transport Any factor which results in a decline in the blood concentration of a hypertonic regulator tends to result in the mobilisation of additional ion transporting capacity. Increased loss of ions resulting from change in permeability or dilution of the medium thus initiates an increase in uptake. The degree of change of blood concentration required to produce maximal transport differs however between fresh water Crustacea and similar forms living in estuarine waters. The crayfish shows some increase in sodium uptake after 1–2% decline in blood concentration and the sites are fully activated by a decrease of some 6–8% (Shaw, 1959b); by contrast the euryhaline isopod *Sphaeroma rugicauda* gradually increases the rate of uptake if acclimatised to media from 80–10% seawater over which range the blood Na concentration falls from about 490 to 250 mM/l (Harris, 1970; *Figure 6.16*).

(c) Sudden dilution of the medium It must be stressed, however, that the gradual increase in uptake rate, linked apparently to blood concentration in *Sphaeroma,* is a feature occurring when the animals have been *acclimatised* to the various media. If by contrast the animals are acclimatised to a high concentration (>150% seawater) and are then suddenly transferred to 2% seawater, the transport rate rises quickly and full capacity is mobilised within 4–5 h, by which time the blood concentration has only fallen to some 500 mM/l sodium. Thus, in the non-steady state, maximal uptake can occur when the blood is still about twice as concentrated as the level at which the same transport rate would be expected in animals after full acclimatisation to 2%

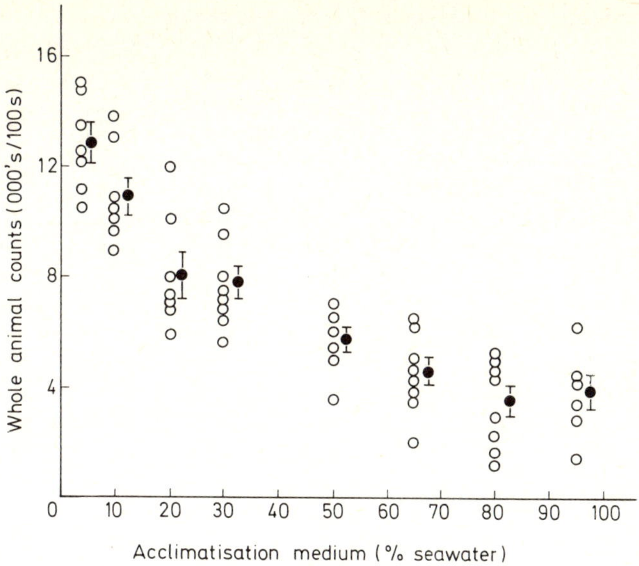

Figure 6.16 The relationship between rate of uptake of ^{22}*Na from 10 mM/l NaCl and the salinity to which* Sphaeroma rugicauda *has been previously acclimatised. (After Harris, 1970; courtesy Pergamon Press Ltd)*

seawater (Harris, 1970). A similar response occurs when the highly euryhaline *Gammarus duebeni* is transferred from a high to low concentration (Lockwood, 1964). This form of 'anticipatory' response on the part of the uptake system must have an invaluable effect, like that of hypotonic urine formation in similar circumstances, in slowing the decline in blood concentration on dilution and so gaining time for osmotic adjustments to be made at the cellular level. Small animals living in niches liable to sudden and extensive salinity changes are particularly liable to suffer rapid changes of blood concentration and it may be expected that such a response may be fairly general in such forms.

The factors initiating the 'anticipatory' response have not been elucidated but could include such parameters as detection of the potential difference or ion gradient across the body surface, rate of change of blood concentration or change in volume of some body compartment. Variation in volume of the whole body can result in changes in transport rate though this does not seem a likely factor in the above response since it would be expected to operate in the opposite sense (*see below*).

(d) The effect of volume on sodium transport Damage responsible for a loss of blood would not result in a drop in blood concentration in isosmotic marine forms. Consequently it is necessary for such animals to have ion and water regulatory systems maintaining volume.

Evidence for the presence of volume monitoring systems has been obtained on *Gammarus duebeni* (Lockwood, 1970) and on the snail *Lymnaea stagnalis* (Greenaway, 1970). In the former, physical removal of blood or decrease in blood concentration effected by placing the animals in isosmotic non-electrolyte results in a subsequent increase in the rate of active sodium uptake. In the snail the depletion of the blood volume initiates a three-fold increase in sodium uptake (Greenaway, 1970).

The inference to be drawn from the response of at least *G. duebeni* is that water accompanies such an ion intake through some form of ion mediated water transport (cf. Diamond, 1965). Even when *G. duebeni* is in a steady state after acclimatisation to seawater (with which medium it is effectively isosmotic), uptake of ions continues at a slow rate. Part of this uptake can possibly be attributed to osmotic inflow produced by blood colloid osmotic pressure, but the remainder appears to be due to active transport processes. Inhibition of part of the sodium uptake with the dye Thionine (3:6 diaminophenthiazine) results in a subsequent equivalent decline in urine volume, implying that ion uptake is also involved in the uptake of water which will subsequently be excreted as urine (Lockwood and Inman, 1973a).

It is interesting to speculate as to whether such a mechanism, evolved initially in marine organisms to transport fluid into the body for volume regulation and urine production, might not have provided the necessary unidirectional transport system on which selection could act to produce mechanisms capable of maintaining the blood hypertonic to dilute media. The presence of such a preadapting feature in marine forms would then go some way towards explaining the frequency with which the capacity to regulate hypertonically in dilute media has evolved in fresh water and brackish water species. More studies are required on the relationship between salt transport and volume regulation in isosmotic marine forms to establish whether the *Gammarus* condition is indeed general to other more fully marine animals.

A necessary requirement for an animal able to maintain its blood hypertonic to dilute media, and also to effect water transport when isosmotic with its medium is to be capable of altering the relative permeability of the body surface to water and inorganic ions. As has already been noted, *Gammarus* does indeed vary the permeability to water in relation to the salinity of the medium.

Nothing is yet known of the way in which the systems controlling volume and concentration of the body fluids interact in euryhaline invertebrates when their requirements conflict. Interesting observations by Greenaway (1970) indicate, however, that when the freshwater snail *Limnaea* is depleted of blood it partly restores volume by permitting net water uptake but full recovery of weight does not occur until sodium intake approximates to water intake.

(e) The effect of moult on ion uptake When some crustaceans moult in seawater there is a marked increase in ion uptake during the period when the body is being expanded. Starting a few hours before ecdysis *Gammarus duebeni* increases the active uptake of sodium to some 20 to 40 times the normal level shown by intermoult animals. The increased uptake declines gradually, returning to the intermoult level some five days after ecdysis

(Lockwood and Andrews, 1969). Water uptake by *Maia* following ecdysis is stopped if chloride ions in the medium are replaced by sulphate suggesting that water uptake is linked to ion transport in this animal also (Dandrifosse, 1966). *Carcinus* drinks extensively at ecdysis implying that, in this case, fluid and ion uptake is largely across the gut wall (Robertson, 1960).

6.2.4 Physical and chemical factors influencing transport rates

6.2.4.1 THE EFFECT OF OTHER CATIONS (H^+, NH_4^+, Ca^{2+} AND K^+)

Seawater is relatively conservative in respect of the major ions. However, admixture with fresh water in estuaries and still more so in special brackish water environments such as mangrove swamps, salt marshes etc. can result in rather extensive variation in pH, nitrogenous materials including ammonia and Ca^{2+}. Such changes might be anticipated to influence the ion transport processes either directly through interference with exchange processes or indirectly via action on the permeability to ions and/or water. Increases in the hydrogen ion content or of ammonium ions decrease sodium uptake. In the presence of 1 mM/l NH_4 or 0.1 mM/l HCl (pH_4) the sodium uptake by crayfish from fresh water is decreased by 70–80%. External NH_4^+ also depresses sodium uptake in *Gammarus pulex* and *G. zaddachi* (Sutcliffe, 1971a).

Detailed understanding of the transport process in epithelial cells is still lacking but the hypothesis presented by Maetz and Garcia Romeu (1964) represents current views on the process and indicates why NH_4^+ and H^+ can interfere with sodium transport. In their view, energy-demanding ion 'pumps' transport sodium and chloride from the lumen of epithelial cells into the blood; the sodium and chloride thus pumped having entered the cell originally largely in exchange for NH_4^+ and HCO_3^- ions. The HCO_3^- is derived from ionisation of carbonic acid and the NH_4^+ from combination of NH_3 (derived from amino acid deamination) with H^+ from the bicarbonate ionisation (*Figure 6.17*). Evidence supporting this concept includes the fact that Diamox, which inhibits carbonic anhydrase, interferes with sodium uptake.

If this model represents the actual transport situation, it would be expected that if NH_4^+ or H^+ levels are raised in the medium the effect would be to inhibit the initial sodium entry into the epithelial cell and so slow down transport into the blood. However, in natural estuarine conditions the NH_4^+ and H^+ levels are probably rarely high enough to have an appreciable effect on ion transport since, as shown by Shaw (1960), the influence of NH_4^+ is lessened as the Na^+ level is raised.

The interaction of calcium with the transport system and its mode of action are more enigmatic since the effect of raising the concentration of calcium in the medium of brackish water organisms and fresh water organisms varies with the species studied. Sodium uptake by *Austropotamobius fluviatilis* is unaffected by concentrations of calcium up to 1 mM/l, but declines somewhat at higher concentrations of Ca^{2+} (Shaw,

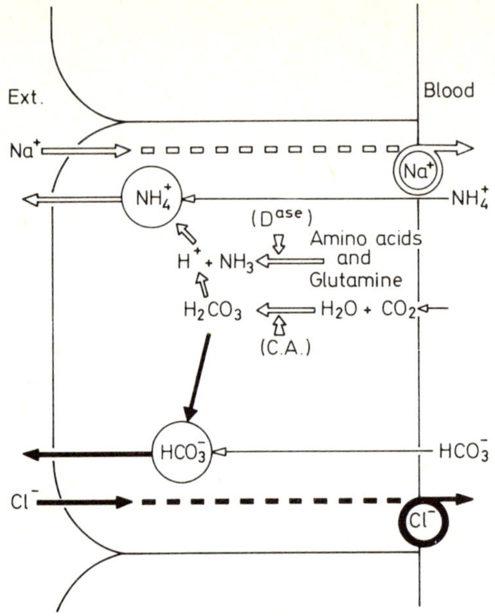

Figure 6.17 A model of sodium and chloride transport across an epithial layer from the medium to the blood C.A. = carbonic anhydrase; Dose = *deamination and deamidation enzymes. (After Maetz and Garcia Romeu, 1964; courtesy J. General Physiology)*

1960). Similarly sodium influx in the fresh water amphipod *Gammarus pulex* and the brackish water species *Gammarus duebeni* is unaffected by Ca^{2+} levels of up to 2 mM/l. However, in another brackish water species, *G. zaddachi,* $CaCl_2$ levels of up to 2–4 mM/l stimulate sodium uptake whilst levels in excess of this depress the uptake. Uptake by *G. pulex* is also depressed by Ca^{2+} in excess of 2 mM/l (Sutcliffe, 1971a). Uptake of sodium by the ammocoete larve of *Lampetra planeri* is enhanced by the presence of Ca^{2+} in the medium (Morris and Bull, 1968). Care must be taken in interpreting the effects of the addition of $CaCl_2$ on sodium uptake as in some cases, including perhaps that of *G. zaddachi* above, it is the effect of the additional chloride rather than the Ca^{2+} ion *per se* which stimulates the increment in sodium uptake (Sutcliffe, 1971a).

The mode of action of Ca^{2+} is uncertain and is in any case probably multiple. If analogy can be drawn with a secretory tissue such as the salivary gland of insects, it appears that Ca^{2+} may increase the permeability of apical membranes to Cl^- and also, acting in conjunction with cyclic AMP, stimulate potassium transport. Furthermore the ion may influence the potential differences and also appears to be involved in a number of other feedback and mediating functions in transport cells (Prince and Berridge, 1972). Prediction of the likely effects of changing the Ca^{2+} concentration of the medium on loss and uptake rates of ions in euryhaline organisms are likely therefore to be of an uncertain value.

6.2.4.2 POTASSIUM

The sodium extrusion mechanism of teleosts in seawater is sensitive to the external K^+ level in some cases, the extrusion slowing in the absence of the ion. In the flounder *Platichthys flexus* the influx of potassium from the medium is equivalent to the calculated net extrusion of sodium ions; the absence of external potassium ion decreases Na^+ extrusion so that the blood Na^+ levels of animals in seawater rises; the addition of K^+ ions to the medium stimulates efflux of sodium (Maetz, 1969). Similarly in the teleost *Dormitator maculatus* removal of external K^+ reduces efflux of sodium (Evans, Mallery and Kravitz, 1973). The K_m value for the influence of potassium on the sodium transport by *Dormitator* is only 2 mM/l and, if the same applies to other euryhaline fish, it would appear that decreasing K^+ levels as seawater is progressively diluted is unlikely to incommode the sodium extrusion system down to the point at which fish reverse the direction of transport and so become independent of external K^+ levels.

At up to 20 times the Na^+ level in the medium, potassium levels do not appear to influence Na^+ transport in the crayfish (Shaw, 1960) and presumably the naturally occurring ratios of this ion to sodium in brackish waters are unlikely to affect sodium transport of other euryhaline species.

6.2.4.3 TEMPERATURE

The rate of transport of inorganic ions, being dependent on metabolic processes, is affected by the level of the ambient temperature. In general a drop in temperature results in a lowering of the transport rate. However, the effect that a decline in temperature has on the blood concentration of hypertonic regulators obviously depends on whether the temperature coefficient for loss of ions is greater or less than that of the uptake system. Two examples will suffice. In *Asellus aquaticus* uptake rate varies directly with temperature whilst loss rate (of sodium) is scarcely affected, consequently the blood concentration declines as the temperature is lowered (Lockwood, 1960). The converse occurs in *Gammarus duebeni* where, the coefficient for loss being apparently greater than that for uptake, the blood concentration tends to rise as the temperature is lowered. A still more complex situation occurs in *Crangon crangon* since in this animal the effect on the blood concentration differs according to the part of the salinity range selected (Weber and Spaargaren, 1970; *Figure 6.18*). Sudden temperature changes at salinities of 10.7‰ and 20.2‰ confirm these differences, the temperature correlation being inverse at the high salinity and direct at the lower.

Differences in the temperature coefficients of loss and uptake do not of course result in animals going permanently out of salt balance, since, if the temperature is altered, any variation in blood concentration will tend to result in alteration in rate of transport. If transport is slowed more than loss by a decline in temperature a drop in blood concentration will ensue and this drop will effect the mobilisation of more transport activity; thus restoring

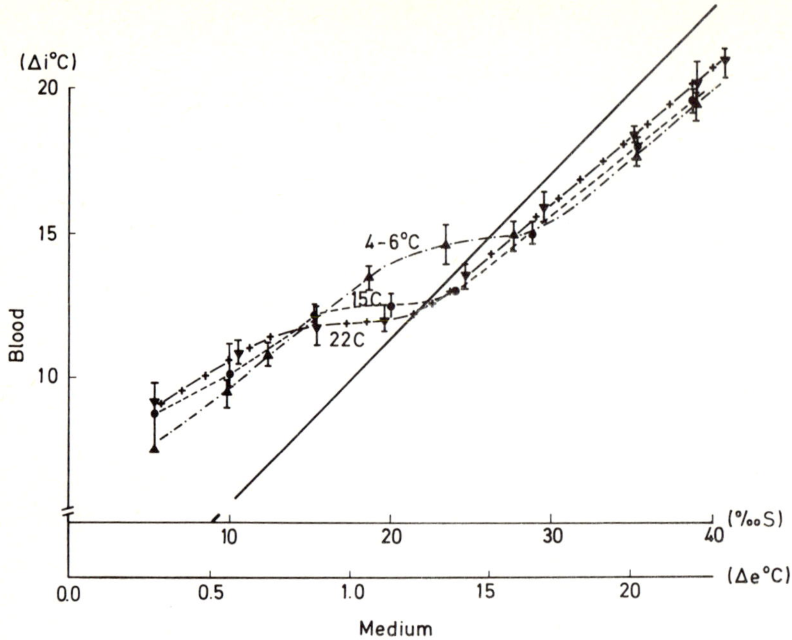

Figure 6.18 The effect of temperature on the concentration of the blood of Crangon crangon *at different salinities. (After Weber and Spaargaren, 1972; courtesy Netherlands J. Sea Research)*

equality of loss and uptake. The degree to which blood concentration changes with temperature will depend on the gearing between change in blood concentration and level of transport (*Figure 6.19*). If a small change in blood concentration excites maximal capacity the blood will tend to be maintained within narrow limits but the overall range of salinity over which such regulation can occur will be relatively short; if a larger decline is necessary to excite a given level of uptake a smaller gradient will be maintained between blood and medium but the work load in replacing ions lost from the body will be decreased and the effect of temperature change will tend to be larger. If such a simple relationship were to be general then it would be anticipated that the change in blood concentration with temperature would be small in fresh water and brackish water animals which mobilise all their transport capacity over a narrow range of blood concentration, e.g. Crayfish, but would be larger in forms having a more gradual increment of transport rate with blood concentration, e.g. *Sphaeroma* (*Figure 6.16*). Unfortunately inadequate information is as yet available on both mobilisation rates and temperature effects to test such a prediction. In any case it is likely that such an effect would apply only in the short term since examination of haemolymph concentration throughout the year indicates that some form of adjustment can occur in the control settings for osmotic concentration of the body fluids. For example, in *Asellus aquaticus* the blood concentration of individuals tends to rise if the temperature of the medium is raised but animals caught in the wild in winter

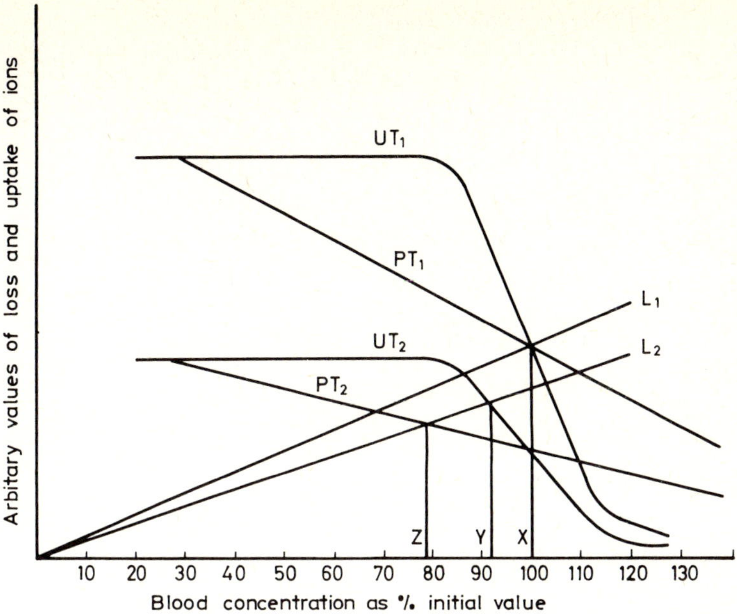

Figure 6.19 Hypothetical model system to illustrate the likely differences that a change in temperature will have on (a) an animal which activates all its transport over a narrow range of blood concentration and (b) an animal with the same maximal potential for transport but more gradual relationship between blood concentration and degree of activation. UT_1 is the curve describing the rate of ion uptake of animal (a) at temperature T_1. UT_2 is the uptake at temperature T_2. L_1 and L_2 are the loss rates corresponding to temperatures T_1 and T_2. PT_1 and PT_2 are the uptake for animal (b) which has a more gradual relationship between transport increment and falling blood concentration. The loss rates of (a) and (b) for a given blood concentration are assumed to be the same. For animal (a) a drop in temperature will decrease the blood concentration from X to Y; animal (b) will experience a larger drop to Z for the same change in temperature before it re-balances loss and uptake

and measured immediately on return to the laboratory are found to have higher blood concentrations than those caught in the summer (Lockwood, 1960). Racial differences may also occur since *Crangon* from the Baltic, where low winter temperatures are found, differ in the effect of temperature on blood concentration from forms studied in Holland (Weber and Spaargaren, 1970; Flügel, 1960).

6.2.5 Affinity of the ion transport system

At low concentrations the rate of active uptake of an ion is influenced by the concentration of the medium (*Figure 6.20*) in a manner similar to that described by the Michaelis–Menten equation for enzyme-substrate reactions:

$$U = K_2\,[C/(K_m + C)]$$

where U is the rate of uptake of ion, K_2 is the maximal transport rate, C is the concentration of the ion in the medium and K_m is the concentration of ion required to give half the maximal transport rate (Shaw, 1959b).

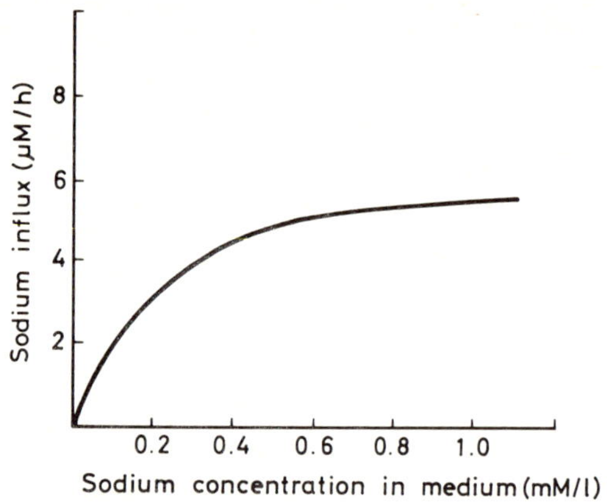

Figure 6.20 The relationship between sodium influx and external concentration of sodium in a single crayfish, showing that the uptake rises asymptotically. (After Shaw, 1959b; courtesy R. J. Skaer)

In a fresh water organism such as the crayfish, *Austropotamobius,* the carrier system involved in transport has a high affinity for sodium ions (low K_m value of 0.20–0.25 mM/l NaCl). Consequently, transport of sodium is tending towards a maximal level at *c.* 1 mM/l in this animal. At media concentrations above this value uptake of sodium will, therefore, be influenced solely by the animal's rate-regulating systems and will be independent of the concentration in the medium.

By contrast with the crayfish, the transport system in *Carcinus* has a relatively high K_m for sodium of some 20 mM/l NaCl. It would seem desirable that the transport rate should not be subject to variations in the concentration of the medium in the normal habitat and, as might be anticipated, one of the features of brackish water animals, especially those liable to exposure to fresh water, has been the evolution of transport systems with low K_m values (*Table 6.17*).

As pointed out by Shaw (1961b) a high affinity transport system may also have advantages in relation to the degree of restriction of ion permeability that must be achieved in order to balance loss and uptake in dilute media. Consider two animals of which one (A) has a K_m of 40 mM/l and the other (B) a K_m of 2.5 mM/l whilst both have the same maximal rate of uptake (K_2) when the transport sites are fully saturated.

At balance, loss is equal to uptake so

$$K_1 (B - C) = L = U = K_2\left(\frac{C}{K_m + C}\right)$$

where L is loss rate, U is uptake rate, B is blood concentration, and C is medium concentration. If the rate of loss of ion from the body is increased by

Table 6.17

	Usual medium	K_m *(Conc. of medium required to give half maximal transport rate)*	*Authority*
Carcinus maenas	Sea and B-W[1]	20 mM/l Na	Shaw (1961)
Mesidotea entomon (Baltic race)	B-W	9 mM/l Na	Croghan and Lockwood (1968)
Marinogammarus finmarchicus	Sea	6–10 mM/l Na	Sutcliffe (1968)
Mesidotea entomon (Lake Mälaren)	F-W[2]	2–3 mM/l Na	Croghan and Lockwood (1968)
Gammarus duebeni	B-W	1.5–2.0 mM/l Na	Sutcliffe (1967)
Gammarus zaddachi	B-W	1.0–1.5 mM/l Na	Sutcliffe (1968)
Gammarus duebeni (celticus)	F-W	0.4 mM/l Na	Sutcliffe and Shaw (1967b)
Gammarus pulex	F-W	0.1–0.15 mM/l Na	Sutcliffe (1967b)
Gammarus lacustris	F-W	0.1–0.15 mM/l Na	Sutcliffe and Shaw (1967a)
Limnaea pereger	F-W	0.25 mM/l Na	Greenaway (1970)
Margaritana margaritana	F-W	0.04 mM/l Na	

[1] B-W=brackish water
[2] F-W=fresh water

changing the permeability constant (K_1) the animal with the high affinity uptake system will be able to balance loss and uptake at a much higher blood concentration than can the other (*Figure 6.21*). It will of course have to expend more energy in maintaining this high blood concentration, but if cell survival is dependent on a high blood concentration the selective advantage of a high affinity transport system will be considerable.

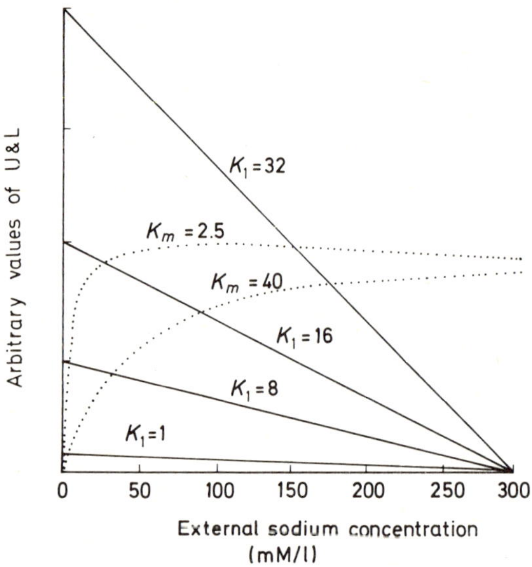

Figure 6.21 The effect of different K_m values on the balance point at various loss rates of sodium. The balance conditions for two hypothetical animals maintaining the same blood sodium concentration (300 mM/l). The straight lines represent various passive loss rates for different values of K_1 in the expression L $K_1(B - C)$. The dotted lines are the uptake rates for two animals, one with a K_m of 2.5 mM/l and the other with a K_m of 40 mM/l. Both have the same maximal uptake rate. U and L are uptake and loss, respectively. (After Shaw, 1961; courtesy R. J. Skaer)

Should the medium concentration fall below the level required to saturate the transport sites the blood concentration is bound to fall. However, provided that the drop in saturation is not too large, balance will be regained at a somewhat lower blood concentration as a result of either (a) decrease in loss rate as the blood concentration declines or (b) through a combination of (a) and an increased mobilisation of transport capacity. Such a mobilisation of additional transport capacity is clearly shown in *Gammarus zaddachi* when uptake is tested over a range of salinities after preacclimation to different salinities (*Figure 6.22*; Sutcliffe, 1968).

Most species normally inhabit media of sufficient concentration to at least half saturate the transport sites but penetration of fresh water at the extreme limit of their salinity tolerance range results in at least some erstwhile estuarine animals living at sodium concentrations well below their K_m. Thus a race of the isopod *Mesidotea* (K_m of 1 to 2 mM/l Na) lives in Lake Vättern

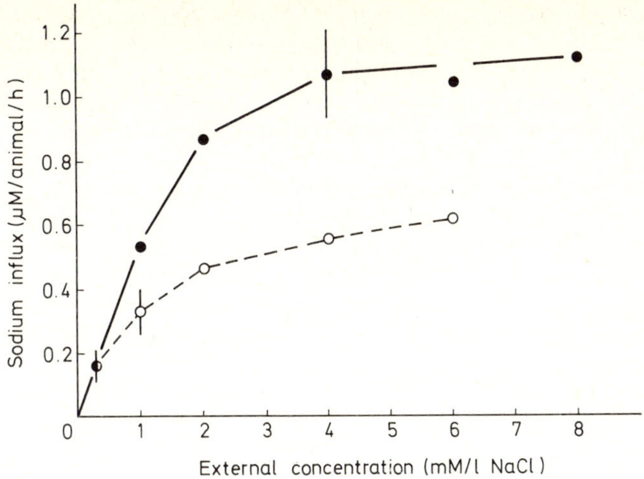

Figure 6.22 The difference in rates of uptake in a range of dilute media between animals (Gammarus zaddachi) *previously acclimatised to a low salinity (closed circles = 0.3 mM/l) and to a higher salinity (open circles = 10 mM/l). (After Sutcliffe, 1968; courtesy R. J. Skaer)*

(250 μM/l Na) (Croghan, P. C. and Lockwood, A.P.M., unpublished data).

At concentrations above their salinity minimum, animals will generally have some transport capacity in reserve which is capable of being mobilised in the event of a decline in blood concentration arising from a subsidiary cause (increased permeability to water or ions or decreased saturation of the ion uptake system). The extent of the decline in blood concentration which will occur in such circumstances will therefore be minimised.

Nevertheless, some doubts remain as to the degree to which the K_m value is a genotypic rather than phenotypic character since Sutcliffe (1971b) has shown that, following the rigorous selection which occurs when brackish water individuals of *G. duebeni* are maintained in fresh water for an extended period (2 years), the survivors (first generation offspring) have a K_m for sodium of *c.* 0.6 mM/l Na, a value which is within the range shown by *G. duebeni celticus* inhabiting fresh water in Ireland. Similarly specimens of *Mesidotea entomon* from Lake Vättern, which has a Na^+ concentration of only 0.25 mM/l, have a markedly lower K_m (1.0–1.5 mM/l) than that of individuals living in Lake Mälaren (0.6 mM/l Na^+). Further studies are required on brackish water animals to ascertain the degree to which the K_m differs in various parts of the species range and also the extent to which the K_m of individuals can be varied on extended exposure to different media.

In view of the apparent ease with which selection over one or at the most two generations, can result in *Gammarus* with K_m values well below the average value for the brackish water stock (Sutcliffe, 1971b) the question may well be asked why, if the potential for low K_m values is present in the parent stock, the lowest obtainable value is not maintained by the population as a whole? Notwithstanding what has been said earlier regarding the apparent desirability of having the rate of transport independent of media concentration it may be that paradoxically a somewhat higher K_m has a practical advantage to the individual in the estuarine context. All animals may be expected to extend their range to the limits of their physiological and biotic capacity and in an estuary, therefore, euryhaline species will tend to penetrate as far towards fresh water as their regulatory mechanisms will permit. However, it would seem improbable that species would voluntarily enter waters which are so dilute during the ebb and low tide that they are exposed to a medium in which, with all transport capacity mobilised, the net loss of salt from the body is liable to drop the concentration to a level deleterious to the cells. Consequently it can be argued that animals will not normally willingly enter water where the net loss is other than slow. However, if such waters are tidal and the animal has a K_m concentration not far below its normal minimal concentration range then, during the raised salinity associated with high tide, uptake will be markedly enhanced as the degree of saturation of the transport sites is increased. Salt lost during the period of low tide, could then be rapidly replaced. The lower the concentration reached relative to the K_m, the greater the enhancement of uptake that will be conferred by a small rise in salinity. Consequently if estuarine animals do not penetrate further than the extent to which they can approximately balance loss and uptake at low tide they will, if the salinity rises with the tide, be assured of the opportunity to replace any losses as the salt concentration rises. No such dramatic increase in uptake at high water would be achieved by an animal with a low K_m and consequently such a form might be more vulnerable to the effects of minor damage if penetrating to the limit of its transport capacity. Of course, any such possible advantage of not possessing a low K_m disappears on colonisation of non-fluctuating salinities making it then advantageous to have as low a K_m as can be obtained.

6.2.6 Racial differences in regulatory capacity

Differences, which are presumably adaptive, have been noted in individuals of a given species taken from areas of differing salinity regimes. *Carcinus* caught in the Baltic (13–18‰) and transferred to 33‰ have a higher blood concentration three days later than North Sea specimens at the same concentration. Longer term adaptation (two weeks) reduces these differences but does not eliminate them (Theede, 1969). Comparison of the closely related forms *Carcinus maenas* from the North Sea and *C. mediterraneus* from the Adriatic also indicate environmentally-linked factors. Mediterranean *Carcinus,* which do not generally experience wide differences in salinity, have larger sodium fluxes and a lower blood concentration after a month in 50% seawater than the northern species which is more exposed to salinity fluctuations (Lucu, C., Siebers, D. and Sperling, K. R., 1972, unpublished data).

A more extreme example of the same general situation is seen in the Arctic Glacial relict isopod, *Mesidotea entomon,* which *inter alia* has colonised the Baltic sea and a number of Swedish Lakes since the last Ice

Age. The lake races of this animal are unusual among fresh water invertebrates in possessing the euryhalinity of the parent stock and they can tolerate salinities at least up to 35‰. The Baltic stock itself cannot however survive in fresh water, the minimum water concentration at which a blood concentration compatible with life can be maintained being some 14 mM/l (Lockwood and Croghan, 1957). As mentioned earlier the tolerance of fresh water by races living in Lake Mälaren and Lake Vättern seems to be based on the possession of a lower ion loss rate, lower K_m value for uptake and a faster maximal rate of ion intake than is usual in the brackish water stock (Croghan and Lockwood, 1968 and unpublished data). It would be premature however to suggest that the Baltic and lake forms of this animal are necessarily genetically distinct since Sutcliffe (1970; 1972) has shown that when *Gammarus duebeni* are kept in Lake Windermere water for two years the animals at the end of the period (probably first generation) differ from the parent brackish water race in much the same way, i.e. lower sodium loss rates and lower K_m.

Such differences could perhaps be accounted for by selection within the natural range of genetic variability within a stock but that this is not necessarily the whole explanation is suggested by observations that salinity tolerance of the same species depends on the salinity in which fertilisation and incubation of the eggs occurs (Kinne, 1953; 1958).

Adult animals are also capable of a measure of adaptation to conditions outside the normal range of tolerance if the salinity change is sufficiently slow. In this context Gross (1961) has observed that the crab *Hemigrapsus oregonensis* in a slowly evaporating saline lagoon survived and maintained effective hypo-osmotic regulation up to a concentration of about 175% seawater, a value markedly higher than that normally tolerated.

An analogy may perhaps be drawn between the above effects and the way in which the usual physiological response of chromatophores in colour regulation may be amplified on long term exposure to a given background by morphological hypertrophy or atrophy of pigment within the cells (cf. Lockwood, 1968).

Morphological change both at a macro level and at the sub-cellular level does appear to play some role in regulation in a number of forms. Thus, the structure of the cells and hydranths of the euryhaline hydroid *Cordylophora* varies according to the external salinity in a way which can be interpreted as being designed to reduce water fluxes when the animal is exposed to dilute media (*Figure 6.23*; Kinne, 1958). At the sub-cellular level, fresh water Crustacea appear to differ from marine forms. Copeland and Fitzjarrel, 1968) have shown that when the blue crab, *Callinectes,* is in dilute media the sub-cuticular surface of the gill epithelial cells has the form of lamellar folds terminating in finger-like processes. These folds are separated from each other by appreciable spaces. The gills of the fresh water *Gammarus pulex* show similar structures (P. Whitfield, unpublished data). By contrast in the marine littoral isopod *Ligia oceanica* the lamellae are broader and consequently the lamella spaces are reduced to narrow channels (Sylvester, 1970). The euryhaline species *G. duebeni* is therefore of interest since there is evidence suggesting that the sub-cuticular surface shows a trend from one

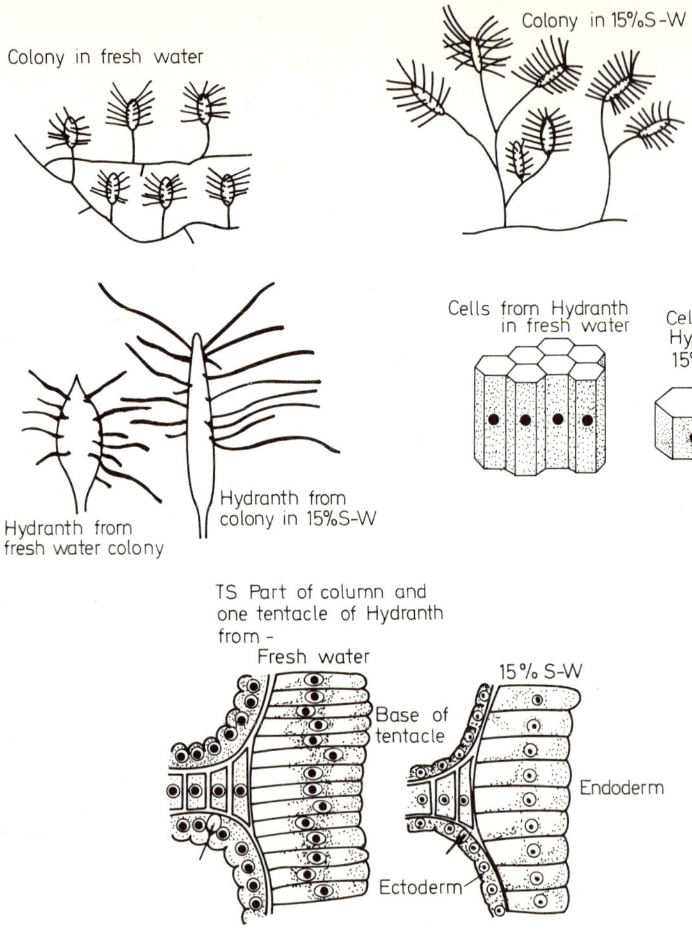

Figure 6.23 Structural differences in the cells and hydranths of Cordylophora *grown in different salinities. (After Lockwood, 1963; from Kinne)*

state to the other during salinity acclimatisation (Lockwood, Inman and Courtenay, 1973), though the precise effect this change may have on ion or water fluxes is at present unclear.

6.2.7 Osmoregulatory work

Active transport of inorganic ions is dependent on energy supplied as ATP. The precise energy cost is open to doubt however. In terms of steady state thermodynamics the minimum work, W, required to transport 1 mol. of sodium across an interface from one concentration to another against a negative potential, V, is given by the expression:

$$W = RT \ln \frac{(\text{Na})_e}{(\text{Na})_i} - VF$$

where R is the gas constant, F is the Faraday 96 500 coulombs/mol., T is the absolute temperature, and $(\text{Na})_e$ and $(\text{Na})_i$ are the sodium concentrations on either side of the interface.

6.2.8 Calculations

Alternatively osmotic work can be estimated from the oxygen consumption associated with transport by making the assumption that 1 mol. of ATP is utilised in the transfer of 3 mol. of sodium (cf. Baker, 1965), that the utilisation of 1 molecule of oxygen produces 6 molecules of ATP and that 1 ml of oxygen is equivalent to 5 cal. Application of both forms of calculation to data on the sodium fluxes of *Mytilus* and *Anodonta* (Potts, 1959) indicates that energy consumption as calculated from the thermodynamic equation is comparable to that indicated by oxygen consumption provided that the change of free energy on hydrolysis of ATP to ADP is taken as equal to 7.6 kcal/mole (Burton, 1973).

It is not always easy, however, to relate the changes in oxygen consumption which occur when an animal is transferred from one medium to another to variations in osmotic work load. Direct correlation is complicated by the following factors:

1. The free energy change of ATP tends to vary with the prevailing ionic conditions (Caldwell, 1968, quoted by Burton, 1973).
2. Animals often become excitable when the salinity of the medium is changed and consequently expend increased energy on physical activity as well as on basal metabolic processes (Gross, 1957a; *see also* Chapter 3).
3. Variations may occur in the rates of processes maintaining cell ionic levels as the blood ionic concentrations change.
4. Enzyme activity may be modified as cell ion levels alter (Lange, 1968b).

Even where physical activity does not show marked alteration the various possible combinations of effects produced by factors (3) and (4) result in widely differing responses. It is easy to see why this should be so. In hypertonic regulators, as the concentration of the medium declines, increased work at the body surface is required to maintain the gradient between blood and medium. However, if the blood concentration is allowed to decline the energy demand at the cellular level to maintain sodium extrusion may be decreased. Theoretically it might, by appropriate lowering of the blood concentration, be possible for an animal to match increased energy demand at the body surface by decreased demand at the cellular level. In practice, differences in such factors as permeability and degree of hypertonicity result in varied changes in oxygen demand, even within the range of physiological competence of the animal. Outside this range, of course, other factors such as the dependence of cellular processes on a limited range of ionic levels begin to affect the overall oxygen demand.

It appears that sometimes increased metabolic demands for the purposes of ion regulation can be met within a constant oxygen uptake by reducing the loading of other functions. Thus *Artemia* maintains a practically constant O_2 uptake over the salinity range 35–140‰ despite the expected increase in osmotic work entailed. Contemporaneously, however, the growth rate and fertility of the females decline (*Table 6.13*; Gilchrist, 1956).

A further complication is produced by the observation that the change in oxygen uptake accompanying salinity change is dependent on the size or age of the individual. Thus, small individuals of the crab *Sesarma plicatum* in 50% seawater have an O_2 uptake of only half that displayed in fresh water; adults by contrast show little difference in O_2 uptake in the two media (Madanmohanrao and Rao, 1962).

Longer term metabolic adjustments also influence O_2 uptake. When *Mytilus* are transferred from 30 to 15‰ the oxygen consumption of gill tissues isolated successively over some weeks shows a gradual increase and eventually is similar to that of mussels collected directly from 15‰ in the wild (Schlieper, 1955), which may imply that long term exposure to given ionic conditions results in enzymic induction producing optimal conditions for energy supply (Lange, 1968a). A consequence of such effects is that in short term experiments the oxygen uptake on transference from one salinity to another will tend to depend on the salinity to which the animal was initially adapted as well as to that to which it is transferred. Dependent upon which of the above features dominates the metabolism, four main categories of response follow change in salinity (Kinne, 1966):

1. Increased metabolic rate on dilution within the physiological range, e.g. *Nereis diversicolor, Gammarus locusta, Carcinus maenas* (Schlieper, 1929b).
2. Increased metabolic rate in both sub-normal and supra-normal salinities, e.g. *Palaemonetes varians* (Lofts, 1956) and *Metapenaeus monoceros* (Rao, 1958).
3. Reduction in oxygen intake in both sub-normal and supra-normal salinities, e.g. *Asterias* (Schlieper, 1929b).
4. Metabolic rate more or less unaffected by salinity variation *Artemia salina* (Gilchrist, 1956), *Theodoxus fluviatilis* (Lumbye, 1958).

The ability to vary oxygen consumption in response to changes in the medium necessitates that the organisms possess a measure of independence of oxygen levels in the water.

6.3 OXYGEN UPTAKE

Any animal living in an environment where the oxygen tension fluctuates must either have a respiratory system capable of maintaining an oxygen uptake suitable for its requirements over a range of external oxygen tensions, or suffer limitation of its activity when a lowering of the tension decreases the O_2 uptake.

In stratified estuaries it is possible for the saline water at the bottom to become isolated and appreciably depleted of oxygen. Similarly estuaries which carry a substantial organic load may also become partially deoxygenated.

Marine benthic but epigean species such as *Homarus* from sub-littoral or inshore waters not normally subjected to lowered O_2 tensions are ill-equipped to respond to conditions of O_2 depletion and their O_2 uptake tends to be directly related to the external oxygen tension at all levels below the equilibration tension in air, i.e. *c.* 150 mm Hg (*Figure 6.24*). Other offshore forms such as actinians, sipunculids, asteroids and echinoids are also generally conformers. By contrast, estuarine and littoral species tend to be 'regulators', maintaining a fairly uniform level of O_2 intake despite some degree of reduction in external O_2 tensions.

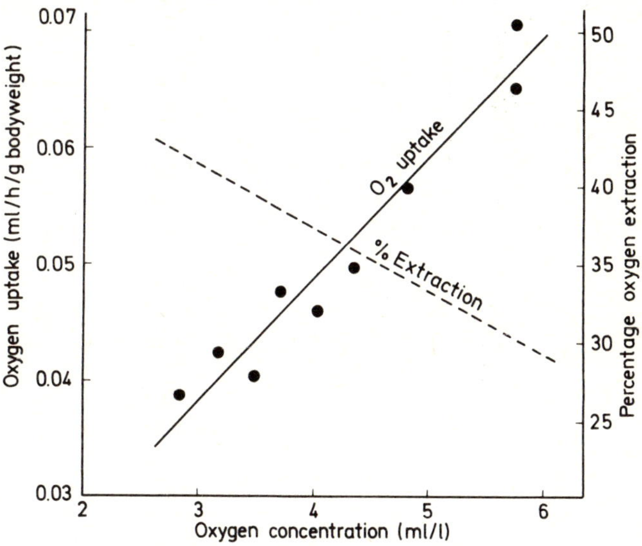

Figure 6.24 The effect of oxygen concentration of the medium on oxygen uptake and the percentage of oxygen extracted by the gills of a lobster. (From Lockwood, 1968; after Thomas, 1954)

The maintenance of O_2 intake by *Carcinus* can be related to the ability of this animal to increase both the ventilation rate and the percentage utilisation of O_2 in the water in the branchial chamber as O_2 tensions in the water decline. The limit of constant intake (critical pressure) is reached when the O_2 tension falls below about 20% (Ayers, 1938). Similarly the barnacle *Balanus amphitrite* regulates down to about 50% saturation at 25°C (Prasada Rao and Ganapati, 1968; *Figure 6.25(a)*). The critical pressure is not constant but varies with temperature and degree of activity

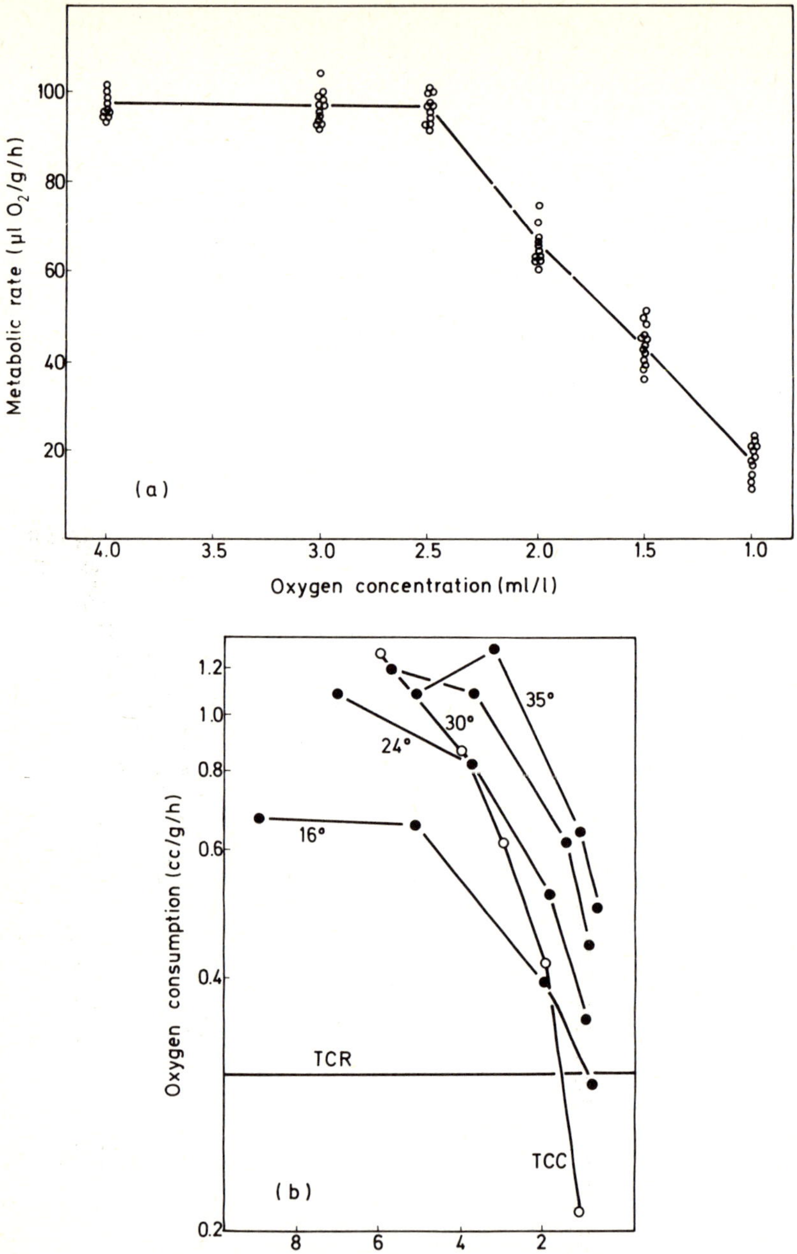

Figure 6.25 Maintenance of oxygen uptake down to a critical external oxygen tension by 'regulators'. (a) O_2 consumption by Balanus amphitrite *as a function of O_2 concentration at 25°C. (After Prasada Rao and Ganaparti, 1968; courtesy Springer-Verlag). (b) The relation between oxygen consumption of* Orconectes immunis *and oxygen concentration at different temperatures. TCR indicates the theoretical curve of a regulator, TCC the theoretical curve of a conformer. (After Wiens and Armitage, 1961; courtesy University of Chicago Press)*

(*Figure 6.25 (b)*)) and at high temperatures the ability to regulate decreases and 'regulators' tend towards the 'conformer' condition. The behavioural responses of some invertebrates also indicate that they are able to detect the oxygen levels in the medium (Farley and Case, 1968; Jansson, 1967).

6.4 REPRODUCTION AND MAINTENANCE OF STATION WITHIN ESTUARIES

Reproduction poses special problems to benthic organisms inhabiting estuaries and is discussed in relation to the rhythmic behaviour of marine animals in Chapter 7. Perhaps the most critical of these are:

1. The salinity tolerance range of larvae is often markedly more restricted than that of adults.
2. The net water flow in estuaries is seaward and hence there is a risk that larval stages will be swept out and lost.

6.4.1 Salinity tolerance of young stages

In the great majority of euryhaline forms the adults can tolerate more dilute media than the young stages; *Carcinus maenas* adults can survive down to 4‰ but the eggs develop only at 28–40‰; *Littorina littorea* adults can live down to about 7–8‰ but the eggs require at least 15‰. Similarly it is found that individuals of both the eelgrass *Zostera marina* and starfish *Asterias rubens* are sterile at the limits of their salinity range in the Baltic; so too is the dab *Pleuronectes limanda* which cannot be fertilised at salinities below 15‰ (Remane and Schlieper, 1971).

A number of species resolve the problems of larval sensitivity to dilution by migrating to sea to breed, e.g. Penaeid prawns, and the crab *Eriocheir sinensis;* others retain the larvae in brood pouches until a late stage of development has been reached. At least in the case of the mysid *Neomysis integer,* the fluid bathing the developing embryos seems to be maintained by the parent within a narrower range of salinity than that pertaining in the medium (Ralph, 1965; *Figure 6.26*).

6.4.2 Factors involved in the maintenance of larval stages in estuaries

Oscillating tidal currents carry planktonic forms backward and forward along estuaries on each tidal cycle. This effect, however, contributes by itself to only a minor potential loss of organisms from estuaries. As Sir Alan Herbert colourfully expressed the point in a debate in the House of Commons on pollution in the River Thames '. . . it takes 30 tides to remove a dead cat from London'. Of more practical importance to planktonic forms are a non-tidal drift seawards at the surface and another drift landwards along the bottom, taken together with modifications in larval behaviour as

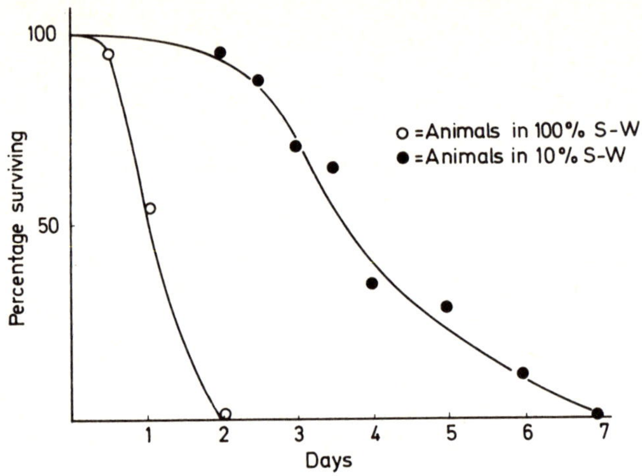

(a)

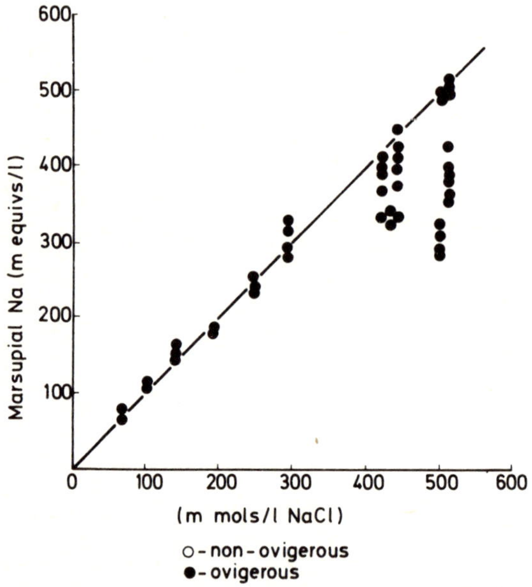

(b)

Figure 6.26 (a) Sensitivity of day-old Neomysis integer *to high salinity. (b) Apparent maintenance of brood pouch medium hypotonic to the environmental salinity at high external concentrations. (After Ralph, 1965)*

they mature (Bousfield, 1955). That larvae do exert an influence on their own distribution is clearly shown by comparison of the distribution of oyster larvae and coal particles in the water at different stages of the tide (*Figure 6.27;* Wood and Hargis, 1971; *see also* Chapters 2 and 7). No correlation is apparent between the distribution of coal and larvae suggesting that the distribution of the latter is determined dynamically.

Adaptations which may contribute to the maintenance of larval stages within estuaries include:

1. Shortening or suppression of free living planktonic stages.
2. Detection and avoidance of low salinities.
3. Responses to changes in hydrostatic pressure.
4. Changes in swimming activity related to the phases of the tidal cycle.
5. Change in depth with age.

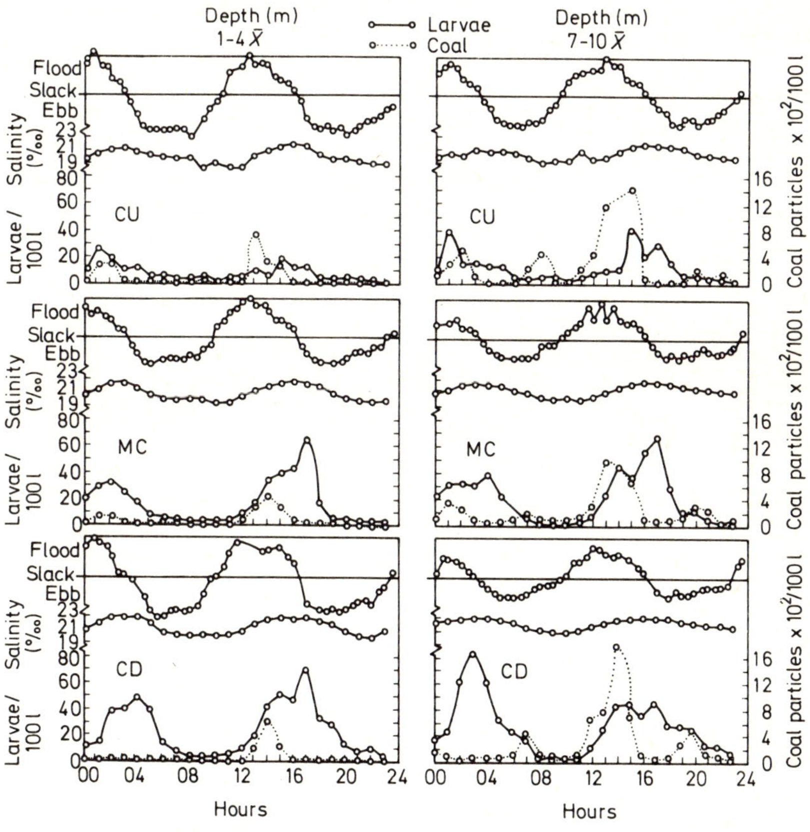

Figure 6.27 Independence of distribution of coal particles and larvae in a tidal estuary. Hourly measurements of flow (uppermost curve), salinity (middle curve) and density of larvae and coal particles (two lowest curves) averaged for three stations CU, MC and CD at depths of 1–4 m (left) and 7–10 m (right). (After Wood and Hargis, 1971; courtesy Cambridge University Press)

6.4.2.1 SHORTENING OF THE LARVAL PHASE

Reduction in the length of time larvae spend in the plankton is a common feature of estuarine organisms. Among bivalves the estuarine *Ostrea* is commonly a member of the plankton for only some 7-14 days, whereas for more fully marine species such as *Arca, Spisula* and *Teredo* the period is nearer 21 days (cf. Loosanoff quoted by Sloan, 1972). Amongst the estuarine annelids the larvae of *Nereis diversicolor* can swim but do not normally enter the plankton, and the same applies to the larvae of *Arenicola marina.* The larval stage of the estuarine nemertine *Lineus ruber* is passed in a gelatinous mass, thus suppressing the planktonic phase. Where larvae of brackish water forms do enter the plankton their behaviour and sensory systems are adapted to ensuring that they remain primarily in landward rather than seaward moving water streams.

6.4.2.2 AVOIDANCE OF LOW SALINITIES

In stratified (salt wedge) types of estuaries there tends to be a layer of fresher water moving seaward over the underlying more saline water. Avoidance of this current may be achieved either actively or passively. The nauplii larvae of *Balanus, Elminius* and *Chthamalus stellatus* are immobilised at concentrations below about 12‰ and consequently tend to sink passively away from dilute surface layers. Copepods such as *Acartia tonsa* show a more positive avoidance of low salinities when they meet an interface between low and high salinity water (Lance, 1965).

In the case of oyster larvae, too, response to salinity may contribute positively towards maintenance in estuaries. Haskin (1964) has shown that the older larvae tend to drop close to the bottom during falling salinities on ebb tides and to rise away from the bottom (and hence tend to be carried landward) on the flooding tide as the salinities rise. Whilst such a mechanism may contribute towards avoiding net movement towards the seaward end of an estuary in stratified regions it would be of doubtful value in retaining organisms in well mixed estuaries. In such regions the response to changes in hydrostatic pressure may play a dominant role in position maintenance.

6.4.2.3 RESPONSES TO CHANGE IN HYDROSTATIC PRESSURE

Many planktonic and free living benthic animals show increase in swimming activity following a rise in the hydrostatic pressure of the medium (Rice, 1964; Knight-Jones and Morgan, 1966; Digby, 1967, 1972; *see also* Chapter 7).

In the context of the estuarine habitat this response may serve the purpose of ensuring that activity of larval forms is maximal at times when the net water movement is in the landward direction.

Field studies on the larvae of *Spionid* annelids (Bird, 1972) suggests that they only move up strongly from the bottom during the period of the high water stand (*Figure 6.28*). Oyster larvae, particularly the older 'eyed' larvae, show a similar tendency (Sloan, 1972; Prytherch, 1928; 1934 in Sloan). It is, however, difficult to be certain that the field response is due to hydrostatic pressure changes alone as the larvae are also sensitive to changes of salinity and light intensity and, in addition, may be subject to tidal rhythms of activity (*see* Chapter 7).

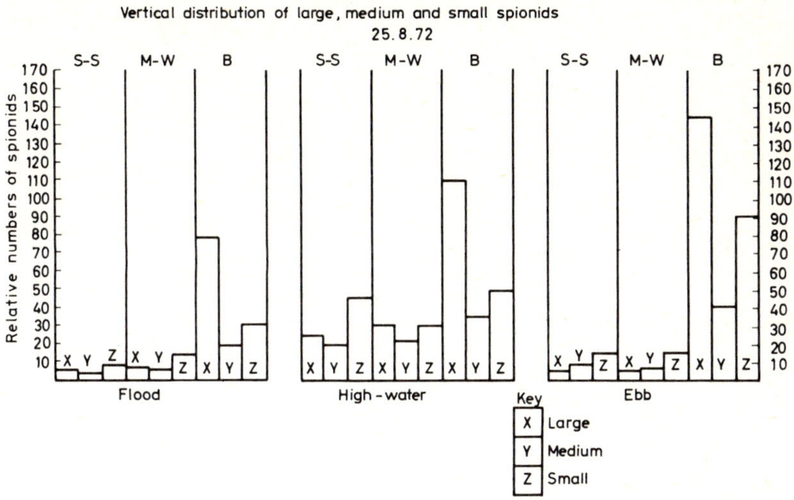

Figure 6.28 Vertical distribution of spionid larvae in Southampton Water during a tidal cycle S-S = subsurface; M-W = mid-water; B = bottom. (After Bird, 1972)

The physiological mechanism underlying sensitivity to changes in hydrostatic pressure remains uncertain but Digby (1972) has postulated an ingenious hypothesis which is compatible with known data. He suggests that certain regions of the body surface of organisms act as semiconductors. Under the influence of the potential difference across the body surface resulting from the active and passive movements of inorganic ions, these semiconductor regions permit electron transfer in the direction inside to out. At the body surface the electrons are discharged in interaction with the medium to produce a thin layer of hydrogen and an alkali reaction in the neighbouring region. Production of the gas layer would tend to polarise the system resulting in a decline in current flow (*Figure 6.29*). Digby suggests that the system would be pressure sensitive, compression of the gas layer exposing more of the semiconductor and so increasing current flow once more. If suitable sensors of current flow are present the pressure change could be detected. Model systems based on concentration cells and semiconducting membranes are indeed pressure sensitive and other points supporting his hypothesis are:

1. On scratching the surface of a prawn a thin gas layer collects in the scratch.

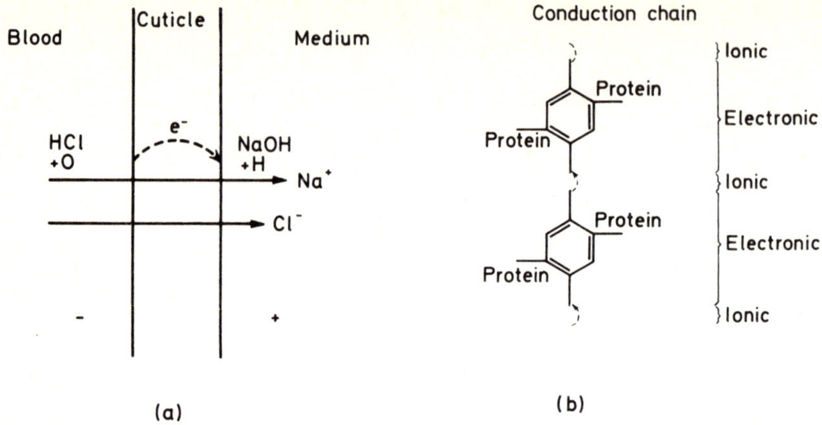

Figure 6.29 (a) Model system for production of a pressure sensitive gas layer in a crustacean. (b) Hypothetical conduction chain in crustacean cuticle, in its simplest form. Electronically conducting semiquinonoid structures stabilised by bonds concerned with tanning alternate with ionic links in the intervening aqueous phase. An applied potential results in current flow through the chain as through a suspension of a granular metallic powder in a saturated solution of its salt. (After Digby, 1972; courtesy Society for Experimental Biology)

2. Ionic detergents such as Cetavlon (dodecamethylammonium bromide) which, having a complex cation and small anion might be expected to be adsorbed on to a negatively charged surface, block the pressure response of Crustacea whilst Teepol (Na and secondary alkylsulphate) does not.
3. It is possible to electroplate the areas of Crustacea which Digby postulates as being semiconductors.
4. H_2O_2 which would be expected to oxidise the H^+ layer abolishes pressure sensitivity.
5. High salinities, which interfere with the potential, also abolish sensitivity.

Tanned cuticle would be expected, from the semiquinonoid structure present, to be a good semiconductor and it is interesting to note that the euryhaline copepods *Temora* and *Centropages,* which are relatively heavily tanned, are markedly more sensitive to pressure change than are less euryhaline forms and less tanned species such as *Acartia clausii* and *Oithona* (Digby, 1967; 1972).

6.4.2.4 CHANGES IN SWIMMING ACTIVITY RELATED TO THE PHASE OF THE TIDAL CYCLE

The adults of a number of estuarine species are known to possess tidal rhythms which affect their activity, e.g. crab *Carcinus maenas* (ambulatory activity) (Naylor and Atkinson, 1972); oyster *Crassostrea virginica* (feeding gape) (Brown, 1954); mud snail *Nassarius obsoletus* (locomotory activity) (Fingerman, 1960).

These rhythms are endogenous, recurring in phase (and advancing 50 minutes daily) with the tides at the site of origin of the organisms even when the animals are maintained in constant conditions. Such rhythms generally damp out within a few days. Their significance is discussed in more detail in Chapter 7.

No specific experiments seem to have been conducted to ascertain whether the larvae of estuarine species also display cycles of activity correlated with the tidal phase and appropriate to the maintenance of their station in the estuary.

6.4.2.5 CHANGE IN DEPTH WITH AGE

Most maturing pelagic larvae of estuarine benthic species tend to become photonegative, geopositive and positively thigmotatic as they approach metamorphosis and consequently an increased proportion of the individuals surviving to the late larval stage will tend to benefit from the backward movement of the lower waters (Bousfield, 1955; cf. *Figure 6.28*).

6.5 SUMMARY AND CONCLUSIONS

Most marine invertebrates are characterised by having a body surface which is relatively permeable to both inorganic ions and water. The body fluids are thus commonly isosmotic with the medium. Urine, which though isosmotic with the blood, usually contributes to the maintenance of such ionic differences between the blood and medium as may occur.

Exposure of the majority of marine species to dilute media is followed by osmotic uptake of water into the body, and subsequently into the cells, resulting in gross swelling in the case of soft bodied forms. Salt loss by diffusion and increased urine flow may mitigate the degree of swelling and declining body fluid concentration reduces the osmotic inflow. In general, however, marine species do not tolerate substantial dilution of the body fluids and few survive more than transitory exposure to media of lower salinity than 50% seawater.

By contrast with their marine relatives euryhaline brackish water species display greater physiological versatility in response to dilution of the medium. Regulation may take one of three forms:

1. Osmotic adjustment at the cellular level only, the body fluids remaining isosmotic with the medium (osmoconformers).
2. Maintenance of the body fluids hypertonic to the medium at low salinities but tending towards isotonicity in salinities of the order of seawater concentration (hypertonic regulators).
3. Hypertonic regulation in dilute media and hypotonic regulation in high salinities (hyper-hypotonic regulators).

The degree of hypertonicity varies widely but tends to be smaller in annelids and molluscs than in the less permeable Crustacea and, in general, is also smaller in species of small body size than in comparable larger forms. As a result of such variation almost all possible gradations occur between osmoconformers and extreme hypertonic regulators. In consequence all regulators must have the capacity to effect some degree of osmotic adjustment at the cellular level in addition to maintaining the blood concentration different from that of the medium.

Regulation of the constancy of cell volume as blood concentration varies necessitates adjustment to the intracellular osmotic concentration. The need to maintain the integrity of the electrical properties of excitable tissues places limitations on the degree to which the concentration of inorganic ions can be varied in cells and generally small organic molecules, principally amino acids, account for half or more of any concentration change. Non-essential amino acids including particularly glycine, glutamic acid, alanine and proline are paramount in osmotic adjustment but the major contributor or contributors tend to vary both with species and the conditions pertaining. Change in amino acid concentration is effected at two levels intracellularly and extra-cellularly. Variation in cellular ion content directly influences enzymes involved in synthesis and degradation of amino acids and also the supply of reducing equivalents utilised in synthesis. Raising cell NaCl levels tends to increase the supply of NADH by reducing other processes utilising this substance, increases amino acid formation and inhibits amino acid breakdown. These intracellular processes are supplemented by the diffusion of proline and alanine out of cells on decline in blood concentration and conversely by the uptake of amino acids from blood when the blood ion concentration rises. The hepatopancreas (Crustacea) deaminates amino acid released into the blood and ammonia from this organ and other cells is released from the body in increased amounts on transference of animals to dilute media and, conversely, in reduced quantities on tranference to high salinities.

It seems improbable that breakdown or formation of intracellular peptide contributes to increasing or decreasing the cell free amino acid pool (at least in Crustacea) but it is possible that variation of haemolymph proteins may act as a source, or sink, of amino acids exchanged across cell surfaces.

Regulators maintain the body fluid concentration hypertonic to dilute media by the active intake of inorganic ions, particularly sodium and chloride, supplemented in some cases by the production of urine hypotonic to the blood. The capacity to transport ions across the body surface has evolved so frequently in non-related groups that there must be a strong implication that the basic process of transepithelial transport is present already in stenohaline marine forms subserving some other purpose than hypertonic regulation. Some evidence suggests that ion uptake is utilised by isosmotic marine forms for volume regulation and to bring into the body some of the fluid subsequently excreted as urine. It is tempting to imagine that hypertrophy of this system coupled with reduction in the permeability of the body surface to water relative to the permeability to ions has repeatedly made hypertonic regulation practicable. As a general consequence of the requirement to restrict osmotic work euryhaline species tend to be less permeable to water and ions than animals restricted to the sea and some estuarine forms can effect changes in the permeability to water according to the salinity they are in.

Various factors influence the rate of ion transport and, where urine hypertonic to the blood is formed, the concentration of the urine. Decline in blood concentration within some specific part of the physiological range generally initiates increased transport capacity, so too does decrease in blood volume and, in Crustacea, moult. Sudden transference from high to low salinity water tends, however, to initiate both increased uptake and production of dilute urine in some Crustacea at much higher blood concentrations than would be expected from steady state experiments. Such 'anticipatory' responses are doubtless of selective advantage to animals inhabiting fluctuating salinities in so far as they will tend to delay change in blood concentration and so permit a longer period for osmotic adjustment at the cellular level.

At low salinities the rate of uptake is also influenced by the affinity of the transport system for ions. The K_m value which relates to this affinity is generally lower in forms from fresh water than in brackish water species.

Temperature increase generally expedites ion transport but the overall effect of a temperature rise on blood concentration is variable since, whilst in some species the temperature coefficient for ion loss is less than that for ion uptake, in others the reverse applies.

Ion transport is an energy demanding process but it is usually difficult to relate changes in the oxygen consumption to varying osmotic loads as salinity is changed because of the variety of effects likely to result from internal ion level changes. In addition to modification of the rate of sodium extrusion from cells and changes in transport at the body surface, O_2 demand may also vary because of alteration in the physical activity of the animals and the activity of enzyme systems within cells unrelated to ion transport or adjustment of cellular osmotic balance.

The requirement to maintain oxygen uptake despite potential fluctuations in both oxygen demand and partial pressure in the medium is reflected in the fact that many estuarine forms are regulators rather than conformers in respect of being able to maintain O_2 uptake despite some measure of drop in external partial pressure of the gas.

The net transport of water in estuaries is seaward and consequently maintenance of station by forms with planktonic larvae poses special problems. These tend to be countered by reducing the length of the free living larval stage and by adaptive responses of the larvae, thus enabling them to avoid the dilute seaward moving water and also to increase swimming actively primarily when the tidal water movements are in a landwards direction.

To conclude, estuarine organisms are adapted behaviourally, physiologically and biochemically not only to wide ranging external conditions but also to respond appropriately to rapid and irregular variation of those conditions. It seems increasingly clear that this breadth and flexibility of response is not based on the development of any fundamentally new processes but rather on the evolutionary adaptation and modification for different roles of processes already present in marine species. Indeed, to close, we may perhaps misquote Pearse (1939)* and aver that 'Heredity offered the means and environment provided the necessity' for the plasticity of response that is the hallmark of the euryhaline organism.

REFERENCES

ABARTI, J. L. and REISCH, D. J. (1972). 'The effects of lowered dissolved oxygen concentrations and salinity on the free amino acid pool of the polychaetous annelid *Neanthes arenaceodentata*', *Bull. S. Californ. Acad. Sci.*, **71,** 32–39

ABBOTT, C. H. (1939). 'Shore isopods; niches occupied, and degrees of transitions towards land life, with special reference to the family Lygididae', *Proc. 7th Pacif. Sci. Cong.*, **3,** 505–511

AKERLUND, G. and FÄNGE, R. (1972). 'Effects of drugs on fluid balance in molluscs', *Proc. Goteborg meeting of the Soc. Exp. Biol.* (Limited circulation)

AUSTIN, D. P. (1973). 'The regulation of intracellular amino-acids in Carcinus maenas. (L.)', Ph.D. Thesis, Newcastle-upon-Tyne

AYERS, J. C. (1938). 'Relationship of habitat to oxygen consumption in certain estuarine crabs', *Ecology,* **19,** 523–527

BAKER, P. F. (1965). 'Phosphorus metabolism of intact crab nerve and its relation to the active transport of ions', *J. Physiol.,* **180,** 383–423

BASSINDALE, R. (1942). 'The distribution of amphipods in the Severn Estuary and Bristol Channel', *J. Anim. Ecol.,* **11,** 131–144

BAXTER, C. F. and ORTIZ, C. L. (1966). 'Amino acids and the maintenance of osmotic equilibrium in brain tissue', *Life Sci.,* **5,** 2321–2329

BAYNE, B. L. (1963). 'Responses of *Mytilus edulis* larvae to increases in hydrostatic pressure', *Nature Lond.,* **198,** 486

BEADLE, L. C. (1943). 'Osmotic regulation and the faunas of inland waters', *Biol. Rev.,* **18,** 172–183

BEADLE, L. C. (1957). 'Comparative physiology: osmotic and ionic regulation in aquatic animals', *Ann. Rev. Physiol.,* **19,** 329–354

BEADLE, L. C. and CRAGG, J. (1940). 'Studies on adaptation to salinity in *Gammarus* species. 1. Regulation of blood and tissues and the problem of adaptation to fresh water', *J. exp. Biol.,* **17,** 153–163

BEDFORD, J. J. (1971). 'Osmoregulation in *Melanopsis trifasciatus.* IV. The possible control of intra-cellular isosmotic regulation', *Comp. Biochem. Physiol.,* **40A,** 1015–1027

BIALASZEWICZ, K. (1933). 'Contribution a l'étude de la composition minerale des liquides nourriciers chez les animaux marins', *Arch. int. Physiol.,* **36,** 41–53

BIRD, E. G. (1972). 'Some aspects of the biology of polychaete larvae in Southampton Water with notes on *Sagitta setosa',* M.Sc. Dissertation, University of Southampton

BOLLETTE-DUGAILLAYS, A. and SCHOFFENIELS, E. (1968). 'Action des ions inorganiques sur l'activite de la dehydrogenase lactique des certains crustacés', *Arch. int. Physiol. Biochem.,* **77,** 493–500

BOUSFIELD, E. L. (1955). 'Ecological control of the occurrence of barnacles in the Miramichi estuary', *Bull. Nat. Mus. Can.,* **137,** 1–65

BORN, J. W. (1968). 'Osmoregulatory capacities of two caridean shrimps *Syncaris pacifica* (Atyidae) and *Palaemon macrodactylus* (Palaemonidae)', *Biol. Bull.,* **134,** 235–244

BRICTEUX-GREGOIRE, S., DUCHATEAU-BOSSON, G., JEUNIAUX, C. and FLORKIN, M. (1962). 'Constituents osmotiquement actifs des muscles du crabs chinois, *Eriocheir sinensis,* adapté à l'eau douce ou à l'eau de mer', *Archs. int. Physiol. Biochem.,* **70,** 273–286

BRONGERSMA-SANDERS, M. (1957). 'Mass mortality in the sea'. In: *Treatise on Marine Ecology and Paleoecology.* Ed. J. W. Hedgpeth. Geological Society of America

BROWN, F. A. (1954). 'Persistent activity rhythms in the oyster', *Am. J. Physiol.,* **178,** 510–514

BRYAN, G. (1960). 'Sodium regulation in the crayfish *Astacus fluviatilis* 1. The normal animal', *J. exp. Biol.,* **37,** 83–89

*'Heredity gave the ability and environment provided the opportunity'. (Pearse, 1939).

BURGER, J. W. (1957). 'The general form of excretion in the lobster, *Homarus*', *Biol. Bull.*, **113**, 207–223

BURTON, R. F. (1973). 'The significance of ionic concentrations in the internal media of animals', *Biol. Rev.*, **48**, 195–231

CALDWELL, P. C. (1968). 'Factors governing movement and distribution of inorganic ions in nerve and muscle', *Physiol. Rev.*, **48**, 1–64

COLE, W. H. (1940). 'The composition of the blood of some marine animals and of the sea water in which they live', *J. Gen. Physiol.*, **23**, 575–584

COPELAND, D. E. and FITZJARREL, A. T. (1968). 'The salt absorbing cells in the gills of the blue crab, *Callinectes sapidus* (Rathbun) with notes on modified mitochondria', *Z. Zellforsch. Mikrosk. Anat.*, **92**, 1–22

CROGHAN, P. C. (1958). 'The osmotic and ionic regulation of *Artemia salina* in various media', *J. exp. Biol.*, **35**, 219–233

CROGHAN, P. C. (1962). 'Competition and methods of osmotic adaptation', *Symp. Soc. Exp. Biol.*, **15**, 156–166

CROGHAN, P. C. and LOCKWOOD, A. P. M. (1968). 'Ionic regulation of the Baltic and freshwater races of the isopod *Mesidotea entomon* (L)', *J. exp. Biol.*, **48**, 141–158

DAINTY, J. and HOUSE, C. R. (1966). 'An examination of the evidence for membrane pores in frog skin', *J. Physiol. Lond.*, **185**, 172–184

DANDRIFOSSE, G. (1966). 'Absorption d'eau au moment de lae mue chez un crustace decapode *Maia squinado', Arch. int. Physiol. Biochem.*, **74**, 329–331

DAVENPORT, J. (1972a). 'Salinity tolerance and preference in the porcelain crabs, *Porcellana platycheles* and *Porcellana longicornis', Mar. Behav. Physiol.;* **1**, 123–138

DAVENPORT, J. (1972b). 'Volume changes shown by some littoral anomuran crustacea', *J. mar. biol. Assoc. U.K.*, **52**, 863–877

DAVENPORT, J. and WANKOWSKI, J. (1973). 'Pre-immersion salinity choice behaviour in *Porcellana platycheles, Mar. Biol.*, **22**, 313–316

DIAMOND, J. M. (1965). 'The mechanism of isotonic water absorption and secretion', *Symp. Soc. exp. Biol.*, **19**, 329–347

DIGBY, P. S. B. (1967). 'Pressure sensitivity and its mechanism in the shallow marine environment', *Symp. Soc. Zool. Lond.*, **19**, 159–188

DIGBY, P. S. B. (1972). 'Detection of small changes in hydrostatic pressure by crustacea and its relation to electrode action in the cuticle', *Symp. Soc. exp. Biol.*, **26**, 445–471

DUCHÂTEAU-BOSSON, G. and FLORKIN, M. (1962). 'Adaptation à l'eau de mer de crabes chinois (*Eriocheir sinensis*) 'présentant, dans le l'eau douce, une valeur élevée de la composante amino acids des muscles', *Arch. internat. Physiol. Biochim.*, **70**, 345–355

DUCHÂTEAU, G., FLORKIN, M. and JEUNIAUX, C. (1959). 'Composante amino acide des tissus chez les Crustacés. I. Composante amino acide des muscles de *Carcinus maenas* L. Lors du passage de l'eau saumâtre et au cours de la mue', *Arch. int. Physiol.*, **67**, 489–500

DUCHÂTEAU-BOSSON, G., JEUNIAUX, C. and FLORKIN, M. (1961). 'Role de l'euryhalinité d'*Arenicola marina* L.', Arch. internat. Physiol. Biochim., **69**, 30–35

DUVAL, M. (1925). 'Recherches physio-chemiques et physiologiques sur le milieu interieur des animaux aquatiques', *Ann. Inst. Oceanogr. Monaco,* **2**, 232–407

EMERSON, D. N. (1968). 'Influence of salinity on ammonia excretion rates and tissue constituents of euryhaline invertebrates', *Comp. Biochem. Physiol.*, **29**, 1115–1133

EVANS, D. H. (1969). 'Studies on the permeability to water of selected marine, freshwater and euryhaline teleosts', *J. exp. Biol.*, **50**, 689–703

EVANS, D. H., MALLERY, C. H. and KRAVITZ, L. (1973). 'Sodium extrusion by a fish acclimated to sea water: physiological and biochemical description of a Na for K exchange system', *J. exp. Biol.*, **58**, 627–636

FARLEY, R. D. and CASE, J. F. (1968). 'Perception of external oxygen by the burrowing shrimp, *Callianassa californiensis* Dana and *C. affinis* Dona', *Biol. Bull.*, **134**, 261–265

FINGERMAN, M. (1960). 'Tidal rhythmicity in marine organisms', *Cold Spring Harb. Symp. Quant. Biol.*, **25**, 481–490

FLORKIN, M. (1962). 'La régulation isosmotique intracellulaire chez les invertebrates marins euryhalins', *Bull. Acad. roy. Belge,* **48**, 687–694

FLORKIN, M. and DUCHÂTEAU, G. (1949). 'Sur l'osmoregulation d'anodonte (*Anodonta cygnaea*)', *Physiologia comp. Oecol.*, **1**, 29–45

FLORKIN, M., DUCHÂTEAU-BOSSON, G., JEUNIAUX, C. and SCHOFFENIELS, E. (1964). 'Sur le mechanisme de la regulation de la concentration intracellulaire en acides amines livre chez *Eriocheir sinensis* au cours de l'adaptation osmotique', *Arch. int. Physiol. Biochem.*, **72,** 892–906

FLORKIN, M. and SCHOFFENIELS, E. (1969). *Molecular Approaches to Ecology.* Academic Press, London

FLÜGEL, H. (1960). 'Über den Einfluss der Temperatur auf die osmotische Resistenz und die Osmoregulation der decapoden Garnele *Crangon crangon* L.' *Kieler Meeresforsch,* **16,** 186–200

FREEL, R. W., MEDLER, S. G. and CLARK, M. E. (1973). 'Solute adjustment in the coelomic fluid and muscle fibres of a euryhaline polychaete *Neanthes succinea* adapted to various salinities', *Biol. Bull.,* **144,** 289–303

FREEMAN, R. F. and RIGLER, F. H. (1957). 'The responses of *Scrobicularia plana* (da Costa) to osmotic pressure changes', *J. mar. biol., Assoc. U.K.,* **36,** 553–563

FRETTER, V. (1955). 'Uptake of radioactive sodium (^{24}Na) by *Nereis diversicolor,* Mueller and *Perinereis cultrifera* Grube', *J. mar. biol. Assoc. U.K.,* **34,** 151–160

GILCHRIST, B. M. (1956). 'The oxygen consumption of *Artemia salina* (L.) in different salinities', *Hydrobiologica,* **8,** 54–65

GILLES, R. (1969). 'Effect of various salts on the activity of enzymes implicated in amino acid metabolism', *Arch. int. Physiol. Biochim.,* **77,** 441–464

GILLES, R. and SCHOFFENIELS, E. (1969). 'Isosmotic regulation in isolated surviving nerves of *Eriocheir sinensis* Milne Edwards', *Comp. Biochem. Physiol.,* **31,** 927–939

GORDON, M. S. (1965). 'Intracellular osmoregulation in skeletal muscle during salinity adaptation in two species of toad', *Biol. Bull.,* **128,** 218–229

GREEN, J. (1968). *The Biology of Estuarine Animals.* Sidgwick and Jackson

GREENAWAY, P. (1970). 'Sodium regulation in the freshwater mollusc *Limnaea stagnalis* (L.) (Gastropoda: Pulmonata)', *J. exp. Biol.,* **53,** 147–163

GROSS, W. J. (1957a). 'A behavioural mechanism for osmotic regulation in a semi-terrestrial crab', *Biol. Bull.,* **113,** 268–274

GROSS, W. J. (1957b). 'An analysis of responses to osmotic stress in selected decapod crustacea', *Biol. Bull.,* **112,** 43–62

GROSS, W. J. (1961). 'Osmotic tolerance and regulation in crabs from a hypersaline lagoon', *Biol. Bull.,* **121,** 290–301

GROSS, W. J. and MARSHALL, L. A. (1960). 'The influence of salinity on the water fluxes of a crab', *Biol. Bull.,* **119,** 440–453

HAEFNER, P. A. and SCHUSTER, C. N. (1964). 'Length increments during terminal moult of the female blue crab, *Callinectes sapidus* in different salinity environments', *Chesapeake Science,* **5,** 114–118

HARRIS, R. R. (1969). 'Free amino acid and haemolymph concentration changes in *Sphaeroma rugicauda* (Isopoda) during adaptation to a dilute salinity', *J. exp. Biol.,* **50,** 319–326

HARRIS, R. R. (1970). 'Sodium uptake in the isopod *Sphaeroma rugicauda* Leach during acclimatization to high and low salinities', *Comp. Biochem. Physiol.,* **32,** 763–773

HASKIN, H. H. (1964). 'The distribution of oyster larvae', *Symp. Soc. exp. mar. Ecol.(Occas. Pub.)',* **2,** 76–80

HAYES, R. R. and PELLUET, D. (1947). 'The inorganic constitution of molluscan blood and muscle', *J. mar. biol. Assoc. U.K.,* **26,** 580–589

HORNE, F. R. (1966). 'Some aspects of ionic regulation in the tadpole shrimp, *Triops longicaudatus', Comp. Biochem. Physiol.,* **19,** 313–316

HYNES, H. B. N. (1954). 'The ecology of *Gammarus duebeni* Lilljeborg, and its occurrence in fresh waters in Western Britain', *J. Anim. Ecol.,* **23,** 38–84

JAECKEL, S. (1952). 'Zur Okologie der Mollusken fauna in der westlichen Ostsee', *Schr. Naturw. ver Schlesw-Holst,* **26,** 18–60

JANSSON, B.-O. (1967). 'The importance of tolerance and preference experiments for the interpretation of mesopsammon field distributions', *Helgoland wiss. Meeresunters,* **15,** 41–58

JEUNIAUX, C., BRICTEUX-GREGOIRE, S. and FLORKIN, M. (1962). 'Regulation osmotique intracellulaire chez *Asterias rubens.* Role du glycocolle et de la taurine', *Cahiers Biol. Mar.,* **3,** 107–113

JEUNIAUX, C., BRICTEUX-GREGOIRE, S. and FLORKIN, M. (1961). 'Contributions des acides aminés libres à la régulation osmotique intracellulaire chez deux crustacés euryhalins, *Leander serratus* E. et *Leander squilla* L.', *Cahiers Biol. Mar.*, **2,** 373–379

JEUNIAUX, C., DUCHÂTEAU-BOSSON, G. and FLORKIN, M. (1961). 'Variation de la composante amino acide des tissus et euryhalinite chez *Perinereis cultrifera* Gr et *Nereis diversicolor* (O. F. Muller)', *J. Biochem.*, **49,** 527–531

JEUNIAUX, C. and FLORKIN, M. (1961). 'Modification de l'excretion azotee du crabe chinois au cours de l'adaptation osmotique', *Arch. int. Physiol. Biochim.*, **69,** 385–386

JØRGENSEN, C. B. and DALES, R. P. (1957). 'The regulation of volume and osmotic regulation in some nereid polychaetes', *Physiol. comp. et Oecol.*, **4,** 357–374

KAMEMOTO, F. I. and ONO, J. K. (1967). 'The effects of eyestalk ligation on salt and water balance in the crayfish, *Procambarus clarkii*', *Am. Zool.*, **7,** 723

KATO, K. N. and KAMEMOTO, F. I. (1969). 'Neuroendocrine involvement in osmoregulation in the grapsid crab, *Metopograpsus messor*', *Comp. Biochem. Physiol.*, **28,** 665–674

KINNE, O. (1953). 'Zur Biologie und Physiologie von *Gammarus duebeni* Lillj', *Z. wiss. Zool.*, **157,** 427–491

KINNE, O. (1958). 'Adaptation to salinity variations — some facts and problems'. In: *Physiological Adaptations.* Ed. C. L. Prosser. *American Physiological Society,* Washington

KINNE, O. (1962). 'Irreversible non-genetic adaptation', *Comp. Biochem. Physiol.*, **5,** 265–282

KINNE, O. (1966). 'Physiological aspects of animal life in estuaries with special reference to salinity', *Netherlands. J. Sea Res.*, **3,** 222–244

KINNE, O. (1967). 'Physiology of estuarine organisms with special reference to salinity and temperature, 525–540. In: *Estuaries.* Ed. G. H. Lauf. *American Association for the Advancement of Science*

KINNE, O. (1970). *Marine Ecology,* **1** and **2.** Wiley-Interscience, London

KNIGHT-JONES, E. W. and MORGAN, E. (1966). 'Responses of marine animals to changes in hydrostatic pressure', *Ocean. and Mar. Biol.*, **4,** 267–299

KOEFORD-JOHNSEN, V. and USSING, H. H. (1953). 'The contribution of diffusion and flow in the passage of D_2O through living membranes. Effect of hypophyseal hormone on anuran skin', *Acta. Physiol. Scand.*, **28,** 60–76

KRISHNAMOORTHI, B. (1963). 'Volume regulation in eggs, larvae and adults of a brackish water polychaete, *Diopatra variabilis* (Southern)', *Proc. Ind. Acad. Sci.*, **58,** 275–289

KRISHNAMOORTHI, B. and KRISHNASWAMI, S. (1966). 'Physiological studies on *Marphysa graveli* Southern; III. Regulation of body fluid concentration', *Zool. Jb. Physiol.*, **72,** 316–326

KRISHNAN, G. (1952). 'On the nephridia of Nereidae in relation to habitat', *Proc. Nat. Acad. Sci. India,* **18,** 241–255

KROGH, A. (1938). 'The active absorption of ions in some freshwater animals', *Z. vergl. Physiol.*, **25,** 335–350

KROGH, A. (1939). *Osmotic regulation in aquatic animals.* Cambridge University Press

LAGERSPETZ, K. and MATTILA, M. (1961). 'Salinity reactions of some fresh and brackish water crustaceans', *Biol. Bull.*, **120,** 44–53

LANCE, J. (1965). 'Respiration and osmotic behaviour of the copepod *Acartia tonsa* in diluted sea water', *Comp. Biochem. Physiol.*, **14,** 155–165

LANG, M. A. and GAINER, H. (1969). 'Volume control by muscle fibres of the Blue crab', *J. Gen. Physiol.*, **53,** 323–341

LANGE, R. (1968a). 'The relation between the oxygen consumption of isolated gill tissues of the common mussel *Mytilus edulis* and salinity', *J. exp. mar. Biol. Ecol.*, **2,** 37–45

LANGE, R. (1968b). 'Isosmotic intracellular regulation', *Nytt. Mag. Zool.*, **16,** 1–13

LANGE, R. (1970). 'Isosmotic intracellular regulation and euryhalinity in marine bivalves', *J. exp. mar. Biol. Ecol.*, **5,** 170–179

LANGE, R. and FUGELLI, K. (1965). 'The osmotic adjustment in euryhaline teleosts the flounder, *Pleuronectes flesus* L. and the three-spined stickleback *Gasterosteus aculeatus* L.', *Comp. Biochem. Physiol.*, **15,** 283–292

LANGE, R. and MOSTAD, A. (1967). 'Cell volume regulation in osmotically adjusting marine animals', *J. exp. mar. Biol. Ecol.*, **1,** 209–219

LILLY, S. J. (1955). 'Osmoregulation and ionic regulation in Hydra', *J. exp. Biol.*, **32,** 423–439

LITTLE, C. (1965). 'The formation of urine by the prosobranch gastropod mollusc *Viviparus viviparus* (Linn)', *J. exp. Biol.*, **43,** 39–54

LITTLE, C. (1972). 'The evolution of kidney function in the Neritacea (Gastropoda, Prosobranchia)', *J. exp. Biol.*, **56,** 249–262

LOCKWOOD, A. P. M. (1959). 'The regulation of the internal sodium concentration of *Asellus aquaticus* in the absence of sodium chloride in the medium', *J. exp. Biol.*, **36,** 556–561

LOCKWOOD, A. P. M. (1960). 'Some effects of temperature and concentration of the medium on the ionic regulation of the isopod *Asellus aquaticus* (L.)', *J. exp. Biol.*, **37,** 614–630

LOCKWOOD, A. P. M. (1961). 'The urine of *Gammarus duebeni* and *G. pulex*', *J. exp. Biol.*, **38,** 647–658

LOCKWOOD, A. P. M. (1962). 'The osmoregulation of crustacea', *Biol. Rev.*, **37,** 257–305

LOCKWOOD, A. P. M. (1964). 'Activation of the sodium uptake system at high blood concentrations in the amphipod *Gammarus duebeni*', *J. exp. Biol.*, **41,** 447–458

LOCKWOOD, A. P. M. (1968). *Aspects of the Physiology of Crustacea.* Oliver and Boyd

LOCKWOOD, A. P. M. (1970). 'The involvement of sodium transport in the volume regulation of the amphipod crustacean *Gammarus duebeni*', *J. exp. Biol.*, **53,** 737–751

LOCKWOOD, A. P. M., (1973). 'Changes in the apparent permeability to water at moult in the amphipod *Gammarus duebeni* and the isopod *Idotea linearis*', *Comp. Biochem. Physiol.*, **44A,** 943–952

LOCKWOOD, A. P. M. and ANDREWS, W. R. H. (1969). 'Active transport and sodium fluxes at moult in the amphipod *Gammarus duebeni*', *J. exp. Biol.*, **51,** 591–605

LOCKWOOD, A. P. M. and CROGHAN, P. C. (1957). 'The chloride regulation of the brackish and freshwater races of *Mesidotea entomon* (L)', J. Exp. Biol., **34,** 253–258

LOCKWOOD, A. P. M. and INMAN, C. B. E. (1973a). 'Water uptake and loss in relation to the salinity of the medium in the amphipod *Gammarus duebeni*', *J. exp. Biol.*, **58,** 149–163

LOCKWOOD, A. P. M. and INMAN, C. B. E. (1973b). 'The blood volume of some amphipod crustaceans in relation to the salinity of the environment they inhabit', *Comp. Biochem. Physiol.*, **44A,** 935–941

LOCKWOOD, A. P. M. and INMAN, C. B. E. (1973c). 'Changes in the apparent permeability to water at moult in the amphipod *Gammarus duebeni* and the isopod *Idotea linearis*', *Comp. Biochem. Physiol.*, **44A,** 943–952

LOCKWOOD, A. P. M., INMAN, C. B. E. and COURTENAY, T. H. (1973). 'The influence of environmental salinity on the water fluxes of the amphipod crustacean *Gammarus duebeni*', *J. exp. Biol.*, **58,** 137–148

LOFTS, B. (1956). 'The effects of salinity changes on the respiratory rate of the prawn, *Palaemonetes varians* (Leach)', *J. exp. Biol.*, **33,** 730–736

LOOSANOFF, V. L. (1949). 'Vertical distribution of Oyster larvae of different ages during the tidal cycle', *Anat. Rec.*, **105,** 591

LUCU, C. (1973). 'Competitive role of calcium in sodium transport in the crab *Carcinus mediterraneus* acclimated to low salinities', *Mar. Biol.*, **18,** 140–145

LUMBYE, J. (1958). 'The oxygen consumption of *Theodoxus fluviatilis* L. and *Potamopyrgus jenkinsi* (Smith) in brackish and fresh water', *Hydrobiologica,* **10,** 245–262

MACKLIN, M., ROMA, T. and DRAKE, K. (1973). 'Water excretion by *Hydra*', *Science,* **179,** 194–195

MADANMOHANRAO, G. and RAO, K. P. (1962). 'Oxygen consumption in a brackish water crustacean, *Sesarma plicatum* (Latreille) and a marine crustacean *Lepas ansifera* L.', *Crustaceana,* **4,** 75–81

MAETZ, J. (1969). 'Sea water teleosts: evidence for a sodium–potassium exchange in the branchial sodium-excreting pump', *Science N.Y.*, **166,** 613–615

MAETZ, J. and GARCIA ROMEU, F. (1964). 'The mechanism of sodium and chloride uptake by the gills of a freshwater fish, *Carassius auratus* II. Evidence for NH_4^+/Na^+ and HCO^-/Cl^- exchanges', *J. gen. Physiol.*, **47,** 1209–1228

MANTEL, L. H. (1968). 'The foregut of *Gecarcinus lateralis* as an organ of salt and water balance', *Am. Zool.*, **8,** 433–442

MARSHALL, P. T. (1968). 'Towards an understanding of the osmo-regulation mechanisms of *Hydra*', *School Sci. Rev.*, **51,** 857–861

MARS, P. (1950). 'Euryhalinite de quelques Mollusques mediterranéen', *Vie et Milieu,* **1,** 441–448

MCLUSKY, D. S. (1968). 'Aspects of osmotic and ionic regulation in *Corophium volutator* (Pallas)', *J. mar. biol. Assoc. U.K.*, **48,** 769–781

MCLUSKY, D. S. (1970a). 'Osmoregulation in *Corophium volutator* — the effect of starvation', *Comp. Biochem. Physiol.*, **35,** 303–306

MCLUSKY, D. S. (1970b). 'Salinity preference in *Corophium volutator', J. mar. biol. Assoc. U.K.*, **50,** 747–752

MORRIS, R. and BULL, J. M. (1968). 'Studies on fresh water osmoregulation in the ammocoete larva of *Lampetra planeri* (Block) II. The effect of de-ionised water and temperature on sodium balance', *J. exp. Biol.*, **48,** 597–609

MOTAIS, R., ISAIA, J., RANKIN, J. C. and MAETZ, J. (1969). 'Adaptive changes of water permeability of the teleostean gill epithelium in relation to salinity', *J. exp. Biol.*, **51,** 529–546

NAGEL, H. (1934). 'Die Ausgaben der Excretionsorgane und der Kiemen bei der Osmoregulation von *Carcinus maenas', Z. vergl. Physiol.*, **21,** 468–491

NAYLOR, E. and ATKINSON, R. J. A. (1972). 'Pressure and the rhythmic behaviour of inshore marine animals', *Symp. Soc. exp. Biol.*, **26,** 395–415

NICOL, E. A. T. (1935). 'The ecology of a salt marsh', *J. mar. biol. Assoc. U.K.*, **20,** 203

ODUM, H. T. (1953). 'Factors controlling marine invasion into Florida fresh waters', *Bull. mar. sci. Gulf Caribb.*, **3,** 134–156

OHSAWA, W. and TSUKUDA, H. (1955). 'Extruding response of the periwinkle, *Nodlittorina granularis* (Gray)', *J. inst. Polytech. Osaka Univ.*, **6,** 71–96

PANTIN, C. F. A. (1931). 'The adaptation of *Gunda ulvae* to salinity', *J. exp. Biol.*, **8,** 63–94

PARRY, G. and POTTS, W. T. W. (1965). 'Sodium balance in the freshwater prawn *Palaemonetes antennarius', J. exp. Biol.*, **42,** 415–421

PEARSE, A. S. (1939). *Animal Ecology,* McGraw Hill Book Co., New York and London

PICKEN, L. E. R. (1937). 'The mechanism of urine formation in invertebrates II. The excretory mechanism in certain mollusca', *J. exp. Biol.*, **14,** 20–34

PIERCE, S. K. and GREENBERG, M. J. (1972). 'The nature of cellular volume regulation in marine bivalves', *J. exp. Biol.*, **57,** 681–692

POTTS, W. T. W. (1959). 'The sodium fluxes in the muscle of a marine and a freshwater lamellibranch', *J. exp. Biol.*, **36,** 676–689

POTTS, W. T. W. and FLEMMING, W. R. (1971). 'The effect of environmental calcium and bovine prolactin on sodium balance in *Fundulus kansae', J. exp. Biol.*, **54,** 63–75

POTTS, W. T. W., FOSTER, M. A., RUDY, P. P. and PARRY HOWELLS, G. (1967). 'Sodium and water balance in the cichlid teleost, *Tilapia mossambica', J. exp. Biol.*, **47,** 461–470

POTTS, W. T. W. and PARRY, G. (1964a). 'Sodium and chloride balance in the prawn *Palaemonetes varians', J. exp. Biol.*, **41,** 591–601

POTTS, W. T. W. and PARRY, G. (1964b). *Osmotic and Ionic Regulation in Animals.* Pergamon, London

PRASADA RAO, G. P. N. and GANAPATI, P. N. (1968). 'Respiration as a function of oxygen concentration in intertidal barnacles', *Mar. Biol.*, **1,** 309–310

PRINCE, W. T. and BERRIDGE, M. J. (1972). 'The role of calcium in the action of 5-hydroxytryptamine and cyclic AMP on salivary glands', *J. exp. Biol.*, **58,** 367–384

PROSSER, C. L., GREEN, W. W. and CHOW, T. S. (1955). 'Ionic and osmotic concentrations in the blood and urine of *Pachygrapsus crassipes* acclimated to different salinities', *Biol. Bull.*, **109,** 99–107

RALPH, R. (1965). 'Some aspects of the ecology and osmotic regulation of *Neomysis integer* Leach', Ph.D. Thesis, University of Southampton

RAMSAY, J. A. (1961). 'The comparative physiology of renal function of invertebrates'. In: *The Cell and the Organism.* Cambridge University Press

RAO, K. P. (1958). 'Oxygen consumption as a function of size and salinity in *Metapenaeus monoceros.* Fab. from marine and brackish water environments', *J. exp. Biol.*, **35,** 307–313

REID, D. M. (1930). 'Salinity interchange between sea water in sand and overflowing freshwater at low tide', *J. mar. biol. Assoc. U.K.*, **16,** 609–614

REID, D. M. (1932). 'Salinity interchange between salt water in sand and overflowing freshwater at low tide. II.', *J. mar. biol. Assoc. U.K.*, **18,** 299–306

REMANE, A. and SCHLIEPER, C. (1971). *Biology of Brackish Water.* John Wiley and Sons. (Translation of *Die Binnengewasser*)

RICE, A. L. (1964). 'Observations on the effects of changes in pressure on the behaviour of some marine animals', *J. mar. biol. Assoc. U.K.*, **44,** 163–175

RICKETTS, E. and CALVIN, J. (1948). *Between Pacific Tides.* 4th Edn. revised J. Hedgpeth. Stanford University Press

RIEGEL, J. A., LOCKWOOD, A. P. M., NORFOLK, J. R. G., BULLEID, N. C. and TAYLOR, P. A. (1974). 'Urinary bladder volume and the reabsorption of water from the urine of crabs', *J. exp. Biol.,* **60,** 167–181

ROBERTSON, J. D. (1939). 'The inorganic composition of body fluids of three marine invertebrates', *J. exp. Biol.,* **16,** 387

ROBERTSON, J. D. (1960). 'Ionic regulation in the crab *Carcinus maenas* (L.) in relation to the moulting cycle', *Comp. Biochem. Physiol.,* **1,** 183–212

ROBERTSON, J. D. (1961). 'Studies on the chemical composition of muscle tissue. II. The abdominal flexor muscles of the lobster, *Nephrops norvegicus* (L.)', *J. exp. Biol.,* **38,** 707–728

ROBERTSON, J. D. (1970). 'Osmotic and ionic regulation in the horseshoe crab, *Limulus polyphemus* (L.)', *Biol. Bull.,* **138,** 157–183

RUDY, P. P. (1966). 'Sodium balance in *Pachygrapsus crassipes', Comp. Biochem. Physiol.,* **18,** 881–907

RUDY, P. P. (1967). 'Water permeability in selected decapod crustacea', *Comp. Biochem. Physiol.,* **22,** 581–589

SALEÉ, M-L. and VIDREQUIN-DELIEGE, M. (1967). 'Nervous control of the permeability characteristics of the isolated skin of the toad *Bufo bufo* L.', *Comp. Biochem. Physiol.,* **23,** 583–597

SCHLIEPER, C. (1929a). 'Die Osmoregulation der Süsswasserkrebse', *Verh. deut. Zool. Ges. Graz.,* **33,** 214–218

SCHLIEPER, C. (1929b). 'Über die Einwerkung niederer Salzkonzentrationen auf maine Organismen', *Z. vergl. Physiol.,* **9,** 478–514

SCHLIEPER, C. 'Über die physiologischen Wirkung des Brackwassers (Nach Versuchen an der Miesmuschel *Mytilus edulis*)', *Kieler Meeresforsch,* **11,** 22–23

SCHOFFENIELS, E. (1960). 'Origine des acides aminés intervenant dans la régulation de la pression osmotique intracellulaire de *Eriocheir sinensis* Milne Edwards', *Arch. int. Physiol. Biochim.,* **68,** 696–697

SCHOFFENIELS, E. (1968). 'The control of intracellular hydrogen transport by inorganic ions', *Arch. int. Physiol. Biochim.,* **76,** 319–343

SEGERSTRALE, S. G. (1969). 'Aspects of the biology of the Baltic Sea, with special reference to the littoral zone'. In: *Cold Water Inshore Marine Biology, Some Regional Aspects,* Symp. Northeastern University

SHAW, J. (1955). 'Ionic regulation in the muscle fibres of *Carcinus maenas.* II. The effect of reduced blood concentration', *J. exp. Biol.,* **32,** 664–680

SHAW, J. (1958a). 'Further studies on ionic regulation in the muscle fibres of *Carcinus maenas', J. exp. Biol.,* **35,** 902–919

SHAW, J. (1958b). 'Osmoregulation in the muscle fibres of *Carcinus maenas', J. exp. Biol.,* **35,** 920–929

SHAW, J. (1959a). 'Salt and water balance in the East African freshwater crab, *Potamon niloticus* (M.EdW)', *J. exp. Biol.,* **36,** 157–176

SHAW, J. (1959b). 'The absorption of sodium ions by the crayfish *Astacus pallipes* Lereboullet. I. The effect of external and internal sodium concentrations', *J. exp. Biol.,* **36,** 126–144

SHAW, J. (1960). 'The absorption of sodium ions by the crayfish *Astacus pallipes* Lereboullet. III. The effect of other cations in the external solution', *J. exp. Biol.,* **37,** 548–556

SHAW, J. (1961a). 'Studies on ionic regulation in *Carcinus maenas.* I. Sodium balance', *J. exp. Biol,,* **38,** 135–152

SHAW, J. (1961b). 'Sodium balance in *Eriocheir sinensis* M.EdW. The adaptation of the crustacea to freshwater', *J. exp. Biol.,* **38,** 153–162

SIEBERS, D. and LUCU, C. (1973). 'Mechanisms of intracellular isosmotic regulation: Extracellular space of the shore crab *Carcinus maenas* in relation to environmental salinity', *Helg. wiss Meeresunters.,* **25,** 199–205

SIEBERS, D., LUCU, C., SPERLING, K. R., and EBERLEIN, K. (1972). 'Kinetics of osmoregulation in the crab *Carcinus maenas', Mar. Biol.,* **17,** 291–303

SKAER, H. C. B. (1974). 'The water balance of a serpulid polychaete, *Mercierella enigmatica* (Fauvel)', *J. exp. Biol.,* **60,** 331–338

SLOAN, N. A. (1972). 'The transport of *Ostrea edulis* in the tidal Beaulieu estuary', M.Sc. Dissertation, University of Southampton

SMITH, P. G. (1969). 'The ionic relations of *Artemia salina* (L.). II. Fluxes of sodium, chloride and water', *J. exp. Biol.*, **51,** 739–757

SMITH, R. I. (1957). 'A note on the tolerance of low salinities by Nereid polychaetes and its relation to temperature and reproductive habit', *Ann. Biol.*, **33,** 93–107

SMITH, R. I. (1967). 'Osmotic regulation and adaptive reduction of water permeability in a brackish water crab *Rhithropanopaeus harrisi* (Brachyura, Xanthidae)', *Biol. Bull.*, **133,** 643–658

SMITH, R. I. (1970a). 'Chloride regulation at low salinities by *Nereis diversicolor* (Annelida, Polychaeta). II. Water fluxes and apparent permeability to water', *J. exp. Biol.*, **53,** 93–100

SMITH, R. I. (1970b). 'Chloride regulation at low salinities by *Nereis diversicolor.* I. Uptake and exchanges of chloride', *J. exp. Biol.*, **53,** 75–92

SMITH, R. I. (1970c). 'Hypo-osmotic urine' in *Nereis diversicolor', J. exp. Biol.*, **53,** 101–108

SMITH, R. I. (1970d). 'The apparent water permeability of *Carcinus maenas* (Crustacea, Brachyura, Portunidae) as a function of salinity', *Biol. Bull.*, **139,** 351–362

SMITH, R. I. and RUDY, P. P. (1972). 'Water exchange in the crab *Hemigrapsus nudus* measured by use of deuterium and tritium oxides as tracers', *Biol. Bull.*, **143,** 234–246

SPAARGAREN, D. H. (1972). 'Osmoregulation in the prawns *Palaemon serratus* and *Lysmata seticaudata* from the Bay of Naples', *Netherlands J. Sea Res.*, **5,** 416–436

STAARLAND, H. (1970). 'Volume regulation in the common whelk *Buccinum undatum* L.', *Comp. Biochem. Physiol.*, **34,** 355–365

STINNAKRE, J. and TAUC, L. (1969). 'Central neuronal response to the activation of osmoreceptors in the osphradium of *Aplysia', J. exp. Biol.*, **51,** 347–361

STONER, L. C. and DUNHAM, P. B. (1970). 'Regulation of cellular osmolarity and volume in *Tetrahymena', J. exp. Biol.*, **53,** 391–399

SUTCLIFFE, D. W. (1967). 'Sodium regulation in the amphipod *Gammarus duebeni* from brackish water and fresh water localities in Britain', *J. exp. Biol.*, **46,** 529–550

SUTCLIFFE, D. W. (1968). 'Sodium regulation and adaptation to freshwater in gammarid crustaceans', *J. exp. Biol.*, **48,** 359–380

SUTCLIFFE, D. W. (1970). 'Experimental populations of *Gammarus duebeni* in freshwater with a low sodium content', *Nature Lond.*, **228,** 875–876

SUTCLIFFE, D. W. (1971a). 'The effect of calcium on sodium influx and loss in *Gammarus* (Amphipoda)', *J. exp. Biol.*, **54,** 485–496

SUTCLIFFE, D. W. (1971b). 'Sodium influx and loss in freshwater and brackish water populations of the amphipod *Gammarus duebeni* Lilljeborg', *J. exp. Biol.*, **54,** 255–268

SUTCLIFFE, D. W. (1972). 'Regulation of water and some ions in Gammarids (Amphipoda). I. *Gammarus duebeni* Lilljeborg from brackish water and fresh water', *J. exp. Biol.*, **55,** 325–344

SUTCLIFFE, D. W. and SHAW, J. (1967a). 'The sodium mechanism in the freshwater amphipod, *Gammarus lacustris* Sars', *J. exp. Biol.*, **46,** 519–528

SUTCLIFFE, D. W. and SHAW, J. (1967b). 'Sodium regulation in the amphipod *Gammarus duebeni* Lilljeborg from freshwater locations in Ireland', *J. exp. Biol.*, **48,** 339–358

SYLVESTER, M. (1970). 'Investigations on the permeable areas of a number of crustacea with special reference to the Isopoda', M.Sc. Thesis, University of Southampton

THEEDE, H. (1969). 'Einige neue Aspekte bei der Osmoregulation von *Carcinus maenas', Mar. Biol.*, **2,** 114–120

THOMAS, A. J. (1954). 'The oxygen uptake of the lobster (*Homarus vulgaris* M.EdW.)', *J. exp. Biol.*, **31,** 228–251

THOMPSON, L. A. (1967). 'Osmotic regulation in the Mexican fresh water crab, *Pseudothelphusa jouyi', Am. Zool.*, **7,** 735

THOMPSON, J. L. and PRITCHARD, A. W. (1969). 'Osmoregulatory capabilities of *Callianassa* and *Upogebia* (Crustacea: Thalassinidea)', *Biol. Bull.*, **136,** 114–129

TODD, M. E. (1964). 'Osmotic balance in *Littorina littorea, L. littoralis* and *L. saxatilis* (Littorinidae)', *Physiol. Zool.*, **37,** 33–44

VAN WEEL, P. B. and CHRISTOFFERSON, J. P. (1966). 'Electrophysiological studies on perception in the antennule of certain crabs', *Physiol. Zool.*, **39,** 317–325

VIRKAR, R. A. (1966). 'The role of free amino-acids in the adaptation to reduced salinity in the sipunculid *Golfingia gouldii', Comp. Biochem. Physiol.*, **18,** 617–625

VIRKAR, R. A. and WEBB, K. L. (1970). 'Free amino acid composition of the soft shelled clam *Mya arenaria* in relation to salinity of the medium', *Comp. Biochem. Physiol.*, **32,** 775–783

WEBB, D. A. (1940). 'Ionic regulation in *Carcinus maenas*', *Proc. roy. Soc. Lond. B.*, **129,** 107–136

WEBBER, H. H. and DEHNEL, P. A. (1968). 'Ion balance in the prosobranch gastropod *Acmaea scutum*', *Comp. Biochem. Physiol.*, **25,** 49–64

WEBER, R. E. and SPAARGAREN, D. H. (1970). 'On the influence of temperature on the osmoregulation of *Crangon crangon* and its significance under estuarine conditions', *Netherlands J. Sea Res.*, **5,** 108–120

WEBER, R. E. and VAN MARREWIJK, W. J. A. (1972). 'Free amino acids and isosmotic intracellular regulation in the shrimp *Crangon crangon*', *Life Sciences*, **11,** 589–595

WERNTZ, H. O. (1963). 'Osmotic regulation in marine and brackish water gammarids (Amphipoda)', *Biol. Bull.*, **124,** 225–239

WIENS, A. W. and ARMITAGE, K. B. (1961). 'The oxygen consumption of the crayfish, *Orconectes immunis* and *Orconectes nais* in response to temperature and to oxygen saturation', *Physiol. Zool.*, **34,** 39–54

WOOD, L. and HARGIS, W. J. (1971). 'Transport of bivalve larvae in a tidal estuary', *Fourth European Marine Biology Symp*. Ed. D. J. Crisp

ZANDEE, D. I. (1966). 'Metabolism in the crayfish *Astacus astacus* (L.). I. Biosynthesis of amino acids', *Arch. int. Physiol. Biochim.*, **74,** 35–44

Seven

Rhythmic behaviour and reproduction in marine animals

E. NAYLOR
Department of Marine Biology, University of Liverpool, Port Erin, Isle of Man

7.1 INTRODUCTION

In developing the main theme of this book, this chapter aims to discuss some aspects of the behavioural physiology of marine animals, particularly in so far as behaviour and reproduction are adaptively related to tidal, daily and seasonal rhythmicity in the marine environment. Arising out of such spectacular events as the spawning of the Palolo worm which, in the Pacific, spawns on the day of the last quarter of the moon in late October, and the spawning of the Californian grunion fish, which rides the waves to the level of the highest high tides of the month, it is not surprising that general observations of lunar effects on marine organisms have for a long time attracted attention (Korringa, 1947, 1957; Fox, 1923, 1956). Equally, the combined effects of solar and lunar (hence tidal) variables in the intertidal zone present widely fluctuating environmental factors against the background of which intriguing rhythmic patterns of behaviour have evolved. Some of the earliest observations of such phenomena were those of Gamble and Keeble (1903) who showed that the small acoelous turbellarian *Convoluta roscoffensis* on sandy beaches in Brittany emerge on the surface during day time low tides when conditions are most suitable for the photosynthetic zooxanthellae which live symbiotically in the turbellarian. Just before the flooding tide covers them, the worms burrow rapidly beneath the sand and avoid being washed away from their preferred zone just below the level of high water neap tides. Subsequent experimental observations by Bohn (1903) and Martin (1907) demonstrated that the *Convoluta* tidal rhythm of emergence persisted for 4–7 days in constant light away from the influence of tides. This fundamental observation, together with a similar report of a spontaneous expansion rhythm in the anemone *Actinia equina* (Bohn and Pieron 1906), led for the first time to the possibility that tidal rhythmicity in marine animals was partially controlled by an internal physiological 'clock' and was not solely in response to environmental changes. The study of such phenomena has developed extensively during the past 20 years, as is reflected in the reviews by Webb and Brown (1959), Fingerman (1960), Enright (1963a), Allen (1966, 1972), Buslé (1969) and Palmer (1973). During this time the concepts of circatidal (*c.* 12.4 h), circalunadian (*c.* 24.8 h), circadian (*c.* 24 h) and similar terms for longer period rhythms have been developed to account for those free running rhythms which are expressed in constant conditions in the laboratory as an approximate match to an environmental geophysical period (Halberg *et al.*, 1959; Neumann, 1969; Palmer, 1973, 1974).

The geophysical periods with which we are mainly concerned are those of the lunar day, which is 24.8 h from moonrise to moonrise, usually resulting in two tidal oscillations 12.4 h apart, and the 24 h solar day. For intertidal organisms these environmental variables interact to produce complex rhythms of light and dark, immersion and emersion, temperature rise and fall, hydrostatic pressure changes and mechanical agitation by waves. Clearly the effects of these variables and the expression of any correlated behavioural rhythmicity will vary from one locality to another depending upon the amplitude of local tides and whether successive tides are of approximately equal amplitude or whether alternate tides are of different amplitude. The effects will also vary in relation to the timing of low spring tides, which occur at different times of day in different localities. Thus, in areas where low spring tides occur at midday and midnight, low shore organisms are exposed to the highest and lowest daily air temperatures, whereas in localities where low spring tides occur at dawn and dusk the effects of exposure to air temperatures are ameliorated.

Further geophysical rhythmicity is imposed on intertidal organisms since the times of high and low tides progress relative to the solar day. High tide coincides with midnight twice during every lunar month thus imposing a semi-lunar or 14-day rhythm upon intertidal organisms, to which they might be expected to show matching physiological rhythmicity. If one considers the interaction of daily, tidal and lunar variables, together with the annual geophysical rhythms of variation in day-length and temperature imposed by the angle of the sun's apparent rotation, perhaps it is not surprising that organisms such as the Palolo worm are able to synchronise their spawning so precisely.

With these general considerations in mind it is useful to consider the problem of rhythmic behaviour in marine animals by attempting to answer a series of questions, namely:

1. Do marine animals in general show behavioural-and physiological rhythms when maintained in constant conditions?
2. What are the properties of such rhythms and how persistent are they?
3. What and where is the physiological clock which controls the approximate period of the circadian or circatidal rhythm being studied?
4. What is the role of environmental variables and how in nature do they effect the accurate phasing of the approximate physiological 'clocks'?

5. Finally, what is the ecological significance and adaptive value of rhythmic behaviour and physiology?

7.2 VERTICAL MIGRATION RHYTHMS IN PLANKTON

Possibly the best known activity rhythms in marine organisms are the daily vertical migrations of plankton (Russell, 1927; Kikuchi, 1930; Cushing, 1951; Banse, 1964; Mauchline and Fisher, 1969). Detailed observations on the diurnal distribution of individual species indicate, for example, that pelagic decapod crustacean species are markedly stratified in the water column during daylight (Foxton 1970). Distributions sometimes overlap but population maxima of congeneric species of genera such as *Sergestes, Gennadas* and *Systellaspis* tend to occur at different depths. At night the species to some extent remain stratified as they migrate upwards, but a greater degree of dispersion occurs than during daytime (*Figure 7.1*).

Some criticism can be levelled at earlier sampling procedures which have sometimes used non-closing nets, made approximate estimations of depth,

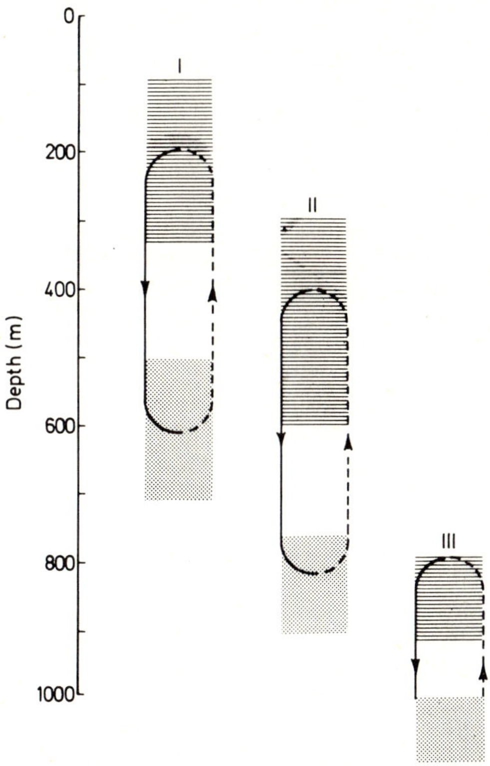

Figure 7.1 Schematic representation of the diurnal pattern of vertical migration of three assemblages of oceanic planktonic species (day distribution–dotted; night distribution–hatched). (After Foxton, 1970; courtesy Cambridge University Press)

or pooled data obtained from several stations separated by time and distance (*see* Woodland 1966; Roe, 1974). Moreover, little work has been carried out on daily migrations of oceanic populations based upon consecutive samples taken at a single station over 24 h at a constant depth. However, recent such round-the-clock sampling confirms daily changes caused by vertical migrations in a wide range of organisms including copepods, ostracods, euphausiids, amphipods, decapods, chaetognaths, siphonophores and fish (Roe, 1974). Vertical migration of this kind appears to be related to food habits and trophic interrelationships, possibly ensuring that populations are maintained in maximum concentrations of prey (Foxton, 1970). Moreover, it seems likely that closely related species are spatially and temporally kept apart, thus reducing competition, as has recently been demonstrated for several pairs of congeneric copepods (Roe, 1974).

Control of these migrations has been partly explained by the suggestion that zooplankton organisms maintain themselves at an optimum level of light intensity (Rose, 1925; Russell, 1927). This 'isolume concept' was supported by observations during the continuous illumination of the arctic summer when the typical migration rhythm was found to be absent (Bogorov, 1946). Indeed there is now considerable evidence that in mesopelagic organisms, particularly those having restricted vertical ranges and associated with sonic scattering layers, there is a strong correlation between the light intensity and their depth of maximum abundance (Clarke, 1966; Boden and Kampa, 1967). Recently Dickson (1972) has supported this view with observations that sonic scattering layers occur deeper in areas of greater ocean transparency. In the Atlantic, light penetration and the extent of migration of sonic scattering layers are greatest in the Sargasso Sea, and least over the Grand Banks and in a tongue of turbid water swept westwards along 20°N from an upwelling centre off W. Africa. Standing station samples at a constant depth (Roe, 1974) also confirm that vertical distributions and migrations of at least some species are ordered by isolumes. Species of decapods, euphausiids, copepods and fish showed a correlation between the time of their migration through a fixed sampling depth of 250 m and their depths of occurrence at a particular time of day. The organisms retained their day depth order by night, deeper living species passing upwards through the sampling point at 250 m later and descending earlier than shallower living forms. So far, only Clarke (1966; 1970) has used a closing net with a deep sea photometer to permit animals and their light regimes to be compared directly. His results again support the notion of layering associated with a particular light level, as evidenced by the distribution of *Euphausia pacifica, Sergestes similis* and the lantern fish *Lampanyctus leucopsarus*.

Temperature gradients have been suggested as possible factors controlling vertical migration and this hypothesis was tested when the relationships between isotherms, isolumes and the vertical distribution of euphausiids was examined by Lewis (1954). Changing levels of occurrence of these organisms were found to show no correlation with isotherms but were positively correlated with isolumes.

Little is known of the effect of hydrostatic pressure on vertical migrations, though Lincoln (1970) has investigated the superimposed effect of hydrostatic pressure on a light-driven vertical migration rhythm in *Daphnia.* In these experiments the animals were induced to migrate up and down by cyclical changes in the overhead light through a gradient steepened by the addition of Indian ink. When the *Daphnia* were subjected to a sharp increase of pressure (*Figure 7.2*) during the course of their migration they immediately spread upwards, while release of pressure caused them to cease movement and sink. The sign of these responses is such that they might be effective in depth-regulation but in these experiments the response was of short duration and was elicited only by pressure increase of more than 2–4

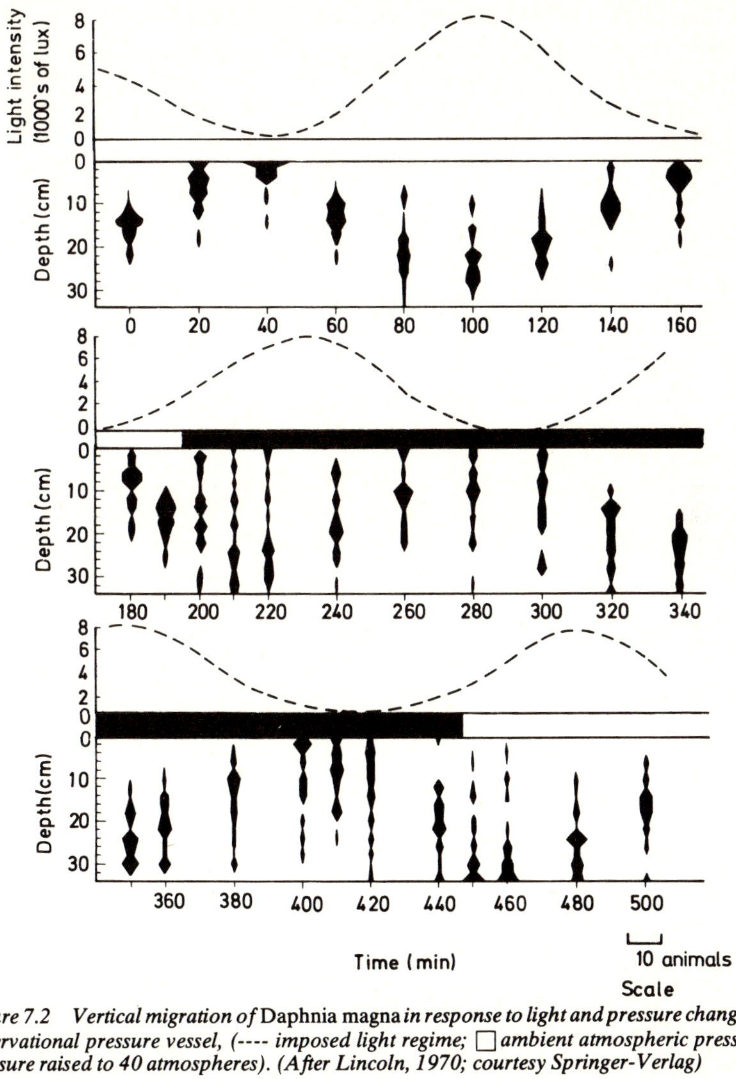

Figure 7.2 Vertical migration of Daphnia magna *in response to light and pressure changes in an observational pressure vessel, (---- imposed light regime; □ ambient atmospheric pressure; ■ pressure raised to 40 atmospheres). (After Lincoln, 1970; courtesy Springer-Verlag)*

atmospheres, equivalent to depth changes of 20–40 m. In view of this, a plankton animal behaving like the fresh-water *Daphnia magna* would clearly accommodate to pressure changes as fast as they develop during vertical swimming. However, some marine species are known to have thresholds of pressure sensitivity which are two orders of magnitude lower than that of *Daphnia* (Naylor and Atkinson, 1972). This taken together with observations that organisms show daily rhythms of sensitivity to pressure (Moore and Corwin, 1956; Lincoln, 1970) and that cycles of pressure change can entrain a persistent rhythm (Naylor and Atkinson 1972), suggest there is clearly scope for an investigation of the effects of pressure on marine zoo-plankton as a factor modifying the levels achieved during vertical migration (Naylor and Atkinson, 1972; Kitching, 1972; *see also* Chapter 6).

Despite the fact that so far light appears to be the main demonstrable factor governing vertical migration in deep sea plankton some other explanation is required to account for the well documented midnight sinking and dawn rise of these organisms (Cushing, 1951). Clarke and Backus (1964) also found that some deep scattering layers overtook each other and the isolumes on their upward and downward migrations, whilst Roe (1974) has demonstrated similar overtaking specifically in fish and copepods. Clearly if midnight sinking and overtaking occur, then not all species can be following an isolume.

Esterly (1917) first demonstrated with the copepod *Acartia* that vertical migration rhythms might be governed by an endogenously controlled rhythm of activity, and Hardy and Paton (1947) found similar evidence for *Calanus*. Along similar lines, Moore and Corwin (1956), studying the daily vertical distribution of siphonophores off Florida, found it necessary to postulate a daily rhythm of responsiveness to light, temperature and depth (pressure) in order to account for their results. More recently Enright and Hamner (1967) have suggested that internal rhythms synchronised by light/dark cycles contribute to the vertical migration rhythms of several crustaceans, while Singarajah, Moyse and Knight-Jones (1967) found an endogenous rhythm in nauplius larvae of *Elminius modestus* and *Balanus balanoides,* which were photonegative at midday and photopositive in the afternoon even in constant conditions. Perhaps the most clear-cut demonstration of endogenous rhythms of vertical swimming is by Harris (1963) in *Calanus* and *Daphnia,* but there is still relatively little experimental evidence of endogenously controlled rhythms of vertical migration in a range of truly planktonic animals.

7.3 BEHAVIOURAL RHYTHMICITY AND POSITION MAINTENANCE IN ESTUARIES

Vertical migration of plankton takes on a greater significance in estuaries where the plankton constituents include larvae of benthic species living in the estuary. As has been mentioned in Chapters 2 and 6 the interaction of tidal flow into an estuary and river flow seawards presents considerable problems relating to the recruitment of larvae to maintain populations of estuarine benthos. It is well known that some estuaries are well stratified in the sense that, despite tidal oscillations, surface water shows a net flow seawards and bottom water shows a net flow inwards. The concept that planktonic animals may utilise the two-layered circulation to alter or maintain their position in such a stratified estuary is generally credited to Nelson (1912).

The problem is well illustrated by the example of the oyster *Crassostrea virginica* in the James River (Virginia), where large populations are self-replenished despite intensive harvesting of adults and the seaward transport of larvae in the surface outflow of river water. The involvement of rhythmic larval behaviour in the process of retention has been demonstrated by Wood and Hargis (1971) (*Figure 7.3*). Lateral swimming is excluded since horizontal tidal currents in the estuary reach 80 cm/s, which is nearly two orders of magnitude faster than the swimming speed of the larvae.

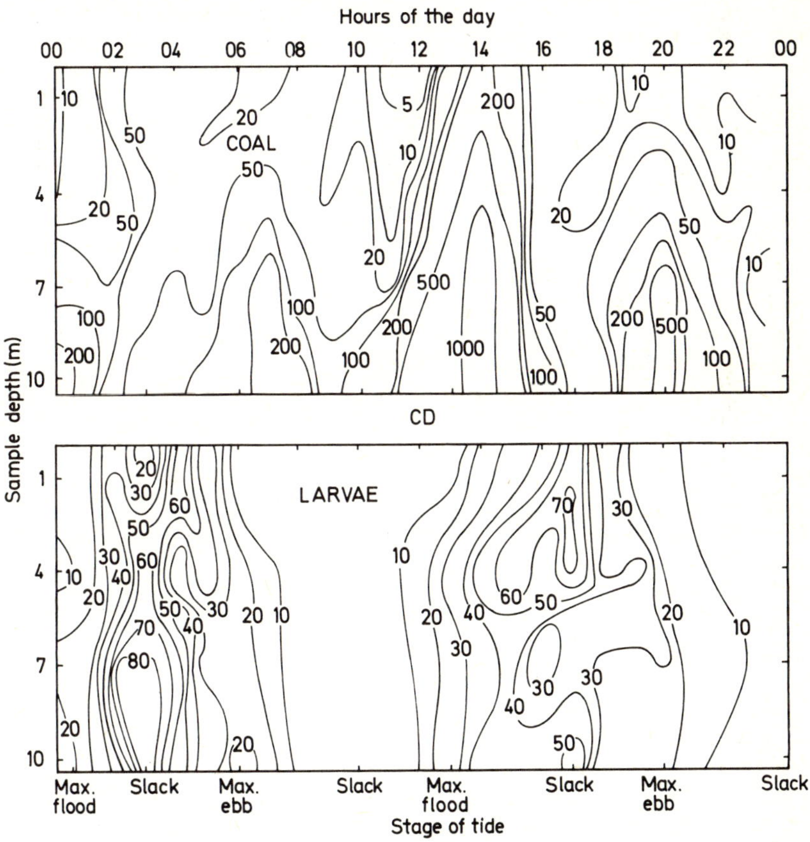

Figure 7.3 Distribution of coal particles (upper) and oyster larvae (lower) in relation to depth and tidal state in the James River, Virginia. Numbers of coal particles show four maxima corresponding to flood and ebb tide, but larvae show only two maxima, related to flood tides. (After Wood and Hargis, 1971; courtesy Cambridge University Press)

However, with a swimming speed of 1 cm/s the larvae could rise vertically through 10 m of water in ¼ h and this would be sufficient to exploit the tidal changes in direction of water flow if swimming took place at tidal periodicity. Round the clock sampling of oyster larvae in the estuary revealed that greatest concentrations of larvae tended to remain on the bottom during the ebbing tide but these moved up into the water column as the tide flooded into the estuary. This was confirmed as a truly active process since inert particles of coal among bottom detritus were agitated upwards into the water column during periods of greatest water movement which occur on the flood and on the ebb. These observations therefore support earlier suggestions (Carriker, 1951; Kunkle, 1957; Haskin, 1964; *see also* Chapter 6) that oyster larvae are retained within an estuary because large numbers show a tidal rhythm of upward swimming on the flood tide.

Since coal particles are carried up the James River, passive transport alone might be sufficient for recruitment in this particular estuary, as Korringa (1957) has earlier suggested. However, there seems little doubt that tidal rhythmicity of swimming occurs in oyster larvae which reinforces the effects of net circulation. It remains to be investigated experimentally whether upward swimming is triggered by increased salinity on the flood as Wood and Hargis (1971) suggest, or whether other external and internal factors are involved. It is likely that differing environmental factors are used as cues dependent upon locality and on the species concerned.

In Florida, as in the James River, where tidal amplitude is small, salinity responses combined with endogenous rhythmicity have been suggested as regulators of the estuarine migrations of the pink shrimp, *Penaeus duorarum* (Hughes, 1969; 1972). This species spawns offshore and the post-larvae move inshore on flood tides at increased salinity, sinking to the bottom when salinity decreases on the ebb. After feeding and growing in estuarine conditions the juvenile shrimps then migrate seawards again, in this case a reduction in salinity on the ebb being followed by downstream swimming. Juveniles resist being carried back into an estuary on the flood tide by exhibiting positive rheotaxis when salinity increases. In localities with extensive tidal oscillations, Knight-Jones and Morgan (1966) have suggested that increased swimming with increased hydrostatic pressure on the rising tide would help in larval recruitment to estuaries. However, pressure responsiveness of this kind is unlikely to operate in the same manner where, as in the James River, tidal rise and fall are small (Naylor and Isaac, 1973).

Apart from vertical migrations of tidal periodicity, it has been suggested that daily migration could be an important retention mechanism for plankton in estuaries with a two-layered circulation (Rogers, 1940). This hypothesis has held wide appeal but it has only recently begun to receive quantitative corroboration from investigations of the estuarine cladoceran *Podon polyphemoides* (Bosch and Taylor, 1973) in Chesapeake Bay where tidal amplitude is low. This cladoceran shows upward migration by day and downward sinking at night. Wind mixing inhibits migration but movement is not impeded by salinity or temperature stratification. The timing of the swimming rhythm coupled with differential sinking speeds combine to ensure that there is no net loss to sea. The downward migration into bottom water, where net flow is inwards, returns individuals which are carried seawards in surface water by day. No studies have been carried out to determine the role of possible endogenous factors in the *Podon* rhythm, which is clearly to a great extent light-dependent; but such behaviour, whether controlled by external or internal factors, probably occurs in other species, allowing them to maintain large populations within the dynamic estuarine environment.

7.4 RHYTHMIC ACTIVITY IN BENTHIC ANIMALS

In contrast to the paucity of experimental studies on the spontaneous rhythmicity of plankton animals, there have been many demonstrations of the rhythmic behaviour of inshore and intertidal organisms in so-called constant conditions. In continuous light, constant temperature and away from the influence of tides many organisms from diatoms to invertebrates and fish show persistent circadian or circatidal rhythms of locomotor activity, ventilation, colour change and respiration (Webb and Brown, 1959; Fingerman, 1960; Enright, 1963a; Allen, 1966 and 1972; Palmer, 1973 and 1974). An early controversy as to whether the rhythms were 'exogenous' or 'endogenous' generated much discussion about the possible role of 'residual periodic variables' such as daily variations in the earth's magnetic field (Brown, 1960; 1972) but this has been countered by a critical appraisal of some of the statistical methods used in analysing for the relationships between biological activity and subtle geophysical phenomena (Cole, 1957; Enright, 1965b; Aschoff, 1965). In addition it seems likely that reported differences in the extent and duration of free-running rhythmicity in intertidal organisms from different localities would be well worthy of investigation in relation to the precise pattern of tidal rhythmicity and the related periodicity of environmental variables in the localities where the organisms were collected.

The hypothesis developed here is that daily and tidal rhythms of behaviour in coastal marine animals are controlled by the interplay of external (exogenous) and internal (endogenous) factors which combine to produce activity at adaptively appropriate times of day. This approach can be illustrated by work on *Carcinus maenas* the common green shore crab which can be seen to move actively between tidemarks at high tide and at night but which remains hidden in crevices at low tide, particularly when low tide occurs during the day. Crabs brought into the laboratory and recorded in actographs at constant temperature and continuous dim light all show rhythmic locomotor behaviour with greatest activity approximating to 'expected' times of high tide and midnight (Naylor, 1958). The rhythms are expressed for at least a week in constant conditions, as confirmed by Blume, Bünning and Müller (1962), indicating a measure of endogenous control by an internal clock mechanism. Crabs rendered arhythmic after several days in constant conditions in the laboratory and then cooled to 4°C for 6 h or more can be shown to re-initiate the tidal rhythm, with peak activity timed from the end of the chilling period (Naylor, 1963). This suggests that tidal rhythmicity is a deep-seated physiological phenomenon in *Carcinus,* which in the study area is subjected to extensive tidal oscillation of up to 10 m.

In contrast *Carcinus maenas* from a non-tidal dock basin in Britain (Naylor, 1960) and *C. mediterraneus* from the relatively non-tidal Mediterranean (Naylor, 1961) all show circadian and not circatidal rhythmicity when recorded in constant conditions and Mediterranean crabs do not respond with tidal rhythmicity when subject to a 6 h cold pulse. However, British crabs from a dock basin which have been away from the influence of tides since the larval stage retain the ability to show tidal rhythmicity after chilling (Naylor, 1963), which suggests that tidal rhythmicity is probably an inherited feature of the physiology of *Carcinus maenas.* This was investigated by rearing crabs from the egg in ambient light/dark in the laboratory (Williams and Naylor, 1967). In continuous dim light, reared crabs show distinct circadian activity with peaks during subjective night. However, tidal rhythmicity was induced in crabs cooled to 4°C for 15 h and then returned to 15°C. It is unlikely that the crabs could have learned the 12.4 h period from the ambient 24 h light cycle or from the 15 h pulse of low temperature, so there is strong support for the view that the ability to show a tidal rhythm is innate. Even stronger evidence for the genetical control of rhythmicity comes from the work of Neumann (1967) on the intertidal midge *Clunio marinus* (*see* p. 420). In these animals hatching takes place under the control of an endogenous semi-lunar rhythm, with peak emergence timed to low spring tides which occur at different times in different geographical localities. Crossbreeding between midges from different localities shows that the differences in emergence times are genetically controlled.

We thus conclude that behavioural rhythms are at least partially controlled by endogenous clock factors which determine the approximate period of the rhythm and result in the expression of the free-running circadian and circa-tidal rhythms in constant conditions. This conclusion conforms with the view of most workers in the field in postulating an escapement-type clock which exists within the organism and generates its own time autonomously. It precludes a non-escapement clock mechanism postulated by Brown, Hastings and Palmer (1970) which receives its timing information solely from periodic environmental variables capable of penetrating so-called constant conditions (*see also* Palmer, 1973; 1974).

With the notion of autonomous clocks determining approximate phase it is now necessary to consider the possible site of the clock(s) and to determine how an apparently deep-seated timing mechanism can be reconciled with the expression of a behavioural rhythm which usually dampens down when animals are maintained in constant conditions. In addition it is important to consider the way in which normal environmental variables impinge upon the organism to act as synchronisers in reinforcing the expressed behavioural rhythm in nature. Also it is necessary to consider the adaptive value of daily rhythmicity, bearing in mind variations in the persistence of rhythms and the emphasis on differing environmental synchronisers in animals from different habitats.

7.4.1 The clock mechanism

Early speculation about the nature of the clock mechanism concentrated particularly upon the so-called temperature-independence of biological rhythms, whereby period and amplitude are relatively similar within the normal range of temperatures experienced by the animal. Indeed, to some extent, these observations have led to the controversy concerning the possible control of biological rhythms by environmental 'residual periodic variables' (*see* p. 401). Now there is evidence that some rhythms are more responsive to temperature change than was previously supposed (*see* p. 408) and in any event the possibility of a temperature-compensated physiological mechanism in invertebrates is also currently less surprising. It could operate, for example, by the close interaction of promoter and inhibitor hormones. The action of hormones as modulators of physiological rhythmicity is well documented in many animals, so perhaps it is not surprising that attempts have been made to assess the role of blood-borne hormones in regulating daily rhythms of behaviour. The experimental approach in these studies is to surgically remove or implant suspected endocrine tissues and most work so far has concerned terrestrial organisms. Hormonal actions have been postulated to explain circadian rhythmicity in a number of species, notably the cockroach *Periplaneta* (Harker, 1960), the cricket *Acheta* (Cymborowski and Dutkowski, 1970) and a scorpion (Rao and Gopalakrishnareddy, 1967), but it should be emphasised that the presence of an autonomous hormonal clock in *Periplaneta* has been questioned by Roberts (1965; 1966) and Brady (1967; 1969) who place greater emphasis on nervous control. Nervous control of rhythmicity in marine organisms will be discussed later.

Among marine animals the role of hormones in controlling rhythmic behaviour has centred on the decapod crustaceans, and has focused particularly on the role of the neuro-endocrine system of the eyestalk. Following early work on fresh water crayfish (Kalmus, 1938; Roberts, 1941 and 1944; Schallek, 1942) in which eyestalk removal resulted in the loss of rhythmicity, similar observations have since been made on the marine crab *Uca* (Edwards, 1950), *Trichodactylus* (Valente and Edwards, 1955), and *Carcinus* (Powell, 1965; Naylor and Williams, 1968) though some evidence of persistent rhythmicity after eyestalk ablation is reported for *Gecarcinus* by Bliss (1962) and a freshwater crayfish by Page and Larimer (1975). In *Uca, Trichodactylus* and *Carcinus* it has been proposed that a hormone inhibiting locomotor activity is produced in the eyestalk neurosecretory system.

In carrying out surgical experiments of this kind it is important to distinguish between the effects of post-operative shock and effects upon a possible rhythmic control centre. This is illustrated in work on *Carcinus* in which eyestalk ablation first causes high activity, followed after a few hours by suppressed activity, but hyperactivity re-establishing itself after a period of 6 days (Naylor and Williams, 1968). Because the tidal rhythm of the shore crab persists for only about 6 days in constant conditions all crabs, with or without eyestalks, tend to be arhythmic by day 6 in the laboratory. However, whereas a period of 6 h at 4°C will re-establish a tidal rhythm in normal animals, eyestalk-ablated crabs after chilling show continuous high activity (Naylor and Williams, 1968). Thus, when the effects of post-operative shock are no longer apparent it can be concluded that eyestalk removal abolishes rhythmicity and promotes overall activity. The severity of the operation itself seems not to be the cause of rhythm abolition since equally severe operations were carried out involving removal of the retinae in other crabs. These control operated animals from which the retinae were removed could also be induced to show rhythmicity by chilling.

Since eyestalk removal is followed not only by a loss of rhythmicity but also by continuous hyperactivity it is reasonable to postulate that the eyestalk neurosecretory system is the site of a rhythmically operative inhibitory factor. That this factor is a blood-borne neuro-hormone is suggested by experiments in which injections of eyestalk extract inhibit activity in normal crabs (Naylor and Williams, 1968). Furthermore, extract from inactive crabs at low tide is more inhibitory than from active crabs at high tide (Naylor, Smith and Williams, 1973).

As a basis for the search for this proposed clock-component in *Carcinus* the distribution of neurosecretory cells on the optic ganglia is described by Smith and Naylor (1972). Axonal transport of neurosecretory granules takes place to the sinus gland which is a neurohaemal organ where release to the blood takes place. Interestingly, the sinus gland itself can be removed by cautery without impairing the ability of the crab to show a tidal rhythm (Naylor, Smith and Williams, 1973), which suggests that neurosecretory material, if involved in the control of rhythmicity, must be released from the damaged axonal endings or peripherally from the neurosecretory cells themselves. However, in *Carcinus* all results so far are consistent with the view that an inhibitory substance is periodically released from the eyestalk neurosecretory system to determine the rhythmic pattern of locomotor behaviour.

In further work on the control of rhythmicity in *Carcinus* recent work has been carried out on rhythms of activity in the nervous system (Arechiga, Huberman and Naylor, 1974; Arechiga and Naylor, 1976). The crabs studied were first kept in light/dark conditions in the laboratory to eliminate the tidal component in their endogenous circadian rhythms of locomotor activity. They were then transferred to continuous dim red light where electrophysiological recordings were made using chronically implanted electrodes for long-term recordings. The response to light of retinal photoreceptors and visual interneurons, the reflex responses of motor neurons to mechanoreceptive stimulation and the spontaneous activity of neurons detecting movements of the body, all show circadian variations, with a phase of high sensitivity at subjective night and low re-activity during subjective daytime. This pattern of nervous activity, therefore, correlates well with the crab's endogenous locomotor rhythms which under these conditions show peak activity during subjective night. Following on the earlier experiments, it has been shown that injection of the eyestalk extract, which inhibits locomotor activity, also suppresses neuronal activity to reproduce the day-phase characteristics of the neuronal rhythm (*Figure 7.4*). The active

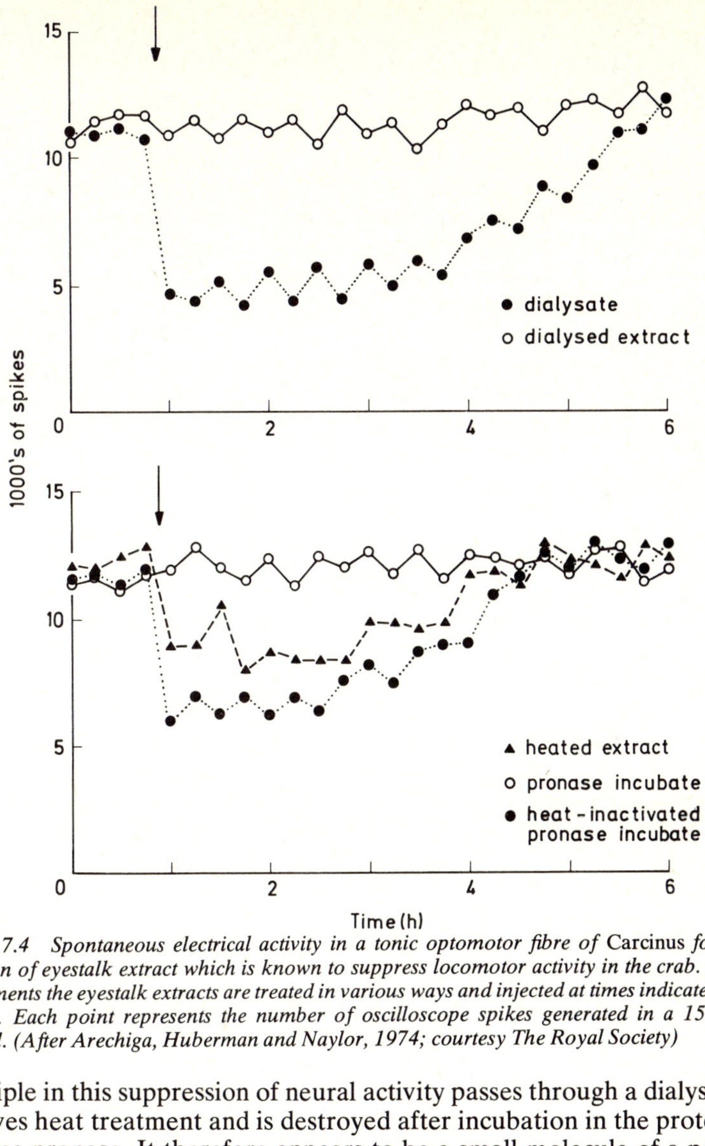

Figure 7.4 Spontaneous electrical activity in a tonic optomotor fibre of Carcinus *following injection of eyestalk extract which is known to suppress locomotor activity in the crab. In these experiments the eyestalk extracts are treated in various ways and injected at times indicated by the arrows. Each point represents the number of oscilloscope spikes generated in a 15 minute interval. (After Arechiga, Huberman and Naylor, 1974; courtesy The Royal Society)*

principle in this suppression of neural activity passes through a dialysis bag, survives heat treatment and is destroyed after incubation in the proteolytic enzyme pronase. It therefore appears to be a small molecule of a peptidic nature (Arechiga, Huberman and Naylor, 1974).

Circadian fluctuations in the responsiveness of sensory elements have also been described in phase with a circadian rhythm of motor activity in a fresh water crayfish (Arechiga and Wiersma, 1969) and a marine decapod *Nephrops* (Arechiga and Bailey 1974). Moreover, the injection of extracts of eyestalk, as well as from other areas of the nervous system, has been found to induce a lowering of neuronal activity, both in intact animals and in isolated nervous structures (Arechiga, Fuentes and Barrera, 1973;

Arechiga, 1974). All these observations, therefore, are consistent with the hypothesis of humoral modulation of nervous activity by a specifically neural or general metabolic inhibitor, giving rise to daily and tidal rhythms of locomotor activity.

So far, in decapod crustaceans, there is no evidence to permit the localisation of an autonomous hormonal clock as has been proposed for the cockroach *Periplaneta americana.* Such a clock was proposed by Harker (1960) who demonstrated that circadian rhythmicity could be induced in an arhythmic cockroach after implantation of the suboesophageal ganglion of a normal animal. An alternative view of the clock mechanism in *Periplaneta* was proposed by Roberts (1965, 1966) and Brady (1967; 1969) who were unable to transfer rhythmicity with implanted ganglia. These authors conclude that a neuro-electrical pacemaker in the optic lobe is more probable than a neuro-humoral system as the basic circadian control mechanism in the cockroach. By analogy, Brady (1974) has suggested that a possible clock site in decapod crustaceans may be within the inner layers of the eyestalk ganglia, where a neuro-electrical pacemaker would be homologous with that proposed for the insect optic lobe. Interestingly, Wells (1937) described a nervous pacemaker in the oesophageal wall controlling short-term contraction rhythms of *Arenicola* and at least two examples are now known for the marine mollusc *Aplysia* in which isolated nervous tissue shows spontaneous circadian rhythmicity. In *Aplysia* the firing of the isolated parabolic burster neuron of the parietovisceral ganglion (Strumwasser, 1967) and the frequency of optic nerve impulses in the isolated eye (Jacklett, 1969) both oscillate with circadian periodicity when kept in darkness. It remains to be seen whether observations of this kind are evidence of a basic neuro-electrical clock, particularly since the neuron recorded from by Strumwasser (1965; 1967) is considered by Frazier *et al.* (1967) to be neurosecretory. In decapods, too, at present it is not known whether locomotor rhythms are maintained solely by cyclical hormone release or whether, as suggested by Page and Larimer (1975), there are neuronal oscillators imposing locomotor rhythmicity axonally via motoneurons, with hormonal influences only modulating the level of activity.

Whilst neural and hormonal elements no doubt intervene in clock control in multicellular organisms, it should be emphasised that the basic clock mechanism probably resides at the cellular level. For example the unicells *Euglena* (Palmer and Round, 1965) and *Gonyaulax* (Sweeney, 1969) show endogenous rhythmicity of burrowing and luminescence, respectively. It is therefore attractive to look for a clock mechanism as a common denominator of cellular organisation. In the dinoflagellate *Gonyaulax* and the parabolic burster cell of *Aplysia,* rhythmicity is associated with changes in membrane potential and cyclical changes in the synthesis of proteins which are, therefore, probably implicated in the cellular clock (Sweeney 1969; Strumwasser, 1971).

Even at the whole organism level it is apparent that one should probably regard control of rhythmicity as a multiple clock phenomenon (Harker, 1958; Naylor, 1960; Palmer, 1973; Pittendrigh, 1974). Such a mechanism

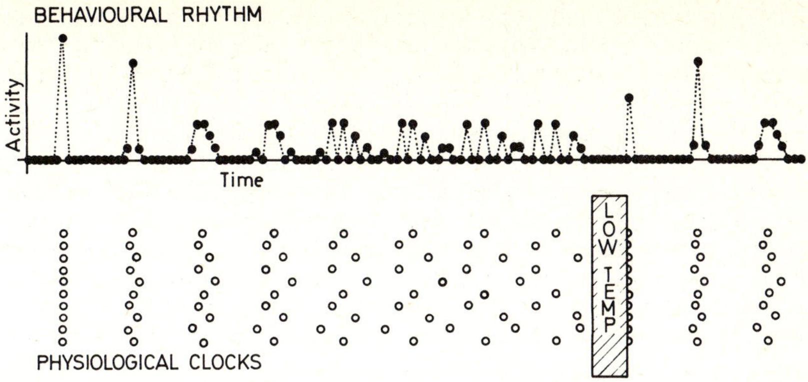

Figure 7.5 Multiple clock model postulating numerous physiological clocks of approximately tidal or circadian periodicity which gradually drift out of phase with each other and result in the loss of the expressed behavioural rhythm in constant conditions. In Nature the clocks would be regularly synchronised by environmental variables and they are here envisaged as being instantaneously resynchronised as the rhythm is re-induced by exposure to low temperature for a few hours, as occurs in the tidal rhythm of Carcinus

appears to be one which permits an explanation of the observed desynchronisation of rhythmicity in organisms in which rhythmicity is clearly deep-seated. Multiple clocks probably at the cellular level and of approximately tidal or circadian period can be envisaged as being in phase when first placed in constant conditions but gradually drifting out of phase in the absence of environmental synchronisers (*Figure 7.5*). Sudden resynchronisation, for example by chilling, can be envisaged as bringing all the clocks back into phase again for the first cycle on return to ambient temperature.

7.4.2 Environmental synchronisation and entrainment

In Nature, accurate phasing of behavioural rhythmicity is maintained by repeated exposure to environmental variables. On the multiple clock model proposed above, environmental variables would continuously adjust the internal clocks of approximate geophysical period, which would otherwise drift out of phase with each other under constant conditions. Responses of the endogenous rhythms to environmental variables can be regarded as synchronisation; repeated exposure to such variables which generates a rhythm that persists in subsequent constant conditions can be regarded as entrainment.

Animals which live between tidemarks are subjected to the widest possible range of environmental factors which vary tidally and diurnally, including periodic immersion, mechanical agitation by waves, hydrostatic pressure, temperature, light/dark, and respiratory gases. These factors show regional and temporal variations according to local tidal amplitude, semi-lunar variations of tidal amplitude, the daily timing of low spring tides, shore aspect, water turbidity and the position of the organism on or below the intertidal zone. An approach to the study of synchronisation and entrainment of the behavioural rhythms of animals in such localities can be illustrated with work on the green crab *Carcinus,* typically found on rocky coasts. Normal environmental synchronisation and entrainment of the *Carcinus* rhythm have been tested using crabs kept in cages anchored on the shore (Williams and Naylor, 1969). Crabs without tidal rhythms kept for 11 days between tidemarks became entrained to a tidal rhythm which persisted in constant conditions in the laboratory. Similar results were obtained with crabs kept below tidemarks suggesting that synchronisation does not depend solely on exposure to air. Evidently, hydrostatic pressure changes associated with tidal rise and fall may also be important. Shorter periods of exposure also entrained a persistent rhythm but two days' exposure between tidemarks was much more effective than the same period below low water mark. This result suggests that cycles of pressure change coupled with cycles of immersion and associated temperature changes are more effective entrainment factors than pressure changes alone.

Field experiments are supported by laboratory studies which first set out to test the effects of temperature oscillations such as would be induced by alternate immersion in cold water at high tide and exposure to warmer air at low tide such as occurs in spring where the field experiments were carried out. Though the rhythm of *Carcinus* is relatively temperature-independent (Naylor, 1963), with its period unaffected in the range 10–25°C, transient changes are seen in amplitude and phase of the first activity peak after a change of temperature. A temperature rise decreases the amplitude and delays the phase of the next peak (Naylor, 1963; Naylor, Atkinson and Williams, 1971). With this in mind, crabs were exposed to simulated tidal cycles of alternating 6 h periods at high and low temperature. With temperature differentials of 7 (13 to 20°C) and 11 (13 to 24°C) during treatment for 5 days, activity was synchronised to the low temperature periods and a clear tidal rhythm was entrained in crabs transferred to a constant temperature room. Crabs continue to show high activity at the times of 'expected' low temperature for at least 3 days (Williams and Naylor, 1969). With a temperature differential of 4 degrees in alternating 6 h periods of 17°C and 13°C, rhythmicity was induced during treatment but this did not persist subsequently at 13°C. However, the combination of an immersion cycle in which crabs were kept for alternating 6 h periods in water at 13°C and air at 17°C entrained a very persistent rhythm (Williams and Naylor, 1969). Differences of 3–4°C do occur between air and water temperatures, particularly in spring and summer in the study locality where low spring tides occur at midday, and so could entrain a tidal rhythm at that time of year in crabs which are periodically stranded at low tide in air.

Experiments to test the effects of hydrostatic pressure on the *Carcinus* rhythm have been carried out by Naylor and Atkinson (1972). Using raised pressures of only up to 0.6 atm above ambient, that is equivalent to about a 6 m tidal amplitude, which is not high for British coasts, arhythmic crabs were subjected to alternating 6 h periods of raised and ambient pressure (*Figure 7.6*). Activity was clearly induced by raised pressure and successful entrainment of a persistent tidal rhythm took place using pressure increases

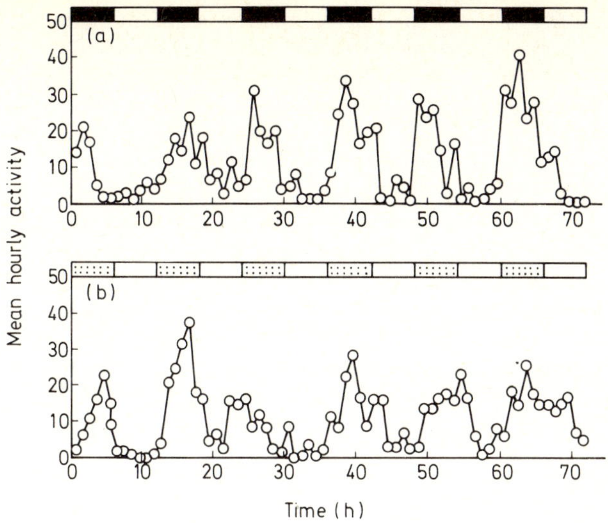

Figure 7.6 Mean hourly activity of six Carcinus *(a) during three days exposure to alternate semi-tidal periods of atmospheric pressure (white bars) and an additional 0.6 atmospheres (black bars), followed by (b) three days at constant atmospheric pressure. Dotted bars in the lower graph indicate periods of 'expected' high pressure which would have occurred if the previous pressure cycles had been continued. (After Naylor and Atkinson, 1972; courtesy J. W. Hannay)*

of as little as 0.1 atm. The degree of persistence of the rhythm at ambient pressure after treatment was linearly related to the duration of the treatment period. These results also indicate that hydrostatic pressure changes of tidal amplitude and period have a marked effect on *Carcinus* at all times of the year in exogenously stimulating locomotor activity at high tide. This synchronisation is carried a step further in entraining an approximate tidal rhythm which persists at subsequent ambient pressure, particularly in autumn (Naylor and Atkinson, 1972).

It is now of interest to assess the relative importance of pressure as one of the variables known to affect the *Carcinus* rhythm, particularly in view of the seasonal variations in the effects of this sensory modality. Seasonal observations show that *Carcinus* usually exhibits a clear-cut rhythm from spring to late autumn (Atkinson and Parsons, 1973). This is also the time when crabs can be most readily collected in the middle reaches of the shore between the levels of high water neaps and low water neaps. In March and December, crabs tend to migrate in with each tide but are less frequently stranded at low tide, perhaps because of low temperatures (Naylor, 1962), and they show little evidence of endogenous rhythmicity. In the coldest months of January and February crabs remain at the lowest levels of the shore, showing little evidence of onshore tidal migrations and no evidence of endogenous rhythmicity in the laboratory. Evidence so far (Naylor and Atkinson, 1972) suggests that after a period of winter inactivity, tidal migrations first begin in spring above a sea temperature of 8°C in the form of exogenous rhythmicity induced and synchronised by the pressure changes of tidal rise and fall. From April to August pressure-induced rhythmicity is reinforced by temperature/immersion cycles associated with the stranding of crabs at low tide. During this period the temperature differential between air and sea temperatures then permits the entrainment of an endogenous rhythm, which is expressed very clearly in constant conditions. In the autumn, temperature differentials would be less effective in entraining the activity rhythm, but it is at this time of year that pressure cycles seem to be at their most effective as an entraining agent of persistent rhythmicity.

The effects of temperature cycles have been little studied as entraining agents for tidal rhythms, though Gibson (1971) had negative results with the shore fish *Blennius pholis* tested in this way. *Blennius* is however presumed to entrain to pressure cycles (Gibson, 1971) as may also be the case with the sand beach isopod *Eurydice pulchra* (Jones and Naylor, 1970). The amphipods *Corophium* (Morgan, 1965) and *Synchelidium* (Enright, 1962), and the pycnogonid *Nymphon gracile* (Morgan, Nelson-Smith and Knight-Jones, 1964; Isaac and Jarvis, 1973) all show exogenous responses to pressure cycles of tidal periodicity but entrainment of their endogenous rhythmicity by this factor has not been demonstrated.

Two isopod species which burrow into surf-beaten sandy shores, emerging to swim and feed on the flood tide, appear to depend upon agitation by wave action as the dominant entraining factor for their swimming rhythm. Thus, the persistent tidal rhythms of *Excirolana* (Enright, 1965a; Klapow, 1972a) and *Eurydice* (Jones and Naylor, 1970) are readily entrained by mechanical stimulation in the laboratory at intervals of 12 h.

Light is clearly an important synchroniser and entraining agent for the circadian components of activity in inshore marine animals. Animals from tidal localities when transferred to non-tidal conditions in normal light/dark cycles often retain the ability to exhibit a tidal rhythm though the recorded pattern is superficially circadian (Naylor, 1960; Webb, 1976; Palmer, 1973). However, representatives of genera which naturally occur in both tidal and non-tidal seas, appear to be predominantly circadian and lose their endogenous tidal rhythmicity in non-tidal conditions. Thus, *Carcinus* (Naylor, 1961) and *Blennius* (Gibson, 1969) from the relatively non-tidal Mediterranean exhibit endogenous rhythms only of circadian periodicity. Similarly, the shrimp *Crangon* which exhibits weak endogenous tidal rhythmicity in British coasts (Al-Adhub and Naylor, 1975) has only very weak circadian periodicity in the tideless Baltic (Hagerman, 1970).

A priori one might expect tidal cycles of light and dark to entrain the tidal component of rhythmicity in inshore species but experiments with *Excirolana* (Enright, 1965a) and *Blennius* (Gibson, 1969) have failed to achieve this. However, animals living in intertidal pools which are not subjected to dramatic temperature changes throughout the tidal cycle, and those living in turbid estuaries, would warrant further investigation in this respect. Darkening at high tide certainly appears to phase the tidal swimming rhythm of the pool-dwelling prawn *Palaemon elegans* in the highly turbid Bristol Channel where maximal tidal amplitude is about 10 m (Rodriguez and Naylor, 1972). In that locality *P. elegans* inhabits pools above the level of high water neap tides. These are reached by the sea every two weeks at the times of spring tides, when the *Palaemon* are high tide active. During neap tides when tides do not reach the pools, the 'tidal' rhythm becomes phase shifted to become a dusk/dawn rhythm. Observations of this kind are of interest in suggesting how tidal rhythms could have evolved from a semi-diurnal dusk/dawn rhythm, or vice versa (Gibson, 1969; Rodriguez and Naylor, 1972).

A further factor which is of interest in the phasing of biological rhythmicity is the possibility that animals may interact with each other to give mutual synchronisation of rhythmicity (Harker, 1964). This has been investigated in the amphipod *Talitrus saltator* which normally lives buried in sand above high tide mark by day and emerges to feed on shore at night utilising a very persistent endogenous circadian clock (Bregazzi and Naylor, 1972). Mixed populations of *Talitrus* were tested in actographs, some with normal periodicity and others in which the spontaneous activity rhythm was re-set artificially to be 12 h out of phase. In constant conditions the two populations combined to maintain separate patterns of activity for at least 10 days without influencing each other. However, there is evidence that mutual synchronisation is possible between *Talitrus* when the phase difference between individual rhythmicity is small, as occurs between single animals when free-running in constant conditions for one or two days. This was demonstrated by recording mid-activity times of batches of sand

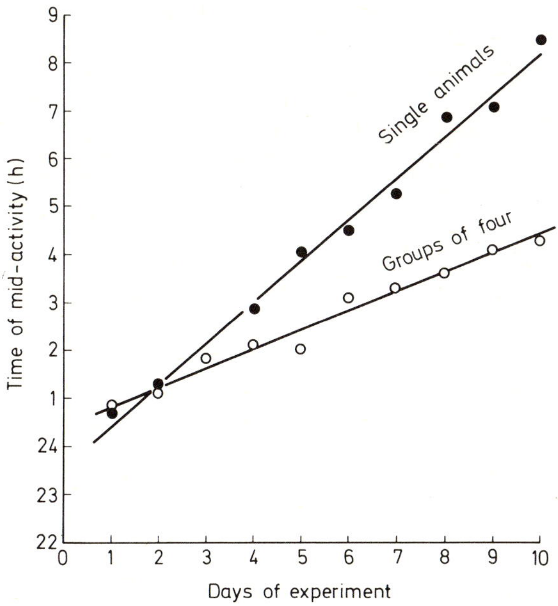

Figure 7.7 Times of mid-activity in the locomotor rhythm of the amphipod Talitrus *kept for 10 days in continuous dim light in the laboratory. Closed circles are the mean values of 15 animals kept singly in actographs; open circles are the mean rates of eight groups of four animals. (After Bregazzi and Naylor, 1972; courtesy R. J. Skaer)*

hoppers recorded singly and in groups. In these experiments the rate of drift of peaks in the free-running rhythm was greater in talitrids recorded singly than in animals recorded in groups (*Figure 7.7*). It is as though those animals which emerge earliest during an activity period synchronise the emergence of other talitrids whose endogenous clocks are running slightly more slowly (Bregazzi and Naylor, 1972).

7.5 ADAPTIVE SIGNIFICANCE OF BEHAVIOURAL RHYTHMS

We can now seek to show how the temporal behaviour of marine animals is adaptively related to the tidal, daily and seasonal rhythmicity of the environment. For planktonic species it has already been suggested that diurnal vertical migrations are probably related to feeding habits in ensuring that animals are maintained in maximum concentrations of prey. In addition it seems likely that differing patterns of vertical migration keep apart closely related species and consequently reduce competition between them. In this way behavioural differences presumably develop in relation to the establishment of isolated populations and permit speciation in plankton communities.

Among inshore and intertidal benthic animals it is perhaps not surprising that locomotor activity is also discontinuous, with active periods of migration, feeding, avoidance of predators, and reproduction, alternating with quiescent periods which may be regarded as 'sleep'. Moreover, the periods of activity would reasonably be expected to vary according to the physiological tolerances of an organism and therefore take place at an adaptively appropriate time. Among crabs, the semi-terrestrial fiddler crab *Uca,* which is an inhabitant of many sandy coastlines, is active mainly at low tide and retires to a burrow at high tide (Barnwell, 1963; 1968), whereas, in contrast, the aquatic green crab *Carcinus* is active mainly at high tide (Naylor, 1958, 1962; Crothers, 1967, 1968). Among supra-littoral forms such as the ghost crab *Ocypode,* some species show behaviour similar to that of *Uca* (Barnwell, 1968), but others are predominantly nocturnal (Jones, 1972), presumably dependent upon whether they forage primarily below high tide mark or above it. Differences of rhythmicity patterns related to zonation are also seen in talitrid amphipods, with *Orchestia gammarella* and *Talitrus saltator* at high water mark showing only circadian rhythmicity, but *Orchestia mediterranea* living somewhat lower down the shore having endogenous rhythms of both circadian and tidal frequency (Wildish, 1970; Bregazzi and Naylor, 1972). Below tidemarks and in non-tidal localities, marine invertebrates (*see* p. 410) and fish (Woodland, 1966) also tend to exhibit predominantly daily, not tidal, patterns of activity.

In view of the overall repeatability of environmental oscillations it is not surprising that the physiological control of temporal behaviour patterns has become deep-seated, even genetically determined (*see* p. 402) as in physiological and structural adaptations. This is particularly so in those organisms for which it is of selective advantage for them to anticipate tidal and daily oscillations rather than rely on direct responses to environmental changes. Thus, the fiddler crab *Uca* returns to its burrow, and often plugs the entrance with a compact ball of sand, in advance of the rising tide and not in response to wetting (Barnwell, 1963, 1968; Palmer, 1973). Similarly the green shore crab *Carcinus* which is particularly mobile at high tide has a selective advantage in avoiding predation by gulls by entering its inactive phase and seeking shelter in a crevice before being exposed to air by the falling tide. Otherwise it might find itself stranded away from the shelter of rocks, pools or a suitable substrate in which to burrow.

Endogenous rhythms of activity and quiescence in intertidal animals are probably also of adaptive value in helping to maintain the characteristic patterns of zonation observed in many species. For example, spontaneous swimming at the times of ebb tide is of considerable ecological advantage in reducing the risk of being stranded high up on the shore, as has been demonstrated for the amphipods *Synchelidium* and *Corophium volutator* (see Enright 1963b; Morgan 1965) and for the pycnogonid *Nymphon gracile* (*see* Morgan, Nelson-Smith and Knight-Jones, 1964; Isaac and Jarvis, 1973). Endogenous rhythmic behaviour patterns also appear to maintain the zonation on the upper shore of the sand-burrowing isopod *Eurydice pulchra* which swims up into the surf as the tide rises (Jones and Naylor, 1970). In some experiments it was found that *Eurydice* did not spontaneously emerge from sand into seawater in laboratory tanks but that nevertheless the animals did show a pronounced circatidal rhythm of swimming when kept in constant conditions without sand. On the basis of these results Jones and Naylor (1970) suggested that emergence from sand in Nature is probably under exogenous control, in response to wave action, and that the endogenous component of the activity rhythm serves to ensure that *Eurydice* stops swimming in anticipation of the fall of tide. Such a mechanism would explain how dense concentrations of *Eurydice* on exposed shores are maintained between MTL and HWN without the isopods being carried offshore by the ebbing tide.

More recently, Fish and Fish (1972) and Alheit and Naylor (1976) have reported some spontaneous emergence of *E. pulchra* from sand, dependent upon the time of year and the time of the month when experiments were carried out. This occurred in the laboratory during the times of high tide, particularly on the days just after highest spring tides, indicating a circasemilunar rhythm of emergence which combines with the circatidal swimming rhythm to induce maximal swimming in the field every two weeks after new and full moon. Such a mechanism ensures that *Eurydice* avoids being stranded on those regions of the upper shore which are not reached by high tides at neaps. In this example, therefore, circatidal and circasemilunar rhythms appear to combine to control the dynamic aspects of zonation in an intertidal species.

Daily patterns of vertical migration have also been proposed as an integral part of the horizontal dispersion mechanisms of pelagic and demersal fish (Woodland, 1966). For example, some Continental Shelf species appear to migrate horizontally by a combination of orientated movements by day when they are close to the bottom and drift by night when they are in mid-water (Jones, 1965). In addition, in elvers and soles in coastal and estuarine waters, passive lateral transport is probably achieved by upward swimming from the sea bed at a particular phase of the tide (Verwey, 1958; Creutzberg, 1961; de Veen, 1967). So far, however, there is little experimental evidence of an endogenous component in the control of these vertical migration rhythms in fish.

Further insight into the adaptive value of endogenous control of rhythmicity can be gained by considering the degree of persistence, as expressed by the maintenance of amplitude and the phasing of the free-running rhythm, in relation to the ecology of the species concerned. For example, it has been suggested by Rodriguez and Naylor (1972) that among intertidal animals the degree of endogeneity of a biological rhythm may be weakest in some surface-living, sessile forms, which are structurally well adapted to withstand a wide range of environmental variables. This is supported by observations on shore barnacles in which the tidal rhythm of valve opening and cirral beat at high tide is purely exogenous. The rhythm occurs in direct response to tidal ebb and flow and does not persist under endogenous control in constant conditions (Southward and Crisp, 1965; Sommer, 1972). In such sessile species which are structurally well adapted to withstand desiccation at low tide, there would clearly be little adaptive value in 'anticipating' closing behaviour as the tide ebbs and a purely exogenous closing response in air would suffice. On the other hand, mobile intertidal species which are active at high tide tend to exhibit endogenous rhythms of locomotor activity which ensure that they remain inactive at low tide by hiding under stones as in *Carcinus* (Naylor, 1958) or burrowing in sand (Jones and Naylor, 1970). Such an activity pattern among mobile shore species can be regarded as a behavioural adaptation which is selected to resist exposure to air at low tide (*see also* Chapter 1). In this context it is of interest that the intertidal pool-dwelling prawn *Palaemon elegans,* which does not risk desiccation at low tide, has only a very weak endogenous component in its tidal activity patterns (Rodriguez and Naylor, 1972). Developing this argument further it is interesting to note that some of the most persistent endogenous rhythms in marine organisms occur in burrowing species, for example, in the high shore amphipod *Talitrus saltator* (Bregazzi and Naylor, 1972) and the sublittoral crab *Goneplax rhomboides* (Atkinson and Naylor, 1973; *Figure 7.8*). It is of considerable selective advantage for these animals to have a pronounced endogenous component in their activity rhythms. Firstly, it permits them to return to their burrows, and, in the case of *Talitrus,* to its preferred narrow zone on the upper shore, in advance of the onset of unfavourable conditions. Moreover, a well developed physiological clock would permit animals to remain in their burrows for one or more cycles without constant reference to environmental variables on the surface and still emerge more or less in synchrony with other members of the population.

Finally, though natural selection may favour endogenously controlled rhythmicity where adaptively appropriate, there would clearly be a considerable disadvantage in fixed patterns of endogenous rhythmicity which are inflexible against the background of seasonal variations in daylength, lunar variations in tidal amplitude and regional variations in tidal

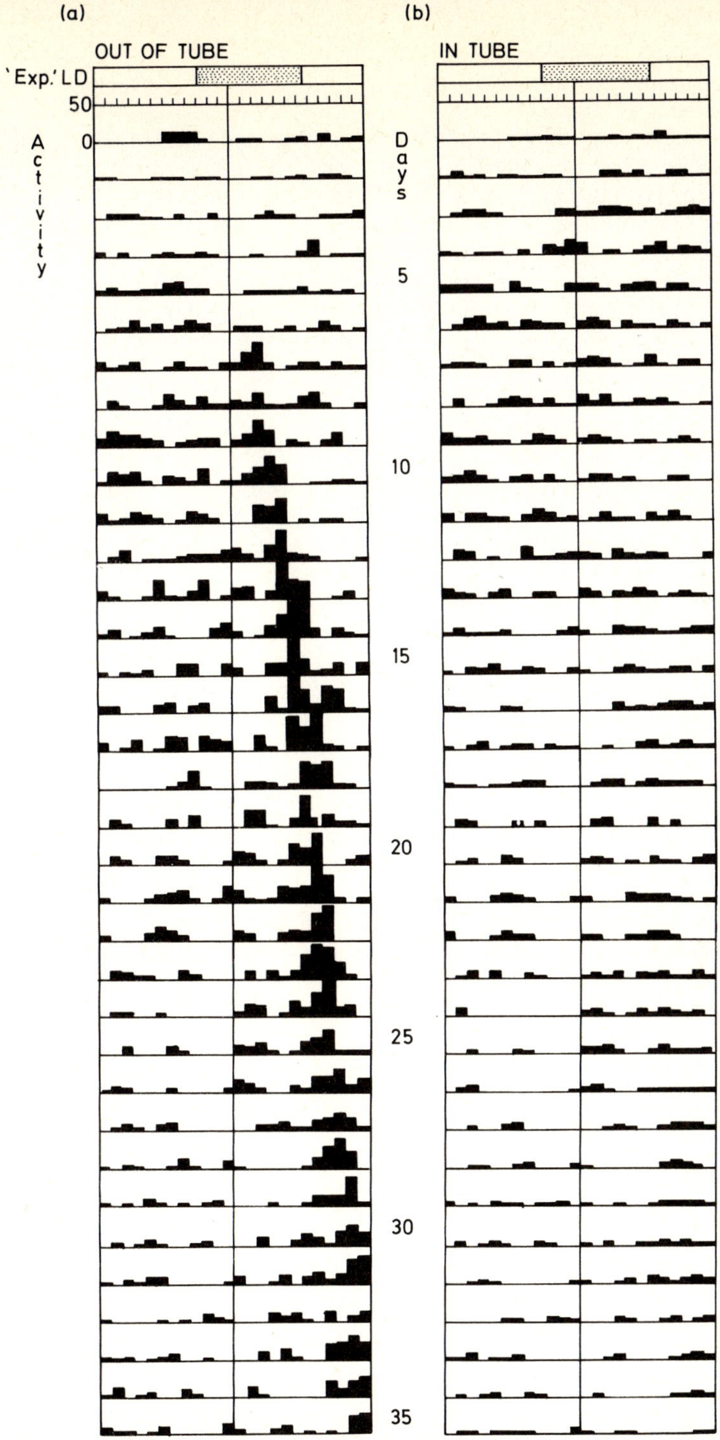

Figure 7.8 Highly persistent circadian rhythm of emergence in the crab Goneplax rhomboides. *Normally resident in sublittoral mud, the crab is provided with a perspex tube as an artificial burrow and maintained in continuous dim light and at constant temperature. 'Out of tube' activity is clearly circadian, initially phased to subjective night. (After Atkinson and Naylor, 1973; courtesy Editors, Helgoländer. wiss. Meeresunters)*

phase. These conflicting demands presumably explain why natural selection has favoured internal physiological clocks which free-run at periods which only approximate to geophysical periodicities. In Nature, the particular pattern of environmental variables on any one day determines the precise phase of the expressed behaviour by modulating the expression of the internal controlled approximate rhythm. In addition, the endogenous component of the rhythm will be entrained to anticipate approximately the return of the next favourable phase of the environmental cycle.

7.6 RHYTHMIC PATTERNS OF REPRODUCTION

Rhythmic fluctuations in the reproductive activities of marine organisms have been known for a long time, but the mode of control of these phenomena is still poorly understood. Annual breeding rhythms are particularly characteristic of mid and high latitude species, in marine invertebrates (Giese, 1959) and fish (Qasim, 1956; Cushing, 1970). There are exceptions but, in general, spawning behaviour is related to seasonal differences of photoperiod, light intensity, temperature and availability of food for the larvae. Low latitude species tend not to have regular spawning seasons but, even among these, there are several good examples of closely synchronised spawning despite the relative temporal uniformity of their environment. Many such rhythms run closely parallel to the lunar cycle, and, as in the wider literature of biological rhythmicity, there has been controversy over the relative importance of environmental and physiological control. In particular, there has been a marked reluctance to accept the possibility of direct control by lunar variables (Korringa, 1957). Early attempts to study these phenomena experimentally were unsuccessful but with more recent work, particularly on polychaetes (Hauenschild, 1960) and dipterans (Neumann, 1968; 1969), it is now well worthwhile to re-assess lunar rhythmicity of breeding against the general background of biological clocks in marine animals.

7.6.1 Adaptive value

Whilst breeding rhythmicity no doubt enhances the possibilities of fertilisation and cross-breeding (Korringa, 1957; Buslé, 1969), there are nevertheless species which do not have rhythmically restricted spawning periods and have no apparent lack of success in their reproductive performance. The serpulid polychaete genus *Spirorbis* has been particularly well studied in this respect, some species showing semi-lunar periodicity and others not (Gee, 1967; Rothlisberg, 1974).

Further insight into the adaptive value of synchronised breeding may be gained by considering the ensuing release of larvae into the plankton. Thus among molluscs, the oyster *Ostrea edulis,* which has a semi-lunar rhythm of reproduction, spawns at the time of spring tides and retains the larvae for about eight days before release takes place during neap tides (Korringa,

1947; Knight-Jones, 1952). Release during the quieter water movements of neap tides probably ensures that the larvae are less likely to be carried out to sea by tidal currents in the oyster creeks. The larvae, however, will achieve adequate dispersal within the creeks and be more likely to pass successfully through the critical change from larval lecithotrophy to planktotrophic habits after settling, during conditions of minimum turbulence and turbidity. Similar semi-lunar rhythmicity with greatest larval abundance at neap tides is shown by the serpulid polychaetes *Spirorbis borealis* (Garbarini, 1936; Knight-Jones, 1951) and *S. marioni* (Rothlisberg, 1974). The advantages of this type of rhythmic behaviour are considered to be the same for *Spirorbis* as for *Ostrea,* but with an additional advantage accruing to *Spirorbis borealis.* The last species settles intertidally and, for such organisms, a further benefit is that settlement at neap tides will avoid the risks of desiccation and starvation which would prevail low on the shore during the extreme ebbs of spring tides (de Silva, 1967).

Clearly, from what has been said so far, the breeding pattern of *Spirorbis* and *Ostrea,* though sometimes referred to as lunar rhythmicity should more strictly be designated as semi-lunar rhythmicity. Though species of both produce abundant larvae in the plankton at the times of waxing and waning moon, there is more likely to be a causal relationship with lunar variations in tidal amplitude than directly with moonlight. The same is probably also true of the classical example of the grunion, *Leuristhes tenuis,* a small atherinid fish which deposits its eggs in the sand of beaches in S. California (Korringa, 1957). The fish ride the waves to the top of the beach to mate and spawn on three or four nights after each full and new moon in summer. For a brief time during a period of one to three hours after the highest spring tides at night the parent fish leave the water for a short while to deposit eggs which then develop before being washed from the sand as young fish when the sand is next covered on the following set of spring tides fourteen days later. Other examples of semi-lunar reproductive rhythmicity are reported from a number of phyla, including the coral *Pollicipora bulbosa* (Marshall and Stephenson, 1933), the swarming polychaete *Platynereis dumerilii* at Concarneau (Korringa, 1947), and in a number of echinoderms such as *Lytechinus variegatus, Mesopilia globulus, Diadema setosum* and *Centrostephanus coronatus* (Pearse, 1972). Among crustaceans, a few decapods also exhibit semi-lunar rhythms of larval release, no doubt reflecting underlying trends of oögenesis and ovulation (Hartnoll, 1976). In this group, semi-lunar rhythms of larval hatching are possibly quite widespread among semiterrestrial forms, especially species of *Uca* and *Gecarcinus* living at levels on the shore reached only by the spring tides. Indeed, in most cases it seems likely that semi-lunar rhythmicity occurs in organisms inhabiting areas where tidal excursions are fairly large and where spawning or larval release takes place most advantageously either at neaps or at spring tides.

Evidence of true lunar reproductive periodicity is known for relatively fewer species but it is reported for example among some populations of the echinoid *Diadema setosum* (Fox, 1923; Yoshida, 1952) and palolo worms such as the Pacific *Eunice viridis* (Korringa, 1957). It is possible that this phenomenon is most likely to occur in localities where tidal amplitude is small and where weekly differences in tidal height are negligible. Thus, whereas the pelagic nuptial swarming of the polychaete *Platynereis dumerilii* occurs fortnightly at neaps near Concarneau where tidal amplitude is great (Korringa, 1947), swarming occurs at new moon periods near Naples where tidal range is small (Hauenschild, 1960). Moreover, for *Platynereis dumerilii* at Naples there is good evidence for the first time in marine animals that lunar periodicity is phased directly by lunar variations in intensity of moonlight at night (*see below*). Interestingly enough, lunar variations in the intensity of moonlight have also been shown to phase the semi-lunar rhythm of emergence of the intertidal midge *Clunio*. Adult *Clunio* can emerge to mate and lay eggs only at low tides and, in some localities, there is good adaptive advantage for them to do so at fourteen day intervals during low spring tides (*see below*).

For the reproductive rhythms discussed so far, their adaptive advantages seem fairly well understood. However, the adaptive value of a remarkable rhythm of larval release in the European lobster *Homarus gammarus* (Ennis, 1973) so far remains unexplained. Berried females hatch their larvae each night during a one-minute period just after dark, a single female releasing batches of larvae each successive night for periods of 2–6 weeks, depending upon water temperature and the size of the animal. The rhythm persists in typical circadian fashion in continuous darkness, indicating some endogenous control which is probably normally synchronised by the exogenous effect of onset of darkness. A feature of this behaviour is that hatching only takes place when the female emerges from her refuge and vibrates the pleopods. Artificial stimulation of the pleopods before and after the time of emergence does not induce hatching which suggests that the developing larvae also have a circadian rhythm of development which is synchronised to the behavioural rhythm of the parent. It remains to investigate the puzzling question of how circadian embryonic development is so finely regulated that small batches of larvae can be hatched night after night over a period as long as six weeks and how hatching is triggered by parental behaviour and changes of environmental light. Indeed this is clearly the kind of fundamental question for which answers must be sought in most of the examples considered so far.

7.6.2 Physiological and environmental control

Owing to the long time-scale of many reproductive rhythms and the associated problems of maintaining experimental animals in controlled environments, it is perhaps understandable that the control of such rhythms is less well understood than, say, circadian and tidal rhythms of locomotor activity. The first well-analysed example was probably that of Hauenschild (1960) working with the polychaete *Platynereis dumerilii* from Naples kept in laboratory cultures. When sexually mature, this species transforms into the 'heteronereis' which swarms at the surface to spawn and eventually die. In normal light/dark cycles in the laboratory the cultures spawn as in the sea, with maxima at new moon (*Figure 7.9*). In continuous light, spawning occurs

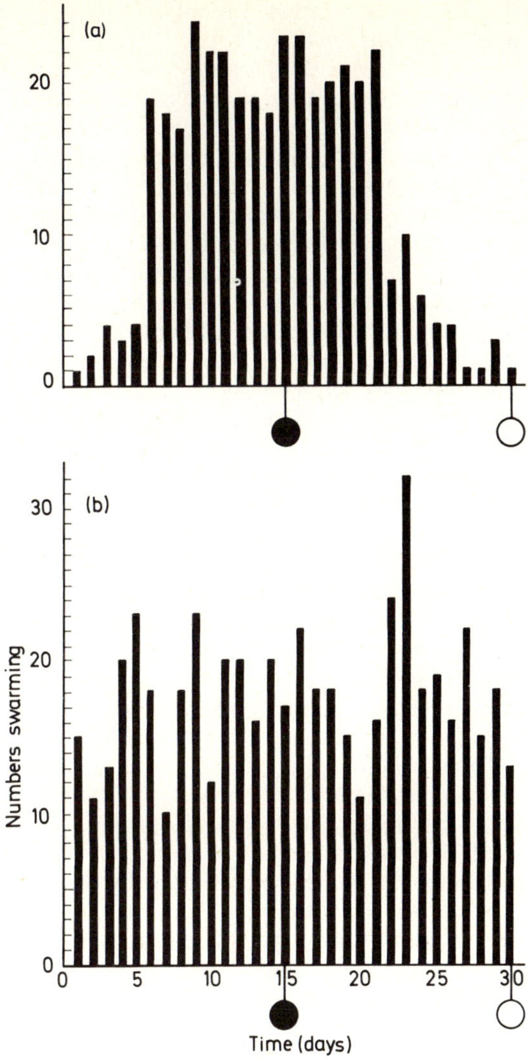

Figure 7.9 Distribution of swarming dates in an average lunar month of heteronereids of Platynereis dumerilii *maintained for one year in the laboratory. (a) 366 swarmings in cultures maintained under natural illumination. (b) 524 swarmings in cultures maintained under continuous artificial light. (After Hauenschild, 1960; courtesy Cold Spring Harbor Laboratory)*

uniformly throughout the month but lunar periodicity can be re-initiated by subjecting the worms to dim light equivalent to moonlight for alternate 12 h periods during 6 days every two weeks. Evidently moonlight serves as the prime environmental synchroniser of the spawning rhythm. The rhythm also appears to have an endogenous component since swarming of *Platynereis* will take place in nature even after a succession of cloudy nights when moonlight is obscured, and an induced lunar rhythm will persist for three months in continuous light in the laboratory.

Other work on the control of long-term rhythmicity has been directed towards the reproductive behaviour of the intertidal midge *Clunio* first reported by Caspers (1951) and subsequently studied experimentally by Neumann (1965; 1966; 1967; 1968). Eggs of this midge are laid between tidemarks, and emergence of adult flies from the pupated larvae must take place at low tide. Copulation between the winged males and wingless females, and subsequent egg-laying, can only take place in a short period of a few hours after emergence. In *Clunio takahashii* from Japan (Hashimoto, 1965) and *C. marinus* in Arctic Europe (Neumann and Honeggar, 1969) egg laying takes place in the mid-tidal zone, and emergence occurs twice a day between the times of high and low tide. In contrast, the intertidal habitat of *Clunio marinus* on most European coasts is restricted to the lowest level of the intertidal zone and is exposed only at low spring tides. In these areas *Clunio* emerges for only a few days every two weeks and does so at about the same time of day, indicating combined semi-lunar and diurnal rhythms of emergence. Cultures of the midge kept in normal light/dark cycles exhibit only 24 hour rhythmicity and hatch at night. However, if the cultures are exposed to dim light of 0.3 lux intensity, equivalent to moonlight during three simulated nights in the laboratory, a semi-lunar rhythm of hatching is promptly re-established (*Figure 7.10*). It should be emphasised that synchronisation in this manner is applicable only to populations in southern Europe. In northern Europe where, owing to irregularities of weather, moonlight is unreliable as a synchroniser, it appears that the diurnal light-dark cycle and a tidal factor are the requisite synchronisers for the *Clunio* rhythm. The unreliability of moonlight as a synchroniser in some localities has also been emphasised by Enright (1972) who demonstrated an endogenous lunar rhythm in the isopod *Excirolana chiltoni.* The tidal activity rhythm of this animal shows a monthly pattern of amplitude modulation which appears to be synchronised by monthly variations in agitation by waves, associated with lunar changes in tidal height. A similar mechanism of control has also been postulated for the semi-lunar rhythm of emergence from sand in the related isopod crustacean *Eurydice pulchra* (Alheit and Naylor, 1976).

In considering the physiological basis of endogenous components of long-term periodicities, one possible mode of control of semi-lunar rhythms is through the interaction of a tidal and a solar day rhythm. Two interacting rhythms of these periodicities would be in phase with each other every 14 or 15 days, thus giving exaggeratedly large peaks of activity which could be the basis of a semi-lunar physiological rhythm (Naylor, 1958; Hauenschild, 1960; Bünning and Müller, 1961). However, such a mechanism would be expected to apply only in localities where tidal excursions are significant. In *Clunio* and *Platynereis* from localities where tidal excursions are negligible, it seems clear that separate endogenous semi-lunar rhythms do occur (Neuman, 1969). In addition, the lunar activity rhythm (Enright, 1972) and a semi-lunar reproductive rhythm (Klapow, 1972b) in *Excirolana* also seem to be based upon truly endogenous long term rhythmic components rather

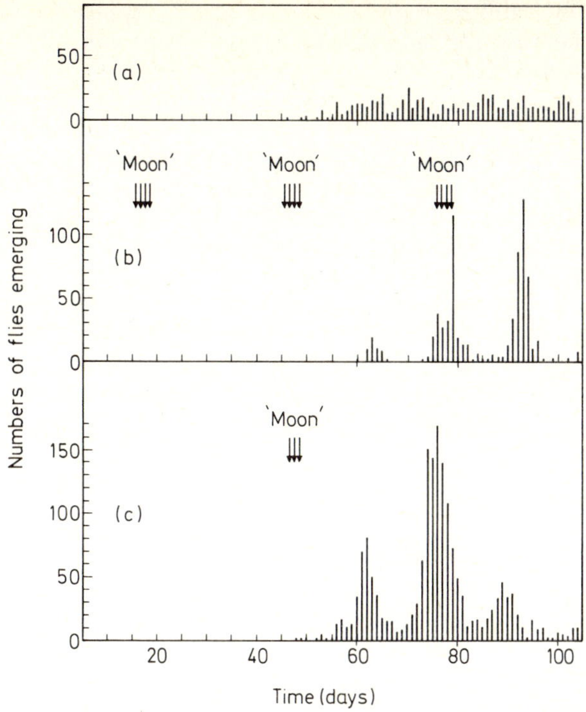

Figure 7.10 Induction of semi-lunar hatching rhythm of Clunio marinus *by artificial moonlight in the laboratory. (a) Controls maintained in a light/dark cycle in the laboratory. (b) Culture exposed to dim light of 0.3 lux intensity ('moonlight') during 4 artificial nights every 28 days. (c) Culture exposed to dim light of 0.3 lux during 3 artificial nights. (After Neumann, 1965; courtesy Editor, Z. Naturforschg.)*

than 'beat' effects of shorter term solar day and lunar day or tidal cycles. For *Clunio* the physiological basis of the semi-lunar rhythm remains unexplained but in *Platynereis* there is evidence from experiments involving extirpation and implantation of tissue, that internal control is effected by a hormonal mechanism. This interpretation relates to the observations on nereid polychaetes as a whole in which gametogenesis and metamorphosis to the heteronereid condition are brought about by reduced secretion of a juvenile hormone produced in the supra-oesophageal ganglia (Clark, 1965). Originally, Hauenschild (1960) identified apparent neurosecretory cells in the posterior region of the prostomium, in which deposition of fuschin-positive cell material took place in synchrony with the lunar cycle, and these cells were thought to be the source of the juvenile hormone and a component of the lunar clock. Further experiments questioned whether these particular cells were truly neurosecretory but these and later experiments (Hauenschild, 1966) suggest that the most promising hypothesis still remains one which postulates an important role for humoral control from neurosecretory cells. Enright (1972) excludes the possibility that a hormonal mechanism controls the lunar rhythm of *Excirolana* and alternative mechanisms may be possible since a 'spontaneous' fortnightly rhythm of neuro-electrical activity has been demonstrated in the isolated parabolic burster cell of *Aplysia* (Strumwasser, 1965). Nevertheless, in view of their long term periodicities, it would not be surprising if hormonal mechanisms prove to be important in the control of semi-lunar and lunar rhythms as has been proposed earlier for tidal and circadian rhythmicity (*see* p. 406).

More general aspects of the control of reproduction in polychaetes are well reviewed by Clark (1965) and Clark and Olive (1973) and need not be expanded here. It is, however, appropriate to conclude this chapter with a brief reference to the precisely timed annual spawning rhythms of palolo worms and to comment on these rhythms in the light of the conclusions reached so far. Detailed experimental work of the kind carried out on *Platynereis dumerilii* has so far not been carried out on palolo worms, particularly on the most accurately synchronised species *Eunice viridis* in the Pacific. However, some information is available for the Atlantic species *Eunice fucata* and, in view of recent work with *Clunio* and *Platynereis,* perhaps it is less surprising now than it appeared over 30 years ago when Clark and Hess (1940) suggested that moonlight was to some extent directly involved. Immature *E. fucata* are photonegative to light intensities greater than 0.01 ft candles and therefore remain in their burrows by day and on moonlit nights. After epitoky the anterior unmodified part remains photonegative but the modified posterior reproductive portion of the worm becomes photopositive to intensities above a threshold of 0.005 ft candles. Spawning, therefore, tends to be inhibited at full moon because the worms remain in their burrows, and at new moon because there is insufficient light to attract the now emerged epitokal region to the surface. At the lunar quarters light intensity is too low to promote photonegative behaviour of the anterior part of the worms, thus the epitokal regions are exposed to light above their threshold of sensitivity, so they break away and swim towards the light at the surface. Separation of the epitokes and their associated mass spawning appears to be reinforced by intense activity created as light intensity increases at dawn. Such a mechanism clearly depends upon all the worms reaching sexual maturity during the two weeks preceding the spawning season in July. It is therefore also necessary to postulate an annual rhythm of maturation and metamorphosis which Clark and Hess (1940) suggest is synchronised by fluctuations of feeding activity, again imposed by lunar cycles of light intensity.

Drawbacks to the mechanism proposed by Clark and Hess (1940) have been put forward (Clark, 1965) notably because there may be slight regional differences in swarming times, swarms sometimes begin to form before sunrise, and swarming may occur when the moon is obscured by cloud or if the worms are kept in darkness for 24 h before swarming is expected. These objections are quite valid if it is envisaged that exogenous factors alone control the rhythm. However, the objections are less valid if one takes the view that the rhythm may be controlled by a combination of endogenous factors determining approximate periodicity and exogenous factors determining the precise phase. With tidal, daily, semi-lunar and lunar rhythms now well documented as being controlled in this way it would not be surprising if the precision of spawning in palolos was at least partly controlled by endogenous lunar periodicity. In Nature this would be triggered by previous lunar cycles and would be more or less accurately expressed at spawning depending upon the eventual combination of internal physiological cycles and environmental parameters at the expected time of spawning. The conclusion seems to be that, as with the control of shorter term activity cycles, marine animals are opportunist in their utilisation of environmental variables, to synchronise their longer term reproductive periodicity. In addition, this has to be judged against the background of whether particular species reproduce once in a lifespan or several times, and whether natural selection has favoured close synchrony of all reproduction in any one year or whether repeated breeding takes place. In the first instance latitudinal differences of temperature, photoperiod and light intensity clearly play a part, but a mosaic of other factors may also intervene. In inshore and intertidal areas subjected to extensive tidal oscillations it is not surprising that physical variables associated with daily and lunar variations in tidal amplitude and phase are important synchronisers. In the open ocean and elsewhere in the absence of detectable tidal oscillations, then clearly solar and lunar variations in light intensity may be the most prominent physical variables. Perhaps the phenomenon of 'lunar periodicity' has indeed moved out of the realms of mysticism and become a testable hypothesis as Hauenschild (1960) predicted.

REFERENCES

AL-ADHUB, A. H. Y. and NAYLOR, E. (1975). 'Emergence rhythms and tidal migrations in the brown shrimp *Crangon crangon* (L.)', *J. mar. biol. Ass. U.K.*, **55**, 801–810

ALHEIT, J. and NAYLOR, E. (1976). 'Behavioural basis of intertidal zonation in *Eurydice pulchra*', *J. exp. mar. Biol. Ecol.* (In the press)

ALLEN, J. A. (1966). 'The rhythms and population dynamics of decapod Crustacea', *Oceanogr. Mar. Biol. Ann. Rev.*, **4**, 247–265

ALLEN, J. A. (1972). 'Recent studies on the rhythms of post-larval decapod Crustacea', *Oceanogr. Mar. Biol. Ann. Rev.*, **10**, 415–436

ARECHIGA, H. (1974). 'Circadian rhythm of sensory input in the crayfish', 517–524. In: *Neurosciences Research Program.* Ed. F. O. Schmitt. M.I.T. Press

ARECHIGA, H. and BAILEY, H. (1974). 'An accurate and simple method to analyse neuronal activity over long periods of time', *Mar. Behav. Physiol.*, **2**, 307–310

ARECHIGA, H., FUENTES, B. and BARRERA, B. (1973). 'Circadian rhythm of responsiveness in the visual system of the crayfish', 402–421. In: *Neurobiology of Invertebrates.* Ed. J. Salanki. Plenum Press, Budapest

ARECHIGA, H., HUBERMAN, A. and NAYLOR, E. (1974). 'Hormonal modulation of circadian neural activity in *Carcinus maenas* (L.)', *Proc. roy. Soc. B.*, **187**, 299–313

ARECHIGA, H. and NAYLOR, E. (1976). 'Endogenous factors in the control of rhythmicity in decapod crustaceans'. In: *Biological rhythms in the marine environment.* Ed. P. de Coursey. (In the press)

ARECHIGA, H. and WIERSMA, C. A. G. (1969). 'Circadian rhythm of responsiveness in crayfish visual units', *J. Neurobiol.*, **1**, 71–85

ASCHOFF, J. (1965). 'Diurnal rhythms', *Ann. Rev. Physiol.*, **25**, 581–600

ATKINSON, R. J. A. and NAYLOR, E. (1973). 'Activity rhythms in some burrowing decapods', *Helgoländer. wiss. Meeresunters.*, **24**, 192–201

ATKINSON, R. J. A. and PARSONS, A. J. (1973). 'Seasonal patterns of migration and locomotor rhythmicity in populations of *Carcinus*', *Neth. J. Sea Res.*, **7,** 81–93

BANSE, K. (1964). 'On the vertical distribution of plankton in the sea', *Progr. Oceanogr.*, **2,** 53–125

BARNWELL, F. H. (1963). 'Observations on daily and tidal rhythms in some fiddler crabs from Equatorial Brazil', *Biol. Bull.*, **125,** 399–415

BARNWELL, F. H. (1968). 'The role of rhythmic systems in the adaptation of fiddler crabs to the intertidal zone', *Am. Zool.*, **8,** 569–583

BLISS, D. E. (1962). 'Neuroendocrine control of locomotor activity in the land crab *Gecarcinus lateralis*', 391–408. In: *Mem. Soc. Endocrinol. No. 12 Neurosecretion.* Ed. H. Heller and R. B. Clark. Academic Press, New York

BLUME, J., BÜNNING, E. and MÜLLER, D. (1962). 'Periodenanalyse von Aktivitätsrhythmen bei *Carcinus maenas*', *Biol. Zentr.*, **81,** (5), 569–573

BODEN, B. P. and KAMPA, E. M. (1967). 'The influence of natural light on the vertical migrations of an animal community in the sea', *Symp. zool. Soc. Lond.*, **19,** 15–20

BOGOROV, B. G. (1946). 'Pecularities of diurnal vertical migrations of zooplankton in polar seas', *J. mar. Res.*, **6** (1), 25–32

BOHN, G. (1903). 'Sur les mouvements oscillatoires des *Convoluta roscoffensis*', *C. r. Acad. Sci. Paris,* **137,** 576–578

BOHN, G. and PIERON, H. (1906). 'Le rhythme des marées et la phénomène de l'anticipation reflexe', *C. r. Soc. Biol. Paris,* **61,** 660–661

BOSCH, H. F. and TAYLOR, W. R. (1973). 'Diurnal vertical migration of an estuarine cladoceran *Podon polyphenoides* in the Chesapeake Bay', *Mar. Biol.*, **19,** 172–181

BRADY, J. (1967). 'Control of the circadian rhythm of activity in the cockroach. II. The role of the sub-oesophageal ganglion and ventral nerve cord', *J. exp. Biol.*, **47,** 165–178

BRADY, J. (1969). 'How are insect circadian rhythms controlled?', *Nature,* **223,** 781–784

BRADY, J. (1974). 'Insect circadian rhythms'. In: *Adv. Insect Physiol.* Ed. J. E. Treherne. Berridge, M. J. and Wigglesworth, **10,** 1-115. Academic Press, London and New York

BREGAZZI, P. K. and NAYLOR, E. (1972). 'The locomotor activity rhythm of *Talitrus saltator* (Montagu)', *J. exp. Biol.*, **57,** 375–391

BROWN, F. A. Jr. (1960). 'Response to pervasive geophysical factors and the biological clock problem', *Cold Spring Harbor Symp. quant. Biol.*, **25,** 57–71

BROWN, F. A. Jr. (1972). 'The "clocks" timing biological rhythms', *Am. Sci.*, **60,** 756–766

BROWN, F. A. Jr., HASTINGS, J. W. and PALMER, J. D. (1970). *The Biological Clock: Two Views.* New York, Academic Press

BRUSLÉ, J. (1969). 'Les rhythmes biologiques chez les invertebres marins', *Ann. Biol.*, **8** (5–6), 281–318

BÜNNING, E. and MÜLLER, D. (1961). 'Wie messen Organismen lunare Zyklen?', *Zeit. Matur.*, **166** (6), 391–395

CARRIKER, M. R. (1951). 'Ecological observations on the distribution of oyster larvae in New Jersey estuaries', *Ecol. Monogr.*, **21,** 19–38

CASPERS, H. (1951). 'Rhythmische Erscheinungen in der Fortpflanzung von *Clunio marinus* (Dipt. Chiron) und das Problem der lunaren Periodizität bei Organismen', *Archiv. f. Hydrobiol.*, **18,** 415–594

CLARK, L. B. and HESS, H. W. (1940). 'Swarming of the Atlantic Palolo worm, *Leodice fucata*', *Carnegie Publ.*, **524,** 21–27

CLARK, R. B. (1965). 'Endocrinology and the reproductive biology of polychaetes', *Oceanogr. Mar. Biol. Ann. Rev.*, **3,** 211–255

CLARK, R. B. and OLIVE, P. J. W. (1973). 'Recent advances in polychaete endocrinology and reproductive biology', *Oceanogr. Mar. Biol. Ann. Rev.*, **11,** 175–222

CLARKE, G. L. and BACKUS, R. H. (1964). 'Interrelations between the vertical migration of deep-scattering layers, bio-luminescence and changes in daylight in the sea', *Bull. Inst. océanogr. Monaco,* **1318,** 1–36

CLARKE, W. D. (1966). 'Bathyphotometric studies of the light regime of organisms of the deep scattering layers', *Gen. Mot. Defence Research Laboratories,* Final Report contract AT (04–3)–584, Santa Barbara, California

CLARKE, W. D. (1970). 'Comparison of different investigative techniques for studying the deep scattering layers', 550–562. In: *Proceedings of an International Symposium on Biological*

Sound Scattering in the Ocean. Ed. G. B. Farquhar. Washington, Maury Centre for Ocean Science

COLE, L. C. (1957). 'Biological clocks in the unicorn', *Science,* **125,** 874

CREUTZBERG, F. (1961). 'Use of tidal streams by migrating elvers (*Anguilla vulgaris* Turt.) in a tidal area', *Neth. J. Sea Res.,* **1,** 257–338

CROTHERS, J. H. (1967). 'The biology of the shore crab *Carcinus maenas* (L.) I. The background anatomy, growth and life history', *Fld. Stud.,* **2** (4), 407–434

CROTHERS, J. H. (1968). 'The biology of the shore crab *Carcinus maenas* (L.) II. The life of the adult crab', *Fld. Stud.,* **2** (5), 579–614

CUSHING, D. H. (1951). 'The vertical migration of planktonic Crustacea', *Biol. Rev.,* **26,** 158–192

CUSHING, D. H. (1970). 'The regularity of the spawning season in some fishes', *J. Cons. int. Explor. Mer.,* **33,** 81–97

CYMBOROWSKI, B. and DUTKOWSKI, A. (1970). 'Circadian changes in RNA synthesis in the neurosecretory cells of the brain and suboesophageal system of *Acheta domesticus', J. Insect Physiol.,* **16,** 341–348

DE SILVA, P. H. D. H. (1967). 'Studies on the biology of Spirorbinae (Polychaeta)', *J. Zool. Lond.,* **152,** 269–279

DE VEEN, J. F. (1967). 'On the phenomenon of soles (*Solea solea* L.) swimming at the surface', *J. Cons. perm. int. Explor. Mer.,* **31,** 207–236

DICKSON, R. R. (1972). 'On the relationship between ocean transparency and the depth of some scattering layers in the North Atlantic', *J. du Conseil,* **34,** 416–422

EDWARDS, G. A. (1950). 'The influence of eyestalk removal on the metabolism of the fiddler crab', *Physiologia comp. Oecol.,* **2,** 34–50

ENNIS, G. P. (1973). 'Endogenous rhythmicity associated with larval hatching in the lobster *Homarus gammarus', J. mar. biol. Ass. U.K.,* **53,** 531–538

ENRIGHT, J. T. (1961). 'Pressure sensitivity of an amphipod', *Science, N.Y.,* **133,** 758–760

ENRIGHT, J. T. (1962). 'Responses of an amphipod to pressure changes', *Comp. Biochem. Physiol.,* **7,** 131–145

ENRIGHT, J. T. (1963a). 'Endogenous tidal and lunar rhythms', *Proc. XVI Int. Congr. Zool.,* Washington D.C., **4,** 355–359

ENRIGHT, J. T. (1963b). 'The tidal rhythm of activity of a sand-beach amphipod', *Z. vergl. Physiol.,* **46,** 276–313

ENRIGHT, J. T. (1965a). 'Entrainment of a tidal rhythm', *Science, N.Y.,* **147,** 864–867

ENRIGHT, J. T. (1965b). 'The search for rhythmicity in biological time-series', *J. theoret. Biol.,* **8,** 426–468

ENRIGHT, J. T. (1972). 'A virtuoso isopod', *J. comp. Physiol.,* **77,** 141–162

ENRIGHT, J. T. and HAMNER, W. M. (1967). 'Vertical diurnal migration and endogenous rhythmicity', *Science, N.Y.,* **157,** 937–941

ESTERLY, C. O. (1917). 'The occurrence of a rhythm in the geotropism of two species of plankton copepods when certain recurring conditions are absent', *Univ. Calif. Publ. Zool.,* **16,** 393–400

FINGERMAN, M. (1960). 'Tidal rhythmicity in marine orgamisms', *Cold Spr. Hbr. Symp. quant. Biol.,* **25,** 481–489

FISH, J. D. and FISH, S. (1972). 'The swimming rhythm of *Eurydice pulchra* and a possible explanation of intertidal migration', *J. exp. mar. Biol. Ecol.,* **8,** 195–200

FOX, H. M. (1923). 'Lunar periodicity in reproduction', *Proc. Roy. Soc. B.,* **95,** 523–550

FOX, H. M. (1956). 'The moon and life', *Proc. roy. Inst. G.B.,* **36,** (163), 310–322

FOXTON, P. (1970). 'The vertical distribution of pelagic decapods (Crustacea: Natantia) collected on the Sond Cruise 1965. II. The Penaeidea and general discussion', *J. mar. biol. Ass. U.K.,* **50,** 961–1000

FRAZIER, W., KANDEL, E. R., KUPFERMANN, I., WAZIRI, R. and COGGLESHILL, R. E. (1967). 'Morphological and functional properties of identified neurones in the abdominal ganglion of *Aplysia californica', J. Neurophysiol.,* **30,** 1288–1351

GAMBLE, F. W. and KEEBLE, F. (1903). 'The bionomics of *Convoluta roscoffensis,* with special reference to its green cells', *Proc. roy. Soc. Lond. B.,* **72,** 93–98

GARBARINI, P. (1933). 'Rhythme d'emission des larves chez *Spirorbis borealis* (Daudin)', *C. r. Soc. Biol. Paris,* **112,** 1204–1205

GARBARINI, P. (1936). 'Rhythme de croissance des et d'incubation des larves chez *Spirorbis borealis* (Daudin)', *C. r. Soc. Biol. Paris,* **122,** 157–158

GEE, J. M. (1967). 'Growth and breeding of *Spirorbis rupestris* (Polychaeta: Serpulidae)', *J. Zool. Lond.,* **152,** 235–244

GIBSON, R. N. (1969). 'Activity rhythm in two species of *Blennius* from the Mediterranean', *Vie Milieu,* **30,** 235–244

GIBSON, R. N. (1971). 'Factors affecting the rhythmic activity of *Blennius pholis* (Teleostei)', *Anim. Behav.,* **19,** 336–343

GIESE, A. C. (1959). 'Comparative physiology: annual reproductive cycles of marine invertebrates', *Ann. Rev. Physiol.,* **21,** 547–576

HAGERMAN, L. (1970). 'Locomotory activity patterns of *Crangon vulgaris* (Fabricus) (Crustacea: Natantia)', *Ophelia,* **8,** 255–266

HALBERG, F., HALBERG, E., BARNUM, C. and BITTNER, J. (1959). 'Physiologic 24-hour periodicity in human beings and mice, the lighting regime and daily routine, 803–873. In: *Photoperiodism and Related Phenomena in Plants and Animals.* Ed. R. B. Withrow. *Amer. Assoc. for the Adv. Sci. Washington D.C.*

HARDY, A. C. and PATON, W. W. (1947). 'Experiments on the vertical migration of plankton animals', *J. mar. biol. Ass. U.K.,* **26,** 467–526

HARKER, J. E. (1958). 'Diurnal rhythms in the animal kingdom', *Biol. Rev.,* **33** (1), 1–52

HARKER, J. E. (1960). 'Endocrine and nervous factors in insect circadian rhythms', *Cold. Spring Harb. Symp. quant. Biol.,* **25,** 279–287

HARKER, J. E. (1964). *The physiology of diurnal rhythms.* Cambridge University Press, London

HARRIS, J. E. (1963). 'The role of endogenous rhythms in vertical migration', *J. mar. biol. Ass. U.K.,* **43,** 153–166

HARTNOLL, R. G. (1976). 'Brachyura'. In: *Reproduction of Marine Invertebrates* **6.** Eds. A. C. Giese, and J. S. Pearse. Academic Press. (In the press)

HASHIMOTO, H. (1965). 'Discovery of *Clunio takahashi* Tokmaga from Japan', *Japan J. Zool.,* **14,** 13–29

HASKIN, H. H. (1964). 'The distribution of oyster larvae'. In: *Symp. Exp. Marine Ecol.* (Occasional Publ.), **2,** 76–80. Narangsett Marine Laboratory

HAUENSCHILD, C. (1960). 'Lunar periodicity', In: *Biological Clocks. Cold Spring Harb. Symp. quant. Biol.* **25,** 491–497

HAUENSCHILD, C. (1966). 'Der hormonele Einfluss des Gehirns auf die sexuelle Entwicklung bei dem Polychaeten *Platynereis dumerilii', Gen. comp. Endocr.,* **6,** 26–73

HUGHES, D. A. (1969). 'Responses to salinity change as a tidal transport mechanism of pink shrimp *Penaeus duorarum', Biol. Bull.,* **136,** 43–53

HUGHES, D. A. (1972). 'On the endogenous control of tide-associated displacements of pink shrimp *Penaeus duorarum', Biol. Bull.,* **142,** 271–281

ISAAC, M. J. and JARVIS, J. H. (1973).'Endogenous tidal rhythmicity in the littoral pycnogonid *Nymphon gracile* (Leach)', *J. exp. mar. Biol. Ecol.,* **13,** 83–96

JACKLETT, J. W. (1969). 'A circadian rhythm of optic nerve impulses recorded in darkness from the isolated eye of *Aplysia', Science,* **164,** 562

JONES, D. A. (1972). 'Aspects of the ecology and behaviour of *Ocypode ceratophthalmus* and *O. kuhlii', J. exp. mar. Biol. Ecol.,* **8,** 31–43

JONES, D. A. and NAYLOR, E. (1970). 'The swimming rhythm of the sand beach isopod *Eurydice pulchra', J. exp. mar. Biol. Ecol.,* **4,** 188–199

JONES, F. R. H. (1965). 'Fish migration and water currents', *Spec. Publs. int. Commn. NW Atlant. Fish,* **6,** 257–266

KALMUS, H. (1938). 'Das Aktogram des Flusskrebses', *Z. verg. Physiol.,* **25,** 798–802

KIKUCHI, K. (1930). 'Diurnal migration of plankton Crustacea', *Q. Rev. Biol.,* **5,** 189–206

KITCHING, J. A. (1972). 'The effects of pressure on organisms: a summary of progress', *Symp. Soc. Exp. Biol.,* **26,** 473–477

KLAPOW, L. A. (1972a). 'Natural and artificial rephasing of a tidal rhythm', *J. comp. Physiol.,* **79,** 233–258

KLAPOW, L. A. (1972b). 'Fortnightly molting and reproductive cycles in the sand-beach isopod *Excirolana chiltoni', Biol. Bull.,* **143,** 568–591

KNIGHT-JONES, E. W. (1951). 'Gregariousness and some other aspects of the setting behaviour of *Spirorbis', J. mar. biol. Ass. U.K.,* **30,** 201–222

KNIGHT-JONES, E. W. (1952). 'Reproduction of oysters in the rivers Crouch and Roach, Essex, during 1947, 1948 and 1949', *Fish. Invest. Ser. II.*, **18** (2), 48 pp

KNIGHT-JONES, E. W. and MORGAN, E. (1966). 'Responses of marine animals to changes in hydrostatic pressure', *Oceanogr. Mar. Biol. Ann. Rev.*, **4,** 267–299

KORRINGA, P. (1947). 'Relations between the moon and periodicity in the breeding of marine animals', *Ecol. monogr.*, **17,** 347–381

KORRINGA, P. (1957). 'Lunar Periodicity', In: *Treatise on Marine Ecology and Paleoecology I: Ecology. Geol. Soc. Amer.*, **67,** 917–934

KUNKLE, D. E. (1957). 'The vertical distribution of oyster larvae in Delaware Bay', *Proc. natn. Shellfish Assoc.*, **48,** 90–91

LEWIS, J. B. (1954). 'The occurrence and vertical distribution of the Euphausiacea of the Florida Current', *Bull. mar. Sci. Gulf Caribb.*, **4,** 265–301

LINCOLN, R. J. (1970). 'A laboratory investigation into the effects of hydrostatic pressure on the vertical migration of planktonic Crustacea', *Mar. Biol.*, **6** (1), 5–11

MARSHALL, S. M. and STEPHENSON, T. A. (1933). 'The breeding of reef animals. II. The corals, Gt. Barrier Reef Exped., 1928–29, *Sci. Rep.*, **3,** 219–245

MARTIN, L. (1907). 'La memoire chez *Convoluta roscoffensis', C. r. hebd. Seanc. Acad. Sci. Paris,* **145,** 555–557

MAUCHLINE, J. and FISHER, L. R. (1969). 'The Biology of Euphausiids'. In: *Advances in Marine Biology,* **7,** 454 pp. Eds. Sir F. S. Russell and Sir M. Yonge. Academic Press, London

MOORE, H. B. and CORWIN, E. G. (1956). 'The effects of temperature, illumination and pressure on the vertical distribution of zooplankton', *Bull. mar. Sci. Gulf Caribb.*, **6,** 273–287

MORGAN, E. (1965). 'The activity rhythm of the amphipod *Corophium volutator* (Pallas) and its possible relationship to changes in hydrostatic pressure associated with the tides', *J. Anim. Ecol.*, **34,** 731–746

MORGAN, E., NELSON-SMITH, A. and KNIGHT-JONES, E. W. (1964). 'Responses of *Nymphon gracile* (Pycnogonida) to pressure cycles of tidal frequency', *J. exp. Biol.*, **41,** 825–836

NAYLOR, E. (1958). 'Tidal and diurnal rhythms of locomotory activity in *Carcinus maenas* L.', *J. exp. Biol.*, **35,** 602–610

NAYLOR, E. (1960). 'Locomotor rhythms in *Carcinus maenas* (L.) from non-tidal conditions', *J. exp. Biol.*, **37,** 481–488

NAYLOR, E. (1961). 'Spontaneous locomotor rhythm in Mediterranean *Carcinus', Publ. Staz. Zool. Napoli,* **32,** 58–63

NAYLOR, E. (1962). 'Seasonal changes in a population of *Carcinus maenas* (L.) in the littoral zone', *J. Anim. Ecol.*, **31,** 601–609

NAYLOR, E. (1963). 'Temperature relationships of the locomotor rhythm of *Carcinus', J. exp. Biol.*, **40,** 669–679

NAYLOR, E. and ATKINSON, R. J. A. (1972). 'Pressure and the rhythmic behaviour of inshore marine animals', *Symp. Soc. exp. Biol.*, **26,** 395–415

NAYLOR, E., ATKINSON, R. J. A. and WILLIAMS, B. G. (1971). 'External factors influencing the tidal rhythm of shore crabs', *Proc. 2nd int. Interdisc. Conf. Cycle Res.*, **2** (2), 173–180

NAYLOR, E. and ISAAC, M. J. (1973). 'Behavioural significance of pressure responses in megalopa larvae of *Callinectes sapidus* and *Macropipus* sp.', *Mar. behav. Physiol.*, **1,** 341–350

NAYLOR, E., SMITH, G. and WILLIAMS, B. G. (1973). 'The role of the eyestalk in the tidal activity rhythm of the shore crab *Carcinus maenas* (L.)', 423–439. In: *Biological rhythms in invertebrates.* Ed. J. Salanki. Plenum Press, Budapest

NAYLOR, E. and WILLIAMS, B. G. (1968). 'Effects of eyestalk removal on rhythmic locomotor activity in *Carcinus', J. exp. Biol.*, **49,** 107–116

NELSON, J. (1912). 'Observations of natural populations of oysters at Barnegat, N.J. in 1911', *New Jers. agri. Exp. Stn.*, **1911,** 271–309

NEUMANN, D. (1965). 'Photoperiodische Steuerung der 15-tägigen lunaren Metamorphose – Periodik von Clunio-Population (Diptera: Chironomidae)', *Z. Naturforschg.*, **20b,** 818–819

NEUMANN, D. (1966). 'Die lunare und tägliche Schlüpfperiodik der Mücke *Clunio', Z. vergl. Physiol.*, **53,** 1–61

NEUMANN, D. (1967). 'Genetic adaptation in emergence time of *Clunio* populations to different tidal conditions', *Helgoländer wiss. Meeresunters.*, **15,** 163–171

NEUMANN, D. (1968). 'Die Steuerung einer semilunaren Schlüpfperiodik mit Hilfe eines Künstlichen Gezeitenzyklus', *Z. vergl. Physiol.*, **60,** 63–78

NEUMANN, D. (1969). 'Die Kombination verschiedener endogener Rhythm bei der zeitlichen Programmierung von Entwicklung und Verhalten', *Oecologia (Berl.),* **3,** 166–183

NEUMANN, D. and HONEGGER, H. W. (1969). 'Adaptations of the intertidal Midge *Clunio* to Arctic conditions', *Oecologia (Berl.),* **3,** 1–13

PAGE, T. L. and LARIMER, J. L. (1975). 'Neural control of circadian rhythmicity in the crayfish. I. The locomotor activity rhythm', *J. comp. Physiol.,* **97,** 59–80

PALMER, J. D. (1973). 'Tidal rhythms: the clock control of the rhythmic physiology of marine organisms', *Biol. Rev.,* **48,** 377–418

PALMER, J. D. (1974). *Biological clocks in marine organisms.* John Wiley & Sons, New York. pp. 173

PALMER, J. D. and ROUND, F. E. (1965). 'Persistent, vertical migration rhythms in benthic microflora. I. The effect of light and temperature on the rhythmic behaviour of *Euglena obtusa', J. mar. biol. Ass. U.K.,* **45,** 567–582

PEARSE, J. S. (1972). 'A monthly reproductive rhythm in the diadematid sea urchin *Centrostephanus coronatus', J. exp. mar. Biol. Ecol.,* **8,** 167–186

PITTENDRIGH, C. S. (1974). 'Circadian oscillations in cells and the circadian organization of multicellular systems', 437–458. In: *The Neurosciences: third study program.* Eds. F. O. Schmitt and F. G. Worden. M.I.T. Press

POWELL, B. L. (1965). 'The hormonal control of the tidal rhythm of locomotory activity in *Carcinus maenas', Gen. comp. Endocrinol.,* **5,** 705

QASIM, S. Z. (1956). 'Time and duration of the spawning season in some marine teleosts in relation to their distribution', *J. Cons. perm. int. Explor. Mer.,* **21,** 144–155

RAO, K. P. and GROPALAKRISHNAREDDY, T. (1967). 'Blood borne factors in circadian rhythms of activity', *Nature Lond.,* **213,** 1047–1048

ROBERTS, S. K. DE F. (1965). 'Photoreception and entrainment of cockroach activity rhythms', *Science, N.Y.,* **148,** 958–959

ROBERTS, S. K. DE F. (1966). 'Circadian activity rhythms in cockroaches. III. The role of endocrine and neural factors', *J. cell. Physiol.,* **67,** 473–486

ROBERTS, T. W. (1941). 'Evidences that hormonal inhibition of locomotion occurs for the crayfish *Cambarus virilis* Hajen', *Anat. Rec. (Suppl.),* **81,** 46–47

ROBERTS, T. W. (1944). 'Light, eyestalk, chemical and certain other factors as regulators of community activity for the crayfish *Cambarus virilis', Ecol. Monogr.,* **14,** 359–373

RODRIGUEZ, G. and NAYLOR, E. (1972). 'Behavioural rhythms in littoral prawns', *J. mar. biol. Ass. U.K.,* **52,** 81–95

ROE, H. S. J. (1974). 'Observations on the diurnal vertical migrations of an oceanic animal community', *Mar. Biol.,* **28,** 99–113

ROGERS, H. M. (1940). 'Occurrence and retention of plankton within the estuary', *J. Fish Res. Bd. Can.,* **5,** 164–171

ROSE, M. (1925). 'Contribution a l'étude de la Biologique du Plankton. Le probleme des migrations verticales journalieres', *Arch. Zool. exp. gén.,* **64,** 387–542

ROTHLISBERG, P. C. (1974). 'Reproduction in *Spirorbis (Spirorbella) marioni* Caullery & Mesnil (Polychaeta, Serpulidae)', *J. exp. mar. Biol. Ecol.,* **15,** 285–297

RUSSELL, F. S. (1927). 'The vertical distribution of plankton in the sea', *Biol. Rev.,* **2,** 213–262

SCHALLEK, W. (1942). 'Some mechanisms controlling locomotor activity in the crayfish', *J. exp. Zool.,* **91,** 155–166

SINGARAJAH, K. V., MOYSE, J. and KNIGHT-JONES, E. W. (1967). 'The effect of feeding upon the phototactic behaviour of cirripede nauplii', *J. exp. mar. Biol. Ecol.,* **1,** 144–153

SMITH, G. and NAYLOR, E. (1972). 'The neurosecretory system of the eyestalk of *Carcinus maenas* (Crustacea: Decapoda)', *J. Zool. Lond.,* **166,** 313–321

SOMMER, H.-H. (1972). 'Endogene und exogene Periodik in der Aktivität eines niederen Krebses (*Balanus balanus* L.)', *Z. vergl. Physiol.,* **76,** 177–192

SOUTHWARD, A. J. and CRISP, D. J. (1965). 'Activity rhythms of barnacles in relation to respiration and feeding', *J. mar. biol. Ass. U.K.,* **45,** 161–185

STRUMWASSER, F. (1965). 'The demonstration and manipulation of a circadian rhythm in a single neuron', 442–462. In: *Circadian Clocks.* Ed. J. Aschoff. North Holland Publishing, Amsterdam

STRUMWASSER, F. (1967). 'Neurophysiological aspects of rhythms', 516. In: *The Neurosciences:*

An Intensive Study Program. Eds. G. C. Quarton, T. Melnechuk, F. O. Schmitt. Rochefeller University Press, New York

STRUMWASSER, F. (1971). 'The cellular basis of behaviour in *Aplysia*', *Psychiat. Res.*, **8,** 237–257

SWEENEY, B. M. (1969). *Rhythmic phenomena in plants.* Academic Press, New York

VALENTE, D. and EDWARDS, G. A. (1955). 'The regulation of the activity rhythm of the crab *Trichodactylus petropolitanus*', *Fac. Filos. Cien. Let. Univ. Sao Paulo,* **207,** 5–12

VERWEY, J. (1958). 'Orientation in migrating marine animals and a comparison with that of other migrants', *Archs. neerl. Zool., Suppl.,* **13,** 418–448

WEBB, H. M. (1976). 'Interactions of diurnal and tidal rhythms'. In: *Biological rhythms in the marine environment* Ed. P. de Coursey. (In the press)

WEBB, H. M. and BROWN, F. A. (1959). 'Timing long-cycle physiological rhythms', *Physiol. Rev.,* **39** (1), 127–161

WELLS, G. P. (1937). 'Studies on the physiology of *Arenicola marina* (L.). I. The pace-maker rôle of the oesophagus, and the action qf adrenaline and acetylcholine, *J. exp. Biol.,* **14,** 117–157

WILDISH, D. J. (1970). 'Locomotory activity rhythms in some littoral *Orchestia*', *J. mar. bioi. Ass. U.K.,* **50,** 241–252

WILLIAMS, B. G. and NAYLOR, E. (1967). 'Spontaneously induced rhythm of tidal periodicity in laboratory-reared *Carcinus*', *J. exp. Biol.,* **47,** 229–234

WILLIAMS, B. G. and NAYLOR, E. (1969). 'Synchronization of the locomotor tidal rhythm of *Carcinus*', *J. exp. Biol.,* **51,** 715–725

WOOD, L. and HARGIS, J. H. (1971). 'Transport of bivalve larvae in a tidal estuary', *Proc. Eur. mar. Biol. Symp.,* **4,** 29–44

WOODLAND, P. M. J. (1966). 'The behaviour of fish in relation to light in the sea', *Oceanogr. Mar. Biol. Ann. Rev.,* **4,** 337–403

YOSHIDA, M. (1952). 'Some observations on the maturation of the sea urchin *Diadema setosum*', *Annotnes zool. Japan,* **25,** 265–271

Eight

Vision in pelagic animals

J. K. BOWMAKER
MRC Vision Unit
Centre for Research on Perception and Cognition,
University of Sussex, Brighton

8.1 INTRODUCTION

In the diverse species that live in the ocean there are a number of convergent evolutionary features that are clearly adaptations of the visual systems of these animals to the specific problems and limitations imposed by the photic environment of the ocean. Some of these features are immediately apparent, such as the large size of the dioptic parts of the eye in relation to the body of many mesopelagic species, the bioluminescence of these animals and the camouflaging silvery flanks exhibited by many fishes and cephalopods. Closer study of the eye reveals further convergent features, such as the structure of the retina, in terms of the arrangement of the visual receptor cells and, perhaps even more striking, the similarity of the maximum absorbance of the visual pigments contained within the receptors of animals living in similar regions of the ocean and presumably having to perform similar visual tasks.

Almost all of these adaptations can be closely correlated with the characteristics of the underwater space light, i.e. to its non-uniform distribution in which the light comes primarily from above, its intensity and spectral range, as well as less easily recognised features such as the degree of polarisation of the light. In this chapter an attempt has been made to summarise the physical limits of underwater light and to describe some of the adaptations found in the animals populating the ocean.

8.2 LIGHT UNDERWATER

Vision underwater is fundamentally different from vision on land in that the visual limits on land are governed by the receiver, the eye, whereas those underwater are limited by the signal, the ambient light. On land the spectral limits of vision are controlled by the spectral sensitivity of the visual pigments within the receptor cells of the retina and by the absorption of the pre-retinal material in the eye, primarily the cornea and lens. Water, however, acts as a monochromator and selectively absorbs ultra-violet and red light so that daylight, after passing through a few metres of water, is reduced to a narrow bandwidth centred on the blue region of the spectrum. In deep water the wavelengths available for vision are restricted to a band of about 150 nm, which is considerably less than the spectral sensitivity band of a single visual pigment.

The blueness of water is, therefore, a property of the absorption of the water. The clearest natural water that has been studied (Smith and Tyler, 1967) is that of Crater Lake, Oregon, that has a maximum transmittance at about 420 nm with a sharp cut-off in the ultra violet below 350 nm and in the red above about 550nm. Dissolved salts have little or no effect on the spectral absorbance of water so that oceanic water, off the continental shelf, similarly transmits the blue wavelengths between 420 and 500 nm, with a maximum transmission at about 475 nm. The transmission of light through water is, however, affected by dissolved and suspended matter such as chlorophyll within plankton and the 'yellow substance' from vegetable decay. Clearly, the effect of this material is more pronounced in estuaries and coastal waters where the water colour may be more green to yellow with a maximum transmission at about 530 nm and even going beyond 570 nm.

The effects of such factors on the attenuation of the downward irradiance of light through the first 25 m or so of water is illustrated by the two extreme water types shown in *Figure 8.1*. The maximum transmission in the clear

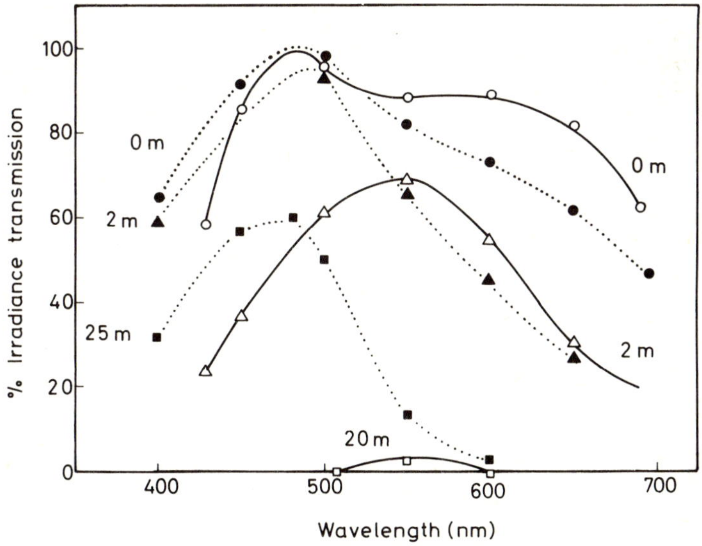

Figure 8.1 Spectral energy distribution of downward irradiance at different depths in the sea. Solid lines in the northern Baltic sea, dotted lines in the eastern Mediterranean Sea. Maximum irradiance brought to 100% for comparison. (After Jerlov, 1970; courtesy John Wiley & Sons)

oceanic water of the Mediterranean Sea occurs at about 470 nm and is only reduced to about 60% of that at the surface in the first 25m. In contrast, in the northern shelf waters of the Baltic, the maximum transmission lies close to 550 nm and the radiance is reduced to less than 5% of that at the surface at 20 m depth. In the clear waters of Crater Lake the irradiance is not reduced to 5% of the surface intensity until a depth of 200 m is reached.

The downward irradiance of light in water is measured as the energy per second falling on a surface from all directions and is measured in W/m^2 and given per unit wavelength or for a specific wavelength interval, i.e. $W/cm^2/nm$. The vertical extinction coefficient k for light passing through water is found from the equation $I/I_0 = e^{-kL}$, where I_0 is the intensity at one depth and I is the intensity at a second deeper depth, L being the distance between the two depths. If the light collecting surface of the photometer used in irradiance measurements collects the flux according to the cosine law ($J_\theta = J_0 \cos \theta$, where J_θ is the radiant intensity of a beam of light at an angle θ from the normal) then the vertical extinction coefficient will equal the diffusion attentuation coefficient K. Ocean water below the first 100 m or so has a high transparency with $k = 0.03$ to 0.04, but in inshore surface water k can be as high as 0.46 to 1.5 in turbid estuaries.

The scattering of light by pure water is of a molecular nature and is related to wavelength according to the Rayleigh Law where scattering increases rapidly from long wavelengths to short wavelengths, being inversely proportional to the fourth power of the wavelength. In the attenuation of underwater light the effect of Rayleigh scattering is small when compared to the effect of suspended particular material which scatters light independently of wavelength. The effect of scattering on the perception of objects underwater is discussed later with reference to the contrast hypothesis for visual pigments.

The distribution of light underwater is not uniform, but comes primarily from above with the angular distribution of the underwater light being dependent on the solar elevation, the degree of cloud cover, the state of the sea, and suspended matter. Refraction at the surface also modifies the distribution of underwater light in that the whole hemisphere of skylight is compressed in the water within a cone of apex angle $2 \times 48.6°$ (fresh water). As a further consequence of refraction, much scattered light travelling upwards is totally reflected at the sea surface and does not escape.

As the depth increases, the light field alters becoming less directional than at the surface, with an approach of the maximum radiance towards zenith. Finally, the space light becomes independent of the surface lighting conditions resulting in an asymptotic radiance distribution which is symmetrical about the vertical (*Figure 8.2*). At this point the downward radiance of the daylight is about 100 to 200 times greater than the upward radiance of scattered light. With increased depth this relationship continues to hold, but both light intensities decrease exponentially at a rate governed by the attenuation coefficient.

A further feature of the underwater spacelight is that it is polarised as a result of Rayleigh scattering and particle scattering, with the degree of maximum polarisation in those lines of sight at about right angles to the

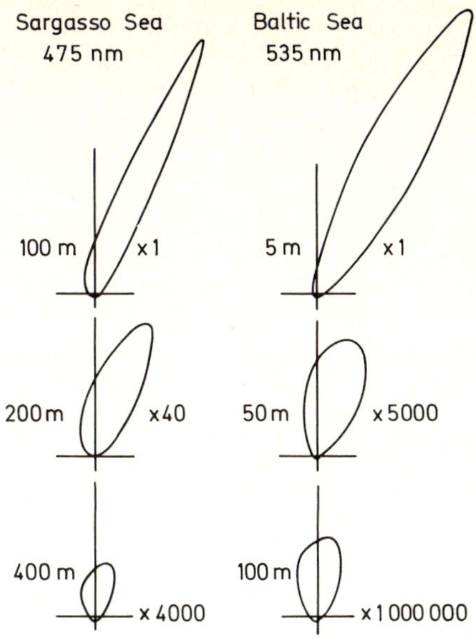

Figure 8.2 Polar diagrams for Sargasso Sea and northern Baltic Sea showing the transformation of the radiance distribution with increase of depth to a final state which is symmetrical around the vertical. (After Jerlov, 1970; courtesy John Wiley & Sons)

direction of maximum radiance, that is the apparent angle of the sun. However, at depth, since the spacelight is permanently symmetrical about the vertical, the plane of maximum polarisation is nearly horizontal.

8.3 VERTICAL ZONATION

From a biological standpoint, the ocean can be divided into three layers, identified by their light and temperature and, therefore, by their flora and fauna. The surface layer, the epipelagic zone, extends down to about 100 to 150 m in clear oceanic water and may be defined as the layer in which photosynthesis can occur and, therefore, represents the level of phytoplankton growth, the euphotic zone. Photosynthesis can occur down to a depth at which the light intensity is reduced to about 1% of that at the surface, i.e. from about 10^5 μW/m^2 to less than 10^3 μW/m^2 (*Figure 8.3*). Although in oceanic water (k = 0.046) this may be greater than 100 m, it may be only 10–30 m in coastal waters (k = 0.46) and reduced to about 3 m in turbid estuaries and harbours.

Below the epipelagic zone in oceanic waters is the permanent thermocline where the water temperature falls from about 20°C to about 4–8°C at 1000 m and where the light level falls from about 1% of that at the surface to what for all intents and purposes may be considered as zero light (of the order of 10^{-11} μW/m^2). Of course, at these depths bioluminescence probably plays a significant part in the total light available, but this will be considered later. In

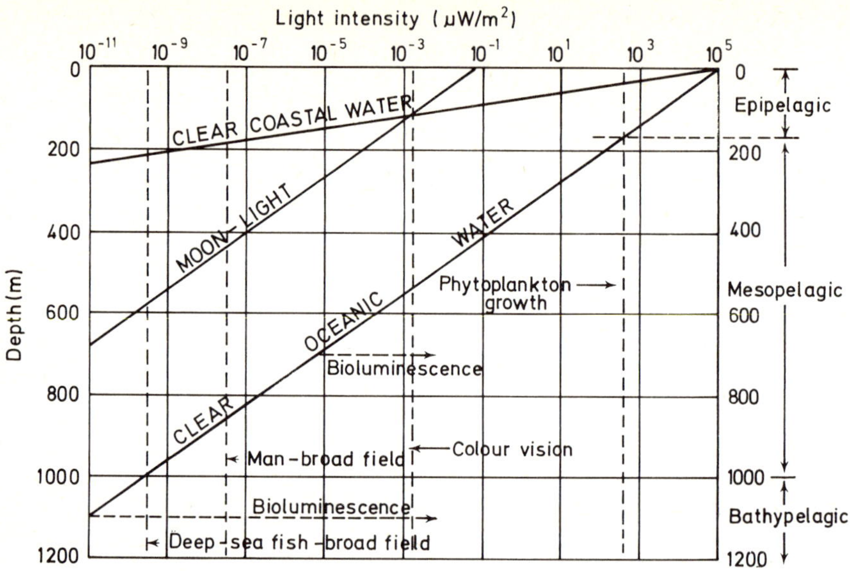

Figure 8.3 Schematic diagram to show the penetration of sunlight into the clearest ocean water and into clear coastal water in relation to minimum intensity values for the vision of man and of certain deep-sea fishes. The approximate minimum values for colour vision in man and for phytoplankton growth are indicated as well as the range of intensities of bioluminescence in the sea. The penetration of moonlight in the clearest ocean water is also shown. (After Clarke and Denton, 1962; courtesy John Wiley & Sons)

this mesopelagic zone the main species of fish belong to the *Myctophidae* (lantern-fishes) and the *Sternoptychidae* (hatchet-fishes).

Below 1000 m in the bathypelagic zone the only light available is that from bioluminescence and there is a very gradual fall in temperature by 2–5°C to the mean depth of the ocean (about 4000 m). This area is dominated by the ceratioids (angler-fishes). These divisions of the ocean are shown diagrammatically in *Figure 8.3*, in which light penetration in coastal and oceanic water is compared with the intensities of bioluminescence and the levels of photopic and scotopic vision for man.

8.4 SCOTOPIC VISION

For an animal to see it must have a means of absorbing and thereby detecting light energy. This is mediated by photosensitive pigments contained within the visual receptor cells of the retina and at low intensities by the rod cells in the retina that contain either of the visual pigments rhodopsin or porphyropsin, based on Vitamin A_1 and Vitamin A_2, respectively. Generally, when visual pigments are extracted from retinae into a solvent such as digitonin, it is found that only one or two pigments can be identified and in the past it has been assumed that these were rod visual pigments. More recently this assumption has been confirmed by the spectral analysis of individual receptor cells using microspectrophotometry, where the absorbance spectrum of a visual pigment can be identified within a specific receptor cell. Extensive studies have been made to identify cone visual pigments in extracts, but apart from some birds such as the turkey and chicken, cone visual pigments have not been satisfactorily demonstrated until very recently (Munz and McFarland, 1975). As a general statement it can be said that in all extracts of visual pigments made in the past from marine fish, it is the rod visual pigments that have been extracted.

Visual pigments are characterised not only by whether they are based on retinol (Vitamin A_1) or on 3-dehydroretinol (Vitamin A_2), but also by the wavelength at which they absorb maximally (λ_{max}). For example, the extracted pigment of the hatchet-fish, *Argyropelecus affinis,* absorbs maximally at 478 nm and, as with the majority of marine fish, the pigment is based on retinal and can be identified as $P478_1$. The remarkable feature of these fish 'rhodopsins' is the spectral range over which they absorb maximally. Although there are only the two prosthetic groups in the visual pigments, the protein moiety (the opsin of the pigment) is species specific and this has resulted in pigments having a range of λ_{max} from 472 nm up to 527 nm in the marine fishes that have so far been studied. This is in marked contrast to the terrestrial vertebrates which have visual pigments restricted to a narrow band from about 493 to 528 nm.

What is the basis for this diversity of visual pigments within the fish? It would appear not to be related directly to the phylogeny of the fish since, even at a generic level, closely related species may have quite different pigments. For example, in the squirrel fishes, *Holocentrus* spp., the visual pigments have λ_{max} ranging from 481 to 502 nm (Munz and McFarland, 1973). However, two general theories, the sensitivity hypothesis and the contrast hypothesis, both based on the functional tasks of vision, have been proposed to account for this diversity of visual pigments.

8.4.1 The sensitivity hypothesis

In early studies on the selective transmission of light by oceanic waters, Clarke, in 1936, noting the selection of blue wavelengths of light, suggested that a shift in the sensitivity of the eyes of deep-sea fish towards shorter wavelengths than the then known visual pigments, absorbing maximally around 500 nm, would be a distinct advantage. Later work has since confirmed this theory, in that deep-sea fish do indeed have visual pigments which in extract have λ_{max} ranging from 472 nm in the deep-sea shark, *Centroscymnus coelolepis,* up to 490 nm in the mesopelagic lantern-fish, *Lampanyctus mexicanus.* Recent studies have shown that the coelacanth, *Latimeria,* and the castor-oil fish, *Ruvettus pretiosus* (Dartnall, 1972), also have visual pigments that absorb maximally at about 473 nm and these rhodopsins are the shortest wavelength rod pigments that have been measured, apart from the extraordinary so-called green rods of the amphibians. As was stated earlier, the maximum transmission of clear oceanic water below about 100 m is at about 475 nm and thus these pigments with λ_{max} around 473 nm are remarkably precise adaptations to the ambient light. The sensitivity hypothesis, viz. that the λ_{max} of a fish's visual pigment is determined by the wavelength of maximum transmission of light in its environment would, therefore, appear to hold for deep-sea fish. Recently some fascinating exceptions amongst deep-sea fish have been reported, but this will be dealt with under bioluminescence.

Munz (1964) studied fish not only from different depths, but also from areas with different spectral irradiances, such as the more green waters of bays and estuaries, and he found that the fish inhabiting these waters possessed pigments absorbing maximally between about 504 and 522 nm and that surface living fish had visual pigments with λ_{max} located around 494 nm. This type of relationship has since been amply confirmed by Dartnall and Lythgoe (1965) and extended to tropical fishes by the recent work of Munz and McFarland (1973). The correlation found between environment and the visual pigments is summarised in *Table 8.1*.

Table 8.1

	Temperate		*Tropical*	
	Range	*Mean (n)*	*Range*	*Mean (n)*
Deep sea	477–490	484 (7)	480–486	483 (12)
Epipelagic	491–499	494 (4)	484–502	492 (129)
Surface (0–5m)	—	—	494–501	497 (34)
Rocky shore[1]	492–505	498 (8)	—	—
English Channel	493–500	497 (6)	—	—
Bays and estuaries	504–512	509 (10)	—	—

[1]Primarily Mediterranean

Although there is clearly a correlation between the visual pigments of fish and their environment, there is not necessarily a correlation between the λ_{max} of the visual pigment and the wavelength of maximum transmission of the water. Dartnall and Lythgoe (1965) found that the visual pigments extracted from fish caught in the Mediterranean clustered around 498 nm and that the rhodopsins from fish living in the English Channel also clustered around 498 nm. However, the water in the Mediterranean (around Malta) is oceanic in type and has a maximum transmission between 470 and 490 nm. In contrast the English Channel is always green or yellow-green (as will be confirmed by many a seasick cross-Channel traveller). According to the sensitivity hypothesis a difference in the visual pigments from fish from these two areas might be expected.

There is a further interesting and somewhat puzzling exception to what seems to be a simple relationship between the environment and rhodopsin λ_{max} and that is in the flying fish, *Cypselurus simus,* which clearly is a surface living fish, but which has a $P475_1$ that would appear to be perfectly adapted for a deep-sea environment. Munz and McFarland (1973) have suggested that, since the fish is preyed on by tuna, it must be able to detect a predator striking from the side or below, that is through the intensely blue water column. The predominant wavelength of upwelling light in oceanic conditions is centred around 460 nm and so a $P475_1$ would provide for high sensitivity with the greatest chance of detecting a dark target against background light. However well this may appear to explain the anomaly of *Cypselurus,* it must be wondered why other surface fish that presumably are also preyed on in a similar manner do not also have blue shifted visual pigments.

If there is a correlation between visual pigments and the environment in the fishes, does it also apply to other marine animals such as crustaceans and mammals? Much less data are available for crustacean visual pigments which are, as with marine fish, based on retinal. Nevertheless, the deep-sea euphausids and shrimps that have been studied have visual pigments which in solution range from a $P462_1$ in *Euphausia pacifica* to $P480_1$ in the bathypelagic shrimp, *Acanthephyra haeckeli,* with the mean of the nine species so far reported being at 470 nm (*see* Goldsmith, 1972). The surface living crustaceans, as with the surface and epipelagic fish, have pigments with λ_{max} grouped around 498 nm, but ranging from 480 nm in the fiddler crab to 516 nm in the pink shrimp, *Penaeus duorarum* (*Table 8.2*).

Table 8.2

	Deep-sea		*Epipelagic*	
Crustacea				
Euphausiacea	462–480	467 (6)	—	—
shrimps	470–480	475 (3)	—	516 (1)
crabs	—	—	480–515	496 (7)
Cephalopods				
Octopus	—	—	470–477	474 (3)
Squid				
Loligo pealii (English Channel)	—	—	—	493 (1)
Todarodes pacificus (Japan Sea-oceanic)	—	—	—	480 (1)
Cuttlefish (inshore)	—	—	486–500	493 (3)
Mammalia				
Mysticeti (inshore surface)	—	—	492–497	(2)
Odontoceti (diving mammals)				
Berardius bairdii	—	481 (1)	—	—
Delphinidae	485–489	486 (8)	—	—

So far all comparisons between the maximum transmission of the water and the maximum absorbance of the visual pigments have been made with the λ_{max} of the pigments determined from extracts. An important question that has arisen is whether the absorbance of a visual pigment in extract is identical to the absorbance of the visual pigment in the intact retina and hence to the scotopic spectral sensitivity of the animal from which the extract is taken. In other words, does removing the pigment from the membrane of the visual receptor, of which it is a constituent part, into a digitonin micelle soluble in water, affect the absorption characteristics of the pigment?

Within the crustaceans there is limited evidence to suggest that this is true. For instance, in the blue crab, *Callinectes sapidus,* which inhabits shallow water, the extracted pigment absorbs maximally at 480 nm, which would be better suited for a deep-water species according to the sensitivity hypothesis. However, the spectral sensitivity of the animal is maximal at about 505 nm. Similarly, in the lobster, *Homarus americanus,* the extracted pigment has a λ_{max} at 515 nm, whereas its spectral sensitivity peaks at about 525 nm. Recent microspectrophotometric measurements on isolated rhabdomes of *Callinectes* (Bruno and Goldsmith, 1974) show a much closer agreement between pigment absorption in the rhabdome and the spectral sensitivity, implying that extraction does in some way alter the absorption characteristics of the visual pigment.

Within the vertebrates there is even less evidence available, but clearly a difference of only a few nanometres between the pigment absorbance in solution and the absorbance in the intact retina could have a considerable effect on the correlation between the spectral maximum of the ambient light and the absorbance of the visual pigment. The data that are available within the vertebrates suggest that there is a close correlation between the spectral absorbance of pigments in solution, the absorbance of the pigment within the visual cells and the scotopic spectral sensitivity of the animal. However, it has been noted recently that at least in the frog, *Rana temporaria,* the λ_{max} of the extracted rhodopsin is at 502 nm, but that the absorbance of the intact retina and of individual rods measured by microspectrophotometry has a maximum absorbance at 505 nm (Bowmaker, Loew and Liebman, 1975). The scotopic spectral sensitivity of the frog has always been accepted as maximal at 502 nm, but a subtle difference of only a few nanometres would be difficult to detect and until further work is carried out in this field the matter must remain in question.

The cetaceans also have visual pigments that appear to be correlated with their environment (*Table 8.2*) (McFarland, 1971). The diving delphinids that have been studied have pigments with λ_{max} at 486 nm, with the exception of *Delphinus delphis* which has a $P489_1$. These pigments lie within the range characteristic of deep-sea fish and are probably an adaptation to the open ocean and diving habits of the dolphins. Similarly, the visual pigments found in the beaked whale, *Berardius bairdii,* absorb maximally at 481 nm and this species is known to dive to depths below 1000 m when harpooned.

The baleen grey whale has a $P497_1$ that correlates well with the non-oceanic coastal and lagoon habits of this species. The humped-backed whale has a $P492_1$ and it seems possible that this may correlate with the seasonal variations in this species' habits. In the summer the animals feed in northern surface waters whereas in winter they migrate to more equatorial waters where the animals do not feed. Is the difference in pigments between odontocetes and baleen whales related to the photic environment of their respective feeding habits? Odontocetes ($P481_1$) feed both in and below the epipelagic zone on fish and cephalopods, whereas the baleen whales

($P492_1$–$P497_1$) feed close to the surface on krill. Further studies of the whales will be needed before this question can be answered satisfactorily.

In the cephalopod molluscs the picture is far less clear. The three octopus that have been studied have visual pigments with λ_{max} ranging from 470 to 477 nm, but these animals tend to be bottom dwellers in relatively shallow water. Within the squid the visual pigment of *Loligo pealli* has a λ_{max} at 493 nm which perhaps might be expected in an epipelagic species, while *Todarodes pacificus* has a $P480_1$. In the cuttle fish the visual pigments range from 486 to 500 nm which again might be predicted for these inshore epipelagic animals. However, the extremely blue shifted pigments of the octopus are difficult to explain in terms of their shallow water environment.

From the mass of data collected above it is clear that the sensitivity hypothesis, though highly satisfactory with respect to deep-sea animals, will not satisfy all of the visual pigments. In seeking an hypothesis to explain the range of visual pigments found in pelagic animals it is necessary to try to determine the visual tasks that an animal has to perform. Is a maximum sensitivity to the ambient light all that is required to perform these tasks? Lythgoe (1966) has suggested that visual contrast might be as important as sensitivity in the evolutionary process and so contribute to the production of the wide range of visual pigments found in fishes.

8.4.2 The contrast hypothesis

Vision underwater can be compared to vision on land in fog, in that it is not low light intensity that prevents distant objects being seen, but rather that the light scattered by water droplets in the fog interposes a light that degradates contrast below the level required for vision. This can be clearly demonstrated by the dipping of car headlights in a fog, which has the effect of decreasing light intensity but increasing the range of vision because of the decrease in the backward scattered light from the headlight beam. Similarly, for a horizontal path of sight underwater, the image-forming light is reduced in the passage between an object and the eye by both absorption and scattering, while simultaneously there is a gain in the brightness from the light scattered into the eye by the intervening water. Such an effect causes a decrease in the apparent radiance contrast of the object and, as the visual range increases, the apparent contrast of the object seen horizontally against an infinite water background decreases exponentially. Further, it will be evident that in turbid water the apparent contrast of an object will be greatly reduced when compared to the same object viewed in clear water.

For an animal underwater, the problems of contrast perception by the eye and contrast degradation by the water are fundamental to its ability to see. Of course, in determining the visual capabilities of an animal, information is required on the light quanta absorbed by the eye, the direction of the object being viewed and the background spacelight. In shallow water, because of the filtering effect of water, light penetrating from above, having a short path from the surface, will have a broader spectral radiance distribution than light travelling horizontally or from below. The absorbance properties of the visual pigment will have a marked effect upon the perception of brightness contrast and hence the range at which an object can be detected through the water. If the λ_{max} of the visual pigment is offset from the maximum water space light radiance it will absorb less light from both the object and its background, but because of the broader spectral radiance of the light reflected from the object, it will absorb more light from the object than from the background. The relative brightness of the object will thus be enhanced and if the object is brighter than the background it will accordingly be seen more easily by an offset visual pigment than if the pigment had a λ_{max} coincident with the maximum water transmission. This is illustrated in *Figure 8.4*.

Lythgoe (1966) has used the theory of contrast perception to account for the apparent discrepancy between the visual pigments of English Channel fish and fish from the Mediterranean. As previously stated, in the English

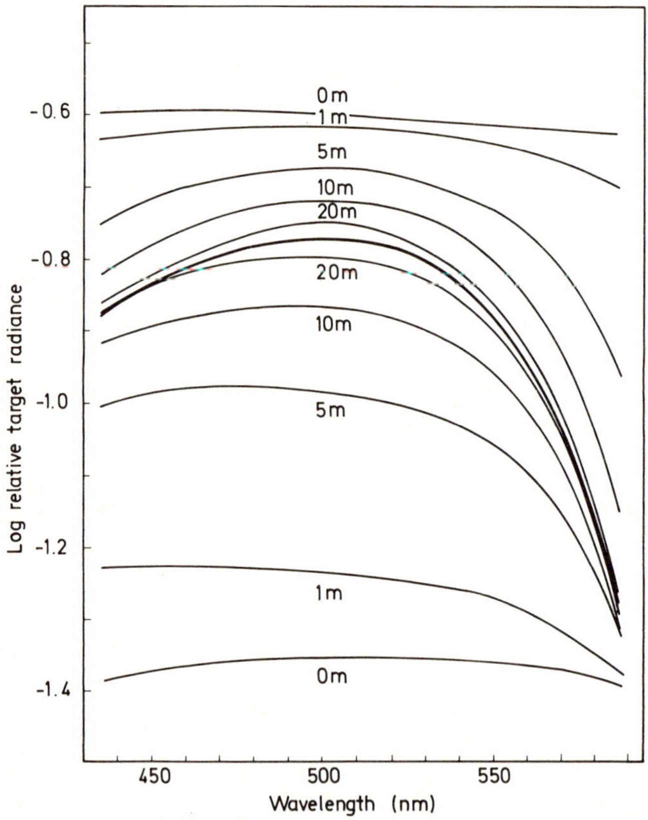

Figure 8.4 The relative spectral radiance of the water background (heavy line) just below the water surface and the apparent spectral radiances of two matt grey targets, one slightly brighter (curves above heavy line) and the other slightly darker (curves below heavy line) than the background at various ranges. Both families of curves approach the water background radiance as the distance increases. (After Lythgoe, 1968; courtesy Pergamon Press Ltd)

Channel, the λ_{max} of the visual pigments from the fish that have been studied is 497 nm, but the maximum transmission in this water is at a considerably longer wavelength in the green at about 530 nm. Similarly, although the visual pigments of fishes from bays and estuaries have λ_{max} around 509 nm, which is slightly longer than those of English Channel fish, the waters in these areas can be green to yellow with a maximum transmission as high as 570 nm. Further, in clear Mediterranean water, the maximum transmission of the water is at about 470 nm, whereas the visual pigments of Mediterranean fish cluster around 498 nm (*see Table 8.1*). There is thus an offset of the λ_{max} of the visual pigments from the wavelength of maximum transmission of the water of from 30 to 60 nm, either towards the blue or the red depending on the environment. Such offset visual pigments will, as illustrated in *Figure 8.4,* permit enhanced contrast perception.

If the contrast hypothesis does explain the diversity of the λ_{max} of the visual pigments found in epipelagic fish, it demands that the necessity of seeing a bright object against a lighted background is the most important visual task for a fish. Even so, any fish with an offset visual pigment will have the benefit of enhanced contrast perception and it would seem that, since vision depends upon both sensitivity and contrast, both of these qualities have functioned in terms of the selective processes that have produced the great diversity of visual pigments.

One of the difficulties with both the sensitivity hypothesis and the contrast hypothesis is that there is little information available as to the spectral radiance present in a given epipelagic environment. Recently, Munz and McFarland (1973) have questioned whether the use of maximum transmission values is a proper estimate of the spectral distribution of the background space light, at least in shallow environments. The space light of surface waters will be dependent both on the maximum transmission of the water and on the properties of the light source. The work of Munz and McFarland (1973) on the spectral radiance present in the surface waters of a coral reef, the behaviour of the fish in this environment and the visual pigments of the reef fishes has produced some interesting conclusions. In the shallow waters of a coral reef the diurnal fishes, as twilight begins, leave the water column and move to the proximity of the cracks and holes in the reef. According to Hobson (1972) this is an ordered and predictable pattern on the part of the various families, some leaving before others. At about the same time the nocturnal species leave their crevices in the reef and prepare to enter the water column. However, there is a quiet period of about 20 min when no fish are seen in the water column and this period coincides with the last few minutes of rapidly falling light levels associated with twilight (*Figure 8.5*).

During twilight the light intensity decreases in terms of quanta between 400 and 700 nm by about 10^4 from sunset to the end of the quiet period. This reduction in intensity induces the photomechanical changes of dark adaptation and the shift from photopic vision to scotopic vision. It is suggested that the 20 min quiet period is a result of the slow dark adaptation processes, i.e. the fish wait close to the reef while they dark adapt to the full scotopic function. A further important change occurring at this time is not

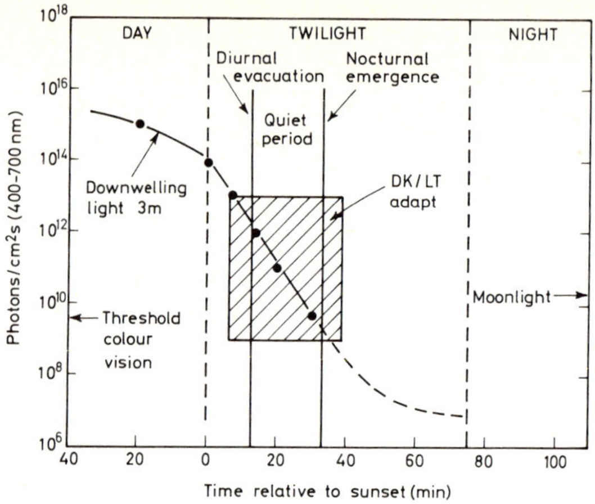

Figure 8.5 Correlation between twilight light levels, retinal dark-light adaptation and the behaviour of coral-reef fishes as night descends. Light intensities are total photons between 400 and 700 nm obtained from spectral irradiance measurements for downwelling light at 3 m beneath the surface. For further details see test. (After Munz and McFarland, 1973; courtesy Pergamon Press Ltd)

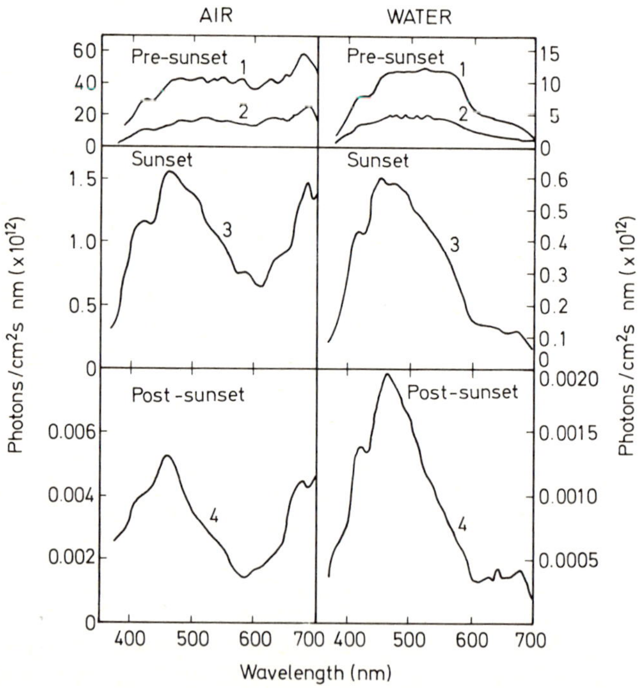

Figure 8.6 Change in spectral curves in air and for downwelling light at 3 m depth during sunset in a coral lagoon. Actual times for curves are: pre-sunset, 1–57 min, 2–26 min, 3–2 min; post-sunset, 4–34 min. (After Munz and McFarland, 1973; courtesy Pergamon Press Ltd)

only in the intensity of the light but also in the spectral irradiance. In daylight the spectral irradiance of sunlight is relatively flat between 450 and 700 nm with a λP_{50} (wavelength which divides the photon distribution between 400-700 nm into equal halves) at 515 nm, 60 min prior to sunset at 3 m depth. During sunset there is a reduction of photons in the yellow-orange (550-650) as a result of the specific absorption by ozone through the increased atmospheric path length owing to the low elevation of the sun. Since the water acts as a red filter, the peak remaining at 700 nm is lost leaving the underwater light with a λP_{50} at about 499 nm, 2 min before sunset, and 487 nm 30 min after sunset (*Figure 8.6*).

In moonlight conditions, however, the λP_{50} shifts back towards the red to about 548 nm and at 3 m depth is above the threshold for cone vision. Similarly, on starry nights the λP_{50} is red shifted, though the intensity will be greatly reduced. It should perhaps be pointed out that the spectral irradiance curves shown in *Figure 8.6* were obtained at 3 m which is very shallow in a reef environment and most species tend to live somewhat deeper.

Just prior to and during the 20 min quiet period, fish predation on a reef reaches a maximum and Hobson (1972) has suggested that the behaviour was '. . . shaped by the threat of crepuscular predators'. In other words, predation can be correlated with the visually 'difficult' period of twilight when a fish's vision is shifting from photopic to scotopic. At this time fish appear to a diver as dark objects against a brighter greyish background and the most successful visual pigment for such detection is onc that correlates with the ambient spacelight, i.e. about 490 nm. This is precisely the case with the coral fishes, since the majority of rod pigments studied absorb maximally between 485 and 497 nm.

It would appear, therefore, that for coral reef fish at least, contrast enhancement, through off-setting, has not been a major selective force in the evolution of these visual pigments. In nocturnal fishes though, the position is somewhat different since during starry nights the ambient light will have a shifted λP_{50} so that a visual pigment with a λ_{max} at about 490 nm will be offset by as much as 50 nm or so; sufficient for contrast enhancement of light objects against a dark background.

8.5 PHOTOPIC VISION IN THE EPIPELAGIC ZONE

During the hours of daylight in the epipelagic zone there will be sufficient intensity in the water space light for photopic vision, or in other words, for the discrimination of spectrally different lights of equal intensity. In terms of the threshold for colour vision in man, colour can be distinguished down to about 500 m in the clearest oceanic waters, but only to about 100 m in clear coastal waters (*Figure 8.3*). Of course, at depths of 500 m the only colour available (excluding bioluminescence) is blue and it is not the intensity that restricts the colour-range visible, but the cut-off filtering effect of the water. In clear oceanic waters the bandwidth of available light to stimulate successfully the three retinal colour receptors, i.e. red, green and blue cones, exists only in the first 30–100 m or so, depending on the water type, after which the spectral range is reduced to the 150 nm between about 375 and 525 nm.

From a purely theoretical standpoint, there is no reason why wavelength discrimination should not be possible even at depths with a very restricted waveband, assuming that the necessary visual pigments and neural networks were available. Light, that to man can only be described as blue in colour, could be divided into any number of 'colours' by an animal with the necessary receptor systems. Of course, at present there is no evidence to suggest that such a system exists.

The bright colours of many tropical fish indicate that they probably have the necessary system for wavelength discrimination. To prove categorically that fish have colour vision is a difficult task, but as Walls stated '. . . no fish has ever been shown not to have colour vision'. Evidence for colour vision in fishes has been obtained from classical behaviour studies carried out at the beginning of the century (for a review, *see* Walls, 1942), but, more recently, physiological data have become available. Colour discrimination is mediated by the cones and, as will be discussed later, the majority of epipelagic fish have cone rich retina. Until very recently, extraction of cone visual pigments has not been successful, but the use of microspectrophotometry, where the absorbance of visual pigments within individual cone cells can be studied, has shown that in the goldfish, for example, three populations of cones exist with λ_{max} at 455, 530 and 625 nm (Leibman, 1972). Evidence has also been obtained by Tomita for the three cone populations in the carp by intra-cellular recordings from individual cones in which the maximum sensitivities were found at 462, 529 and 611 nm; a close correlation with the measurements from microspectrophotometry.

Further physiological evidence has been obtained for colour vision from electrical potentials, the *S* potentials, recorded from the inner nuclear layer of the retina. These potentials are intra-cellular and are generated in the large horizontal cells found in this region of the retina. The *S* potentials can be divided into two major types from their response patterns to spectral light. Those exhibiting only a hyperpolarising response to all wavelengths are termed luminosity types (L response) and those which respond with a polarity that is wavelength dependent are termed the chromaticity type (C response). Both the L- and C-types can be further subdivided by the wavelengths that cause maximum polarity changes.

Most *S* potential studies have been performed on photopically adapted retinae, though it would appear that both rods and cones can contribute to the response. Certainly rods can cause *S* potentials since the nocturnal neko shark, which has a pure rod retina, gives L-type responses with a maximum sensitivity at 494 nm (Tamura and Niwa, 1967), which corresponds with the rhodopsins commonly found in epipelagic fish. It has been suggested that species that show no C responses, but only L responses are colour blind. However, *Eugerres plumieri* (Laufer and Millan, 1970), a marine fish inhabiting shallow tropical lagoons and coastal waters to a depth of 5 m, has three cone populations, as measured by microspectrophotometry, with λ_{max} at 470, 568 and 604 nm. L-type *S* potentials have been recorded from this species with maximum responses at 476, 568 and 606 nm, which indicates that there is probably no mixing of the signals between receptors containing different photopigments, unlike species that exhibit C-type potentials. The term 'luminosity' type potentials is perhaps not a useful term with respect to this fish since, presumably, the three L-type responses of *Eugerres* contribute to colour coding. Similar bimodal and trimodal responses have been recorded from the carp, again suggesting more than a simple brightness detecting system.

C-type *S* potentials have been divided into three general classes, one is depolarised to red and hyperpolarised to green (R/G) or vice versa; another class is depolarised to green and hyperpolarised to blue (G/B) or vice versa; and a third is depolarised to red and blue and hyperpolarised to green (R,B/G), but the reverse has not been reported. The type of C responses found are dependent on the species of the fish studied. In the surface living *Mugilidae* both L and C responses are found with variations of all three of the C-type responses (*Figure 8.7*). However, in the *Serranidae* and *Centropomidae* only one or two types of C responses were identified along with L-type responses. In a recent survey of 10 species of fishes (Tamura and Niwa, 1967), including two elasmobranchs, seven species including a sting ray exhibited both C and L responses, whereas the other three species responded only with L-type potentials even though two of these, the chidae and black porgy, have mixed retinae, the third species being the neko shark. Such variability may be related to the cone

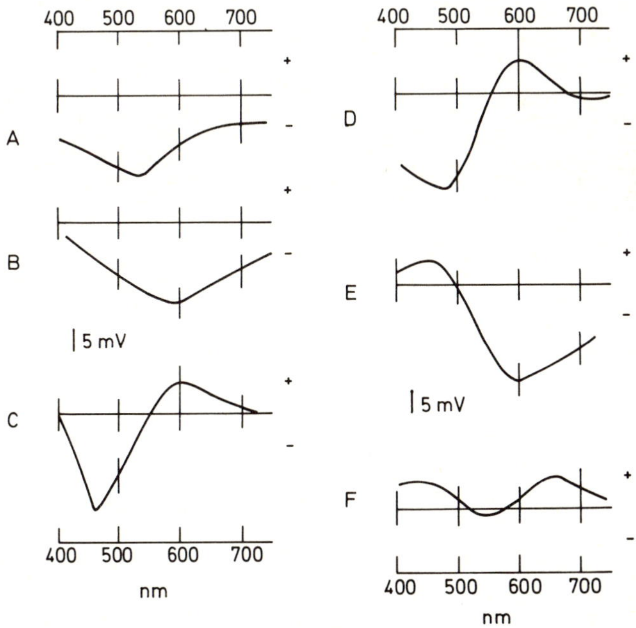

Figure 8.7 S-potentials from the retina of Mugil cephalaus. *A and B, L-type responses with maxima at about 540 and 600 nm, respectively. C to F, C-type responses. C, orange +ve with blue −ve; D, orange +ve with blue and deep red −ve; E, blue +ve with orange −ve; F, blue and red +ve with green/yellow −ve. (After Tamura and Niwa, 1967; courtesy Pergamon Press Ltd)*

populations of the different species in that a species with only two populations of cones might have few types of *S* potentials.

Very recently Munz and McFarland (1975) have successfully demonstrated the presence of cone pigments in extracts of visual pigments from a number of pelagic fish and have been able to correlate these findings with the photic environment of the fish and to their behaviour (McFarland and Munz, 1975a, b). From the data they concluded that the evolution of colour vision was probably related to the enhancement of visual contrast against a monochromatic background, as proposed by Walls (1942). To illustrate the hypothesis, they use two examples of diurnal predators: the mahi mahi (*Coryphaena hippurus*), which is limited to the top surface 15 m and usually feeds within the upper 6 m and, therefore, has its main visual axis orientated along the horizontal line of sight with well developed forward binocularity and, in contrast, the skipjack tuna (*Katsuwontus pelamis*), which lives down to 70 m and feeds at depth or on surface prey by attacking upwards from deeper water. It thus has a line of sight orientated upwards and forwards and will have to detect objects silhouetted against a bright downwelling light, unlike mahi mahi whose prey will be contrasted against the blue background of the water space light which will be less bright than the downwelling surface light. From the contrast hypothesis proposed by Lythgoe (1966) and discussed above, it might be predicted that the tuna would have a blue/green

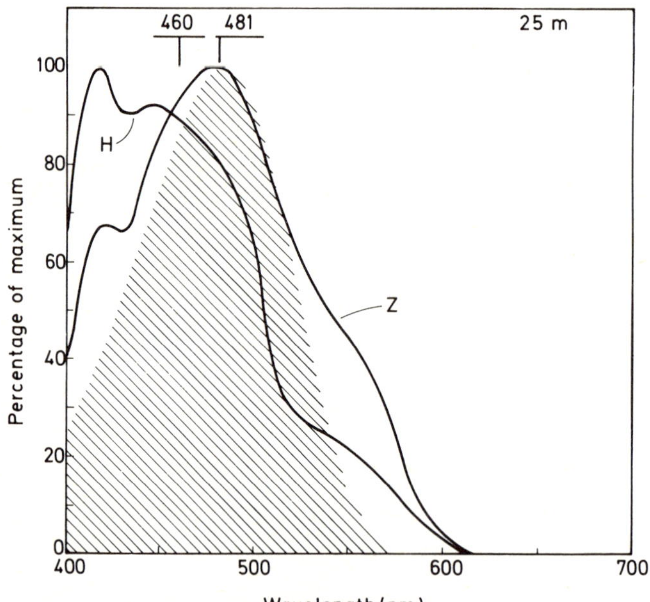

Figure 8.8 Comparison of the background radiance spectra at 25 m depth (heavy lines; Z = zenith and H = horizontal line of sight) and the absorbance spectrum of visual pigment P483 of the skipjack (area covered by diagonal lines). Radiance and absorbance spectra have been scaled to the same maximum. The λP_{50} *values of the horizontal (460 nm) and zenith (481 nm) radiance spectra are indicated. (After McFarland and Munz, 1975b; courtesy Pergamon Press Ltd)*

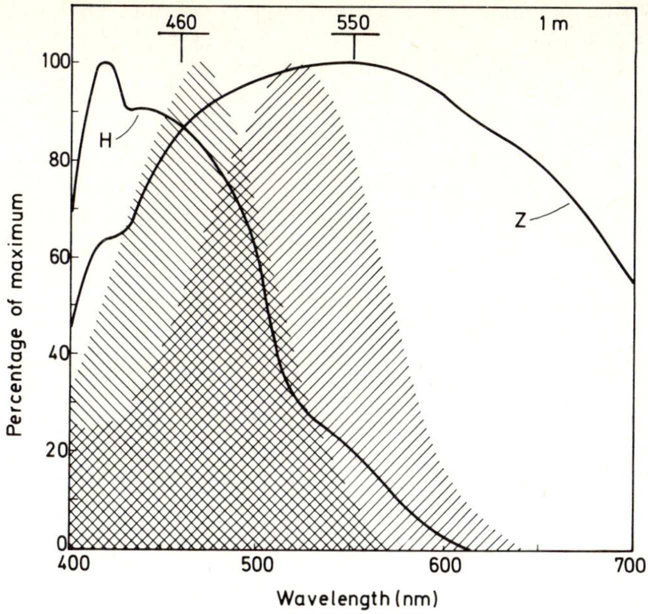

Figure 8.9 Comparison of the background radiance spectra at 1 m depth (heavy lines; Z = zenith and H = horizontal line of sight) and the absorbance spectra of two visual pigments of the mahi mahi (areas covered by diagonal lines). The blue sensitive pigment (P469) is to the left of the more red-sensitive P521, and they overlap. The middle pigment P499 has been omitted for clarity of the figure. Radiance and absorbance spectra have been scaled to the same maximum. The λP_{50} values of the horizontal (460 nm) and zenith (550 nm) radiance spectra are indicated. (After McFarland and Munz, 1975b; courtesy Pergamon Press Ltd)

absorbing pigment that matched the maximum transmission of the water, while mahi mahi would have an offset pigment to enhance the contrast of its prey.

In the skipjack tuna the retinal extracts contained only a $P483_1$, similar to other tuna studied. This pigment matches the 'blue' photic environment of the tuna in all its fields of view including downwelling light which will lack sufficient yellow and green light to require multiple visual pigments. This is illustrated in *Figure 8.8*. Although the tuna has a duplex retina it is probable that the P483 is found within both the rods and the cones. Support for a single visual pigment can be found from the electrophysiological studies of Tamura, Hanyu and Niwa (1972) who demonstrated the presence of only L-type *S* potentials in tuna retinae with a maximum response around 490 nm. No evidence for chromaticity-type responses was found and they concluded that the tunas were probably colour blind.

In contrast, the pigment extracts of the mahi mahi were found to have at least three visual pigments, $P521_1$, $P499_1$ and $P469_1$, and it would seem likely that the P521 and P469 are cone pigments and that the P499 is present in cones and in the rods. The downwelling light close to the surface will be relatively rich in green and yellow light (*Figure 8.9*) and this will be reflected from the silvery flanks of fishes that the mahi mahi preys on and will be seen against the predominantly blue or blue-green horizontal space light (*Figure 8.9*). Thus the P521, which is the most abundant pigment in extracts of light-adapted fishes, is offset from the background space light and is suited to detect a bright object against the horizontal background by enhancing the apparent contrast of the object. The other two pigments are matched or offset pigments depending on the depth and line of sight. Near the surface the P499 is probably matching the horizontal space light and the P469 will be offset to shorter wavelengths, while at depth the position will be reversed with the P469 more closely matched to the horizontal and downward lines of sight (*Figure 8.9*). In other words, the fish is beautifully adapted to detect bright or dark objects in any line of sight or at any depth at which the fish normally lives by seeing the object with maximum contrast against the background.

All of the physiological evidence, although demonstrating the high probability of colour vision in fishes, yields little information about the actual visual capabilities of light adapted fish. To obtain such information behavioural methods must be employed, involving either trained or innate responses to light. However, the form of the spectral sensitivity curves obtained from such experiments depend on the type of visual task set for the fish. An example of three such behaviourally determined sensitivity curves for the freshwater rudd, *Scardinius erythrophthalmus,* are shown in *Figure 8.10.* The form of the sensitivity curves seems to reflect the sensitivities of

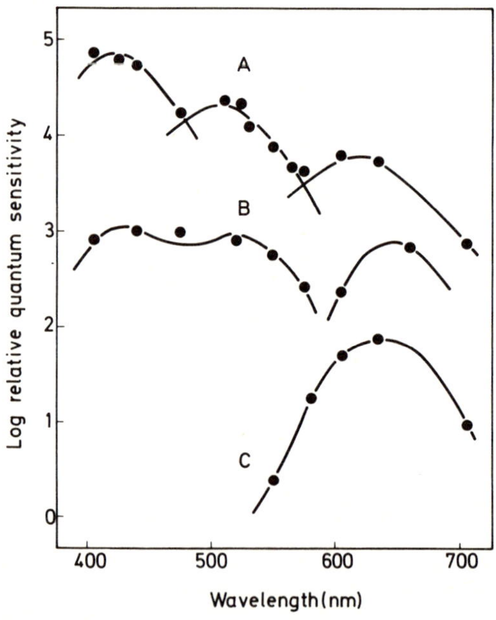

Figure 8.10 Light-adapted spectral sensitivity curves of the rudd, Scardinius erythrophthalmus, *obtained by three behavioural methods. A, two choice training method; B, Pavlovian conditioning of activity to large diffuse stimuli flashed overhead; C, innate orientation responses to bars of light passing intermittently overhead. (After Lythgoe and Northmore, 1973; courtesy Hilger (Adam) Ltd)*

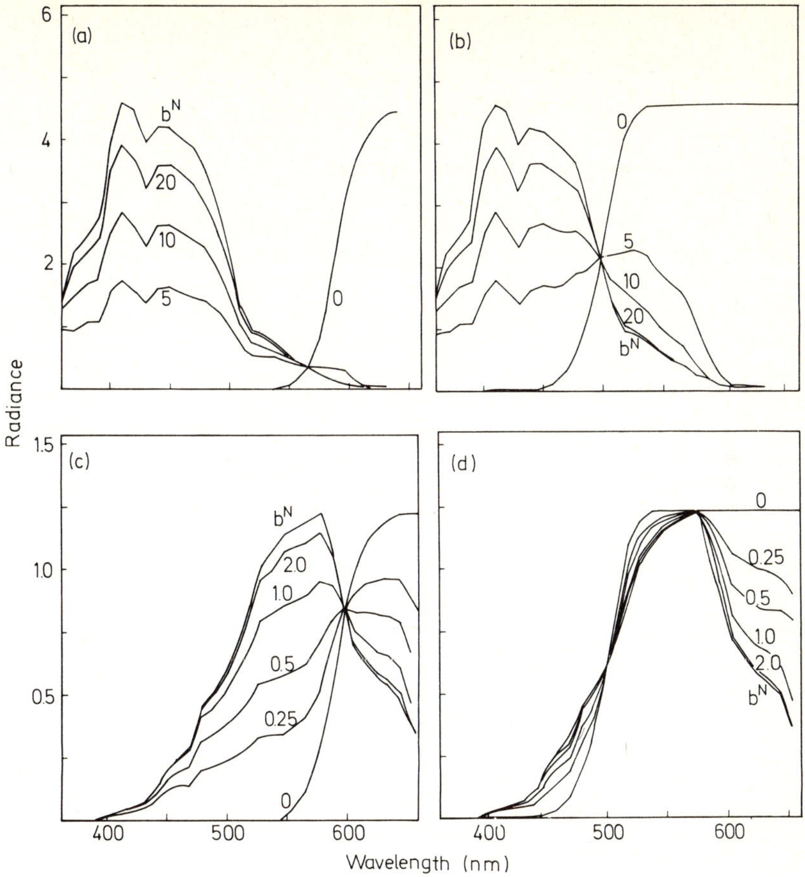

Figure 8.11 The change in spectral radiance of a yellow and a red object as they recede horizontally from the eye in blue (Gulf Stream) water and green (reservoir) water. b^N represents the spectral radiance of the water background. Distance in metres. (a) Red in blue water; (b) yellow in blue water; (c) red in green water; (d) yellow in green water. (After Lythgoe and Northmore, 1973; courtesy Hilger (Adam) Ltd)

the three receptor types whose λ_{max} are well spaced out along the spectrum. The variability of the results probably lies in the different processing channels present in the visual system being used for specific acts and it is possible that the ability of the fish to discriminate colour is not only related to the pigments of the cones, but also the visual tasks that it has to perform.

The colours that can be distinguished at different depths and at varying ranges underwater are greatly affected by the natural colour of the water. As depth increases and the bandwidth of the ambient light decreases, any colours produced by selective reflection that are outside this bandwidth are irrelevant to vision. Thus a red object will appear black in blue water since only the short wavelengths can penetrate the water and it is these that the red object selectively absorbs. In contrast, where the spectral reflectance changes rapidly with wavelength in the region of maximum light transmission, the object will appear different in hue to its background. Thus yellow and blue objects in clear blue water such as the open ocean would be more visible in green coastal or estuarine water (*Figure 8.11*). Further, Lythgoe and Northmore (1973) have shown that as a general rule yellow can always be seen at greater depths than red in blue water and vice versa in green water.

As an illustration of the importance of these colour effects, many inshore fish which live in green or yellow-green water have bright red patches that are used behaviourally, such as in the lumpsucker, *Cyclopterus lumpus,* where the red belly of the fish intensifies during the mating season. Similarly, as might be expected, in the clear blue waters around coral reefs many of the fish have yellow markings, such as *Chaetodon lunula,* which intensifies its yellow markings in agonistic display.

Fish living in the surface layers of the ocean can be divided behaviourally, as with terrestrial animals, into diurnal, nocturnal and crepuscular species. In diurnal fishes living in the epipelagic zone, in which it is reasonable to assume that acute vision plays an important part in their behaviour pattern, the cones within the retina are arranged in two basic types of mosaics. One pattern consists of rows of parallel double cones, alternating in some fish groups with rows of single cones, while the second pattern is composed of square units with double cones surrounding single cones (*see* Engström, 1963). In these retinae there is a very high density of cones, when compared with nocturnal species, ranging as high as 40 000/mm^2.

In a recent survey of reef fishes (Munz and McFarland, 1973) it has been shown that in diurnal feeders with a tendency to eat small items such as coral polyps and plankton where high visual acuity is necessary, the cone density in restricted areas of the retina can be much higher. In the wrasse, *Thalassoma* and *Bodianus,* values in excess of 100 000/mm^2 were found in the dorsal retina which correlate with their habit of cruising slightly above the reef substrate.

Herbivorous diurnal fishes also possess high cone densities and, although their feeding behaviour might not require such a high visual acuity, it would provide the maximum ability to detect the motion of predator species. In fact, it has been observed that during daylight, predators tend to ignore their prey and likewise the prey tend to be unconcerned about the presence of their predators; a behaviour consistent with their high visual acuity.

As might be expected, typical nocturnal fishes possess few cones, in the range of 3000/mm^2 up to about 9000/mm^2. In these species the mosaics seen in the cones of diurnal species tend to break down leaving a more random arrangement of visual cells. Vision in these fish is restricted to scotopic levels mediated by the rods which predominate over the cones.

In crepuscular predators, Munz and McFarland (1973) have shown that the number of cones present falls somewhere between those found in diurnal and nocturnal fishes. Thus in the carangid, *Carangoides ajax,* the number was about 30 000/mm^2, while in *Epinephelus merra,* the number was reduced to 24 000/mm^2. A further difference noted in the cones was the increase in size of the outer segments as compared to those of diurnal fishes, though the cones still appeared to have a similar ratio to the bipolar cells as found in diurnal fishes. Munz and McFarland suggested that with the reduced number of enlarged cones and little summation, the crepuscular feeder sacrifices high visual acuity, but gains in the capacity of the photopic system for a high quantum catch per unit receptor cell. This will be of considerable advantage to the fish during twilight since the large cones will increase the probability of detecting prey and will also be able to track the movement of the object across the retina because of the low summation to the bipolar cell and ganglion cells. Conversely, the animal will be at a disadvantage during the day and night which correlates with their tendency to ignore prey during these times. In daylight their visual acuity will be less than that of the diurnal feeders while at night their sensitivity will be below that of the nocturnal feeders.

8.6 THE EYE OF FISHES

Having described the visual conditions under water and the visual pigments that have evolved to detect objects in the light that is available, consideration must be given to the adaptations of the structure of the eye to underwater vision. Because of the high refractive index of water, the cornea is not available as a major refracting surface as it is in terrestrial vertebrates, but refraction is achieved through a spherical crystalline lens. The lens of fish and cephalopods forms an image that is clear of spherical and chromatic aberrations apparently by being composed of layers of continuously varying refractive index from 1.53 in the centre to a value close to that of water at the periphery. With such a lens and the large aperture (*f*/0.8), the eye is well adapted for detecting weak and small sources of light. In a theoretical, perfectly optically adjusted teleostean eye, the retina should form a hemispherical surface concentric with the spherical lens such that the ratio of the radius of the eye to the radius of the lens is 2.55 (Matthiessen's ratio).

8.6.1 Yellow lens and cornea

In many surface living diurnal fishes the lens has a yellow colouring which transmits light in the green to red part of the spectrum, but absorbs blue light with a sharp cut-off at about 400 nm. In bottom dwelling and deeper living fishes the lens tends not to be so yellow and can transmit light below 400 nm. However, in *Lepidorhombus bosci,* living below 100 m, the lens is transparent down to 310 nm, but *Chlorophthalmus agassizi,* which also is found below 100 m, has a cut-off point at 440 nm. Denton (1956) has suggested that since there is no ultra-violet light at depth the cut-off point of the lens is not significant, but that in surface fishes the nocturnal forms have lenses transparent to the ultra-violet while in predatory fishes the lenses tend to absorb these wavelengths.

The cephalopods also exhibit a similar relationship in that deep-sea squid have lenses transparent to ultra-violet light, while species that live in surface waters, such as *Onychoteuthis banksi,* have yellow lenses with a cut-off at about 430 nm. The *Histioteuthidae* is a group of squid which have one eye much larger than the other and the lens of the large eye is yellow in colour while that of the small eye is colourless. These squid migrate from the surface down to below 1000 m and it has been suggested that the large eye is adapted to surface vision, while the small eye is for deep water vision (Denton and Warren, 1968).

Many surface living teleosts also have a yellow colouring in the cornea which extends over the dorsal region of the cornea leaving the ventral section relatively clear. Surface living fishes are exposed to very large differences in light intensity between that penetrating downwards from the surface and the scattered light coming from below. The existence of the yellow dorsal 'eye shade' absorbing light preferentially from above will tend to even out this difference, though in *Coris julis* the optical density difference between the top and bottom of the cornea is only 0.9 log units or less, so that there will still be a considerable difference in retinal illumination (Moreland and Lythgoe, 1968).

8.6.2 Tubular eyes

In deep-sea fish, to quote Walls, '. . . everything possible has been done to increase the sensitivity of the eye to light'. The pupil and lens are relatively and absolutely enlarged, the cones have been eliminated from the retina (though it appears that there are some exceptions) and the rods have been stretched to great lengths and enormously multiplied.

In the majority of deep-sea species the eyeball maintains the normal form, but may attain a great size relative to the size of the head. However, there is a limit to the relative volume an eye could increase to without encroaching into other cephalic structures. In a number of fish this has been overcome by the development of tubular eyes. In such eyes the iris is reduced, with a main retina situated at the end of the tube and continuing over the sides of the tube to form an accessory retina (*Figure 8.12(a)*). Such eyes are found in eleven families, but are not related either to the form or the mode of life or to the regimen of the owners. They are a clear example of convergent evolution in that tubular eyes have been independently acquired in lineages that have evolved under the demands of similar environmental conditions.

As can be seen from *Figure 8.12(b),* the tubular eye is only a section of a large normal eye in which Matthiessen's ratio holds true, though the lens is nearly doubled in size from that expected in a theoretical fish eye with a retina of similar area to the main retina of the tubular eye. This has the effect of doubling the focal distance of the lens and radius of the retinal image, thus increasing the area of the retinal image by a factor of four. Using a tubular eye it is possible, therefore, to obtain a much higher resolving power of the main retina, though at the expense of any optical adjustment of the remaining accessory retina that will not be able to form an image. It should be pointed out that the illumination of the retina will be the same in either a small or a large eye.

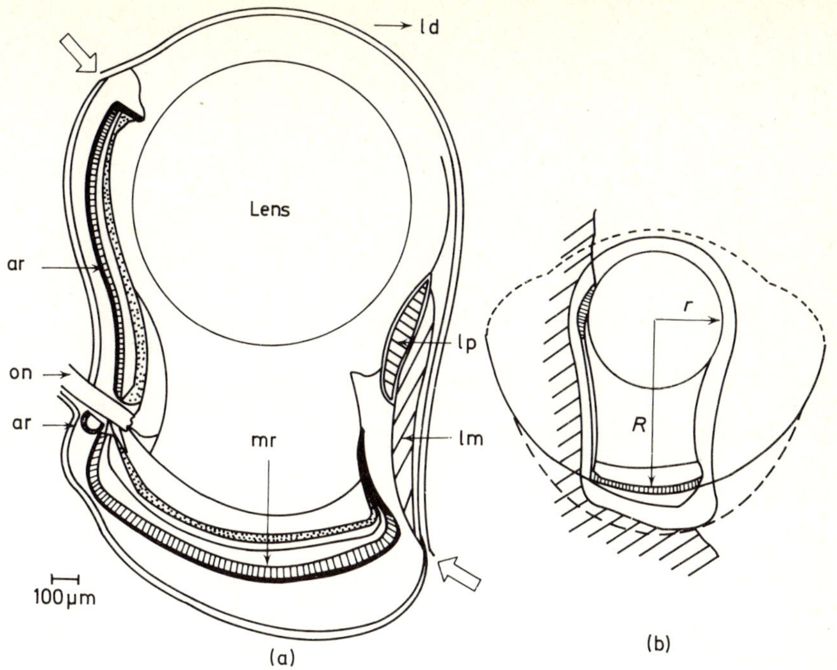

Figure 8.12 *(a) Diagram of a section through the dorsally directed tubular eye of* Scopelarchus guentheri. *Thick arrows point at limbus cornea. ar, accessory retina; ld, laterad; lm, lens muscle; lp, lens-pad; mr, main retina; on, optic nerve. (After Munk, 1966; courtesy Editor, Dana Reports). (b) Tubular eye of* Argyropelecus *superimposed upon outline (dotted) of a normally shaped eye of the same lens size where R = 2.55r. (After Walls, 1942; courtesy Cranbrook Institute of Sciences)*

Tubular eyes instil a further advantage in that they develop with the main axis of the two eyes parallel, either pointing anteriorly or dorsally. The fish thus achieve a high degree of binocularity that will give a better judgment of distance as well as probably achieving even more sensitivity. The tubular eye is also specialised for binocular vision in having an area temporalis or a fovea temporalis with a large rostral aphakic aperture anterior to the lens. In species where there is not a specific area, the temporal part of the retina is better developed in terms of an increased number of acromeres and the aphakic aperture is combined with sighting grooves in front of the eyes. Deep-sea fish are one of the few examples of animals with a pure rod area and not the typical photopic cone area of diurnal animals. Such an area may be of use if bioluminescent flashes merge to give a continuous background of light.

It has been demonstrated that in human vision the lowest illumination visible to the dark adapted eye is less by about 10% for binocular vision than for monocular vision. However, having tubular eyes with the main axis parallel reduces the field of view considerably which led Weale (1955) to ask whether 'binocularity in deep-sea fish was worth the price paid for it in terms of increased vulnerability because of the reduced visual field'. As he pointed out, mesopelagic and bathypelagic fish live in a light intensity range where light is at a premium and that intermediate to the monocular and binocular thresholds of vision is a finite intensity range where fused binocular vision is clearly an advantage. 'It is better to see a small field than not to see a large one.'

8.6.3 Retinal diverticula

A further interesting, if not confusing, feature of many tubular eyes is the presence of retinal diverticula. These are extensions from the main eye usually having a clear region of sclera through which to receive light. They may make up partially for the loss of visual field associated with tubular eyes. In *Rhynchohyalus natalensis* and *Opisthoproctus soleatus* the tubular eyes are dorsally directed, but they have a laterally directed diverticulum (*Figure 8.13(a)*), while in *Winteria telescopa,* which has rostrally and slightly dorsally directed eyes, the diverticulum is located rostrolaterally with a caudal window. The exact function of these diverticula is difficult to ascertain since *Gigantura,* which has rostrally directed eyes, has ventrally located diverticula that can only receive light via the roof of the mouth. However, many

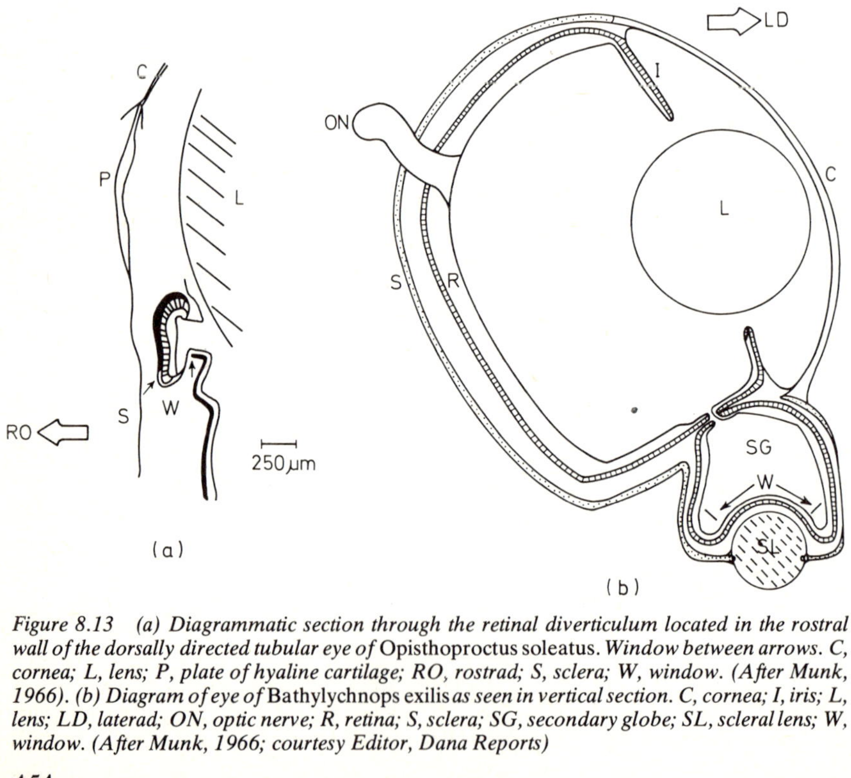

Figure 8.13 (a) Diagrammatic section through the retinal diverticulum located in the rostral wall of the dorsally directed tubular eye of Opisthoproctus soleatus. *Window between arrows. C, cornea; L, lens; P, plate of hyaline cartilage; RO, rostrad; S, sclera; W, window. (After Munk, 1966). (b) Diagram of eye of* Bathylychnops exilis *as seen in vertical section. C, cornea; I, iris; L, lens; LD, laterad; ON, optic nerve; R, retina; S, sclera; SG, secondary globe; SL, scleral lens; W, window. (After Munk, 1966; courtesy Editor, Dana Reports)*

tubular-eyed fishes do not have diverticula, yet their occurrence in the distantly related *Opisthoproctidae* and the *Giganturidae* suggests some common functional value.

In dealing with retinal diverticula, it is worth a moment to comment on the strange eye structure of the argentinoid, *Bathylychnops exilis.* It has a basically normal main eye that looks dorsally at an angle of about 35° to the perpendicular, but budded off from this ventrally is a diverticulum which is ventrally and slightly caudally directed. Unlike the diverticulum of tubular eyes, that of *Bathylychnops* has all the essential parts of an eye, including an approximately spherical lens derived from the scleral layers of the eye, that may perhaps concentrate light even to the extent of forming a crude image on the retina of the diverticulum (*Figure 8.13(b)*). Marshall has suggested that this diverticulum, which is provided with muscles, may be able to move over an arc below the main eye in order to follow luminescent organisms.

8.6.4 The deep-sea retina

Apart from these modifications in the basic eye design, what other methods are there for increasing the sensitivity of the eye? Denton and Warren (1957) pointed out that it is the efficiency with which the retina absorbs light quanta incident on it that is of the first importance. Clearly, at depth where light is at a premium, cones will be of little use and thus most species of deep-sea fish that have been examined have pure-rod retinae. To this, however, there is a notable exception, that of the alepisauroid, *Omosudis lowei,* which is a deep-sea fish with an almost pure cone retina according to Munk (1966), though the cones do have acromeres that are only slightly tapered. In the closely related species *Evermannella indica* there are also rod shaped acromeres, although the inner segments of the visual cells are more closely identified as cones. The transmutation theory of Walls (1942) suggests that from morphological studies of the reptilean retina, there was a systematic evolutionary relationship, a phylogenetic transmutation of visual cell types from cones found in diurnal lizards, through the intermediate cells of the nocturnal lizards to the rods of the nocturnal geckos. Munk is of the opinion that the retinae of *Omosudis* and *Evermannella* have cones which are in the process of transmutation to rods and that these fishes may have originated from species with cone rich retinae, but that have adapted themselves to the deep-sea environment by such a transmutation. In view of the fascinating problems of the visual pigments of the geckos in relation to the transmutation theory (for review, *see* Crescitelli, 1972), a study of the pigments of these deep-sea fish would be of great interest in adding physiological evidence to the morphological data of Munk.

A further means of increasing the quantal absorbing properties of the eye is to increase the amount of visual pigment within the receptor cells. In studies by Denton and his co-workers (Denton and Warren, 1957; Denton and Nicol, 1964), it has been demonstrated that in deep-sea teleosts the optical density of the visual pigment was as high as 1.0 or more, i.e. the pigment would absorb about 90% of the blue-green light incident upon it.

This may be compared to that of the human rod in which the optical density of rhodopsin is about 0.15, which will absorb only about 30% of the incident light, giving the deep-sea fish a three-fold advantage. Denton and Nicol (1964) have also shown that there is a reasonable correlation between the length of the rod outer segment and the density of the visual pigment. Thus, in deep-sea fish one would expect to find long rod acromeres.

In a number of deep-sea fishes the pure rod retinae have two or more regularly superposed layers of equally long acromeres, viz. *Bathylagus* spp., *Bathylychnops exilis, Winteria telescopa, Astronesthes niger* (Figure 8.14). These layers of rod acromeres occur within several groups of teleosts. In the argentinoids, *Winteria,* there are three layers of acromeres with an overall length of 86 μm, while *Bathylychnops* has up to six layers. However, in *Opisthoproctus* and *Rhynchohyalus* there is only a single layer of acromeres about 36 μm long. In the diverticulum of these species the acromeres are reduced to 7 μm. The greatest depth of acromeres so far recorded is in the area temporalis of the argentinoid *Bathylagus pacificus* where there are six layers with an overall length of 200 μm. These layers are reduced to three with an overall length of 70 μm in the central part of the fundusretina. In comparison, in the clupeoid, *Platytroctegen mirus,* the foveal rod acromeres

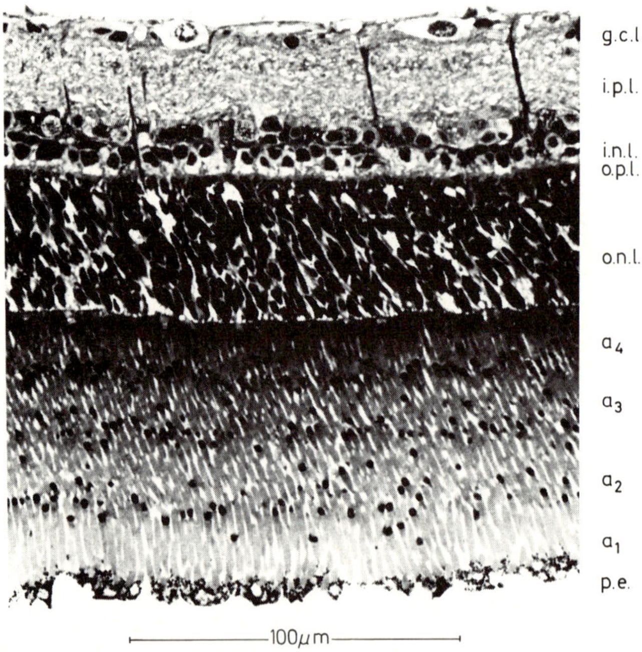

Figure 8.14 Photomicrograph of a section of deep-sea fish retina showing 4 layers of rod acromeres of Astronesthes niger. *The well stained inner segments of the rods clearly show the multibanked outer segments. p.e., pigment epithelium; a_1–a_4, layers of rod acromeres with dark stained inner segments; o.n.l., outer nuclear layer; o.p.l., outer plexiform layer; i.n.l., inner nuclear layer; i.p.l., inner plexiform layer; g.c.l., ganglion cell layer. (By kind permission of N. A. Locket)*

reached a length of 200 μm with only a single layer. Such a length of acromere will, according to the relationship demonstrated by Denton, have an optical density approaching 2.0 which would absorb about 99% of the light incident upon it.

A further effect of increasing the optical density of the visual pigment is to considerably broaden the absorptance* spectrum of the pigment. As shown in *Figure 8.15(a),* as the optical density increases the absorptance of the pigment flattens over the peak maximum absorbing region so that a pigment with an optical density of 2.0 will absorb 90% or more of the incident light over a spectral range of approximately 100 nm. Thus not only is the pigment highly efficient at absorbing light quanta at its λ_{max}, but also over a considerable spectral range on either side. In fact, a $P480_1$, a pigment typical of deep-sea fish with an optical density of 2.0, will absorb 90% or more of the incident light over the spectral range from about 425 to 522 nm. Similarly, a $P480_1$ with an optical density of 1.0 will absorb 85% or more of the incident light from about 453 to 504 nm (*Figure 8.15(b)*).

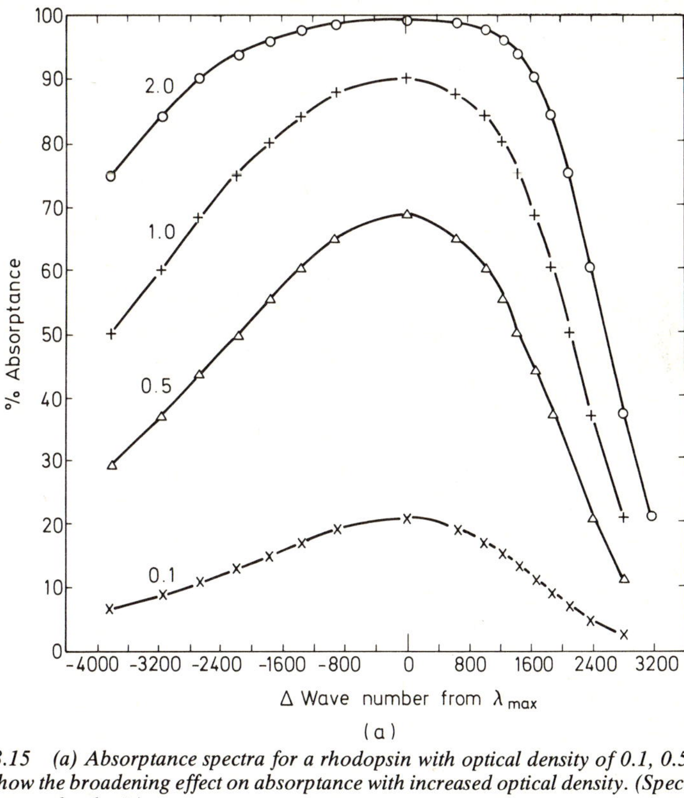

Figure 8.15 (a) Absorptance spectra for a rhodopsin with optical density of 0.1, 0.5, 1.0 and 2.0, to show the broadening effect on absorptance with increased optical density. (Spectra drawn on a wavenumber basis).

**Absorptance* is defined as the fraction of incident light absorbed by the pigment, i.e. $(I_i - I_t)/I_i$, where I_i is the incident light and I_t the transmitted light and is to be distinguished from *absorbance,* or optical density, defined as $\log I_i/I_t$. Absorbance spectra have shapes independent of concentration whereas absorptance spectra become broader with increasing concentration.

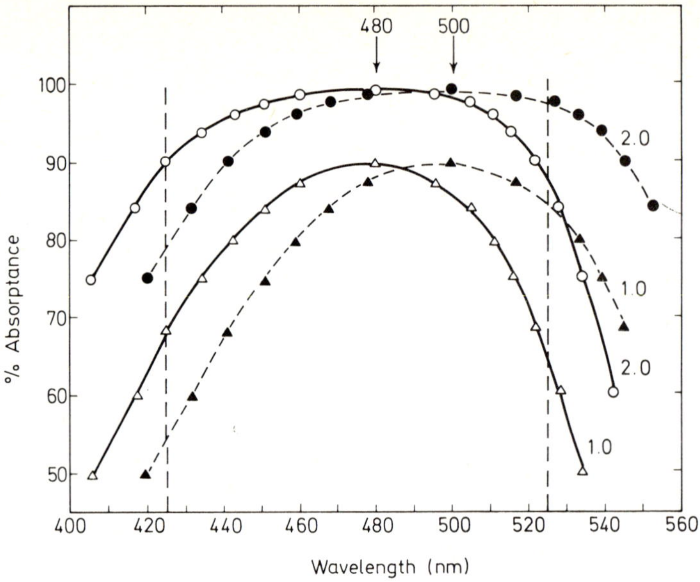

(b)

Figure 8.15 (b) Absorptance spectra of $P480_1$ (open symbols and $P500_1$ (closed symbols) of optical density 1.0 and 2.0, compared to the spectral window of light (between vertical dashed lines) available at depth in the ocean to illustrate the advantage of a $P480_1$ over a $P500_1$

The presence of visual pigments with optical densities as high as those of deep-sea fish has an interesting effect on the sensitivity hypothesis. The hypothesis suggests that the λ_{max} of the pigment is blue shifted to increase its sensitivity to the ambient light at depth, but a visual pigment with a λ_{max} at 500 nm and an optical density of 1.0 will absorb 87.9% of the incident light at 480 nm as compared to 90% absorptance by a $P480_1$. If the λ_{max} is determined by natural selection it must be assumed that the 2% difference in the absorptance of light is highly advantageous with respect of the survival of the fish. However, the spectral range from 425 to 528 nm (90% or more absorptance for a $P480_1$ with an optical density of 2.0) is precisely the envelope of spectral light available at depth in the ocean. As can be seen from *Figure 8.15(b)*, although the λ_{max} is not important in terms of absorptance at 480 nm, it is significant in matching the total absorptance of the pigment to the spectral range of the ambient light, an important consideration in an environment where light is at a premium.

A further fascinating feature of some deep-sea fish retinae has been described by Locket (1970). In the tubular-eyed alepisauroid fish, *Scopelarchus*, the main retina is divided into two sections. Anteriorly the retina is similar to other deep-sea retinae, but in the posterior region the receptor cells are grouped together in bunches of about 23 cells which are surrounded by projections of the pigment epithelial cells. In the projections surrounding the receptors are flat crystals presumably of guanine which are arranged parallel to the surface of the cell and with their long axis running along the length of the surface. The crystals are about 65 nm thick and arranged so that they will give maximum reflectance at about 476 nm (see later in the discussion of silvery surfaces in fishes). This wavelength is coincident with the spectral maximum of light at depth in the ocean and with the λ_{max} of deep-sea fish rhodopsins, though no data are available for the rhodopsin of *Scopelarchus* itself.

As a result of the isolating effect of the tapetum each group of 23 cells can be considered as a macro-receptor some 35 μm across and spaced in a lattice of 46 μm between centres. Locket (1970) further found that at the level of the inner segment of the receptors, all the cells were interconnected by tight junctions, suggesting the possibility that the cells function as a single unit. Such a system, with grouped receptors surrounded by a reflecting surface so that any light passing through the retina which is not absorbed by the visual pigment will be reflected back into the outer segments, and in which the individual receptor cells are linked together, will have a much increased sensitivity over single receptors, while the lattice of the macro-receptors may also permit some type of crude form discrimination.

A further way of increasing the sensitivity of the retina, albeit with a considerable decrease in the resolving power, is by increasing the summation of adjacent visual cells connected to the bipolar cells and hence to the ganglion cells in the retina. However, counts made by Munk (1966) do not show conclusively whether this occurs, though it is possible that insufficient numbers of teleosts have been studied with satisfactory care.

All of the above discussion has dealt exclusively with teleostean eyes, but in many of the cartilagenous fishes the problem has been overcome in a different way. In many chondrichthys a tapetum lucidum is present that consists of reflecting plates containing guanine crystals. A tapetum is also present in many bony fishes and has been shown to occur in 28 families of *Holostei* and *Teleostei*. Several different types have been identified consisting of lipid and pteridine containing structures as well as guanine crystal formations (Nicol, Arnott and Best, 1973).

Denton and Nicol (1964) have shown that the guanine plates of elasmobranchs are orientated around the eye in such a way as to be perpendicular to the incident light, in order that any light that is not absorbed by the visual cells in its double passage through the retina will either be reflected directly back out of the eye or absorbed by the melanophores located in the back of the iris (*Figure 8.16(a)*). If stray light were reflected on to other parts of the retina it would have the effect of diminishing the sharpness of the visual image. The retinae of most elasmobranchs are rod dominated and to increase the sensitivity of the eye to the dim light at depth in the ocean, instead of increasing the length of the rod acromeres or by layering them, the tapetum doubles the effective length of the rod outer segment. Denton and Nicol (1964) have measured the spectral reflectivity of the tapeta of a number of elasmobranchs and found that over the spectral range 400 to 600 nm the reflectivity is reasonably uniform and as high as 80 to 90%. The maximum reflectivity occurs in the region of 480 to 500 nm and is, therefore, in the spectral region of the maximum absorbance of the rhodopsins found in deep-sea fish. (The

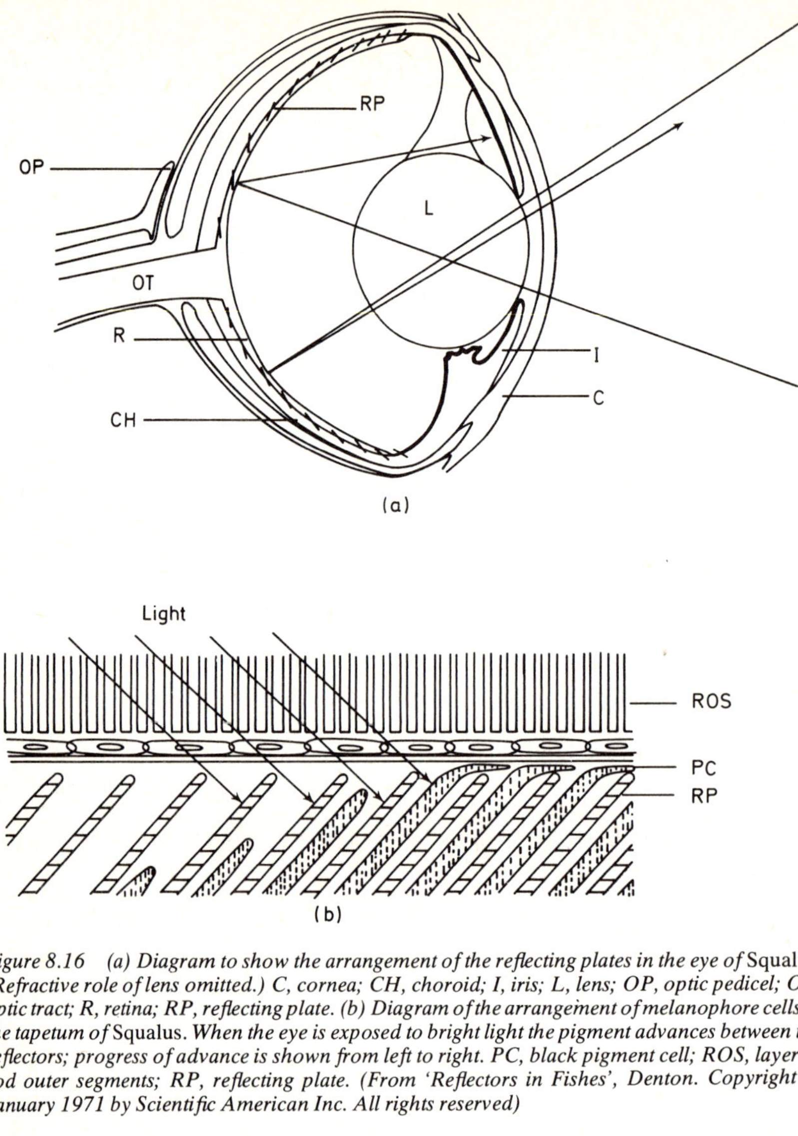

Figure 8.16 (a) Diagram to show the arrangement of the reflecting plates in the eye of Squalus. *(Refractive role of lens omitted.) C, cornea; CH, choroid; I, iris; L, lens; OP, optic pedicel; OT, optic tract; R, retina; RP, reflecting plate. (b) Diagram of the arrangement of melanophore cells in the tapetum of* Squalus. *When the eye is exposed to bright light the pigment advances between the reflectors; progress of advance is shown from left to right. PC, black pigment cell; ROS, layer of rod outer segments; RP, reflecting plate. (From 'Reflectors in Fishes', Denton. Copyright © January 1971 by Scientific American Inc. All rights reserved)*

properties of the guanine reflecting plates are discussed later with respect to silvery sided fishes.)

In the surface living elasmobranch, *Squalus acanthus,* the optical density of the visual pigment is about 0.22, with the outer segment length of 28 μm. In the deep-sea sharks, *Centroscymnus coelolepis, Centrophorus squamosus* and *Deania calcea,* the outer segment lengths were 45, 48 and 43 μm, respectively with the optical density of the visual pigment ranging from 0.60 in *Deania* to 0.47 in *Centrophorus.* These values are low when compared to deep-sea teleosts such as *Winteria,* with acromeres of 86 μm and *Bathylagus* with 200 μm of acromere layers. However, the 90% reflectivity of the elasmobranch tapetum will almost double the effective length of the acromeres so that the light absorbed will increase from about 70% of the incident light up to about 90%, which is similar to many deep-sea teleosts.

A problem that is associated with the tapetum lucidum is that in bright light conditions the light reflected out of the eye by the tapetum will cause 'eyeshine', making the fish conspicuous to both predator and prey. To prevent this the fish has a screening device consisting of melanophores located behind the reflecting plates (*Figure 8.16(b)*). In bright light the melanophores migrate in between the plates where they will absorb the incident light that has passed through the retina and prevent its reflection out of the eye.

8.7 POLARISED LIGHT

A feature of underwater light that at depth becomes uniform is the plane of polarisation of the light. In clear oceanic water the maximum degree of polarisation is between 20 and 60% and it might be expected that animals living in this environment would be adapted to utilise the electric vector of the polarised light. According to Waterman (1966), specific effects of polarised light have been reported in twenty-six species of crustaceans and a number of cephalopod molluscs.

As with having to isolate colour discrimination from intensity discrimination, it is necessary to assess whether an animal can consistently discriminate direction and intensity of illumination from polarisation. To separate these two responses can be extremely difficult because artifacts resulting from differential reflection and refraction as well as differential scattering can convert patterns of simple polarised irradiance into highly complex patterns including intensity distributions. Nevertheless, it has been shown that many crustaceans and cephalopods can perceive the plane of linearly polarised light as a distinct stimulus parameter.

Polarised light can be detected by crustaceans and cephalopods as a result of the basic arrangement of their eyes. In the compound eye one ommatidium (*Figure 8.17*) is the functional unit in image perception but contains, in the usual seven retinular cells, independent components that can detect other visual parameters such as polarisation. Light detection including *e*-vector detection is restricted to the rhabdomeres consisting of closely packed stacks of microvilli which extend axially from the retinular cells and it is the dichroism of the visual pigment molecules contained within these microvilli which provides the molecular basis for the detection of polarised light. As in the vertebrate receptor cell where the visual pigment molecules are aligned with their major dichroic axis in a predominantly transverse plane, the visual pigment in the microvilli of invertebrate receptors has its dichroic axis aligned parallel to the long axis of the microvilli which are, in turn, closely parallel to one another. Such an arrangement will form at the cellular level a unit dichroic analyser with the

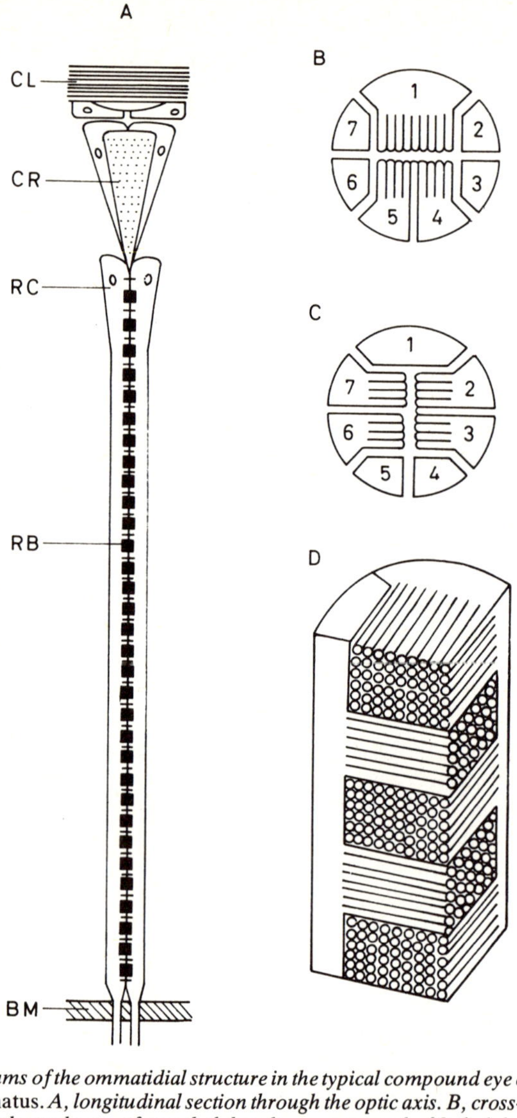

Figure 8.17 Diagrams of the ommatidial structure in the typical compound eye of the swimming crab, Callinectes ornatus. *A, longitudinal section through the optic axis. B, cross-section through the retinula showing the make-up of one rhabdom layer composed of 3 rhabdomeres; a double sized one from retinular cell 1 and two regular quarter rhabdomeres from cells 4 and 5. C, cross-section of an adjacent rhabdom with their microvilli orientated at 90° to those in the adjacent layer. The rhabdomeres are derived from the other four retinular cells 2, 3, 6 and 7. D, stereo-diagram showing rhabdom-layered structure with regular closed packed microvilli with their long axes all parallel in one set of alternate layers and perpendicular to their counterparts in the other set. BM, basilar membrane; CL, corneal lens; CR, crystalline cone; RB, rhabdom; RC, retinular cell. (After Eguchi and Waterman, 1966; courtesy Pergamon Press Ltd)*

maximum optical density to photons vibrating in the direction parallel to the microvillus.

In most of the crustaceans and cephalopods the microvilli in all rhabdomeres are orientated in only two directions at right angles to each other. In selective adaptation experiments it has been shown that the maximum sensitivity to polarised light is in the same direction as the microvilli observed in electron microscopy and these directions correspond with the vertical and horizontal axes of the animal's normal spatial orientation. The seven retinular cells of a single decapod ommatidium are divided into two sub-groups of four and three cells respectively so that *e*-vector detection depends on a two channel system consisting of a pair of dichroic analysers with their major transmitting axes perpendicular to each other, determined by the two directions of microvillus orientation (*Figure 8.17*). A similar retinular pattern has been identified in the cephalopods.

The action spectra for polarotaxis have been measured in few animals, but in *Daphnia* (Waterman, 1966), there is a significant response between 360 and 580 nm with a peak sensitivity at about 440 nm having a relatively sharp fall off on either side, but with a second response shoulder in the blue-green at about 500 nm. The λ_{max} at 440 nm is close to the λ_{max} of natural polarisation of clear blue sky which is at about 460 nm. However, underwater polarisation is not very sensitive to wavelength of maximum transmission of water. The visual action spectra for phototaxis in *Daphnia* have a peak in the region of 530 to 540 nm, so that clearly phototaxis and polarotaxis are governed by different visual channels involving cells with different wavelengths of maximal sensitivity. How these features are related to visual pigment absorption and to neuronal interactions is at present unknown and there is clearly scope for further research in this field.

Although there is very clear evidence for orientation behaviour in response to polarised light within the invertebrates, there is little evidence for such responses in the fishes. The vertebrate eye is not adapted for the detection of polarised light and could only be used for such detection if a polarising filter were present. In some fishes, such as the herring, it has been shown that the adipose eye-lid is birefringent (Blaxter and Jones, 1967) and may act as a polarising filter, though the ability of the filter to analyse or polarise light is weak and thus any detection of polarised light is probably inefficient. However, Lythgoe and Hemmings (1967) have shown that selective absorption of polarised patterns of underwater light can aid in extending the visual range.

Although underwater space light is plane polarised most natural objects tend to depolarise the light reflected from them such that if an object is viewed horizontally underwater through a rotating polarising filter the apparent brightness of the background will fluctuate more than the object. As was discussed when dealing with the contrast hypothesis, when the inherent contrast is at a maximum, the apparent contrast of an object will fall to the level of perception at a greater range than when the inherent contrast is at a minimum. Thus if the inherent contrast is increased by the use of a polarising filter an object would be visible at a greater range than if viewed without the filter. Such a situation would clearly have selective advantages, but no evidence is available to suggest that fish actually utilise their adipose eye-lids in such a way.

8.8 BODY CAMOUFLAGE — SILVERY SIDED FISHES

Having considered how a fish can improve its chances of detecting objects in the water under the limiting light conditions, space must be given to the opposing problem that faces an animal in this environment and that is 'how not to be visually detected', i.e. body camouflage. It is not the purpose of this chapter to discuss the individual body colourations such as are found in reef fish, but rather to discuss the general condition of pelagic fish. One of the most striking features of epipelagic and mesopelagic fish is the silvery sheen that covers the sides of the body and it is this that is used to merge the fish into its background.

To make an object invisible it is necessary that the light reflected by the surface of the object be identical in brightness and spectral distribution to that of the ambient light coming from behind the object. As has been pointed out the ambient light underwater is primarily directed downwards from the surface and is symmetrical about a vertical plane, but that diffuse light will be scattered upwards such that the ratio of the relative radiance of light at a point directed downwards to light directed upwards is approximately 200:1. Thus an object viewed from above will, if a perfect mirror, reflect about 200 times that of the background radiance and will be, therefore, highly visible. To be invisible from this direction the object must in some way reduce the reflectance of the surface. Considering the vertical sides of a square object, an observer below and to the side will be unable to detect the object if the side of the object acts as a plane mirror, as is shown in *Figure 8.18(a)*. Clearly, an observer directly below an object looking upwards will see the silhouette of the object against the bright downward directed radiance. No system of surface mirrors will be able to remove this problem.

A fish is able to reduce the area of its silhouette by modifying its body shape. A fish of circular cross section will cast a much larger shadow than a fish of the same cross-sectional area, but flattened in the vertical plane (*Figure 8.18(b)* and (c)). However, to be a good swimmer, a fish requires a circular cross section and so many fish have compromised their cross section as shown in *Figure 8.18(d)* and arranged their reflecting plates more closely to the vertical than to the sides of the body. Even so, the ventrally inclined surfaces of the fish will still project the reflected light over a wider area than the incident light, thus appearing darker than the background. To reduce reflectivity upwards from the dorsal surface of the fish, the vertically orientated plates in that region will allow light to pass between individual plates and be absorbed by the dark pigment layers in the dermis to such an extent that the reflected light from the surface will match the upwelling background radiance (*Figure 8.18(d)*).

The position is further complicated though by the tapering of the fish's body from behind the head towards the tail. Over the region of the body the

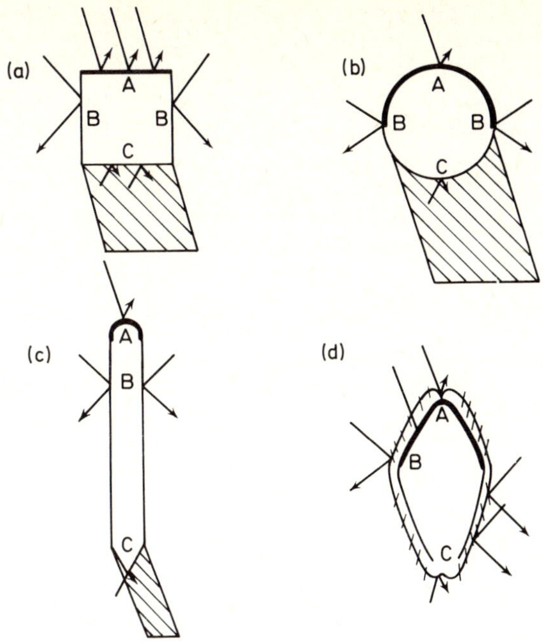

Figure 8.18 The reflection of light from objects of different cross-sectional shape, but of similar area. (A) Light of high intensity from above absorbed by the pigmentation of the dorsal surface. (B) Light of less intensity from the side is reflected by the mirrored lateral surfaces. (C) Light of low intensity coming from below insufficient to overcome shadow. The square and circular cross-sections cast a much greater shadow than the flattened shape and the cross-section of the fish illustrates how the problem of shadow is partially overcome. For full details see text. (Modified from 'Reflectors in Fishes', Denton. Copyright © January 1971 by Scientific American Inc. All rights reserved)

plates, though vertical, are arranged so that their reflecting surfaces face posteriorly while the platelets on the head region face anteriorly. This arrangement has the effect that for an observer below and behind the fish the ratio of reflected light to incident light will be closer to unity so that the fish will be a better match for the background. The fish will, of course, still be clearly visible from directly below. In terms of the visual field of a fish such an arrangement is desirable since, although the visual fields of the fish's eyes overlap anteriorly, there are blind areas behind the fish and it is from this direction that the fish is well camouflaged.

The reflectors in fish, whether silvery scales, the tapetum lucidum of elasmobranchs or the reflectors of the complex photophores of luminescent fish, are composed of alternate layers of high and low refractive index. The layers of high refractive index are made of crystals ranging in shape from oblongs to needles composed of guanine and hypoxanthine with a refractive index of 1.83. These layers are separated by regions of low refractive index 1.33 composed of cytoplasm.

Theoretical studies have shown that the highest reflectivity can be obtained at a given wavelength λ_0, together with the widest waveband of high reflectivity, if the alternating layers of high and low refractive index have an optical thickness (the actual thickness times the refractive index) of ¼ λ_o. In the herring the plates in the lateral scales are about 70 nm thick giving an optical thickness of 128 nm which will give a maximum reflectivity at 512 nm. Similarly, in the horse mackerel, *Trachurus trachurus,* the green reflecting plates range from 66 to 86 nm in thickness giving a mean value of 556 nm at which maximum reflectivity will occur (Denton and Land, 1971).

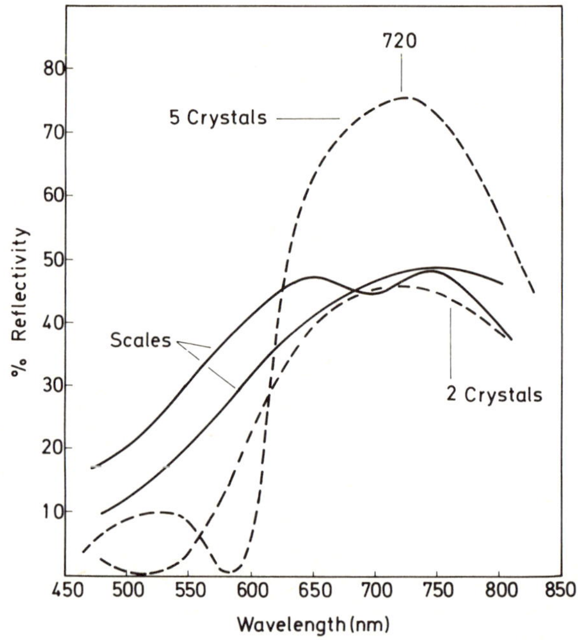

Figure 8.19 Spectral reflectivity of two scales (full lines) from the most ventral line of scales of juvenile Clupea sprattus *compared to the theoretical reflectivity of 2 and 5 stacks of crystals (dashed lines) whose individual optical thickness gives maximum reflectivity at 720 nm. (After Denton and Land, 1971; courtesy The Royal Society)*

As the number of layers in a platelet increases the reflectivity increases and an ideal stack of only five crystals will reflect up to 75% of the light that strikes it over a spectral range covering more than a third of the visible spectrum (*Figure 8.19*). Stacks of guanine and cytoplasm reflect well through a spectral range of over $\lambda_o \pm 10\%$, where λ_o is the ideal wavelength. However, in the spurdog, *Squalus acanthias,* and the dogfish, *Scyliorhinus canicula,* reflectivity of the tapetum lucidum is from 60 to 90% over the entire visible spectrum. This is possibly due to a random distribution of the thickness of either the guanine or the cytoplasm, though more probably to a systematic change in the thickness of the layers through the stack. In the tapetum of *S. canicula,* the reflectivity peaks at about 520 nm and the thickness of the layers varies from 66 to 80 nm, giving a mean value for the theoretical maximum reflectivity of 534 nm. Similarly, in *Squalus acanthias* the peak reflectivity has been measured at 470 nm and the reflecting layers have a mean thickness of 66 nm which will give a (theoretical) maximum reflectivity at about 483 nm.

The colour reflected by a stack of crystals is not due to the absorption of light, but to interference colours. In a single fish scale, viewed in white light, several bright regions of contrasting colours can be seen, but on the fish the scales overlap so that light which passes one layer will be reflected by another. In this way the final reflected light is composed of many wavelengths and thus appears silvery.

In the cephalopods silvery reflecting layers are found around the eyes and ink sacs and, in oceanic squid, along the flanks and, as in teleosts, as reflecting layers in photophores. However, the reflecting layers are somewhat different from fish in not having guanine crystals. The high refractive index layers have a refractive index of 1.56 in *Loligo forbesi* and *Sepia elegans* and this is compatible with chitin, though as yet no chemical tests have been carried out. Nevertheless, the same ¼ wave plate system occurs such that in the reflectors in the eyelids of *Sepia elegans* the layers have a thickness of 82 to 94 nm, giving an ideal reflected wavelength in the region of 550 nm. In *Loligo,* the green reflectors at the side of the eye have layers 82 to 113 nm thick with a maximum reflectivity around 580 nm, while the red reflectors of the eyelid are thicker ranging from 102 to 137 nm with a peak reflectivity at about 770 nm (Denton and Land, 1971).

Amongst mesopelagic fish silvery flanks are found within the gonostomatids, the hatchet-fish and the lantern-fishes. According to Marshall (1971) more than 100 of the some 750 species of mesopelagic fish have developed silvery flanks and most of these fish have small mouths and feed on zooplankton. Fish not possessing such silvery sides are usually dark coloured or black and include the elasmobranchs which tend to be predator species. At night many of the silvery sided fish will spend hours feeding in the upper waters where flashes of luminescence will cause them to expose their mirror-like sides. Black-skinned predators do not suffer from this drawback. Similarly, the mid-water predacious squid are also dark bodied.

Body colouration in the deep-sea crustaceans also gives an illustration of selective pressures within the environment. Most are red coloured which, in view of the monochromatic blue light available at depth in the ocean, will make them almost invisible since little or no light will be reflected from them.

8.9 BIOLUMINESCENCE

The problems of seeing and not being seen in the mesopelagic regions of the ocean are related not only to eye structure and body camouflage, but, as has been briefly referred to previously, also to bioluminescence, perhaps the most striking feature of marine life.

At depths where only weak surface light is received, bioluminescence contributes a significant portion of the total light present. In general, bioluminescence can be recorded at all depths investigated at night and, during the day, at depths where daylight does not interfere. At night, in the Atlantic off New York, for example, the frequency of luminescent flashes reached a maximum at two distinct depths (Clarke and Hubbard, 1959). At about 100 m the flashes reached over 260 per min and at 900 m there was a secondary maximum of 90 flashes per min, though flashes were recorded down to a depth of 3750 m. During the day, flashes at a rate of 110 per min were recorded at 900 m. The brightest flashes measured were in the order of 10^{-3} $\mu W/cm^2$ and lasted for up to one second, but could overlap to give continuous light for up to 10 s. The greatest depth at which bioluminescence has been recorded is 7200 m.

Efforts to photograph the organisms responsible for luminescence have revealed few macroscopic animals which suggests that the layering in the ocean recorded in luminescence studies is due chiefly to very small organisms. It has also been shown that nearly all of the luminescent organisms in the surface waters and at depth could be pumped through 240 μm aperture netting. Thus, only bacteria, dinoflagellates or radiolarians could cause the luminescence and, in face, dinoflagellates are the only planktonic organism common enough to explain the ubiquity of luminescence in the ocean (for review, *see* Tett and Kally, 1973).

The identification of luminescent 'layers' in the ocean indicates the presence of different populations of bioluminescent organisms at various depths, but the factors that dictate these layers are not easy to define. All that can be said is that bioluminescence is greatest in and near the euphotic zone because of the dinoflagellate populations and that there is usually some layering of luminescent organisms at greater depths.

The significance of dinoflagellate bioluminescence in terms of an adaptive function is difficult to explain. Because of the considerable cellular organisation required for the control of luminescence that clearly implies an evolutionary selectivity, the luminescence must have some survival value. Since the peak of the luminescence spectrum is at 480 nm, which corresponds to the wavelength of maximum transmission of light in oceanic water and also the maximum sensitivity of the visual pigments of a number of marine animals, one result of the luminescence of dinoflagellates is to allow visual responses by other organisms. One feature of concentrations of dinoflagellates whose luminescence may be stimulated by contact is that a larger organism passing through such a population will leave a streak of light behind it that will accurately trace its passage.

So far as is known, luminescence in fishes is restricted to the marine species, both elasmobranchs and teleosts. It is also found in the cephalopods and crustaceans. According to Harvey (1952) some two-thirds of all the species of fishes found in mesopelagic waters exhibit bioluminescence and these fishes add up to about 90% of the total fish population found in this region. In catches of mesopelagic fish taken off Bermuda, luminescent cyclothones accounted for 82% of the individual fishes with the myctophids (lantern-fish) making up the next 10%. Similar figures have been obtained from the eastern Pacific.

The light organs of mesopelagic fish occur in a great variety of locations, but are generally found on the ventral side of the animals. In many *Isospondylii* the photophores are regularly arranged in rows along the lower surface of the body, e.g. *Cyclothone* and the lantern-fish. In the angler-fishes (*Caratioidea*) all but two of the eighty odd species have a luminous gland possessed by the females and carried on a tentacle formed from the dorsal fin rays (illicium). Some of the stomiatoid fish have a large light organ behind each eye, while luminous organs can also be found on the jaws or even within the mouth as in the stomiatoid, *Dactylostomias*.

The structure of photophores is very variable from simple forms consisting of a mass of photocytes with or without a mantle of pigment cells (*Figure 8.20 (a)*), to highly complex tubular structures having dioptric accessories of lenses, reflectors and sometimes with filters. The simple photophores are found in selachians and also superficially in the dermis of many stomiatoid fishes. In *Chauliodus* the whole body is covered with several thousand photophores causing the whole body to glow. The more complex photophores are found close to the eyes of many stomiatoid fish and also make up the ventral photophores. Some complex photophores, such as the sub-ocular light organ of the stomiatoid, *Astronesthes,* have musculature that can rotate the entire photophore into a pigment lined pocket so as to cut off the light emission (*Figure 8.20(b)*).

The reflectors found in complex photophores, such as in *Porichthys,* are composed of cells lying tangentially to the curvature of the photophore and these cells contain platelets of guanine arranged in piles parallel to the surface of the reflector and are similar to the tapetum lucidum of elasmobranch eyes and the silvery flanks of fishes.

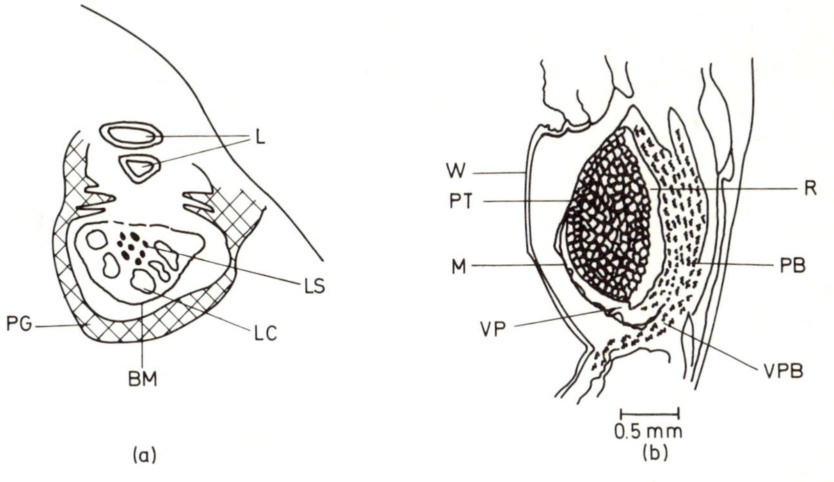

Figure 8.20 (a) Diagrammatic section through the simple photophore of a shark, Spinax niger. *BM, basement membrane; L, lens cells; LC, luminous cells; LS, luminous secretions; PG, melanophores. (Modified from Nicol, 1969). (b) Diagrammatic transverse section through the subocular light organ of* Astronesthes richardsoni. *M, muscle; PB, pigment backing; PT, photogenic tissue; R, reflector; VP, ventral pocket; VPB, ventral pigment; W, clear window. (After Nicol, 1969; courtesy Academic Press)*

The luminescence produced by the photophores can be generalised as a blue-green or blue light with a peak emission about 470 nm with half of the energy lying between about 435 and 530 nm. Harvey has listed the colours from photophores, but relatively few spectral emission curves are available. Those for *Myctophum punctatum* (a lantern-fish) and the euphausid, *Euphasia pacificus,* are shown in *Figure 8.21* together with the absorbance spectrum for the rhodopsin extracted from the eyes of *Myctophum* which has a λ_{max} at about 485 nm. It is clear that the general emission spectrum of luminescence is matched to the maximum transmission wavelength of oceanic water, which is at about 475 nm and similarly matched to the absorbance spectrum of deep-sea rhodopsins which range from 477 to 490 nm.

Although the luminescence of marine animals can be generalised as blue-green, many animals emit light ranging from blue through to deep red and these variations are brought about by coloured filters covering the photophores. One such example is the small deep-sea squid, *Lycoteuthis diadema,* that is found at depths around 2500 m. This animal displays a

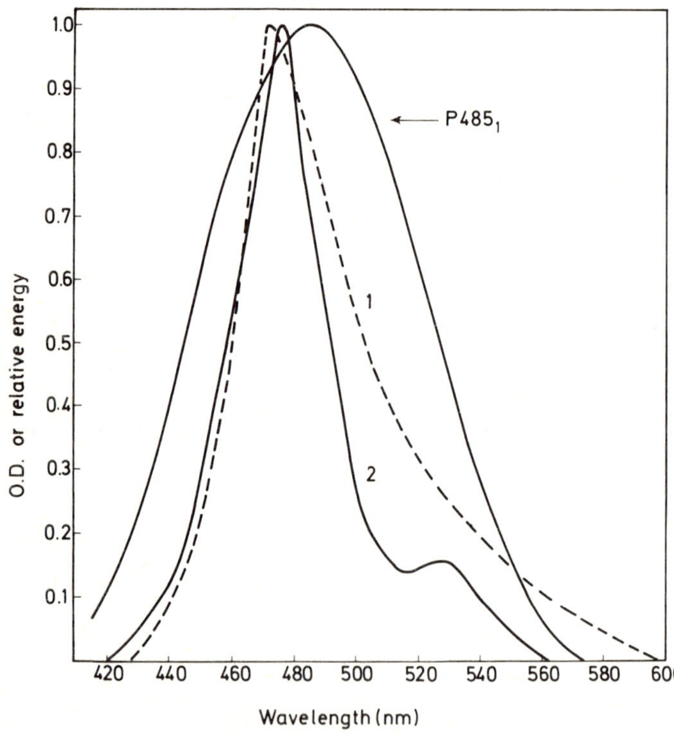

Figure 8.21 Spectral emission curves for the bioluminescence of Myctophum punctatum *(dashed line, 1) (Nicol, 1960) and* Euphasia pacificus *(solid line, 2) (Kampa and Boden, 1957), compared with the absorption spectrum of the P485$_1$ of* Myctophum *(Denton and Warren, 1957). Curves normalised to optical density or relative energy of 1.0*

variety of lights described by Chun as follows: 'The middle organs of the eye shone with ultra-marine light, the lateral ones with a pearly sheen. Those towards the front of the lower surface gave out a ruby-red light, while those behind were snow white or pearly, except the median one which was sky blue'. This is certainly a fine array of lights for a creature only about 10 cm long!

Recently Denton and his colleagues (Denton, Gilpin-Brown and Wright, 1970) have reported that the mesopelagic fish, *Pachystomias,* emits, from photophores close to the eye, bright flashes of red light that are produced by a filter of red tissue. In this species the maximum retinal absorbance is not around 485 nm as in most deep-sea fishes, but at 575 nm with an optical density close to 1.0. *Pachystomias* is thus highly adapted to its predacious existance as most deep-sea fish are highly insensitive to red light, though their degree of insensitivity would depend on the broadness of the spectral emission of the photophore. *Pachystomias* will, however, be exceptionally sensitive to the bioluminescence from others of the same species.

In addition O'Day and Fernandez (1974) have identified two visual pigments in *Aristostomias scintillans* (*Malacosteidae*), one absorbing at about 551 nm and based on 3-dehydroretinal and a second absorbing at 526 nm, but based on retinal. *Aristostomias* is similar to *Pachystomias* in having a red-light emitting suborbital photophore, but in addition, it has a postorbital green-emitting photophore. Clearly its two visual pigments are beautifully matched to these lights with the lower wavelength pigment being satisfactory for detecting the blue space light and other blue-green bioluminescence.

With the knowledge of the close correlation between the light emission and the visual pigment absorbance of *Pachystomias* and *Aristostomias,* it is interesting to speculate about the squid *Lycoteuthis.* Does it, too, like *Pachystomias,* have a red sensitive pigment in order to recognise members of its own species, or is the 'ruby-red' light for other predacious species to see and to avoid? Unfortunately, information of this kind is not available and little is known about the absorption properties of the visual pigments of deep-sea squid.

Denton has suggested the the red light of *Pachystomias* may be used as a type of 'snooperscope' so that they can see their prey without being seen. Such a suggestion requires that the light emitted can be directed into a beam. Such a situation has been seen to occur in a stomiatoid fish. According to reports, '. . . a 9–12 in fish was seen feeding at night on krill by directing two beams of strong blue light directly forward for a distance of two feet. The fish, lying 2–6 ft below the surface and at an angle of 35–40° from the horizontal, would snap at the euphasids caught in its "head lights" '.

It was mentioned earlier that many of the mesopelagic fish have rows of ventrally directed photophores, especially marked in the hatchet-fishes. Clarke (1963) has suggested that the function of these photophores is to obliterate the shadow cast by the animal in the downward radiating ambient light. As was described, by the careful use of reflecting guanine plates, a silvery sided fish can make itself almost invisible from all angles other than from directly below. If the ventral photophores do function to diminish the fish's shadow, then the light they produce must match in spectral range, intensity and angular distribution the ambient light radiating downwards.

Denton, Gilpin-Brown and Wright (1972) have shown that the light produced by the ventral photophores have to pass through filters which ensure that the light emitted matches the waveband of the daylight that penetrates to the depth at which the fish live, that is, with a maximum energy at about 485 nm.

The hatchet-fish, *Argyropelecus,* lives in the daytime between 450 and 600 m and the intensity of light measured by a photometer facing directly upwards at this depth on a cloudy day is about 10^{-11} W/cm^2 (at 550 m) and that this decreases by a factor of 10 for every 60 m increase in depth. Denton, Gilpin-Brown and Wright (1972) have measured the intensity of light produced by *Argyropelecus* and the maximum radiances given were about 10^{-11} W/sterad/cm^2 of projected surface area. Clearly the light intensity through the depth from 450 to 600 m will have a 1000-fold range so that animals must be able to vary their light intensity emitted and indeed the intensity produced varies from fish to fish.

Denton, Gilpin-Brown and Wright (1972) also studied the stomiatoid fish, *Chauliodus sloani,* and measured an intensity of light from a single specimen as about 4×10^{-13} W/sterad/cm^2 of projected surface area. Although this is less than the radiance of *Argyropelecus, Chauliodus* lives at a greater depth during the daytime where the lower intensity will be sufficient to match the ambient downwelling light.

If these fish do use their photophores as a means of obliterating their shadow, the fish must be able to monitor both the ambient downwelling light and the intensity of its own luminescence. The mechanisms involved in this control system are not known at present, though some recent work has indicated a possible means (Lawry, 1974). In the lantern-fish, *Tarletonbeania crenularis,* there is a supra-orbital photophore which emits a blue-green light in a ventral direction and this light, together with the downwelling daylight, can pass by refraction through the lens and via an aphakic space, ventral to the lens, on to the ventral retina. The supra-orbital photophore is innervated by a branch of the supra-orbital nerve and it is suggested that the fish is able to compare the intensity of the downwelling light with that of the photophore and then adjust the luminescence of the photophore to be equal to the day-light. If the ventral photophores are similarly adjusted, the ventral body outline will be camouflaged maximally.

In *Figure 8.22(a)* is shown the light producing organ of *Argyropelecus* which is screened with a filter through which the light must pass before entering the ventrally directed reflecting tube. The reflecting tube has an inside surface that is fully silvered, while the outside surface is only partially silvered. As shown schematically in *Figure 8.22(b),* such a structure will have the effect of emitting the greatest intensity of light downwards with the lowest intensity horizontally which theoretically will match exactly the ambient radiance. Recently Denton, Gilpin-Brown and Wright (1972) have succeeded in measuring the angular distribution of this light for both *Argyropelecus* and *Chauliodus* in both the longitudinal plane, i.e. from head to tail through the long axis of the fish, and transversely from side to side

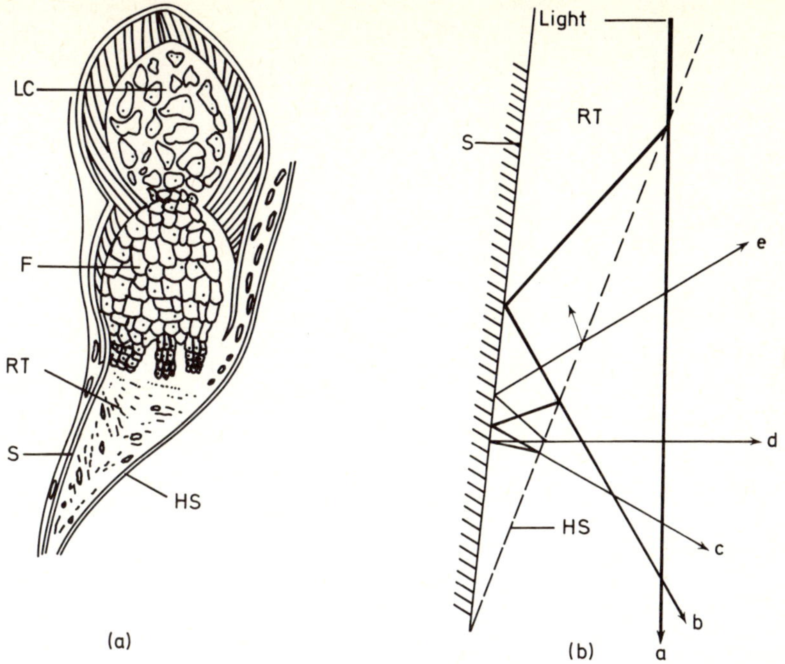

Figure 8.22 (a) Diagrammatic section through the ventral photophore of Argyropelecus affinis. *F, filter; HS, half-silvered outside surface; LC, light producing chamber; RT, reflecting tube; S, fully silvered inside surface. (After Marshall, 1954; courtesy N. B. Marshall). (b) Schematic of the light path through the reflecting tube of the photophore to show the distribution of light diminishing in intensity from a to e. HS, half-silvered outside surface; RT, reflecting tube; S, fully silvered inside surface. (From 'Reflectors in Fishes', Denton. Copyright © January 1971 by Scientific American Inc. All rights reserved)*

across the body of the fish. As shown in *Figure 8.23,* the angular distribution of luminance produced by the fish is a very close match to that of the ambient daylight radiance at the depth at which the fish lives.

Taking all of these factors, that is spectral distribution, intensity and angular distribution, the close match between the luminance emitted by the fish and the daylight at the depth at which the fish lives clearly supports the original hypothesis of Frazer (1962) and Clarke (1963), that the fish can use its bioluminescence to obliterate the shadow that would otherwise be cast in the ambient daylight.

A further function of bioluminescence is that of intraspecific recognition. The species of lantern-fish can be distinguished by their lateral photophore patterns and being a shoaling species they could also keep together by flashing their lights. As was stated earlier, the coloured ocular light organs of some stomiatoid fish could also act as species recognition signs. In the *Myrotophidae* the pattern of their lateral light organs is the same in the two sexes of a species, but in many species there is a sexual difference in the arrangement of photophores on the dorsal and ventral surfaces close to the

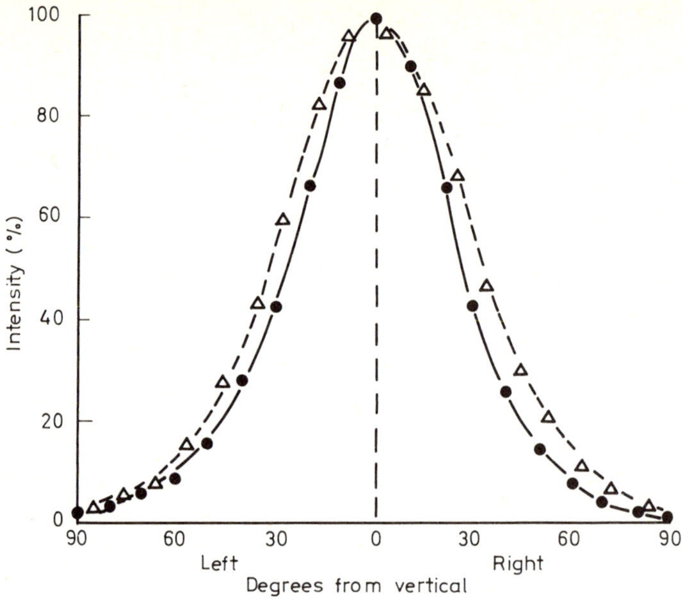

Figure 8.23 Angular distribution of light in the transverse plane produced by Chauliodus sloani (△); Argyropelecus affinis (●). *The continuous and dashed curves are computed curves for daylight in water at depth. (After Denton* et al., *1972; courtesy The Royal Society)*

caudal peduncle. Usually the male has the more powerfully developed display.

Similarly, within the *Melanostomiatidae* and *Idiacanthidae* there is a notable difference in the development of the cheek organs between the sexes. In the males the cheek organ is relatively enormous in comparison to that of the female even though in *Idiacanthus* the male is only about one-sixth the size of the female. Likewise, in the ceratioid fish (angler-fish) the females have luminous lures which are not present in the smaller males. Use of luminescence as a warning signal has already been mentioned, but an interesting observation by Beebe (1935) is of importance in this respect. He noted from the bathyscope that the lateral photophores of the lantern-fishes, when switched off, faded slowly leaving the impression of the fish, while the much brighter caudal lights could be flashed to leave the viewing eye temporarily blinded by the intensity and he suggested that this would confuse a predator and allow the lantern-fish to escape. Amusingly, Beebe noted that a living specimen of *Myctophum affine* kept in an aquarium flashed its caudal photophores in response to the low light emission of a luminous watch dial — surely not a sexual response!

A further use of luminescence as a warning has been postulated by Nicol (1967). In solitary fish he has suggested that the fish may become evenly spaced by having their territories limited by being able to see the warning photophores of another individual.

Mention has already been made of the luminescent lures of the female angler-fishes and presumably the function of these photophores and those located actually within the mouth of some stomiatoids is to attract prey. The structure of the lure in ceratioids is very variable and complex. In *Gigantactis macronema* the illicium is some four times the length of the body, whereas in *Ceratias holboelli* the lure is attached to a moveable basal bone which can be moved within skin folds and drawn towards the mouth. In the stomiatoid *Chauliodus* there are about 350 small photophores arranged on the roof of the mouth and on the ventral and inner surface of the eyeball. It has been suggested that when the fish opens its mouth nearby crustaceans would dart towards the lighted gape.

Whatever the function of photophores, the light emitted can only be of adaptive value if it can be directly perceived by other organisms. It is, therefore, necessary to have some estimate as to the visibility of luminescent flashes in the ocean. A small source, such as a single photophore or a dinoflagellate, at some distance from a detector can be treated as a point source so that the irradiance E in W/m^2, measured at a distance s metres from a source of radiant intensity I in W $sterad^{-1}$ is given by $E = I/s^2$, so long as the receiving surface is at right angles to the direction of the source. In the case of multiple sources such as a fish or euphausid the luminescence can be dealt with by treating each photophore as a separate point source.

In the copepods the intensity of the photophores at 1 m range from 0.05×10^{-9} to 21.4×10^{-9} W/m^2, but are generally less than 10^{-9} W/m^2, and these flashes last from about 0.1 up to 6 s. Similar values have been recorded in the euphausids as well as in the fishes. Nicol (1958) has made estimates as to the distance the ctenophore, *Boröe*, could be detected by the human eye in clear oceanic water if it had a transparency of 99%/m or 90%/m and arrived at distance of 120 and 41 m, respectively. Nicol measured the intensity of the luminescence of *Boröe* as $0.17–0.85 \times 10^{-9}$ W/m^2. However, these estimates of distance are certainly too high since under natural conditions Clarke found that an artificial source 1000 times brighter than *Boröe* was visible to only 56 m in natural water with a transmission of 97%/m (Clarke and Denton, 1962). Oceanic water more typically has a transmission closer to 95%/m and particle scattering of light from a point source will play a greater role in visibility than the transparency of the water so that photophores of the intensities measured are probably only visible for a few metres.

8.10 SUMMARY

Visual adaptations of pelagic animals can be divided most easily into two groups, those exhibited by surface living species where light is not at a premium and those exhibited by the deeper living species where light is greatly restricted both in intensity and in spectral range, but where the majority of animals carry their own illumination produced from photophores. A marine animal, just as any other animal in its environment, has a dual task of perceiving its surroundings and thereby detecting both prey and predator and also of being camouflaged so that it is not easily detected visually, but yet is recognisable by members of its own species.

In the surface layers of the ocean during daylight photopic conditions prevail and it appears most probable that many species inhabiting this zone have colour vision. As suggested by Walls (1942) the function of colour vision is probably to enhance the contrast of an object against the background. However, to test this hypothesis data on the histology of the retina, the absorbance spectra of the visual pigments, the photic environment of the fish and the visually dominated behavioural tasks performed by the fish are required. It is only recently that these data have become available and it would appear from the work of McFarland and Munz (1975b) that the photopic visual pigments of diurnal fish can indeed be shown to be adapted to the function of contrast enhancement in relation to the specific visual tasks of the fish. It is probable that such correlations will also be found within the marine mammals, cephalopods and crustaceans that share this environment with the fish.

To counter these finely tuned visual systems, the animals in the epipelagic and mesopelagic zones of the ocean have evolved both their body shape and colouring to become less easily visible. Of course, there are obvious exceptions such as the beautifully coloured and exotically shaped tropical-reef fish, but in general fish have compromised between the circular cross section suited for rapid movement and the laterally flattened shape best suited to avoid detection from below. In addition, the flanks of many mid-water fish are covered with silvery scales so orientated as to mimic the background space light when seen from all directions except from below where no arrangements of plates can camouflage the body silhouette. However, as has been shown in the section on bioluminescence, all is not lost since many deep-sea fish have rows of downwardly directed photophores that are under nervous control so that they can be adjusted to match exactly the downwelling light in intensity, spectral characteristics and angular distribution.

Deep-sea fish are, perhaps, the most highly adapted fish in the visual sense in that almost every possible means has been employed to increase the visual sensitivity of the eye except in some cases where the fish has given up vision as a useful sense and possesses only degenerate eyes. To increase sensitivity, fish (such as stomiatoids and myctophids) have enlarged dioptic parts designed to collect and pass light on to a retina that is itself modified to increase its sensitivity, features best displayed possibly in the bizarre tubular eyes of many deep-sea fish. Sensitivity has been increased by having binocular vision and receptor cells packed closely together with long outer segments or layers of acromeres to give a high density of absorbing pigment. The visual pigments of many of these fish have λ_{max} matching the maximum wavelength of transmission of light at depth in the ocean and the dominant blue-green bioluminescence produced by animals in these regions.

Biologically produced light, exhibited by a high percentage of the deep-sea population, from dinoflagellates to fish, is used either for illumination to see with, identification patterns to be recognised by, lures to attract prey with or as camouflage. In the past few years it has become apparent that a number of deep-sea fish such as malacosteoids have taken advantage of the dim monochromatic space light by evolving photophores and visual pigments with maximum wavelength emission and absorbance outside the spectral range of the space light, perhaps most beautifully illustrated by *Aristostomias* which has visual pigments absorbing close to 550 and 520 nm and photophores emitting red and green light. It thus possesses its own specific signalling system that is probably undetectable by other deep-sea species.

The study of visual adaptations of pelagic animals has now reached an exciting stage since it is possible in a limited number of species to collate the earlier anatomical data and limited information of scotopic visual pigments and photophore emission with the recent data available on photopic pigments, quantitative data on bioluminescence and the characteristics of the underwater space light in a given environment. Nevertheless, it is a field of study that is wide open to future research since in general little is known either of the visual tasks pelagic animals have to perform or of their visual physiology and this is especially true of the deep-sea species.

REFERENCES

BEEBE, W. (1935). *Half Mile Down.* John Lane, London

BLAXTER, J. H. S. and JONES, M. P. (1967). 'The development of the retina and retino-motor responses in the herring', *J. mar. biol. Assoc. U.K.,* **47,** 677–697

BOWMAKER, J. K., LOEW, E. R. and LIEBMAN, P. A. (1975). 'Variation in the λ_{max} of rhodopsin from individual frogs', *Vision Res.,* **154,** 997–1003

BRUNO, M. S. and GOLDSMITH, T. H. (1974). 'Rhodopsin of the blue crab *callinectes:* evidence for absorption differences *in vitro* and *in vivo', Vision Res.,* **14,** 653–658

CLARKE, G. L. (1936). 'On the depth at which fishes can see', *Ecology,* **17,** 452–456

CLARKE, G. L. and DENTON, E. J. (1962). 'Light and Animal Life', 456–468. In: *The Sea,* **I.** Ed. M. N. Hill. John Wiley & Sons, New York

CLARKE, G. L. and HUBBARD, C. J. (1959). 'Quantitative records of the luminescent flashing of oceanic animals at great depth', *Limnol. Oceanog.,* **4,** 163–180

CLARKE, W. D. (1963). 'Function of bioluminescence in mesopelagic organisms', *Nature Lond.,* **198,** 1244–1246

CRESCITELLI, F. (1972). 'The visual cells and visual pigments of the vertebrate eye'. In: *Handbook of Sensory Physiology, VII/1.* Ed. H. J. A. Dartnall. Springer-Verlag, Berlin

DARTNALL, H. J. A. (1972). 'Visual pigments of the Coelacanth', *Nature Lond.,* **239,** 341–342

DARTNALL, H. J. A. and LYTHGOE, J. N. (1965). 'The spectral clustering of visual pigments', *Vision Res.,* **5,** 81–100

DENTON, E. J. (1956). 'Recherches sur l'absorption de la lumière par le cristallin des poissons', *Bull. Inst. Océanog. Monaco.,* **1071,** 1–10

DENTON, E. J. (1971). 'Reflectors in Fishes', *Sci. Am.,* **224,** 65–72

DENTON, E. J., GILPIN-BROWN, J. B. and WRIGHT, P. G. (1970). 'On the "filter" in the photophores of mesopelagic fish and on a fish emitting red light and especially sensitive to red light', *J. Physiol.,* **208,** 72

DENTON, E. J., GILPIN-BROWN, J. B. and WRIGHT, P. G. (1972). 'The angular distribution of the light produced by some mesopelagic fish in relation to their camouflage', *Proc. roy. Soc. London B.,* **182,** 145–158

DENTON, E. J. and LAND, M. F. (1971). 'Mechanism of reflexion in silvery layers of fish and cephalopods', *Proc. roy. Soc. London B.,* **178,** 43–61

DENTON, E. J. and NICOL, J. A. C. (1964). 'The chorioidal tapeta of some cartilaginous fishes (Chondrichthyes)', *J. mar. biol. Assoc. U.K.,* **44,** 219–258

DENTON, E. J. and WARREN, F. J. (1957). 'Photosensitive pigments in the retinae of deep-sea fish', *J. mar. biol. Assoc. U.K.,* **43,** 65–70

DENTON, E. J. and WARREN, F. J. (1968). 'Eyes of *Histioteuthidae*', *Nature Lond.*, **219,** 400–401

EGUCHI, E. and WATERMAN, T. H. (1966). 'Fine structure patterns in crustacean rhabdoms'. In: *The functional organization of the compound eye.* Ed. C. G. Bernhard. Pergamon Press, Oxford

ENGSTRÖM, K. (1963). 'Cone types and cone arrangements in teleost retinae', *Acta Zool.*, **44,** 179–243

FRAZER, J. (1962). *Nature Adrift.* Fowlis, London

GOLDSMITH, T. H. (1972). 'The natural history of Invertebrate visual pigments'. In: *Handbook of Sensory Physiology VII/I. Ed. H. J. A. Dartnall. Springer-Verlag, Berlin*

GOURAS, P. (1972). 'S-Potentials'. In: *Handbook of Sensory Physiology VII/2.* Ed. M. G. F. Fuortes. Springer-Verlag, Berlin

HARVEY, E. N. (1952). *Bioluminescence.* Academic Press, New York

HOBSON, E. S. (1972). 'Activity of Hawaiian reef-fishes during the evening and morning transitions between daylight and darkness', *Fish Bull. Nat. Mar. Fish. Ser.*, **70,** 715–740

JERLOV, N. G. (1970). 'Light—General Introduction', 95–102. In: *Marine Ecology* **1,** pt. 1. Ed. O. Kinne. John Wiley & Sons Ltd., London

KAMPA, E. M. and BODEN, B. P. (1957). 'Light generation in a sonic scattering layer', *Deep-sea Res.*, **4,** 73–92

LAUFER, M. and MILLAN, E. (1970). 'Spectral analysis of L-type S-potentials and their relation to photopigment absorption in a fish *(Eugerres plumieri)* retina', *Vision Res.*, **10,** 237–252

LAWRY, J. V. (1974). 'Lantern fish compare downwelling light and bioluminescence', *Nature Lond.*, **247,** 155–157

LIEBMAN, P. A. (1972). 'Microspectrophotometry of photoreceptors'. In: *Handbook of Sensory Physiology VII/1.* Ed. H. J. A. Dartnall. Springer-Verlag, Berlin

LOCKET, N. A. (1970). 'Deep-sea fish retina', *Br. med. Bull.*, **26,** 107–111

LYTHGOE, J. N. (1966). 'Visual pigments and underwater vision'. In: *Light as an ecological factor.* Eds. R. Bainbridge, G. C. Evans and O. Rackham. Blackwell, Oxford

LYTHGOE, J. N. (1968). 'Visual pigments and visual range underwater,' *Vision Res.*, **8,** 997–1012

LYTHGOE, J. N. (1972). 'The adaptation of visual pigments to the photic environment'. In: *Handbook of Sensory Physiology VII/1.* Ed. H. J. A. Dartnall. Springer-Verlag, Berlin

LYTHGOE, J. N. and HEMMINGS, C. C. (1967). 'Polarized light and underwater vision'. *Nature Lond.*, **213,** 893–894

LYTHGOE, J. N. and NORTHMORE, D. P. M. (1973). 'Colours underwater', 77–98. In: *Colour '73, the 2nd Congress of the International Colour Ass.* Adam Hilger, London

MARSHALL, N. B. (1954). *Aspects of Deep-sea biology.* Hutchinsons, London

MARSHALL, N. B. (1971). *Explorations in the Life of fishes.* Harvard University Press, Cambridge, Mass. Oxford University Press, London

McFARLAND, W. N. (1971). 'Cetacean visual pigments', *Vision Res.*, **11,** 1065–1076

McFARLAND, W. N. and MUNZ, F. W. (1975a). 'The photic environment of clear tropical seas during the day', *Vision Res.*, **15,** 1063–1070

McFARLAND, W. N. and MUNZ, F. W. (1975b). 'The evolution of photopic visual pigments in fishes', *Vision Res.*, **15,** 1071–1080

MORELAND, J. D. and LYTHGOE, J. N. (1968). 'Yellow corneas in fishes', *Vision Res.*, **8,** 1377–1380

MUNK, O. (1966). 'Ocular anatomy of some deep-sea teleosts', *Dana-Report,* **70,** 1–62

MUNZ, F. W. (1974). 'The visual pigments of epipelagic and rocky shore fishes', *Vision Res.*, **4,** 441–454

MUNZ, F. W. and MCFARLAND, W. N. (1973). 'The significance of spectral position in the rhodopsin of tropical marine fish', *Vision Res.*, **13,** 1829–1874

MUNZ, F. W. and MCFARLAND, W. N. (1975). 'Presumptive cone pigments extracted from tropical marine fishes', *Vision Res.*, **15,** 1045–1062

NICOL, J. A. C. (1958). 'Observations on luminescence in pelagic animals,' *J. mar. biol. Assoc. U.K.*, **37,** 705–752

NICOL, J. A. C. (1960). 'Spectral composition of the light of the lantern-fish, *Myctophum punctatum*', *J. mar. biol. Assoc. U.K.*, **39,** 27–32

NICOL, J. A. C. (1967). 'The luminescence of fishes', *Symp. zool. Soc. London.*, **(19),** 27–55

NICOL, J. A. C. (1969). 'Bioluminescence', 355–400. In: *Fish Physiology* **III.** Eds. W. S. Hoar and D. J. Randall. Academic Press, New York and London

NICOL, J. A. C., ARNOTT, H. J. and BEST, A. C. G. (1973). 'Tapeta lucida in bony fishes *(Actinopterygii)* a survey', *Can. J. Zool.,* **51,** 69–81

O'DAY, W. T. and FERNANDEZ, H. R. (1974). *'Aristostomias scintillans (Malacosteidae):* a deep-sea fish with visual pigments apparently adapted to its own bioluminescence', *Vision Res.,* **14,** 545–550

SMITH, R. C. and TYLER, J. E. (1967). 'Optical properties of clear oceanic water', *J. Opt. Soc. Am.,* **57,** 589–595

TAMURA, T., HANYU, I. and NIWA, H. (1972). 'Spectral sensitivity and colour vision in skipjack tuna and related species', *Bull. Japan Soc. Sci. Fish.,* **38,** 799–802

TAMURA, T. and NIWA, H. (1967). 'Spectral sensitivity and colour vision of fish as indicated by S-potential', *Comp. Biochem. Physiol.,* **22,** 745–754

TETT, P. B. and KELLY, M. G. (1973). 'Marine Bioluminescence', *Oceanogr. Mar. Biol. Ann. Rev.,* **11,** 89–173

TOMITA, T., KANEKO, A., MORAKAMI, M. and PAUTLER, E. L. (1967). 'Spectral response curves of single cones in the carp', *Vision Res.,* **7,** 519–531

WALLS, G. L. (1942). *The Vertebrate Eye and Its Adaptive Radiation.* Cranbrook Institute of Sciences, Bloomfield Hills, Michigan

WATERMAN, T. H. (1966). 'Polarotaxis and Primary Photoreceptor events in Crustacea', 493–511. In: *The Functional Organization of the Compound Eye.* Ed. C. G. Bernhard. Pergamon Press, Oxford

WATERMAN, T. H. and HARCH, K. W. (1966). 'Mechanisms of polarized light perception', *Science,* **154,** 467–475

WEALE, R. A. (1955). 'Binocular vision and deep-sea fish', *Nature Lond.,* **175,** 996

Nine

Biochemical adaptations to pressure

G. N. SOMERO
Scripps Institution of Oceanography, La Jolla, California

P. W. HOCHACHKA
Department of Zoology, University of British Columbia, Vancouver

9.1 INTRODUCTION

The effects of hydrostatic pressure on biochemical structures and processes have been studied more in an abstract than in a real-world context. Because of the logistic and technical difficulties entailed in examining the effects of elevated hydrostatic pressures on marine organisms, a large percentage of the high pressure biochemistry which has been done has utilised materials from terrestrial organisms. In addition, many of the study systems used have not even employed biomolecules, but instead have utilised simplified model compounds such as amino acid side-chain analogues.

However, the tendency to examine high pressure effects on systems which differ greatly, especially in their complexity, from marine organisms must not be viewed entirely as an illustration of experimental naïveté. Most studies of high pressure effects on biological or biological-like systems have not been performed in order to shed light on the mechanisms by which deep-sea and vertically migrating marine forms adapt to large and/or variable pressures. Instead, the majority of biochemists and biophysicists who perform high pressure studies do so using pressure as a valuable tool for elucidating the properties of proteins, nucleic acids and aqueous solutions. What environmentally-oriented biochemists can gain from the results of these studies is less an appreciation of how marine organisms cope with pressure than a glimpse of the nature of high pressure stress and, in addition, at least some inkling of the adaptive strategies marine organisms might employ to adjust their cellular chemistry to either extremes of pressure or large-scale changes in pressure.

The achievements which have been made by biochemists and biophysicists in their studies of simplified model compound systems and biomolecules from one-atmosphere-adapted organisms, when combined with the recent advances which have been made in deep-sea collection technology, appear to poise the study of biochemical adaptation to high pressures by marine organisms in a 'take-off' phase of growth. What seems to be required is a set of questions to serve as guides to this growth and, in addition, a set of cautions concerning the experimental conditions which must be realised if experimental work is to reveal the nature of pressure effects in actual living systems. A major purpose of this essay is to suggest what we feel are promising areas for future study of pressure adaptation. In addition, we hope to illustrate the nature of the experimental design requirements which will be necessary if the expansion of pressure studies from simplified, abstract systems is to be successfully extended to what, for marine biologists, is the 'real world'.

9.2 THE BASIC EFFECTS OF HYDROSTATIC PRESSURE ON BIOLOGICAL SYSTEMS

In the marine environment two sources of pressure stress exist. Deep-sea forms experience extremes of *absolute* pressure which are of sufficient magnitude to exert profound effects on cellular structures and processes. Organisms which migrate vertically through the water column, either on a diurnal basis or during transitions between different stages of the life cycle as is discussed in Chapters 5 and 6, may encounter large *changes* in pressure. In both cases an extremely diverse array of structural and functional features of the cell can be adversely affected, and at first glance a marine biologist might well despair of ever finding a common denominator to appreciate and analyse these varied pressure effects. Fortunately, a simple common denominator for evaluating pressure effects does exist. The physical basis of all pressure effects is volume changes, and the three equations given below describe how the volume changes, which occur during chemical reactions and during the formation of activated complexes, determine the effects of pressure on equilibrium states and reaction velocities, respectively.

$$\Delta H = \Delta E + P\Delta V \quad (1)$$
$$\Delta G^\circ = \Delta E - T\Delta S + P\Delta V \quad (2)$$
$$\Delta G^\ddagger = \Delta E^\ddagger - T\Delta S^\ddagger + P\Delta V^\ddagger \quad (3)$$

The first equation states that the net enthalpy (H) change which occurs during a chemical reaction or activation process is equal to the change in the total internal energy (E) of the system plus the pressure-volume work which is performed ($P\Delta V$). Since the thermodynamic equilibrium of a reaction is determined by the ΔG° of the reaction, we can expand equation (1) to describe the effects of pressure on the equilibrium of a chemical reaction, as shown by equation (2). It is clear from this equation that, if a chemical reaction involves a volume increase of the system as reactants are converted to products, increases in hydrostatic pressure will tend to shift the equilibrium of the reaction towards the initial reactants. Conversely, if ΔV is negative, increasing the pressure on the system will reduce the value of ΔG°

and thus favour products over reactants. It should be stressed at this early point in this chapter that the volume of the *system* is what matters. As we shall see in more detail later in this chapter, *the volume changes which accompany a chemical reaction or an activation process often are due less to changes in the volumes of the chemical reactants themselves than to changes in the structure and volume of the surrounding water of the system.*

Volume changes not only affect the pressure sensitivity of equilibria, but in addition determine the effect of pressure on the rates at which equilibria are attained. Equation (3) expresses the effects of changes in the internal energy, the entropy ($\Delta S^{\ddagger}$), and pressure-volume changes on the free energy of activation ($\Delta G^{\ddagger}$) of a chemical reaction. The superscript ‡ ('double daggers') indicates that the thermodynamic quantities pertain to the energy changes involved in going from the ground (unactivated) state to the high-energy transition state (the activated complex). Since $\Delta G^{\ddagger}$ is the thermodynamic parameter which determines how rapidly equilibrium is attained, the volume changes which occur during the formation of the activated complex will affect the rates of chemical reactions. If $\Delta V^{\ddagger}$ is zero, the reaction rate will be pressure-insensitive. A reaction with a positive $\Delta V^{\ddagger}$ will be pressure inhibited, and a reaction with a negative $\Delta V^{\ddagger}$ will be pressure activated (excluding such effects as pressure denaturation of the enzyme, of course).

The magnitudes of pressure effects on equilibrium positions and reaction rates can be calculated using equations (4) and (5), respectively.

$$\left(\frac{\partial \ln K}{\partial P}\right)_T = \frac{-\Delta V}{RT} \tag{4}$$

$$k_p = k_o e^{-P\Delta V^{\ddagger}/RT} \tag{5}$$

Equation (4) relates the effect of a change in pressure, with temperature (T) held constant, on the equilibrium constant (K) of a chemical reaction which occurs with a volume change ΔV. R is the gas constant equal to 82.07 atm.cm^3/mole °K, and T is the absolute temperature in degrees Kelvin.

Equation (5) expresses the relationship between the reaction velocity constant (k) and the change in pressure for a reaction with activation volume of $\Delta V^{\ddagger}$. k_o can represent the velocity constant at one atmosphere pressure; k_p is the velocity constant at a different pressure of P atmospheres. For enzyme-catalysed reactions this equation pertains only under conditions of saturating substrate concentrations. When the enzyme is not functioning at its maximal velocity (V_{max}), the volume changes which accompany substrate binding will also affect the pressure-dependence of reaction velocity. Equations describing pressure effects on enzymic reaction velocities, where both binding and activation volumes are involved, are given by Laidler (1951).

Given the above theory, it is apparent that the first task in determining how changes in pressure are apt to affect biochemical structures and processes must be the elucidation of the signs and the absolute values of the volume changes which occur during the course of enzymic reactions and during the formation or disruption of biological structures, e.g. the higher orders of protein structure. Because these volume changes are of such importance, we shall discuss them in some detail; they form the foundation on which this chapter, and all treatments of pressure effects, must rest.

Table 9.1 lists the signs of the volume changes which accompany chemical reactions involving charged species. The reactants involved may be low molecular weight compounds or macromolecules. Note the important generalisation that whenever a net increase in the number of charged species occurs, a decrease in the volume of the system (reactants plus water) results. The basis of this charge-dependence of solution volume is, to a very great extent, the effect which charged species have on water structure and volume. Electrostriction of water molecules around a charged species leads to shrinkage of the solution, since water in a tightly-organised hydration sphere is likely to occupy less volume than so-called 'bulk' water.

Table 9.1 VOLUME CHANGES IN REACTIONS WHICH INVOLVE CHARGED SPECIES

Reaction type	*Signs of volume change*
$XY \rightarrow X^+ + Y^-$	Negative
$X^+ + Y^- \rightarrow XY$	Positive
$X^+ + Y^+ \rightarrow XY^{+2}$	Negative
$X^+ + Y^- \rightarrow X^+Y^-$	Positive
$Y^- + RX \rightarrow YR + X^-$	Approximately zero ΔV
$R_3\mathrm{N} + R'X \rightarrow R_3R'\mathrm{N}^+X^-$	Negative

Because of the vast number of biochemical reactions in which charged species are involved, it seems very probable that water-ion-pressure interactions will pose significant problems for deep-sea and vertically-migrating marine organisms. Increases in pressure will tend to favour dissociation of weak acids and bases, of ion pairs etc., with concomitant alterations of cellular pH and ionic compositions. For example, the pH of seawater, which is buffered largely by a bicarbonate system, decreases from near 8.10 to 7.87 as pressure is increased from 1 to 1100 atmospheres at a temperature of 0°C (ZoBell, 1970). Buffering systems in the cellular and extracellular fluids, while far more complex than the seawater buffering system, may also exhibit biologically significant pressure sensitivities. Ion pair dissociations may also pose problems for marine forms. For example, the formation of the Mg-ATP complex (the form of ATP which is utilised in most enzymic phosphorylation reactions) occurs with a volume change of +22 cm^3/mole under certain *in vitro* conditions (Rainford, Noguchi and Morales, 1965). Increases in pressure would thus be expected to dissociate this ion pair, with the possible result that intracellular levels of Mg-ATP would fall to suboptimal ranges unless compensatory adaptations, e.g. higher intracellular Mg^{2+} concentrations, occurred.

Uncharged molecules, both polar and non-polar, may also exert very significant effects on water structure and solution volume. Of singular importance in pressure-volume relationships in biological systems is the influences which non-polar amino acid side-chains have on water structure (solution volume). One of the major 'driving forces' responsible for the formation of protein quaternary and tertiary structures is the class of non-polar interactions termed 'hydrophobic interactions'. These interactions between non-polar amino acid side-chains such as those of valine, isoleucine and phenylalanine stem from the thermodynamic favourability of removal of these non-polar groups from the aqueous phase to a non-polar environment. This non-polar environment is provided by the clustering hydrophobic side-chains themselves. Thus, current models of protein structure picture an internal concentration of non-polar side-chains and the exposure on the protein surface of many of the charged (acidic and basic) amino acid residues.

It has been proposed that a major locus of pressure sensitivity derives from the volume changes which, on the basis of model compound studies (*see Table 9.2*), would be predicted to occur when the 'buried' hydrophobic amino acid side-chains are thrust into water. Model compound studies using highly simplified and highly dilute organic analogues of amino acid side-chains have shown that the transfer of an organic, non-polar molecule from an organic phase to an aqueous phase is accompanied by a substantial *decrease* in the volume of the system. It is thought that the non-polar molecule is accommodated in the aqueous phase via formation of a dense clathrate of water molecules around the hydrophobic compound (*see* Brandts, 1967). The water molecules surrounding the hydrophobic

Table 9.2 IMPORTANT SOURCES OF VOLUME CHANGES ASSOCIATED WITH WEAK INTERACTIONS IN BIOLOGICAL SYSTEMS (MODIFIED AFTER LOW AND SOMERO, 1975A)

Process	*Volume change* (cm^3/mole)
Hydrogen bond formation[2]	−(3–5)
Hydrophobic interactions[1]	
CH_4 in hexane → CH_4 in water[3]	−22.7
C_6H_6 (pure liquid) → C_6H_6 in water[3]	− 6.2
H_2O (pure) → H_2O (dilute in 1,1,1 trichloroethane)[4]	+ 4.3
H_2O (pure) → H_2O (dilute in CCl_4)[4]	+13.6
Ionic Interactions[1]	
Lysine (neutral) → Lysine (+)[2]	−26.4
Acetic acid → Acetate + H^+[2]	−11.8
Glutamic acid → Glutamate + H^+[2]	−12.7
Mg-ATP complex → ATP + Mg^{2+}[5]	−22
Change in exposure of polar group[1]	
Methanol in CCl_4 → Methanol in H_2O[6]	− 7.1
Ethanol in CCl_4 → Ethanol in H_2O[6]	− 4.9
n-propanol in CCl_4 → *n*-propanol in H_2O[6]	− 6.4
Helix-coil transition[7]	+ 1

[1]In these model studies, the transfer of, for example, an amino acid side-chain analogue between a non-polar, organic phase and water is analogised to the exposure of the side-chain during denaturation or other type of conformational change
[2]Suzuki and Taniguchi (1972)
[3]Kauzmann (1959)
[4]Masterton and Seiler (1968)
[5]Rainford, Noguchi and Morales (1965)
[6]Values calculated from Duboc (1969) and Friedman and Scheraga (1965)
[7]Noguchi (1966)

molecule (or amino acid side-chain) occupy a smaller volume than bulk water.

The magnitudes of the volume changes which occur when a non-polar species is transferred from an organic phase into water are large enough to pose severe threats to protein structure (*Table 9.2*). For example, if a protein contained ten buried non-polar side-chains, and if the exposure of these side-chains to water led to volume decreases of the order noted for model compound studies (up to 20 cm^3/mole in the case of many side-chain analogues), then the unfolding of the protein could lead to volume reductions of the order of 200 cm^3/mole. If this volume change is inserted into equation (4), one finds that pressures well within the marine range would lead to virtually total denaturation of the protein (Hochachka and Somero, 1973). In fact, if one extrapolates quantitatively from model compound studies such as those described in *Table 9.2* to actual biomolecules, it becomes difficult to understand how proteins could exist in a native state at abyssal pressures. One must therefore conclude that either (a) deep-sea organisms maintain native protein structures through mechanisms different from those utilised by terrestrial or shallow-water organisms, or (b) extrapolating from model compound studies of hydrophobic molecules to the 'real world' is not justified, at least in a strictly quantitative manner.

Recent experimental results from more biologically realistic model compound studies and from enzyme denaturation experiments suggest that the second alternative listed above is correct. The conclusions resulting from simple model compound experiments may be valid within the realm of physical organic chemistry, but these conclusions cannot be extrapolated quantitatively to macromolecular systems. Bøje and Hvidt (1972) and Masterton and Seiler (1968) have criticised earlier model compound studies on the basis of their overly simplified approach to the analysis of macromolecular phenomena. These authors argue convincingly that little can be said about protein-pressure interactions on the basis of studies of exceedingly dilute solutions of very low molecular weight organic molecules. 'Real' biopolymers such as enzymes are (a) very large, and (b) contain non-polar residues which are closely juxtaposed and by no means in 'infinitely dilute' concentration. Such concentrated non-polar groups may affect water structure very differently from highly dilute organic compounds. Bøje and Hvidt (1972) have shown conclusively that model compounds which mimic the concentrated, closely juxtaposed hydrophobic side-chains found in proteins affect water differently from small, dilute non-polar molecules. In fact, they discovered that concentrated groups of hydrophobic residues could lead to small *positive* volume changes when these molecules were transferred to water. Bøje and Hvidt (1972) suggest that when a protein unfolds in aqueous solution, what is presented to the aqueous phase is not an infinitely dilute solution of small non-polar moities, but rather a concentrated front of hydrophobic groups. Relativistically, it seems more accurate to regard the interactions between the exposed hydrophobic side-chains and water as a transfer reaction in which water is being added to a concentrated organic phase. Transfers of this type can lead to *increases* in the volume of the system (*Table 9.2*; Masterton and Seiler, 1968). Thus, as we shall discuss in more detail later, the views of biochemists and biophysicists concerning pressure effects on protein structure are now undergoing a rapid evolution.

The other class of weak bond which is important in stabilising the higher orders of macromolecular structure is hydrogen bonding. Again in this case great uncertainty remains about the volume changes which result when, for example, amino acid residues hydrogen bond among themselves instead of with the cellular water. Suzuki and Taniguchi (1972) (*Table 9.2*) suggest, on the basis of model compound studies, that the formation of intra-polypeptide hydrogen bonding during the formation of helical structures leads to a volume decrease relative to the situation which pertains when the amino acids are hydrogen bonding to the surrounding water. If these conclusions are correct for 'real' proteins, then the helical structure of an enzyme may help make the enzyme resistant to pressure denaturation.

A final class of basic pressure effects to consider involves the interactions among long-chain hydrocarbons such as those found in lipid molecules. Here we are not considering transfers of hydrophobic molecules or side-chains between organic (non-polar) and aqueous phases, but instead we are examining how pressure affects the physical properties of large aggregates of non-polar molecules. As *Table 9.3* reveals, increases in hydrostatic pressure have large effects on the physical state of long-chain hydrocarbon compounds. The van der Waals attractions which exist among the side-chains are stabilised by high pressures since the application of increased pressure to such a system is apt to align more closely the long aliphatic chains, thus permitting tighter bonding among them. The most important biological implication of this pressure effect is in the case of membrane structure, where the physical state of the lipids of the membrane plays a major role in establishing the functional properties of the membrane.

Our aim in the above paragraphs is to enable the reader to achieve an overview of the physical and chemical bases of pressure effects on living systems. We shall now examine certain of the biological systems which have been studied using hydrostatic pressure as an experimental variable. In the discussions which follow we shall attempt to suggest answers to the following questions in each case: (a) What is the type and the magnitude of pressure

Table 9.3 THE EFFECT OF HYDROSTATIC PRESSURE ON THE MELTING TEMPERATURES OF LONG-CHAIN HYDROCARBON COMPOUNDS (DATA FROM WEALE, 1967)

Compound	*Pressure* (atm)	*Melting temperature* (°C)
n-C_{12}	1	−10
	1000	15
n-C_{18}	1	27
	1000	50
n-C_{24}	1	50
	1000	70

stress on the biological system under consideration, and do the stresses observed seem consistent with the predictions of model compound experiments? (b) What are the observed, or possible, avenues of adaptation which are, or could be, utilised to compensate for adverse pressure effects? (c) What experimental approaches seem most promising for elucidating the actual effects of pressure, and the adaptations to pressure, which occur in marine organisms?

9.3 PRESSURE STRESSES AND PRESSURE ADAPTATIONS IN BIOLOGICAL SYSTEMS

9.3.1 Pressure effects on dissociation phenomena

One of the few cases in which the results of model compound studies can be extrapolated more or less quantitatively to biological systems is in the case of pressure effects on dissociation processes. While there does exist a good possibility that the highly structured water of the cell can affect dissociation processes differently from the way in which relatively unstructured water affects these reactions, there are reasonable grounds for believing that at least in the case of simple dissociation reactions involving acids, bases and ion pairs the results of model compound studies can provide us with a fair picture of what occurs within the cell.

Several types of dissociation processes would be predicted to serve as critical loci of pressure stress. These processes include: (a) acid-base dissociations; (b) ion pair equilibria, involving such important complexes as Mg-ATP, and ion-ATPase complexes; and (c) macromolecular dissociations, for example, those which might be involved in the binding of proteins to membrane surfaces through electrostatic interactions (which of course entail charge neutralisations).

Pressure can strongly enhance the dissociation of weak acids (*Table 9.2*). In the absence of any counteracting influence on acid dissociation, one would expect to find that the pH values of deep-sea organisms' cells are at least a few tenths of a pH unit lower than the values characteristic of terrestrial or shallow water species. However, the dissociation of weak acids (and water) is also temperature dependent. The low temperatures characteristic of the deep-sea may therefore counteract the influence of pressure on acid-base dissociations. Similar temperature effects could counteract the influences of pressure on other dissociation reactions, e.g. those involving Mg-ATP complexes. Until we have measurements of intracellular pH values, of ion pair concentrations etc., we cannot frame any final conclusions about the importance of pressure on dissociation effects in deep-sea organisms. Furthermore, we can only raise educated guesses as to how these organisms could adapt to pressure stresses on dissociation processes. Might the concentrations of ions such as Mg^{2+} be elevated, as we have previously suggested? Might the buffering systems used by deep-sea forms differ qualitatively and quantitatively from those of terrestrial and shallow water organisms? Might proteins be bound to ribosomal and membrane structures by non-electrostatic means in deep-sea forms? Do the pH optima of enzymes differ between deep-sea species and shallow and terrestrial species? These are some of the questions which deserve close study by physiologists and biochemists interested in high pressure adaptation.

9.3.2 Pressure effects on protein structure

There are five levels of protein structure:

1. Primary structure, the sequence of covalently-linked amino acid residues which comprise the polypeptide chain.
2. Secondary structure, the α-helical and β-pleated sheet regions which owe their stability to hydrogen bonding among amino acid residues.
3. Tertiary structure ('conformation'), which is the manner in which the polypeptide chain folds upon itself, with weak bonds such as hydrophobic interactions providing a major amount of the stabilisation free energy.
4. Quaternary structure, the aggregation state of multi-subunit proteins.
5. Quintinary structure, which refers to the complexes many proteins form with other large molecules or molecular aggregates (ribosomes, enzyme complexes, membranes).

Of these five levels of structure, the four highest levels might all be expected to exhibit pressure-sensitivities. It seems very unlikely that hydrostatic pressure would favour disruption of peptide bonds under biological pressures (up to perhaps 1400 atmospheres). Although as we will see pressure can sharply affect the translational processes involved in polypeptide synthesis, the primary structure of a polypeptide chain is probably quite pressure stable once the molecule is synthesised.

Pressure effects on secondary structure are not well understood. The data of *Table 9.2* suggest that hydrogen bonding, such as is involved in stabilising α-helical and β-pleated sheet regions of a protein, is stabilised at high pressures. Thus, the only 'danger' we can envisage resulting from pressure effects on secondary structure would result from the formation of too stable a protein structure. If this notion seems paradoxical to the reader, it should be recalled that enzymes owe much of their catalytic efficiency and regulatory sensitivity to the ability of polypeptide chains to alter their conformations (*see* Hochachka and Somero, 1973; Chapters 3 and 5). A protein which is extremely stable might have a very long half-life, but because of this great structural rigidity it might be a very poor catalyst and regulator. Thus, to the extent that pressure leads to extremely rigid protein conformations, it might adversely affect enzyme function. However, since hydrophobic interactions play such a major role in stabilising tertiary and quaternary structures of proteins, pressure enhancement of hydrogen bond stability may be compensated by pressure destabilisation of hydrophobic interactions. The opposing effects of elevated pressures on these two classes of weak interactions may therefore lead to an adaptive balancing of pressure effects. A similar phenomenon may occur in the case of temperature effects on protein structure, where again hydrogen bonding and hydrophobic interactions are affected differently by changes in temperature (Somero, 1975; Chapter 3).

In the case of protein tertiary structure, which is stabilised largely by hydrophobic interactions, the 'threats' posed by extremes of pressure have undergone a devaluation in recent years. As we discussed earlier, the more closely model compound studies approach the real world of protein molecules, the smaller are the observed volume changes which accompany 'denaturation' type reactions. The most recent studies of denaturation volume changes strongly support the predictions made by Bøje and Hvidt (1972) to the effect that the unfolding of proteins will be accompanied by smaller changes in volume than those which would be expected on the basis of solvation of dilute solutions of amino acid side-chain analogues. Brandts, Oliveira and Westort (1970) observed that the unfolding of ribonuclease was accompanied by volume changes ranging between −5 and −45 cm^3/mole, the precise value depending on conditions of assay pH and temperature — an important point we shall return to later. Zipp and Kauzmann (1973) observed volume changes of between approximately 50 and 100 cm^3/mole during denaturation of whale myoglobin.

These recent, highly refined measurements of denaturation volume changes make two important points for our analysis of pressure effects on marine organisms. First, even under the *in vitro* conditions employed in these studies, conditions in which pH, ionic strength and protein content were very different from intracellular conditions, the volume changes accompanying loss of tertiary structure were relatively small compared to the changes which would have been predicted on the basis of simplified model systems. In short, pressure poses much less of a danger to the stability of tertiary structure than seems to be generally realised.

The second important finding of these studies is that the pressure sensitivity of protein conformation is markedly dependent on the solution conditions (pH, temperature, ionic strength, ionic composition) experienced by the protein. Thus, an important note of caution which shall be sounded throughout this chapter: extrapolation from artificial *in vitro* conditions to real, *in situ* conditions is a step fraught with dangers.

Quaternary structure, like tertiary structure, may rely heavily on hydrophobic interactions. And, as in the case of tertiary structure, early hypothesising about pressure effects on quaternary structure was based on the observed volume changes in simplified model compound experiments. These data, of course, suggested that the quaternary structures of enzymes would be exceedingly pressure sensitive.

Initial studies of the pressure sensitivities of multimeric enzymes seemed to bear out the predictions of extreme pressure sensitivity for quaternary structure. For example, Penniston (1971) predicted that deep-sea organisms might lack multi-subunit enzymes owing to the pressure lability (of catalytic activity) he observed when he subjected multimeric enzymes (from terrestrial organisms) to high pressures. Penniston found that the activities of all of the multimeric enzymes were pressure-inhibited, while monomeric enzymes were either not affected or were pressure-activated.

Direct observations of pressure effects on subunit aggregation also suggest that quaternary structure may be extremely pressure labile. For example, Josephs and Harrington (1967, 1968) found that the hydrostatic pressures generated in the ultracentrifuge were sufficient to disrupt the quaternary structures of some proteins (*see also* Harrington, 1975). Thus, under conditions of several hundred atmospheres pressure, conditions well within the range experienced by marine organisms, pressure is seen to exert a profound effect on macromolecular structure.

However, not all studies of multimeric enzymes under pressure have found extreme pressure sensitivities for these catalysts. Lactate dehydrogenases and pyruvate kinases from deep-sea and shallow water fishes were all found to withstand pressures of several hundred atmospheres under *in vitro* assay conditions (Low and Somero, 1975a). Studies of other multimeric enzymes from deep-sea, shallow water and terrestrial species have also yielded data which suggest that quaternary structure is, for many multimeric proteins, quite pressure insensitive (*see* Hochachka, 1971).

As in the case of denaturation experiments, studies of enzymic activity under pressure have shown that the microenvironment of the enzyme is markedly important in establishing the response of the catalyst to pressure. For example, pyruvate kinase exhibits decreased pressure effects on reaction velocity as the salt concentration is raised from sub-physiological to physiological concentrations (Low and Somero, 1975a, b). Although this effect of the solute environment on this tetrameric enzyme probably does not involve changes in quaternary structure (Low and Somero, 1975b, c), there are good examples of the extent to which changes in the microenvironment of an enzyme can affect subunit aggregation.

Perhaps the classic example in the literature of a high pressure disruption of protein structure is the breakdown of the polymeric structure of F-actin to yield G-actin monomers (Ikkai and Ooi, 1966). High pressure favours the loss of polymeric (quaternary) structure, at least under certain *in vitro* conditions. In the absence of ATP, the equilibrium was shifted strongly in favour of G-actin at a pressure of 1500 kg/cm^2 (1400 atmospheres). Taken at its face value, this finding suggests that deep-sea organisms could have serious problems in assembling muscle proteins under the habitat conditions they experience*. However, a partial restoration of the normal intracellular conditions present in the muscle greatly alters the pressure sensitivity of the polymerisation process. When ATP is present in the *in vitro* system in physiological amounts, pressure denaturation was not observed until pressure was increased to 2500 kg/cm^2 (2300 atmospheres). If the F-actin

*It has been suggested that the length of F-actin polymers in deep-sea organisms might be shorter than in species living at lower pressures if the effect of pressure on the F-actin/G-actin equilibrium is critical in establishing polymer length (Herman and Dreizen, 1971). In fact, the length of skeletal muscle sarcomeres in the deep-sea fish, *Coryphaenoides,* is somewhat less than in other vertebrates (Herman and Dreizen, 1971). However, an alternative mechanism for controlling F-actin lengths is known: the muscle protein termed beta-actinin (Muruyama, 1966) seems to set the limit of polymerisation of G-actin monomers into F-actin filaments. It is not known if in deep-sea fish this protein favours an F-actin polymer of different length from the F-actin of vertebrates adapted to lower pressures.

polymer is similarly pressure-insensitive *in vivo,* it is clear that no organism would ever experience pressure denaturation of this protein.

Another example of the importance of examining pressure effects *in vitro* using experimental conditions which approximate as closely as possible the *in vivo* conditions experienced by the enzyme is given by Meyagawa (1965). He observed that the alpha-amylase of *B. subtilis* is inactivated at pressures exceeding 500 atmospheres when calcium ion is absent from the medium. In the presence of calcium, the enzyme is stable at pressures up to 3000 atmospheres. This observation agrees with the finding of Flügel and Schlieper (1970) that the presence of excess calcium in seawater can reduce the pressure sensitivities of whole marine organisms.

The limitations of *in vitro* experiments make such whole organism studies especially valuable and interesting. Fortunately, there have been a number of other studies of pressure effects on living cells. Of particular interest has been the effect of pressure on microtubular systems. Zimmerman (1970) observed that microtubular-based structures such as the mitotic spindles are readily pressure-disrupted in eggs of the sea urchin, *Arbacia.* Pressurisation to 680 atmospheres for one minute was sufficient to disrupt the mitotic apparatus. An effect of this type might well be instrumental in establishing the distribution limits of benthic marine organisms.

More recent studies of pressure effects on microtubular structures *in situ* and on microtubular assembly/disassembly equilibria *in vitro* have tended to produce conflicting results. O'Conner, Houston and Samson (1974) found that neuronal microtubules from the frog *Rana pipiens* were not dissociated by pressures up to 10 000 psi (approximately 680 atmospheres). Studies using intact cells and *in vitro* microtubular preparations yielded identical results. In contrast to these findings, Salmon (1975) observed that neuronal microtubules isolated from rabbit brain were reversibly depolymerised by pressures in this same range. The apparent disagreement between these two sets of data may derive from two sources: the experimental organisms used (ectothermic frogs and homeothermic mammals) and the *in vitro* assay conditions used. In the low cell temperature frog, microtubular assembly may involve a different balance of forces (hydrophobic, ionic) than in the case of the high cell temperature rabbit. In the case of the two *in vitro* assay systems used by the two groups of workers, adenosine-triphosphate (ATP) was used in one case (Salmon) and guanosine-triphosphate (GTP) was used in the other (O'Conner *et al.*). The observed differences in GTP and ATP effects on microtubular assembly (Salmon, 1975) again raises a word of caution concerning the danger of artifacts in studies using artificial systems.

In conjunction with discussion of pressure effects on microtubular systems, mention should be made of a rather analogous system which involves the reversible, pressure-sensitive polymerisation of sickle cell haemoglobin (Hb-S) molecules into long 'cables' (Murayama and Hasegawa, 1969). Hb-S differs from 'normal' (i.e. the most common) human Hb by only a single amino acid residue: a valyl residue replaces a glutamyl residue at position 6 of the beta-chain of Hb (*Figure 9.1*). This amino acid substitution permits the formation of a hydrophobic interaction between valyl residues (1) and (6) (*Figure 9.1*), and the resulting

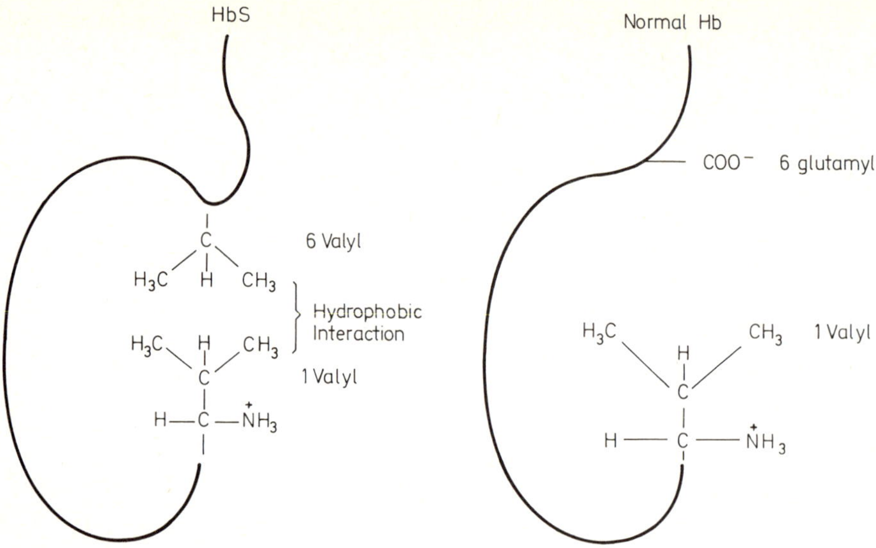

Figure 9.1 Schematic representation of the hydrophobic interaction between valyl residues 1 and 6 of the beta chain of sickle-cell haemoglobin (HbS). In normal Hb, the 6 position is occupied by a charged glutamyl residue. (From Hochachka and Somero, 1973; modified after Murayama, 1966; courtesy W. B. Saunders)

conformational change in the Hb molecule permits the Hb-S molecules to aggregate in long filaments which bear a certain resemblance to microtubules. The transition from soluble Hb-S to insoluble Hb-S filaments is, of course, a classic example of a sol to gel transformation.

The volume changes which accompany the formation of the Hb-S gel are large. Between 1 and 50 atmospheres pressure and at a temperature of 37°C, a positive volume change of approximately 400 cm^3/mole occurs during polymerisation. Over this range of pressures, any increase in pressure leads to polymer breakdown (to the sol state). Between 50 and 150 atmospheres pressure, the volume change in the sol to gel transition is approximately –500 cm^3/mole. Pressure increases over this higher pressure range therefore favour the formation of the gel state.

These findings have a good deal of relevance for our discussion of pressure effects on marine organisms. First, it is obvious that relatively small increases in hydrostatic pressure, e.g. from 1 to 150 atmospheres are able to lead to large changes in the polymerisation state of molecular ensembles. If the polymerisation processes, e.g. those that occur during formation of microtubular systems and contractile systems, of marine organisms are comparably pressure sensitive, then many marine organisms might experience severe pressure stresses as they migrate through the water column. We can only suggest that the Hb-S sol-gel interconversion is atypically pressure sensitive and/or other factors such as pH and ionic strength can greatly reduce the pressure sensitivities of such processes *in vivo*. A second point raised by the Hb-S data is that only minimal changes in the amino acid composition of a protein are necessary to greatly alter its pressure sensitivity. We can view this finding as offering potential adaptive mechanisms for the marine organism which is moving through a wide range of depths. Thus, during colonisation of the deep-sea, perhaps only slight changes in amino acid composition would be necessary to change the pressure sensitivities of biological structures and processes.

Pressure adaptations could involve changes in other factors besides the amino acid compositions of proteins, as we have earlier suggested in the case of ion-pair effects. Here we proposed that adverse effects on ion pair formation could be offset by raising the concentrations of the ions. Blaxter *et al.* (1971) have reported that the freezing point depressions of body fluids of deep-sea fishes are higher than those of shallow water marine teleosts. This observation may indicate that deep-sea fishes have raised ionic concentrations as a pressure-adaptive response. One can further argue, in this connection, that marine invertebrates, which are isosmotic to seawater, are pre-adapted for coping with changes in pressure, at least to the extent that high ionic contents dampen pressure effects. (We will see later how important such ionic effects are in the case of catalytic rate adaptations to pressure.)

The reduction of the size of volume changes associated with biochemical reactions could be achieved by several mechanisms. A model system showing how the volume changes which occur during formation of quaternary structures might be reduced is provided by the G-actin polymerisation reaction. In this reaction the G-actin monomer, which is covalently bound to one molecule of ATP, releases ADP and Pi as it joins a growing F-actin polymer. As we discussed above, the effect of pressure on the G-actin/F-actin equilibrium is greatly reduced in the presence of ATP. Indeed, one would expect that the release of two charged species during the polymerisation process would create a favourable volume change (*Table 9.1*). This volume decrease resulting from electrostriction of water around the ADP and Pi ions might largely offset the volume increase which is caused by the removal of water from the interacting surfaces of the G-actin subunits. As a general rule, therefore, we suggest that whenever a polymerisation reaction is accompanied by a volume increase caused by release of bound water from the polymerising subunits, a coupled release of a charged molecule could 'titrate' this volume change to a much lower value. The reader may recall an analogous argument raised in the discussion of temperature effects, wherein the temperature sensitivity of a process could be reduced by coupling two reactions with equal and oppositely signed enthalpy changes.

One potential source of volume adjustment which we have not yet considered involves the free space or void volume which exists within a folded polypeptide chain. Assarsson and Eirich (1968) have stressed that packing large particles together leads to a larger void volume than that which results from packing the same number of large particles in a solution of solvent molecules. Thus when bulky, hydrophobic side chains are buried within the folded polypeptide chain, they may occupy a larger volume than when they are exposed to the surrounding water. Denaturation may largely eliminate this void volume. However, the quantitative importance of this volume effect on denaturation equilibria is not known.

Of relevance in the context of adaptation mechanisms is the possibility that enzymes could pack their hydrophobic residues into smaller volumes. For example, amino acid changes might facilitate more compact structures if less bulky non-polar side-chains were substituted for bulky residues. In the case of quaternary structure, it is conceivable that during the polymerisation reaction, subunit–subunit interactions might lead to changes in tertiary structure which reduce the void volume among buried non-polar side-chains. We know of no data bearing on either of these potential mechanisms of high pressure adaptation.

To summarise what we regard as the major points of the foregoing discussion, we need only say that both theoretical and experimental approaches to pressure effects on protein structure must be made with extreme caution. Model compound studies are useful guides in some cases; in others they may lead the biologist into erroneous extrapolation. Even more misleading is the discovery of *in vitro* effects which do not occur *in vivo*. We have seen, and will find again in our later discussion, that the local environment in which a protein is functioning can exert a major effect on the structural and functional properties of the protein with regard to pressure effects. Thus the pressure-oriented biochemist is faced with major 'uncertainty principles' as he attempts to work from simplified systems back to the real world. We believe that the rate of progress in unravelling the effects of hydrostatic pressure on biological systems and in discerning the adaptive strategies used to compensate for pressure stresses will be most dependent on the ingenuity used by the investigator to reproduce, or avoid destroying, the particular conditions of pH, ionic strength, ionic composition, cellular compartmentalisation etc. which characterise the local environment of the macromolecule under study.

9.3.3 Pressure effects on membranes

A discussion of pressure effects on protein quintinary structure can best be dealt with in the context of biomembranes, since the ways in which proteins are incorporated into larger cellular structures are well illustrated in the case of cellular membranes. Furthermore, it is very clear that pressure can exert profound effects on membrane-related or membrane-based functions such as transport (Landau, 1970; Paul and Morita, 1971; Pequeux, 1972). Thus, we shall examine in some detail both known and hypothetical patterns of interaction between hydrostatic pressure and the different classes of membrane proteins.

Singer and Nicolson (1972) have categorised membrane proteins into two groups. The 'peripheral' proteins appear to be plated on to the external surfaces of membranes. Their attachment to the membrane surfaces is thought to involve electrostatic interactions between the charged phosphate 'heads' of the membrane phospholipids and surface charges on the protein. Since the binding of peripheral membrane proteins to the membrane phospholipid bilayer is dependent on electrostatic interactions, i.e. on charge neutralisations, we might predict that increases in pressure would disrupt the binding of proteins to the membrane surface.

The second class of membrane proteins are the 'integral' proteins, proteins which are incorporated partially or entirely into the non-polar region of the phospholipid bilayer. Integral proteins appear to have oily surfaces (Singer and Nicolson, 1972), and these proteins, therefore, are most likely held within the membrane by hydrophobic interactions. Whereas it is not clear whether increases in pressure will tend to dissociate the integral proteins from the interior of the membrane, it does seem very likely that pressure- and temperature-dependent changes in the physical state and viscosity of the membrane lipids will affect the integral proteins (*Table 9.3*). For example, if pressure increases (or temperature decreases) greatly increase the viscosity of the fatty acid side-chains, perhaps even causing them to change from a 'liquid crystalline' to solid state, the ability of integral proteins to undergo necessary changes in conformation and in translation through the membrance (Singer and Nicolson, 1972) may be impaired. As we emphasised earlier, a system which has great thermodynamic stability or structural rigidity may prevent the many changes in molecular shape and position which are required for efficient catalysis and regulation.

To our knowledge no one has studied membrane proteins from abyssal organisms. We have no information on the susceptibility of peripheral proteins to pressure dissociation. If pressure does disrupt the electrostatic interactions which hold these proteins on the membrane surface, perhaps a deep-sea organism would benefit from peripheral proteins which are held to the membrane surface by covalent bonds, e.g. disulphide bridges. Pressure effects on integral proteins are also poorly understood. While it is clear that membrane transport can be blocked by increases in pressure, it is not known if this effect is due to (a) inactivation of an integral protein involved in transport, (b) changes in the viscosity or physical state of the lipid bilayer, (c) blocking of the enzymic reaction *per se* owing to unfavourable volume changes during the reaction, e.g. during the activation event; or (d) one or more other causes.

Changes in the fatty acid compositions of membrane lipids are well known in the case of temperature adaptation (*see* Chapter 3). Since decreases in temperature and increases in hydrostatic pressure have similar effects on the physical state and viscosity of lipids, one might predict that deep-sea organisms will adapt to high pressures in much the same way as low temperature ectotherms have adapted to low temperatures: the degree of saturation of phospholipid fatty acid chains will be reduced.

A comparison of deep and shallow water marine ectotherms is rendered difficult, in a logistic sense, by the fact that surface temperatures are generally much higher than abyssal temperatures, especially in the oceanic regions where deep collections are made. We know of only a single study (Patton, 1975) in which deep-sea organisms have been compared with surface organisms which experience a similar thermal regime. Patton compared the fatty acid composition of brain phospholipids of deep-sea and

Antarctic (surface) fishes and found essentially identical fatty acid compositions. The imposition of high pressures on an already cold-stressed system did not seem to promote further reductions in fatty acid saturation. His findings seem to suggest that temperature is a more severe stress than hydrostatic pressure in the case of membrane physical state effects. However, a survey of additional deep-sea organisms would be desirable before any inductive generalisations concerning this phenomenon are attempted.

9.3.4 Pressure effects on catalytic activations

In the preceding sections we have dealt almost exclusively with pressure effects on chemical equilibria, e.g. equilibria between associated and dissociated protein subunits. We now wish to extend our treatment to a consideration of the ways in which enzymic rates are affected by pressure.

A basic strategy of pressure adaptation would seem to be a uniform reduction in the absolute values of the $\Delta V^{\ddagger}$'s of enzymic reactions. If all $\Delta V^{\ddagger}$'s are reduced to zero, all reactions would be pressure-insensitive (excluding effects arising from volume changes during substrate binding and product release, as discussed in Section 9.3.5). One of the strongest arguments in favour of this adaptive strategy is based on considerations of how changes in pressure might affect multi-enzyme pathways and metabolic branchpoints (where two or more enzymes compete for a common metabolic intermediate). Consider, for example, a metabolic branchpoint at which three enzymes compete for a common substrate. If each enzymic reaction has a very different $\Delta V^{\ddagger}$ value from the other two reactions, a change in pressure is apt to exert a large change on the relative amounts of substrate being drawn into each of the three competing pathways. For instance, if enzyme (1) has a large negative $\Delta V^{\ddagger}$ value associated with its reaction, relative to the $\Delta V^{\ddagger}$ values of enzymic reactions (2) and (3), then an increase in pressure will shift the allocation of the common substrate strongly in favour of enzyme (1). What we witness in such a case is a wresting of metabolic control away from the cell by the external environment. This will in general prove to be an adverse situation, since changes in the relative demands for the products of the three competing pathways are much more likely to arise from changes in the metabolic state of the cell than from changes in hydrostatic pressure.

A comparable situation obtains in the case of a single metabolic pathway in which the activities of all contributing enzymes must be closely coordinated. Control of an entire metabolic pathway is generally vested in one or two key regulatory enzymes which are situated either at the top of the pathway (at the first reaction which is unique to the pathway) or at metabolic branchpoints further along the pathway. For example, phosphofructokinase is a regulator acting at the top of the glycolytic sequence, and pyruvate kinase is a secondary control site located at the phosphoenolpyruvate branchpoint.

If a reaction which is normally non-regulatory is highly pressure sensitive, a change in pressure could shift control from the usual control sites to this non-regulatory enzyme. If the non-regulatory enzyme is strongly inhibited by increased pressure, it may block the activity of the entire pathway under conditions where the normal regulatory switches are fully open, i.e. under conditions where the cell requires the products of the pathway. Such a blockage will have a second deleterious effect in addition to depriving the cell of needed metabolic products: the levels of metabolic intermediates formed in reactions above the blocked enzyme may rise exponentially. Since many metabolic intermediates are highly reactive, large increases in their concentrations likely would lead to serious side-reactions which follow rules of mass action rather than the rules of close control *via* metabolic regulation (*see* Atkinson, 1969). It therefore seems imperative that control does not pass from regulatory sites to non-regulatory sites as a result of pressure changes. Reductions in activation volumes seem a potentially important mechanism for insuring that such regulatory upsets do not occur.

These theoretical considerations raise a number of questions which can be examined empirically. First, are the enzymes of deep-sea and vertically migrating marine organisms characterised by lower $\Delta V^{\ddagger}$ values than the homologous (or analogous) enzymes of terrestrial and shallow water species? Second, if the answer to the first question is negative, are there ways in which the local environment, in which the enzyme functions, can be modified to reduce activation volumes?

Table 9.4 contains data bearing on the first question. For at least the few enzymes which have been studied, there is no apparent reduction in the size of $\Delta V^{\ddagger}$ in high pressure adapted species. Interestingly, however, the size of the activation volume does correlate with the species adaptation temperature, as discussed in Chapter 3. The size of the activation volume may provide a measure of the magnitude of the conformational change which accompanies catalytic activation, and temperature may play a dominant role

Table 9.4 ACTIVATION VOLUMES ($\Delta V^{\ddagger}$) FOR LACTATE DEHYDROGENASE AND PYRUVATE KINASE REACTIONS OF DIFFERENT MARINE FISHES (DATA FROM LOW AND SOMERO, 1975 A, B)

	$\Delta V^{\ddagger}$ (cm^3/mole)
Lactate dehydrogenase	
Coryphaenoides acrolepis (rattail)	−3.93
Trematomus borchgrevinki (Antarctic)	−0.43
Hypoglossus stenolepis (halibut)	−0.23
Pyruvate kinase[1]	
Coryphaenoides acrolepis	
0.08 M KCl	23.7
0.08 M NH_4Cl	38.8
Trematomus borchgrevinki	
0.08 M KCl	11.0
0.08 M NH_4Cl	7.6
0.08 M NaCl	54.3

[1]Assays were conducted in the presence of saturating concentration of substrate (phosphoenolpyruvate) and varying ionic compositions and ionic strengths

in establishing the nature of these conformational changes (Low and Somero, 1975b; Somero, 1975).

The answer to the second question raised above, namely are there other ways of reducing activation volumes, is affirmative, as the data of *Figure 9.2* illustrate. As we learned in the case of protein polymerisation reactions, the ionic environment of the enzyme can exert an extremely important effect on the pressure sensitivity of the process. For all of the pyruvate kinase enzymes we examined (Low and Somero, 1975a), increases in potassium ion concentration led to reductions in $\Delta V^{\ddagger}$ values. It can be noted that at physiological potassium concentrations the activation volumes of the three pyruvate kinase reactions are between one-sixth and one-third the values observed at low potassium levels. The marked effect of this single ion on the $\Delta V^{\ddagger}$ of these reactions raises the question as to how much further the $\Delta V^{\ddagger}$ values might be reduced if other substances normally present in the local environment of the enzyme were added to the *in vitro* assay mixture! Some suggestion of the complexity of effects which must occur *in vivo* is given by the data of *Table 9.4*. Both the type of salt and the concentration of salt are able to influence the $\Delta V^{\ddagger}$ value. (A more detailed description of these salt effects, and a mechanistic explanation of the mode of action of the different inorganic cations is given in Low and Somero, 1975b, c).

There are few other data available in the literature on salt effects on enzymic rates and activation volumes. Becker and Evans (1969) found that in the case of beta-galactosidase of *E. coli,* the potassium-activated enzyme was pressure-inhibited while the sodium-activated enzyme was pressure-activated. These effects are the opposite of those observed for pyruvate kinase. For pig liver malate dehydrogenase, both sodium and potassium ion

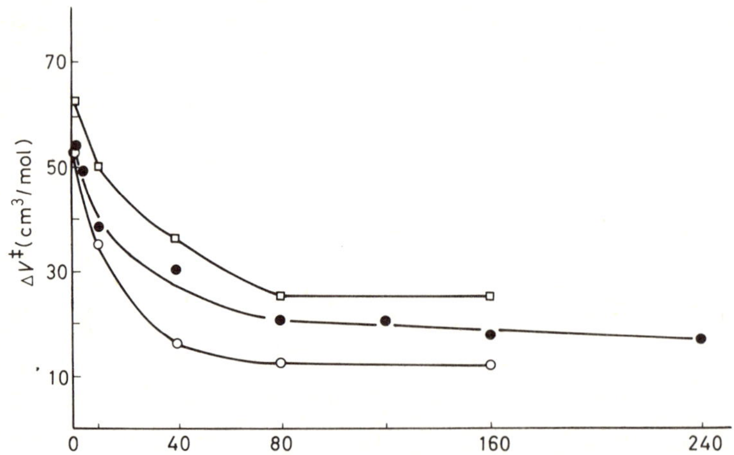

Figure 9.2 The effect of varying KCl concentrations on the activation volume ($\Delta V^{\ddagger}$) of pyruvate kinase reactions catalysed by pyruvate kinases from three marine fishes: Coryphaenoides acrolepis (□); Trematomus borchgrevinki (O); Scorpaena gutatta (●). *(Data from Low and Somero, 1975a)*

are capable of reducing the absolute value of the activation volume (Low and Somero, 1975b). Neville and Eyring (1972) have also reported a sodium dependence of activation volume (lysozyme).

The observed effects of salt concentration and composition on activation volumes, especially our findings that salt concentrations in the upper portions of the physiological range may greatly reduce the pressure sensitivities of reaction velocities, again raise the possibility that the high salt contents of marine invertebrates pre-adapt these organisms for existence under conditions of high and/or variable pressure. Similarly, the elevated salt compositions which may characterise certain deep-sea fishes (Blaxter *et al.*, 1971) may serve an important function in reducing pressure effects on catalytic activation steps.

9.3.5 Pressure effects on enzyme-ligand interactions

Under cellular conditions the velocities of enzymic reactions are determined by at least two factors: (a) the catalytic efficiency of the enzyme, as measured by the free energy of activation of the reaction it catalyses (or by the moles of substrate the enzyme can convert to product per unit time); and (b) the degree to which the catalytic site(s) of the enzyme are saturated with substrate(s). Metabolic regulation is known to depend far more highly on the second class of effects. Under most conditions virtually all enzymes function at rates well below their maximal velocities, for substrate levels in the cell normally do not exceed the magnitudes of the Michaelis constants (K_m values) of enzymes, i.e. substrate levels are usually less than half as great as the concentrations necessary to fully saturate the catalytic sites. Increases in enzymic activity under intracellular conditions in response to positive modulators are generally due to modulator-induced increases in the apparent affinity between enzymes and substrates. Negative modulators generally retard the rates of enzymic activity by making substrate binding less favourable.

Owing to the fact that interactions between enzymes and ligands (substrates and modulators) are dependent on weak chemical bonds such as hydrophobic interactions, hydrogen bonds and electrostatic (Coulombic) interactions, pressure is apt to have important effects on catalytic velocities and metabolic regulation even if, as we have suggested is possible, activation volumes can be held at quite low levels. It therefore seems advantageous for deep-sea and, especially, vertically migrating marine organisms to reduce the volume changes which occur during ligand binding. These volume reductions, which will be reflected in relatively pressure-independent K_m, K_a and K_i values (which represent the half-saturating concentrations of substrates, activators and inhibitors, respectively), will reduce the pressure sensitivity of enzymic reaction velocities and, more importantly, will render metabolic regulation less susceptible to the effect of pressure changes.

Currently available data (*Figure 9.3, Tables 9.5* and *9.6*) indicate that important pressure adaptations have occurred in binding phenomena. Different classes of enzymes and ligand-binding site interactions appear to

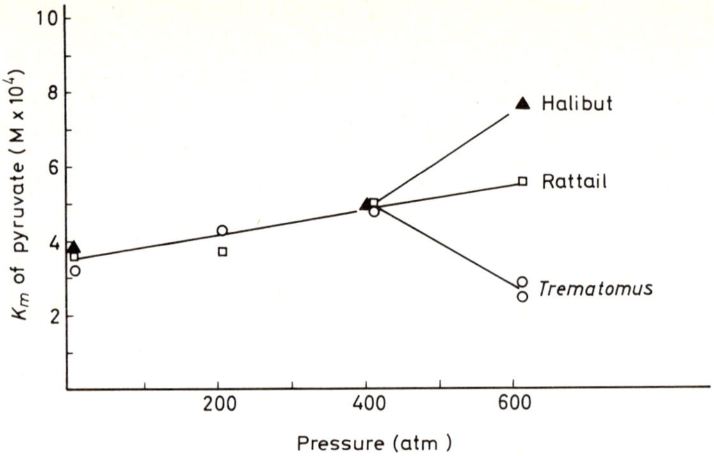

Figure 9.3 The effect of pressure on the apparent Michaelis constant (K_m) of pyruvate for lactate dehydrogenases of three marine fishes: the halibut (Hypoglussus stenolepis); Trematomus borchgrevinki, *an Antarctic species; and the rattail* (Coryphaenoides acrolepis) *a deep benthic species. (Data from Low and Somero, 1975a; courtesy Pergamon Press Ltd)*

differ in their pressure sensitivities. For pyruvate kinase (PK), apparent K_m of PEP values seem to be highly conserved at physiological pressures. The PK's of deep-sea and shallow water marine fishes display highly similar affinities for PEP at their respective adaptation pressures, even though at any one pressure the apparent K_m values may vary widely (*Table 9.5*). A similar conservation in substrate binding abilities among species has been observed in the case of temperature adaptation (Chapter 3). The different pressure sensitivities of a number of regulatory properties of PK's from a shallow water, a deepwater fish, and a midwater fish are given in *Table 9.6*. The vertically-migrating midwater species' PK appears especially insensitive to pressure changes.

Lactate dehydrogenases (LDH's) from deepwater and shallow water fishes are similar in their pressure-K_m (pyruvate) characteristics, at least at pressures up to 408 atmospheres (*Figure 9.3*). At higher pressures, however,

Table 9.5 THE EFFECTS OF PRESSURE ON THE APPARENT MICHAELIS CONSTANT (K_m) OF PHOSPHOENOLPYRUVATE (PEP) FOR PYRUVATE KINASES FROM FOUR SPECIES OF MARINE FISHES. ALL ASSAYS WERE CONDUCTED AT 5°C, UNDER THE ASSAY CONDITIONS DESCRIBED BY LOW AND SOMERO (1975A)

Species (habitat)	*K_m of PEP (X 10^5 M)* 1 atm	204 atm	408 atm
Trematomus borchgrevinki (shallow, Antarctic)	3.5	4.7	5.8
Coryphaenoides acrolepis (deep benthic)	2.2	2.9	3.7
Sebastolobus altivelis (deep benthic)	2.6	2.7	4.5
Scorpaena gutatta (shallow, temperate)	4.8	1.0	4.5

Table 9.6 THE INFLUENCE OF PRESSURE ON THE CATALYTIC AND REGULATORY PROPERTIES OF PYRUVATE KINASES FROM FISHES INHABITING DIFFERENT REGIONS OF THE WATER COLUMN (AFTER HOCHACHKA AND SOMERO, 1973)

Enzyme function	*Pressure effect* *Coryphaenoides (deep water)*	*Ectreposebastes (mid-water)*	*Trout (surface)*
K_m of PEP	small increase	no effect	large effect
K_m of PEP in presence of FDP (enzyme activator)	small decrease	no effect	large effect
K_m of ADP	small increase	no effect	large increase
K_i of ATP	no effect	no effect	large increase
FDP reversal of ATP inhibition	large increase	no effect	no effect

the enzyme of the deep-sea fish, *Coryphaenoides acrolepis,* did not display a break in the pressure-versus-K_m curve as was observed for two LDH's from shallow water fishes. Recent field observations suggest that *Coryphaenoides acrolepis* may traverse a wide depth range (R. Rosenblatt, personal communication), and thus a pressure-insensitive substrate binding ability would be highly adaptive.

For a third enzyme, fructosediphosphatase (FDPase), major differences were noted between the homologues of the enzyme from a surface fish (the rainbow trout) and a deep-sea fish (*Coryphaenoides*). While both enzymes displayed increased V_{max} values at elevated pressures, the trout FDPase was strongly inhibited at low substrate concentrations in contrast to the *Coryphaenoides* enzyme which showed only a slight rise in the apparent K_m of FDP with increasing pressure (*see* Hochachka and Somero, 1973). These data suggest that the volume change which occurs during FDP binding to FDPase can be varied significantly during evolutionary adaptation to high pressures. The mechanism of this reduction in binding volume is not known.

The effects of pressure on enzyme-modulator interactions may also differ among homologues of a given enzyme. The results presented in *Table 9.6* indicate that pyruvate kinase from the deep-sea fish, *Coryphaenoides,* has a much lower pressure sensitivity in its regulatory functions than the homologous enzyme from the rainbow trout. Similar differences have been reported for the regulatory properties of FDPase variants from deep and surface fishes (Hochachka and Somero, 1973).

When we begin to consider the possible mechanisms which might be instrumental in reducing the volume changes which accompany enzyme-ligand binding, we soon realise that an important constraint is imposed on the system: the chemical structures of the substrates and modulators cannot be varied, so any adaptations must be the 'responsibility' of either the enzyme itself or of the local environment in which the enzyme functions.

Adaptive changes in the enzyme could be of several types. First, selection could favour enzymes which possess the ability to 'titrate' the volume changes which result from ligand binding. For example, if ligand binding involves charge neutralisation (with a volume increase caused by release of electrostricted water; *Table 9.1*), the enzyme might expose a charged group to water elsewhere on the enzyme surface to 'titrate' the volume change which occurs as a result of events at the ligand binding site. Similarly, changes in the void volume of the enzyme might be used to compensate for volume changes resulting from ligand binding. These conformational mechanisms would seem to supply adequate raw material for adaptive adjustments in ligand binding volumes.

Another adaptive mechanism for adjusting ligand binding volumes entails changing the amino acid composition of ligand binding sites in such a way that the numbers and types of weak interactions between enzyme and ligand involve only small volume changes. Adaptations of this category have been discussed by Hochachka (1974) for the nervous system enzyme acetylcholinesterase (AChE), which catalyses the reaction:

$$\underset{\text{acetylcholine (ACh)}}{CH_3-\underset{\underset{CH_3}{|}}{\overset{\overset{CH_3}{|}}{N^+}}-CH_2-CH_2-O-\overset{\overset{O}{\|}}{C}-CH_3} + H_2O = \text{choline} + \text{acetate} + H^+$$

The ACh binding site of AChE is composed of two sub-sites: (a) an 'anionic site' which is of primary importance in binding the ACh molecule to the enzyme; and (b) an 'esteratic site' which is the locus at which hydrolysis of the ACh molecule occurs (*Figure 9.4*).

The types of weak interaction which occur between enzyme and substrate at the anionic site make AChE-ACh complex formation pressure and temperature sensitive. Electrostatic (Coulombic) interactions between the positively charged quaternary ammonium group and the dissociated carboxyl group of the anionic site will be stabilised by low temperature and

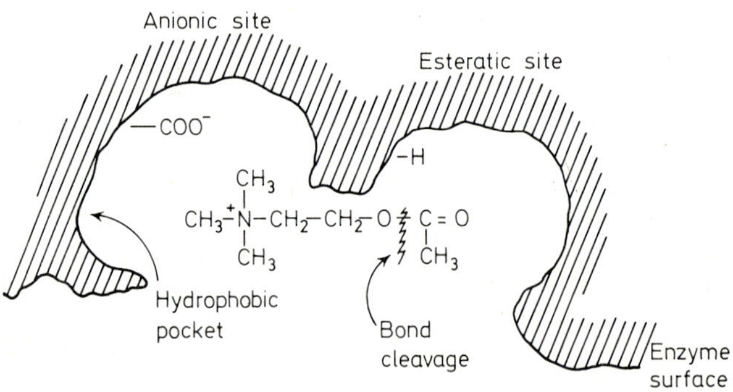

Figure 9.4 A schematic representation of acetylcholinesterase, showing the acetylcholine (ACh) binding site. The major portion of the stabilising energy holding the AChE-ACh complex intact comes from the hydrophobic interactions between the methyl (CH_3) groups of ACh and the hydrophobic amino acid residues found in the hydrophobic 'pocket' of the 'anionic site'. Splitting of the bond between the choline and acetate moieties occurs at the 'esteratic site'. (After Hochachka and Somero, 1973; courtesy W. B. Saunders)

disrupted by high pressures — at least according to the predictions of model compound studies (*Table 9.1*). The hydrophobic interactions between the methyl groups of ACh and the non-polar amino acid side-chains which lie within the hydrophobic pocket of the anionic site may also be temperature and pressure sensitive, with low temperatures and high pressures leading to disruption of the enzyme-substrate complex. We might add, parenthetically, that the predictions based on model compound studies, which have used highly dilute low molecular weight non-polar molecules, may be more valid for enzyme-ligand interactions than for protein denaturation processes, since substrates are present at very low concentrations within the cell and, of course, substrates such as ACh are of low molecular weight and thus do not present a concentrated front of non-polar moieties to the aqueous phase as do proteins which are unfolding and exposing buried hydrophobic residues.

The nature of these pressure effects and the possible interspecific differences in ACh binding among homologues of AChE from different fishes were investigated using substrate analogues and ACh inhibitors which might be expected to differ from ACh in their binding thermodynamics. For example, the carbon analogue of ACh, 3, 3 dimethylbutyl acetate

$$\begin{array}{ccccccccccccc} & & CH_3 & & & & & & & & O & & \\ & & | & & & & & & & & \| & & \\ CH^3 & — & C & — & CH_2 & - & CH_2 & - & O & - & C & - & CH_3 \\ & & | & & & & & & & & & & \\ & & CH_3 & & & & & & & & & & \end{array}$$

is identical to ACh except that a carbon atom has replaced the nitrogen atom to which the methyl groups are attached. Binding of this substrate analogue will not involve electrostatic interactions, and enzyme-'substrate' complex stability will be due almost entirely to hydrophobic interactions. Kinetic studies with 3, 3 dimethylbutyl acetate, using purified AChE from the electric eel (Hochachka, 1974), showed that as the assay temperature is lowered from 35 to 2°C the apparent K_m of this substrate analogue increases by over ten-fold. This finding is entirely consistent with predictions based on model compound studies (Brandts, 1967). Increases in pressure from 1 to approximately 400 atmospheres also led to a large increase in the apparent K_m of the analogue. This result too is consistent with the results of model compound studies which use small, dilute organic molecules.

The effects of temperature and pressure on the electrostatic interactions between ACh and AChE were estimated using inhibitors which compete with ACh at the anionic site. For simple substituted ammonium ions such as dimethyl ammonium, binding is determined largely by electrostatic interactions between the quaternary ammonium nitrogen and the negatively charged group of the anionic site (Froede and Wilson, 1972). For electric eel AChE, the binding of such a competitive inhibitor (as measured by the apparent K_i of inhibitor binding) is facilitated by low temperatures and high pressures. The latter result is of course not consistent with the predictions of model compound studies. At present no explanation of this anomalous result is possible.

These observations, made with an AChE from a shallow water fish, clearly define the 'problems' which ACh enzymes of deep-sea and vertically migrating marine organisms would encounter. The predicted inhibition of AChE activity owing to reduced ACh binding ability at high pressures could be partially or even fully offset if deep-sea organisms maintained relatively high concentrations of AChE in their nervous tissues. This type of 'quantitative' compensation to environmental stresses has already been shown to play an important role in temperature compensation processes (*see* Chapter 3). Alternatively, adaptation to high pressures might lead to the development over evolutionary time periods of a 'better' variant of AChE, i.e. an enzyme with a substrate binding site that exhibits reduced sensitivity to pressure.

The findings of a study of AChE from a deep water fish, *Antimora rostrata,* suggest that both adaptational strategies can be utilised, albeit modifications of the substrate binding site seem of greater significance (Hochachka, Storey and Baldwin, 1975). ACh binding by this high-pressure-adapted enzyme is enhanced by elevated pressures and reduced temperatures. This observation suggests that the importance of hydrophobic interactions may be significantly reduced in the *Antimora* enzyme, and that electrostatic interactions may play the major role in stabilising the ACh-AChE complex. If the latter condition does obtain, one must somehow account for the fact that a charge neutralisation process can be pressure-enhanced (as was found for binding of the inhibitor, dimethyl ammonium chloride). One hypothetical explanation for these 'anomalous' charge neutralisation-pressure interactions can be based on considerations of ion effects on water structure. Ammonium ion and substituted ammonium ion are classed as 'water destructuring ions' (*see* Wiggins, 1971). In solution, a destructuring ion may disrupt water–water interactions and can promote an increase in the volume of the aqueous system. When a destructuring ion is bound to an enzyme surface, its effects on water structure may be eliminated or at least greatly reduced. Thus, the binding of ACh or a similar ion to AChE may be accompanied by a reordering (and contraction) of a sufficient number of water molecules to make the net volume change negative.

Finally, let us consider briefly the types of amino acid substitutions in the anionic site which could promote reduced hydrophobic dependence and increased reliance on electrostatic interactions. Simply by reducing the number of hydrophobic amino acid side-chains protruding into the hydrophobic pocket of the anionic site an AChE would lower its hydrophobic bonding ability and increase its capacity to bind ACh electrostatically. Removal of non-polar amino acid side-chains from the anionic site would facilitate entry of water into this site, and this would enhance the ease with which the –COOH group within the hydrophobic pocket could dissociate. Alternatively, the pK of the –COOH group might be lowered by utilising a different acidic amino acid.

Whether or not modifications in the amino acid composition of ligand binding sites occur during adaptation to high and/or variable pressures can only be ascertained when these sites are isolated in pure form and the amino acid residues are sequenced. *A priori,* it is difficult to predict how important an adaptive mechanism binding site modification might be. Indeed, it is not clear how accessible such an adaptive approach can be. Thus, in contrast to ACh which has both charged and non-polar components, most metabolic intermediates are relatively non-polar and bind exclusively through electrostatic interactions or hydrogen bonds. If binding of the ligand to the surface of the enzyme is via only one class of weak bond, then a sharp constraint is placed on adaptation via changes in the amino acid composition of the ligand binding site. In such cases the adjustment of binding volumes may require conformational changes, such as those discussed above, in which the volume change that occurs locally at the ligand binding site is 'titrated' by a volume change resulting from either altered side-chain exposures to water or changes in the void volume of the enzyme.

9.3.6 Pressure effects on transcription and translation

The magnitude of the stress an environmental factor imposes on a biological system often is directly proportional to the complexity of the system. Thus, as we have stated above, branchpoint enzymes may be a particularly acute site of pressure perturbation, since the proper control of metabolism at these loci involves interactions among numerous proteins and small molecules. The same considerations lead one to predict that the reactions involved in gene expression, namely the processes of transcription (mRNA synthesis) and translation (polypeptide synthesis on polysomes), will also be extremely pressure sensitive. Available data suggest that this expectation is fully realised.

Pressure effects on transcription and translation have been investigated in several organisms, most of which, unfortunately, are adapted to terrestrial pressures (Landau, 1970; Zimmerman, 1970). Landau (1970) found that HeLa cells (human origin) and *E. coli* display similar pressure sensitivities in translational events. For example, in HeLa cells there was no inhibition of translation up to pressures of approximately 270 atmospheres. As pressure was increased to 544 atmospheres, gradual inhibition of translation was noted, and at higher pressures translation was blocked completely. Transcription was inhibited increasingly as pressure was raised above one atmosphere, but some mRNA synthesis was observed even up to 680 atmospheres. On the basis of these and other data (Zimmerman, 1970), we can conclude that both transcription and translation are blocked by elevated pressures, and that the latter reactions are more sensitive than the former.

In recent studies of the steps which might be critical in the pressure blockage of translation, evidence has accumulated which implicates the binding of the amino acid-tRNA complex to the ribosome as the singly most pressure-sensitive event (Schwarz and Landau, 1972). The activation volume change for this reaction has been calculated to be approximately 100 cm^3/mole (Schwarz and Landau, 1972). The overall translational process exhibits a pressure-sensitivity consistent with a volume change of this magnitude. Arnold and Albright (1971) have also observed pressure inhibition of peptide bond formation, so pressure may stress a number of events in the translational process. And, of course, in different species, different steps may be the most pressure-sensitive. Finally, it should be pointed out that many recent studies, including those cited above, have used cell-free *E. coli* protein synthetic systems. Thus, the many cautions we have voiced concerning the importance of a natural milieu around the macromolecules under study should again be recalled.

Fortunately, we can cite at least one study in which pressure effects on *in vivo* protein synthesis were examined. Zimmerman (1970) pressure-shocked intact protozoans and sea urchin embryos and examined polysome profiles from these and control cells. Pressure-shocked cells lacked the heavy polysome fraction, indicating a block to translation. The polysomes of *Tetrahymena pyriformis* were more pressure-sensitive than those of the sea urchin, *Arbacia.* Since the latter species experiences pressure changes during its life, the observed differences could be adaptive. However, recalling what we said earlier about the influences of ion concentration on the pressure sensitivities of enzymic reactions, we can also propose that the observed difference between the marine and freshwater invertebrates might have been due to the different ionic strengths of their intracellular fluids. The marine form, with its higher cellular ion content, may be inherently pressure adapted.

9.3.7 Mechanisms for sensing changes in pressure

Biochemical adaptations to the environment often appear to be 'last resort' responses which an organism must make when it is unable behaviourally to avoid or reduce an environmental stress (Hochachka and Somero, 1973). Behavioural adaptations, e.g. migrations, are ultimately dependent on sensitive mechanisms for detecting changes in the magnitude of an environmental parameter. In the case of certain marine invertebrates, pressure-sensing mechanisms appear to reach their zenith. For example, Enright (1961, 1962) has reported that the intertidal amphipod *Synchelidium* is able to detect pressure changes of less than 0.01 atmospheres. Such extremely high sensitivity to pressure changes may enable an organism to select the proper region of the water column.

The physical and chemical bases of pressure reception in these organisms and in other marine invertebrates which display comparable abilities to detect pressure changes (Digby, 1972) are not well understood. Digby (1972; *see also* Chapter 6) has proposed a mechanism for pressure detection which involves subtle changes in the electrode characteristics of the cuticle. He proposes that an extremely thin layer of hydrogen gas is present at or near the cuticle surface, and changes in pressure affect the volume of this gas layer, which in turn alters the electrode characteristics of the cuticle.

Further understanding of these pressure-sensing mechanisms will likely make an important contribution to the biophysics of energy transducing systems.

9.4 CONCLUDING COMMENTS

The current status of high pressure research with marine organisms might be described as follows: the biological observations summarised in the recent volumes edited by Sleigh and MacDonald (1972) and Zimmerman (1970) have outlined fairly well the major effects of high pressures and variable pressures on a number of morphological and physiological systems. However, molecular interpretations of these pressure effects are incomplete. We are still a long way from appreciating in detail (a) how pressure affects macromolecular structure and function, and (b) how deep-sea and vertically migrating organisms have had to modify their cellular chemistry to reduce or eliminate adverse effects of pressure.

We feel that progress in elucidating the mechanisms of pressure stress and pressure adaptation will depend on progress along several fronts and the close integration of advances made in several disciplines. Development of better *in situ* capturing and holding facilities will be an especially critical advance, since many of the uncertainties about pressure effects derive from difficulties in obtaining deep-sea organisms in good condition. Recent *in situ* respiration studies of *Coryphaenoides acrolepis* by Smith and Hessler (1974) represent an important step in such biologically meaningful studies of abyssal forms. The studies of mesopelagic fish respiration under controlled laboratory conditions by Meek and Childress (1973) also point the way towards better, biologically realistic approaches to the study of pressure-adapted marine organisms. Incidentally, both of these studies showed that deep-sea fishes had significantly lower oxygen consumption rates than shallow water fishes, a finding which currently lacks a biochemical explanation.

Progress in elucidating pressure effects and mechanisms of pressure adaptation will also depend on advances made by the 'pure' biophysicist and biochemist, especially those scientists who are successful in predicting the precise magnitudes of volume changes under cellular conditions. Success at the molecular level, as well as in physiological studies, will in large measure be determined by how innovatively the scientist can overcome the 'uncertainty principles' inherent in his or her work. That is to say, those workers who will make the greatest contribution towards elucidating the pressure relationships of marine organisms will be those who most successfully re-create the natural environment of their study system, be it a macromolecule or a whole organism, and avoid the pitfalls which we have shown to lie in the path of research which fails to consider the complex web of factors which interact to establish the pressure sensitivities of living systems.

REFERENCES

ARNOLD, R. M. and ALBRIGHT, L. J. (1971). 'Hydrostatic pressure effects on the translational stages of protein synthesis in a cell-free system in *Escherichia coli*', *Biochem. Biophys. Res. Commun.*, **238,** 347–354

ASSARSSON, P. and EIRICH, F. R. (1968). 'Properties of amides in aqueous solution. I.A.

Viscosity and density changes of amide-water systems. B. An analysis of volume deficiencies of mixtures bases on molecular size differences (mixing of hard spheres)', *J. Phys. Chem.*, **72,** 2710–2719

ATKINSON, D. E. (1969). 'Limitation of metabolite concentrations and the conservation of solvent capacity in the living cell', 29–43. In: *Current Topics in Cellular Regulation.* Eds. B. L. Horecker and E. B. Stadtman. Academic Press, New York

BECKER, V. E. and EVANS, H. J. (1969). 'The influence of monovalent cations and hydrostatic pressure on B-galactosidase activity', *Biochim. Biophys. Acta,* **191,** 95–104

BLAXTER, J. H. S., WARDLE, C. S. and ROBERTS, B. L. (1971). 'Aspects of the circulatory physiology and muscle systems of deepsea fish', *J. mar. biol. Ass. U.K.,* **51,** 991–1006

BØJE, L. and HVIDT, A. (1972). 'Volume effects in aqueous solutions of macromolecules containing non-polar groups', *Biopolymers,* **11,** 2357–2364

BRANDTS, J. F. (1967). 'Heat effects on proteins and enzymes', 25–72. In: *Thermobiology.* Ed. A. H. Rose. Academic Press, New York

BRANDTS, J. F., OLIVEIRA, R. J. and WESTORT, C. (1970). 'Thermodynamics of protein denaturation. Effect of pressure on the denaturation of ribonuclease A', *Biochem. (A.C.S.),* **9,** 1038–1047

DIGBY, P. S. (1972). 'Detection of small changes in hydrostatic pressure by crustacea and its relation to electrode action in the cuticle', 445–472. In: *The Effects of Pressure on Living Organisms, Symp. Soc. Exp. Biol.* (XXVI). Ed. M. A. Sleigh and A. G. MacDonald. Academic Press, New York

DUBOC, C. (1969). 'Relations entre grandeurs d'excès relatives de solutions binaires d'alcohols aliphatiques — tétrachlorure de carbone et différence entre le volume molaire du soluté á dilution infinie', *Bull. Soc. Chim. biol.,* **7,** 2260–2270

ENRIGHT, J. T. (1961). 'Pressure sensitivity of an amphipod', *Science,* **133,** 758–760

ENRIGHT, J. T. (1962). 'Responses of an amphipod to pressure changes', *Comp. Biochem. Physiol.* **7,** 131–145

FLÜGEL, H. and SCHLIEPER, C. (1970). 'The effects of pressure on marine invertebrates and fish', 211–234. In: *High Pressure Effects on Cellular Processes.* Ed. A. M. Zimmerman. Academic Press, New York

FRIEDMAN, M. E. and SCHERAGA, H. A. (1965). 'Volume changes in hydrocarbon-water systems. Partial molar volumes of alcohol-water solutions', *J. Phys. Chem.,* **69,** 3795–3800

FROEDE, H. C. and WILSON, I. B. (1972). 'Acetylcholinesterase', 89–114. In: *The Enzymes* **5.** Ed. P. Boyer. Academic Press, New York

HARRINGTON, W. F. (1975). 'The effects of pressure in ultracentrifugation of interacting systems', *Fractions,* **(1),** 10–18

HERMAN, L. and DREIZEN, P. (1971). 'Electron microscopic studies of skeletal and cardiac muscle of a benthic fish. I. Myofibrillar structure in resting and contracted muscle', *Am. Zool.,* **11,** 543–557

HOCHACHKA, P. W. (1971). 'Pressure effects on biochemical systems of abyssal fishes. The 1970 Alpha Helix expedition to the Galapagos Archipelago', *Am. Zool.,* **11** (3), 401–576

HOCHACHKA, P. W. (1974). 'Temperature and pressure adaptation of the binding site of acetylcholinesterase', *Biochem. J.,* **143,** 535–539

HOCHACHKA, P. W., STOREY, K. B. and BALDWIN, J. (1975). 'Design of acetylcholinesterase for its physical environment', *Comp. Biochem. Physiol.,* **52B,** 13–18

HOCHACHKA, P. W. and SOMERO, G. N. (1973). *Strategies of Biochemical Adaptation.* W. B. Saunders and Co., Philadelphia. 358 pp

IKKAI, T. and OOI, T. (1966). 'The effects of pressure on F-G transformation of Actin', *Biochem.,* **5,** 1551–1560

JOSEPHS, R. and HARRINGTON, W. F. (1967). 'An unusual pressure dependence for a reversibly associating protein system: sedimentation studies on myosin', *Proc. Nat. Acad. Sci. (U.S.),* **58,** 1587–1594

JOSEPHS, R. and HARRINGTON, W. F. (1968). 'On the stability of myosin filaments', *Biochem. (A.C.S.),* **7,** 2834–2847

KAUZMANN, W. (1959). 'Some factors in the interpretation of protein denaturation', *Adv. Prot. Chem.,* **14,** 1–63

LAIDLER, K. J. (1951). 'The influence of pressure on the rates of biological reactions', *Arch. Biochem.,* **30,** 226–236

LANDAU, J. V. (1970). 'Hydrostatic pressure on the biosynthesis of macromolecules', 45–70. In:

High Pressure Effects on Cellular Processes. Ed. A. M. Zimmerman. Academic Press, New York

LOW, P. S. and SOMERO, G. N. (1975a). 'Pressure effects on enzyme structure and function *in vitro* and under simulated *in vivo* conditions', *Comp. Biochem. Physiol.*, **52B,** 67–74

LOW, P. S. and SOMERO, G. N. (1975b). 'Activation volumes in enzymic catalysis: Their sources and modification by low-molecular-weight solutes', *Proc. Nat. Acad. Sci. (U.S.).* **72,** 3014–3018

LOW, P. S. and SOMERO, G. N. (1975c). 'Protein hydration changes during catalysis: A new mechanism of enzymic rate-enhancement and ion activation/inhibition of catalysis', *Proc. Nat. Acad. Sci. (U.S.).* **72,** 3305–3309

MARUYAMA, K. (1965). 'A new protein-factor hindering network formation of F-actin in solution', *Biochem. Biophys. Acta,* **94,** 208–225

MASTERTON, W. L. and SEILER, H. K. (1968). 'Apparent and partial molal volumes of water in organic solvents', *J. phys. Chem. Wash.,* **72,** 4257–4262

MEEK, R. P. and CHILDRESS, J. J. (1973). 'Respiration and the effect of pressure in the mesopelagic fish *Anoplogaster cornuta* (Beryciformes)', *Deep-sea Res.,* **20,** 1111–1118

MEYAGAWA, K. (1965). 'Reactivation of pressure-inactivated-amylase of *Bacillus subtilis* under moderate pressure', *Arch. Biochem. Biophys.,* **110,** 432–437

MURAYAMA, M. (1966). 'Molecular mechanism of red cell "sickling",' *Science,* **153,** 1667–1671

MURAYAMA, M. and HASEGAWA, F. (1969). 'Effect of hydrostatic pressure on the aggregation reaction of human sickle cell hemoglobin at 37°C', *Fed. Proc.,* **28,** 536

NEVILLE, W. M. and EYRING, H. (1972). 'Hydrostatic pressure and ionic strength effects on the kinetics of lysozyme', *Proc. Nat. Acad. Sci. (U.S.)* **69,** 2417–2419

NOGUCHI, H. (1966). 'Studies of the helix-coil transition of poly-L-lysine in film and solution', *Biopolymers,* **4,** 1105–1113

O'CONNER, T. M., HOUSTON, L. L. and SAMSON, F. (1974). 'Stability of neuronal microtubules to high pressure *in vivo* and *in vitro*', *Proc. Nat. Acad. Sci. (U.S.),* **71,** 4198–4202

PATTON, J. S. (1975). 'The effect of temperature and pressure on phospholipid and triglyceride fatty acids of fish white muscle: a comparison of deepwater and surface marine species', *Comp. Biochem. Physiol.,* **52B,** 105–110

PAUL, K. L. and MORITA, R. Y. (1971). 'Effects of hydrostatic pressure and temperature on the uptake and respiration of amino acids by a facultatively psychrophilic marine bacterium', *J. Bacteriol.,* **108,** 835–843

PENNISTON, J. T. (1971). 'High hydrostatic pressure and enzymic activity: inhibition of multimeric enzymes by dissociation', *Arch. Biochem. Biophys.,* **142,** 322–332

PÉQUEUX, A. (1972). 'Hydrostatic pressure and membrane permeability', 483–484. In: *The Effects of Pressure on Organisms. Symp. Soc. Exper. Biol.* (XXVI). Ed. M. A. Sleigh and A. G. MacDonald. Academic Press, New York

RAINFORD, P., NOGUCHI, H. and MORALES, M. (1965). 'Hydrostatic pressure and the contractile system', *Biochem. (A.C.S.),* **4,** 1958–1965

SALMON, E. D. (1975). 'Pressure-induced depolymerization of brain microtubules *in vitro*', *Science,* **189,** 884–886

SCHWARTZ, J. R. and LANDAU, J. V. (1972). 'Inhibition of cell-free protein synthesis by hydrostatic pressure', *J. Biochem.,* **112,** 1222–1227

SINGER, S. J. and NICOLSON, G. L. (1972). 'The fluid mosaic model of the structure of cell membranes', *Science,* **175,** 720–731

SLEIGH, M. A. and MACDONALD, A. G. (1972). *The Effects of Pressure on Living Organisms. Symp. Soc. Exper. Biol.* (XXVI). Academic Press, New York

SMITH, K. L. and HESSLER, R. R. (1974). 'Respiration of benthopelagic fishes: *in situ* measurements at 1230 meters', *Science,* **184,** 72–73

SOMERO, G. N. (1975). 'Temperature as a selective factor in protein evolution: the adaptational strategy of "compromise" ', *J. exp. Zool.,* **194,** 175–188

SUZUKI, K. and TANIGUCHI, Y. (1972). 'Effect of pressure on biopolymers and model systems', 103–124. In: *The Effects of Pressure on Living Organisms. Symp. Soc. Exper. Biol.* (XXVI). Ed. M. A. Sleigh and A. G. MacDonald. Academic Press, New York

WEALE, K. E. (1967). *Chemical Reactions at High Pressures.* Spon. Ltd., London. 349 pp

WIGGINS, P. M. (1971). 'Water structure as a determinant of ion distribution in living tissue', *J. theoret. Biol.,* **32,** 131–146

ZIMMERMAN, A. M. (1970). *High Pressure Effects on Cellular Processes.* Academic Press, New York. 324 pp

ZIPP, A. and KAUZMANN, W. (1973). 'Pressure denaturation of metmyoglobin', *Biochem. (A.C.S.),* **12,** 4217–4228

ZOBELL, C. E. (1970). 'Pressure effects on morphology and life processes of bacteria', 85–130. In: *High Pressure Effects on Cellular Processes.* Ed. A. M. Zimmerman. Academic Press, New York

Author index

Subject index